Neurosurgical Diseases

An Evidence-Based Approach to Guide Practice

Leon T. Lai, MBBS, PhD, FRACS
Associate Professor of Neurological Surgery
Department of Surgery
Monash University;
Head of Cerebrovascular Surgery and Skull Base Neurosurgeon
Department of Neurosurgery
Monash Health
Melbourne, Australia

Cristian Gragnaniello, MD, PhD
Assistant Professor of Neurological Surgery
Department of Neurological Surgery
University of Texas Health Science Center at San Antonio
San Antonio, Texas, USA

149 illustrations

Thieme
New York • Stuttgart • Delhi • Rio de Janeiro

Library of Congress Cataloging-in-Publication Data is available with the publisher.

Important note: Medicine is an ever-changing science undergoing continual development. Research and clinical experience are continually expanding our knowledge, in particular our knowledge of proper treatment and drug therapy. Insofar as this book mentions any dosage or application, readers may rest assured that the authors, editors, and publishers have made every effort to ensure that such references are in accordance with **the state of knowledge at the time of production of the book**.

Nevertheless, this does not involve, imply, or express any guarantee or responsibility on the part of the publishers in respect to any dosage instructions and forms of applications stated in the book. **Every user is requested to examine carefully** the manufacturers' leaflets accompanying each drug and to check, if necessary, in consultation with a physician or specialist, whether the dosage schedules mentioned therein or the contraindications stated by the manufacturers differ from the statements made in the present book. Such examination is particularly important with drugs that are either rarely used or have been newly released on the market. Every dosage schedule or every form of application used is entirely at the user's own risk and responsibility. The authors and publishers request every user to report to the publishers any discrepancies or inaccuracies noticed. If errors in this work are found after publication, errata will be posted at www.thieme.com on the product description page.

Some of the product names, patents, and registered designs referred to in this book are in fact registered trademarks or proprietary names even though specific reference to this fact is not always made in the text. Therefore, the appearance of a name without designation as proprietary is not to be construed as a representation by the publisher that it is in the public domain.

Thieme addresses people of all gender identities equally. We encourage our authors to use gender-neutral or gender-equal expressions wherever the context allows.

Thieme Medical Publishers, Inc.
333 Seventh Avenue, 18th Floor,
New York, NY 10001, USA
+www.thieme.com
+1 800 782 3488, customerservice@thieme.com

Cover design: © Thieme
Cover image source: Stamp © konstantant/stock.adobe.com,
Head Foreground © Erica Guilane-Nachez/stock.adobe.com,
Brain © User Ancheta Wis on en.wikipedia,
Public domain, via Wikimedia Commons,
Skull © Di Ieva A, Lee JM, Cusimano MD.
Handbook of Skull Base Surgery. 1st ed. Thieme; 2016
Typesetting by TNQ Technologies, India

Printed in Germany by Beltz Grafische Betriebe   5 4 3 2 1

ISBN: 978-1-68420-051-1

Also available as an e-book:
eISBN (PDF): 978-1-68420-052-8
eISBN (epub): 978-1-63853-639-0

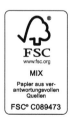

This book is dedicated to our patients and their families, who are our greatest clinical teachers. They impart in us the highs and lows of neurosurgery and the importance of humility in everyday practice.

To our mentors, who have poured so much into us and made us see hope.

Leon T. Lai, MBBS, PhD, FRACS
Cristian Gragnaniello, MD, PhD

Contents

Foreword

Perhaps obvious to most but worth restating, evidence-based neurosurgery is one of the most important pillars upon which to build a decision on management pathways. In no other discipline of medicine is a wrong decision fraught with a greater potential for immediate and catastrophic outcome. A neurosurgeon does not have to think for long before he or she can recall a life lost, a person damaged by deficit or pain, or a family devastated from a neurosurgical procedure performed or withheld. The performance of a procedure can be demonstrated by honest audit and other methods of monitoring competence. This can be judged by the patient, the surgeon, the surgeon's peers, and other work colleagues. A neurosurgeon should rightly feel proud of a more than competent performance. A good and proud performer of a procedure can influence a patient by body language, attitudes, reputation, and exuding confidence that the recommended decision should be followed. This persuasive influence on patients may be for good or bad. Performance of surgery is just one aspect of a good decision. It is also apt to apply the maxim that it is not only being busy that counts, but also what you are busy about. The best performance without support from evidence is nothing more than charlatan behavior. This was excusable in the early days of the barber surgeon, when so little was known, but inexcusable if good-quality evidence runs contrary to the pathway chosen.

Ascertaining the best evidence is a complex problem. There has been a recent belief that unless there is a randomized controlled trial of significant quality there is no evidence. This is not the real world nor is it even true.

Neurosurgery often deals with diseases that do not lend themselves to randomized controlled trials for many reasons: the conditions are often rare; the manifestations may be complex; there are a range of outcomes; innovations of treatment may occur during the trial; the difficulty of randomizing patients with the potential for immediate, permanent, significant consequences; the time scale of measuring results may be too long for most trial designs; multiple treatment options need to be considered; the outcomes are not related to predictable biological performance, such as a medication, but dependent on the uncertainties of teams of people in a social system; and the results may not be able to be applied generally. Then there is the biostatistics, now so complex that close collaboration with a biostatistician is essential to interpret journal articles.

Evidence-based decisions take into account the difficulties in amassing information and take the best evidence available and attempt to extract an honest interpretation that will help guide the decision makers. Leon T. Lai and Cristian Gragnaniello, both from the earliest days in their neurosurgical careers, have pursued expertise in evidence-based neurosurgery. They have put together a book of collaborators, who are experts in their fields, which is a synthesis of the best evidence. This book, made for the practitioner of brain surgery and those involved in management pathways, will give a basis for confidently considering management pathways. In the end, the complex decision, based on best evidence, can be made clearly and concisely.

Michael Kerin Morgan, AO, DSc, MD, MMedEd,
MBBS, FRACS
Professor of Cerebrovascular Neurosurgery
Department of Clinical Medicine
Macquarie University
Sydney, Australia

Preface

Effective delivery of care involves understanding the natural history of the disease and the evidence behind available treatment options. Although conventional paradigms based on pathophysiology and clinical experience are necessary as premises in evidence-based practice, they alone are inadequate to guide clinical decision making. We live in great times for science, where new information that becomes available continues to expand our insights. Disease management changes rapidly with technological advancement and so does the available evidence in the literature. It becomes imperative, therefore, to know and understand not only the latest treatment modalities but also one that better balances the natural history, risks, and outcomes.

Most published textbooks provide us with broad guidelines and indications on how to treat certain conditions. At times these are based on the confrontation between experts in different techniques, their algorithms, and results. There are limited texts that discuss treatment of conditions affecting the CNS, "contextualizing" the natural history and evidence of the different treatment modalities, to help guide the decision makers.

This book covers cranial pathologies commonly encountered in clinical neurosurgery practice. It aims to provide a structured approach to evidence-based neurosurgery, combined with experts' opinions and experience to facilitate the translation of evidence into practice. Each chapter follows a uniform format for ease of reading, including an introduction to the topic, the natural history, treatment options, and authors' recommendation. It integrates clinical expertise and judgment, understanding of patient's preferences and values, and the best available research evidence to provide a framework for patient care.

We hope that you will enjoy reading this text as much as we enjoyed preparing it.

Leon T. Lai, MBBS, PhD, FRACS
Cristian Gragnaniello, MD, PhD

Acknowledgments

We would like to thank Dr. Anthea O'Neill, who provided endless hours of systematic literature research in the preparation of this book.

We are also thankful to our families for their unrelenting patience, understanding, and devotion.

Leon T. Lai, MBBS, PhD, FRACS
Cristian Gragnaniello, MD, PhD

Contributors

Amal Abou-Hamden, MBBS, BMedSc (Hons), FRACS
Senior Consultant Neurosurgeon
Department of Neurosurgery
The Royal Adelaide Hospital
Adelaide, Australia;
Clinical Associate Professor
Department of Surgery
The University of Adelaide
Adelaide, Australia

Hugo Andrade-Barazarte, MD, PhD
Associate Professor in Neurosurgery
Department of Neurosurgery
Juha Hernesniemi International Center for Neurosurgery
Henan People's Provincial Hospital
University of Zhengzhou
Zhengzhou, China

Mohammed Awad, BSc, MBChB, MPhil, FRCS(SN), FRACS
Neurosurgeon
Department of Neurosurgery
Royal Melbourne Hospital
Melbourne, Victoria, Australia

Weixing Bai, MD
Interventional Neurosurgeon
Department of Neurosurgery
Juha Hernesniemi International Center for Neurosurgery
Henan People's Provincial Hospital
University of Zhengzhou
Zhengzhou, China

David Bervini, MD, MAdvSurg
Attending Neurosurgeon
Department of Neurosurgery
Inselspital
Bern University Hospital
Bern, Switzerland

Arnold Bok, MBChB, MMed, FCSSA, FRACS
Neurosurgeon
Department of Neurosurgery
Auckland City Hospital
Auckland, New Zealand

Sarah Cain, MBBS, BSc (Hons)
Registrar
Department of Neurosurgery
Royal Melbourne Hospital
Melbourne, Victoria, Australia

Mendel Castle-Kirszbaum, MBBS (Hons)
Registrar
Department of Neurosurgery
Monash Health
Melbourne, Australia

Zhongcan Cheng, MD
Department of Neurosurgery
Juha Hernesniemi International Center for Neurosurgery
Henan People's Provincial Hospital
University of Zhengzhou
Zhengzhou, China

Jordan Elizabeth Cory, BSc, MBBS, GradDip Surgical Anatomy
Registrar
Department of Neurosurgery
Royal Melbourne Hospital
Melbourne, Victoria, Australia

Ruben Dammers, MD, PhD
Neurosurgeon
Department of Neurosurgery
Erasmus Medical Centre
Erasmus MC Stroke Centre
Rotterdam, The Netherlands

Helen V. Danesh-Meyer, MBChB, MD, FRANZCO, PhD
Head of Academic Glaucoma and Neuro-ophthalmology;
Sir William and Lady Stevenson
    Professor of Ophthalmology
Department of Ophthalmology
University of Auckland
Auckland, New Zealand

Bryden H. Dawes, MS, FRACS
Neurosurgeon
Department of Neurosurgery
St Vincent's Hospital
Melbourne, Australia

Vincent Dodson, MD
Resident
Department of Neurological Surgery
Rutgers New Jersey Medical School
Newark, New Jersey, USA

Katharine J. Drummond, AM, MBBS, MD, FRACS
Director of Neurosurgery
Department of Surgery
Royal Melbourne Hospital
University of Melbourne
Parkville, Victoria, Australia

Guangmin Duan, MD
Neurosurgeon
Department of Neurosurgery
Juha Hernesniemi International Center for Neurosurgery
Henan People's Provincial Hospital
University of Zhengzhou
Zhengzhou, China

Behzad Eftekhar, MD, MPH, FRACS, MAdvSurg, AFRACMA
Professor of Neurosurgery
Head of Department
Department of Neurosurgery
Nepean Hospital
The University of Sydney
New South Wales, Australia

Jean Anderson Eloy, MD, FACS
Professor of Otolaryngology
Department of Otolaryngology – Head and Neck Surgery
Rutgers New Jersey Medical School
Newark, New Jersey, USA;
Center for Skull Base and Pituitary Surgery
Neurological Institute of New Jersey
Rutgers New Jersey Medical School
Newark, New Jersey, USA;
Department of Neurological Surgery
Rutgers New Jersey Medical School
Newark, New Jersey, USA;
Department of Otolaryngology and Facial Plastic Surgery
Saint Barnabas Medical Center – RWJ Barnabas Health
Livingston, New Jersey, USA

Felix Goehre, MD PhD
Neurosurgeon
Department of Neurosurgery
BG Klinikum Bergmannstrost Halle
Halle, Germany

Tony Goldschlager, MBBS, DCH, PhD, FRACS
Neurosurgeon
Department of Neurosurgery
Monash Health
Melbourne, Australia;
Associate Professor
Department of Surgery
Monash University
Melbourne, Australia

Augusto Gonzalvo, MD, FRACS
Associate Professor of Neurosurgery
Department of Neurosurgery
Austin Health
Melbourne, Victoria, Australia;
The University of Melbourne,
Melbourne, Victoria, Australia

Cristian Gragnaniello, MD, PhD
Assistant Professor of Neurological Surgery
Department of Neurological Surgery
University of Texas Health Science Center at San Antonio
San Antonio, Texas, USA

Aye Aye Gyi, MPhil, PhD
Research Officer
Department of Neurosurgery
The Royal Adelaide Hospital
Adelaide, Australia

Juha Hernesniemi, MD, PhD
Professor of Neurological Surgery
Department of Neurosurgery
Juha Hernesniemi International Center for Neurosurgery
Henan People's Provincial Hospital
University of Zhengzhou
Zhengzhou, China

Dana C. Holl, MSc
Registrar
Department of Neurosurgery
Erasmus Medical Center
Erasmus MC Stroke Center
Rotterdam, The Netherlands

Bob Homapour, FRCS(SN) MSc
Neurosurgeon
Department of Neurosurgery
Monash Health
Melbourne, Australia

Stephen Honeybul, FRCS (SN), FRACS
Consultant Neurosurgeon
Statewide Director of Neurosurgery Western Australia;
Head of Department
Department of Neurosurgery
Sir Charles Gairdner Hospital and Royal Perth Hospital
Western Australia, Australia

Wayne D. Hsuen, MD
Assistant Professor
Department of Otolaryngology – Head and Neck Surgery
Rutgers New Jersey Medical School
Newark, New Jersey, USA;
Center for Skull Base and Pituitary Surgery
Neurological Institute of New Jersey
Rutgers New Jersey Medical School
Newark, New Jersey, USA;
Department of Otolaryngology and Facial Plastic Surgery
Saint Barnabas Medical Center – RWJ Barnabas Health
Livingston, New Jersey, USA

Helen Huang, MBBS (Hons), BMedSc (Hons)
Registrar
Department of Neurosurgery
Monash Health
Melbourne, Australia

Benjamin H.M. Hunn, MBBS, DPhil
Registrar
Department of Neurosurgery
Royal Melbourne Hospital
Melbourne, Victoria, Australia

Behnam Rezai Jahromi, MD
Resident
Department of Neurosurgery
Helsinki University Hospital and University of Helsinki
Helsinki, Finland

Jordan Jones
Registrar
Department of Neurosurgery
Royal Melbourne Hospital
Melbourne, Victoria, Australia;
Department of Surgery
University of Melbourne
Melbourne, Australia

Fareed Jumah, MD
Postdoctoral Research Fellow
Department of Neurosurgery
Rutgers-Robert Wood Johnson Medical School and
    University Hospital
New Brunswick, New Jersey, USA

Andranik Kahramanian, MD, MBMSc, BMedSci (Hons I)
Registrar
Department of Neurosurgery
Royal Melbourne Hospital
Melbourne, Victoria, Australia

Bhadrakant Kavar, MBChB, FCS, FRACS
Neurosurgeon
Department of Neurosurgery
Royal Melbourne Hospital;
Honorary Lecturer
University of Melbourne
Melbourne, Victoria, Australia

Andrew H. Kaye, MBBS, MD, FRACS
Professor
Department of Neurosurgery
Hadassah Hebrew University
Jerusalem, Israel;
Department of Surgery
University of Melbourne
Melbourne, Australia

James A.J. King, MBBS, PhD, FRACS
Consultant Neurosurgeon, Director of Training, and
    Head of Pituitary Surgery
Department of Neurosurgery
Royal Melbourne Hospital
Melbourne, Victoria, Australia;
Department of Surgery
University of Melbourne
Melbourne, Australia

Juri Kivelev, MD PhD
Neurosurgeon
Department of Neurosurgery
Turku University Hospital
Turku, Finland

Angelos G. Kolias, PhD, FRCS
Neurosurgeon
Department of Neurosurgery
Addenbrooke's Hospital;
Cambridge University Hospitals NHS Foundation Trust
NIHR Global Health Research Group on Neurotrauma
University of Cambridge
Cambridge, UK

Chien Yew Kow, MBBS
Registrar
Department of Neurosurgery
Auckland City Hospital
Auckland, New Zealand

Leon T. Lai, MBBS, PhD, FRACS
Associate Professor of Neurological Surgery
Department of Surgery
Monash University
Melbourne, Australia;
Head of Cerebrovascular Surgery and Skull Base
    Neurosurgeon
Department of Neurosurgery
Monash Health
Melbourne, Australia

Tianxiao Li, MD
Department of Neurosurgery
Juha Hernesniemi International Center for Neurosurgery
Henan People's Provincial Hospital
University of Zhengzhou
Zhengzhou, China

Rebecca J. Limb, BMBS, BMedSci
Registrar
Department of Neurosurgery
Monash Health
Melbourne, Australia

James K. Liu, MD
Professor of Neurological Surgery;
Director, Cerebrovascular/Skull Base & Pituitary Surgery;
Co-Director, Endoscopic Skull Base Surgery Program
Neurological Institute of New Jersey
Rutgers New Jersey Medical School
Newark, New Jersey, USA

Kevin Liu, MBChB
Neuro-ophthalmology Clinical Research Fellow
Department of Ophthalmology
University of Auckland
Auckland, New Zealand

Neil Majmundar, MD
Chief Resident
Department of Neurological Surgery
Rutgers New Jersey Medical School
Newark, New Jersey, USA

Basant K. Misra, MBBS, MS, MCh, DNB, PDC
Consultant Neurosurgeon;
Head of the Department
Department of Neurosurgery & Gamma Knife Surgery
P D Hinduja National Hospital & Medical Research Centre
Veer Savarkar Marg, Mumbai, India

Michael Kerin Morgan, AO, DSc, MD, MMedEd, MBBS, FRACS
Professor of Cerebrovascular Neurosurgery
Department of Clinical Medicine
Macquarie University
Sydney, New South Wales, Australia

Andrew Morokoff, MBBS, PhD, FRACS
Associate Professor
Department of Neurosurgery
Royal Melbourne Hospital
Melbourne, Victoria, Australia;
Department of Surgery
University of Melbourne
Melbourne, Australia

Michael J. Mulcahy, BMed, MSc (Surgical Science), MS (Neurosurgery)
Registrar
University of Newcastle
Australia

Anil Nanda, MD, MPH, FACS
Professor and Chairman
Department of Neurosurgery
Rutgers-Robert Wood Johnson Medical School and
   University Hospital
New Brunswick, New Jersey, USA

Vinayak Narayan, MD
Fellow
Department of Neurosurgery
Rutgers-Robert Wood Johnson Medical School and
   University Hospital
New Brunswick, New Jersey, USA

Mika Niemela, MD PhD
Professor of Neurological Surgery
Department of Neurosurgery
Helsinki University Hospital
Helsinki, Finland

Anthea H. O'Neill, MBBS, MPH
Registrar
Department of Neurosurgery
Monash Medical Centre
Melbourne, Australia

Nirav J. Patel, MD, MA
Assistant Professor of Neurosurgery
Department of Neurosurgery
Harvard Medical School, Brigham and Women's Hospital,
Neurosciences Centre
Boston, Massachusetts, USA

Adrian Praeger, MBBS BA Dip. Ant. FRACS
Neurosurgeon
Department of Neurosurgery
Monash Hospital
Melbourne, Australia

Harshad R. Purandare, MBBS, MS, MCh
Consultant Neurosurgeon
Jupiter Hospital
Eastern Express Highway
Thane, Maharashtra, India

Bharath Raju, MD, MCh
Postdoctoral Research Fellow
Department of Neurosurgery
Rutgers-Robert Wood Johnson Medical
   School and University Hospital
New Brunswick, New Jersey, USA

Jaakko Rinne, MD PhD
Professor of Neurological Surgery
Department of Neurosurgery
Turku University Hospital
Turku, Finland

Jonathan Rychen, MD
Attending Neurosurgeon
Department of Neurosurgery
University Hospital of Basel
Basel, Switzerland

Zhiyuan Sheng, MD
Resident
Department of Neurosurgery
Juha Hernesniemi International Center for Neurosurgery
Henan People's Provincial Hospital
University of Zhengzhou
Zhengzhou, China

Michael A. Silva, MD
Neurosurgeon
Department of Neurosurgery
University of Miami Miller School of Medicine
Jackson Memorial Hospital
Miami, Florida, USA

Darius Tan, MBBS, MSc
Registrar
Department of Neurosurgery
Monash Health
Melbourne, Australia

Peter Teddy, DPhil, FRACS, FFPMANZCA
Clinical Professor
Department of Neurosurgery
Royal Melbourne Hospital
University of Melbourne
Melbourne, Victoria, Australia

Ivan Timofeev, PhD, FRCS
Consultant Neurosurgeon
Department of Neurosurgery
Department of Clinical Neurosciences
University of Cambridge,
Cambridge, UK

Zhao Tongyuan, MD
Juha Hernesniemi International Center for Neurosurgery
Henan Provincial People's Hospital
University of Zhengzhou
Zhengzhou, China

Jorn Van Der Veken, MD
Neurosurgery Fellow
Department of Neurosurgery
The Royal Adelaide Hospital
Adelaide, Australia

Samuel Wreghitt, MBChB
Registrar
Department of Neurosurgery
Austin Health
Melbourne, Victoria, Australia

Chris Xenos, FRACS
Neurosurgeon
Department of Neurosurgery
Monash Health
Melbourne, Australia

Jiangyu Xue, MD
Department of Intervention
Juha Hernesniemi International Center for Neurosurgery
Henan Provincial People's Hospital
University of Zhengzhou
Zhengzhou, China

Ajmal Zemmar, MD, PhD
Department of Neurosurgery
Juha Hernesniemi International Center for Neurosurgery
Henan People's Provincial Hospital
University of Zhengzhou
Zhengzhou, China

1 Natural History and Management Options of Recurrent Glioblastoma

Benjamin H.M. Hunn and Katharine J. Drummond

Abstract

Glioblastoma (GBM) is the most common primary brain cancer in adults and carries a dismal prognosis. At first diagnosis, the standard of care for GBM is maximal safe resection, with subsequent radiotherapy and chemotherapy, a regimen that extends survival by months to years. Unfortunately, recurrence is inevitable and occurs, on average, 7.8 months after initial diagnosis. There is no standard of care for the treatment of recurrent disease and median survival is just 6.4 months. Younger patients, those with a higher performance status, and those with less diffuse disease may have extended survival. Delineating true tumor recurrence from "pseudoprogression" is critical. At GBM recurrence, no available salvage treatment has been clearly shown to improve survival. Retrospective analysis of repeat resection suggests improved survival; however, prospective data are lacking. Resection of recurrent GBM may be performed to relieve mass effect, or to gain tissue for further investigations, particularly for clinical trials of targeted agents. Surgery to prolong survival should be performed rarely, in younger patients with good performance status and tumor in a favorable location. Consensus expert opinion suggests that the benefit of reirradiation is higher when there is a greater disease-free interval since initial radiotherapy, and if GBM recurs in a noneloquent location. Stereotactic radiosurgery is also an unproven option for discrete recurrent GBM. No chemotherapy has been demonstrated to improve survival in recurrent GBM, but bevacizumab is frequently used and may control symptoms. Given treatment of recurrent GBM has a poor evidence base with little to commend any specific treatment, clinical trials are encouraged.

Keywords: glioblastoma, recurrence, surgery, systematic review

1.1 Introduction

Glioblastoma (GBM) is a World Health Organization (WHO) grade IV malignant tumor of presumed neuroglial origin and conveys an overall poor prognosis (▶ Fig. 1.1).[1] It is the most common primary brain cancer in adults, with an estimated incidence of between 3 and 5 cases per 100,000 person-year.[1,2,7] GBM may occur de novo (primary), or arise from a lower-grade astrocytoma (secondary). Primary GBM accounts for over 90% of cases and has a slight male preponderance (1.3 times higher) with affected individuals generally older at presentation (mean age: 60 years).[2,3] Secondary GBM are less common and affect younger patients (mean age: 30–50 years) with no clear sex predilection.[2,4,5,6]

Mutations in the genes encoding isocitrate dehydrogenase 1 and 2 (*IDH1* and *IDH2*) are now used to separate primary from secondary GBM; *IDH* wild-type tumors are synonymous with primary GBM, whereas *IDH* mutations signify secondary GBM.[9] In general, *IDH* mutant GBM is associated with longer survival.[5]

Primary GBM is further characterized by deletions of chromosome 10, amplification of the epidermal growth factor receptor (*EGFR*) gene, and mutations of the phosphate and tensin homolog (*PTEN*) tumor suppressor gene.[10] Secondary GBM commonly acquires *TP53* mutations as part of progression from lower-grade astrocytoma.[11] Methylation of the promoter of the deoxyribonucleic acid (DNA) repair gene O[6]-methylguanine-DNA methyltransferase (*MGMT*) is a positive prognostic factor in both primary and secondary GBM.[12]

Since 2005, the mainstay treatment at diagnosis involves maximal safe resection (or biopsy) with concurrent radiotherapy and temozolomide chemotherapy followed by adjuvant temozolomide chemotherapy. Surgery is performed to obtain tissue diagnosis, relieve mass effect, improve vasogenic edema, facilitate tolerance to adjuvant therapy, and provide additional tissue for research and clinical trial inclusion. Complete resection of GBM is difficult because of the inherent infiltrative nature of the disease, and the extent of resection (EOR) largely depends on the proximity of eloquent functional brain tissue. In general, resection of all contrast-enhancing tissue seen on the preoperative magnetic resonance imaging (MRI) is the accepted standard. A meta-analysis of 41,117 GBM patients demonstrated that increased EOR at first operation positively correlated with longer progression-free and overall survival,[15] notwithstanding the inherent limitations of selection bias and retrospective data. Some authors have attempted to derive a prognostic threshold for EOR; typically, the best outcomes are seen after 70 to 80% resection.[16,17] One randomized prospective trial demonstrates that survival is correlated with the initial EOR, where 5-aminolevulinic acid was used to guide tumor resection.[14]

Efficacy of radiotherapy in prolonging survival in GBM is well established. A meta-analysis of six randomized controlled trials demonstrated that radiotherapy reduces risk of death within 1 year by 19%.[18] Efficacy of temozolomide chemotherapy primarily comes from the Stupp study, which showed the addition of temozolomide to standard surgery and radiotherapy increased the number of patients surviving 2 years from 10.4 to 26.5%.[19] Extended analysis of these patients demonstrated temozolomide increased survival after 5 years from 1.9 to 9.8%.[12]

GBM recurrence is inevitable, with recurrence within 2 cm of the original tumor margin in 90% of patients.[8,13] The therapeutic approach to recurrent GBM is less well defined. This chapter examined published literature on the natural history of recurrent GBM and available treatment options and recommendations.

1.2 Selected Papers on the Natural History of Recurrent Glioblastoma

- Michaelsen SR, Christensen IJ, Grunnet K, et al. Clinical variables serve as prognostic factors in a model for survival

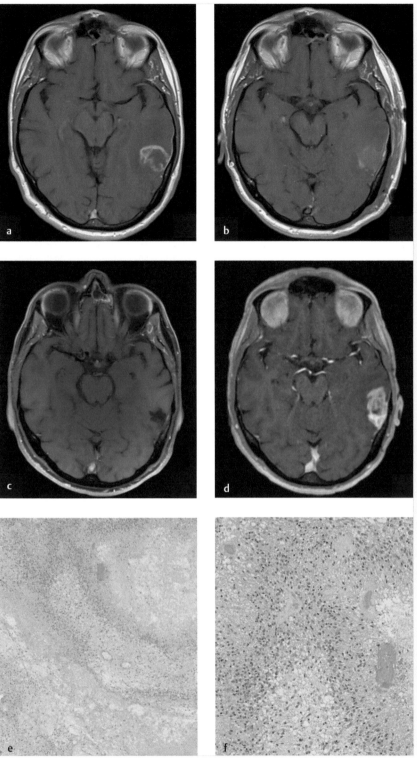

Fig. 1.1 Radiological and histological features of recurrent glioblastoma. **(a)** Contrast-enhanced T1-weighted axial magnetic resonance imaging (MRI) scan of left posterior temporal glioblastoma at diagnosis. **(b)** Contrast-enhanced T1-weighted axial MRI scan on the first postoperative day following resection of the tumor. **(c)** Contrast-enhanced T1-weighted axial MRI scan performed 12 months following initial resection of the tumor showing no recurrence. **(d)** Contrast-enhanced T1-weighted axial MRI scan performed 21 months following initial resection, demonstrating recurrent left temporal glioblastoma at the margin of the resection. **(e)** Low-power and **(f)** high-power hematoxylin and eosin stained photomicrographs of recurrent glioblastoma demonstrating extensive necrosis, pseudopalisading of malignant nuclei and proliferation of endothelial cells. Thanks to Dr. Tewhiti Rogers (Royal Melbourne Hospital) for assistance with photomicrographs.

from glioblastoma multiforme: an observational study of a cohort of consecutive non-selected patients from a single institution. BMC Cancer 2013;13(1):402.
- van Linde ME, Brahm CG, de Witt Hamer PC, et al. Treatment outcome of patients with recurrent glioblastoma multiforme: a retrospective multicenter analysis. J Neurooncol 2017;135(1):183–192.
- Bette S, Barz M, Huber T, et al. Retrospective analysis of radiological recurrence patterns in glioblastoma, their

prognostic value and association to postoperative infarct volume. Sci Rep 2018;8(1):4561.

1.3 The Natural History of Recurrent Glioblastoma

Recurrent GBM is invariably associated with substantial morbidity and mortality. A summary of studies that examine the

Table 1.1 Summary of studies examining the natural history of recurrent glioblastoma

Study	Study period	Patients	Female (%)	Age (y)	Time to recurrence (mo)	OS all patients (mo)	OS no treatment (mo)	OS salvage treatment (mo)
Kappelle et al[31]	1994–1998	63	25.4	46[a]	9.8[b]	NA	NA	8.3[c]
Hau et al[30]	1997–2001	168	38.7	55[a]	6.0[b]	7.5	2.3	8.3
Stupp et al[12][d]	2000–2002	287	35.5	56[a]	6.9	6.2	NA	6.2
Ciammella et al[28]	2007–2012	83	44.6	NA	9.0[b]	7.7	2.5	9.5[e]
De Bonis et al[29]	2002–2008	76	43.4	59[f]	NA	7.0	5.0	14.0[g]
Michaelsen et al[33]	2005–2010	199	35.6[h]	59[a,h]	8.0	5.9	NA	NA
McNamara et al[32]	2004–2011	584	37.8	59[a]	7.8	NA	NA	7.1[i]
Amini et al[26]	2007–2014	60	41.7	57[a]	9.5	5.3[b]	NA	NA
Socha et al[35]	2010–2013	84	45.2	>50[j]	4.0	3.8	2.3	5.8
Parakh et al[34]	2006–2008	194	33.5	61[a,b]	7.0	5.0[b]	3.0	7.0
Azoulay et al[27]	2005–2012	188	37.8	58[a]	7.4	6.6	7.0[k]	10.3[i,k]
van Linde et al[36]	2005–2014	299	32.4	58[b,f]	14.2[b]	6.5	3.1	8.5
Summary (median, range)		2,285	37.8 (25.4–45.2)	58.0 (46.0–61.0)	7.8 (4.0–14.2)	6.4 (3.8–7.7)	3.0 (2.3–7.0)	8.3 (5.8–14.0)

Abbreviations: NA; not available; OS, overall survival following recurrence.
[a]Median.
[b]Calculated from reported data.
[c]Procarbazine, lomustine and vincristine (PCV) chemotherapy as salvage treatment.
[d]Radiotherapy and temozolomide cohort.
[e]Radiotherapy as salvage treatment.
[f]Mean.
[g]Surgery and chemotherapy as salvage treatment.
[h]Refers to entire study cohort of which 199/225 suffered recurrence.
[i]Repeat operation as salvage treatment.
[j]Data not given in study; all patients were older than 50 years.
[k]Survival for no treatment/salvage subgroups reported as a case/control subset.

natural history of recurrent GBM is provided in ▶ Table 1.1 (▶ Fig. 1.2). These data demonstrate that GBM typically recurs within 4 to 14 months of diagnosis, either during or after first-line treatment. If recurrent GBM is untreated, death occurs within 2 to 7 months, although there is likely to be strong selection bias in those studies that suggest that treatment may prolong survival (overall survival: 5.8–14.0 months).

The key prognostic factors to consider at tumor recurrence include the following (▶ Fig. 1.2):
- Age: Younger patients have improved survival.[33,36]
- Performance status: In general, higher performance status at recurrence predicts improved survival.[33,37,38,39,40]
- Extent of disease: Local recurrence is associated with a better prognosis than diffuse disease. Evidences of ventricular contact and ependymal spread are poor prognostic factors.[36,39,40]
- Presence of neurological symptoms: Symptomatic recurrence correlates with a poor prognosis (median survival: 3 months), compared to 10 months for radiologic recurrence.[26]
- Secondary GBM: In one of the few reports to distinguish between primary and secondary GBM, Da Fonseca et al demonstrated increased survival time in six patients with secondary GBM in their series of 89 GBM patients, although it must be noted that patients with secondary GBM were almost 20 years younger.[41] A separate analysis by Mandel et al was underpowered to detect any difference between patients based on IDH status.[42] Further research should examine the impact of IDH mutations on the natural history of recurrent GBM.

It is critical to delineate true tumor progression from "pseudoprogression," which represents treatment response. This determination is important as it will ultimately affect treatment options. Typically, pseudoprogression occurs in the first 12 weeks following completion of chemoradiotherapy, in 15 to 30% of patients.[20,21,22,23] Most pseudoprogression (67%) is asymptomatic, whereas most true progression (67%) is symptomatic.[20]

To guide separation between true progression and pseudoprogression, the Response Assessment in Neuro-Oncology (RANO) criteria were developed (▶ Table 1.2); these supersede the older MacDonald criteria.[24] In general, the RANO criteria dictate that progressive disease should be diagnosed if any of the following is observed at any time:
- Development of a new lesion outside of the radiation field.
- Histological evidence of progression.

In addition, progressive disease should be diagnosed if any of the following occurs more than 12 weeks following cessation of chemoradiotherapy:
- Increase in volume of gadolinium-enhancing tumor of ≥ 25%.
- Increase in T2 or fluid-attenuated inversion recovery (FLAIR) signal extent.
- Worsening of clinical state attributable to GBM.

A modification of the RANO criteria adapted for use in the context of immunological therapies (iRANO) has also been developed, to allow for delayed effects of immunotherapeutic agents and the development of treatment effects that mimic progressive disease.[25]

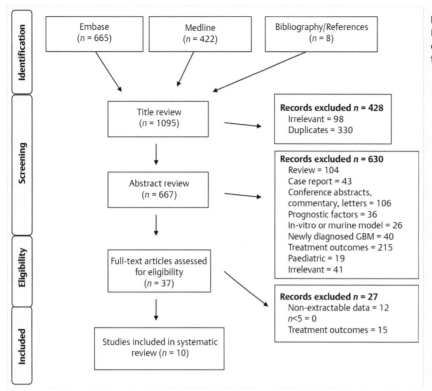

Fig. 1.2 Preferred Reporting Items for Systematic Reviews and Meta-Analyses (PRISMA) chart demonstrating the systematic search process for the natural history of recurrent glioblastoma.

Table 1.2 Summary of the response assessment in neuro-oncology (RANO) criteria

	Complete response	Partial response	Stable disease	Progressive disease
Criteria required	*All* of the following:	*All* of the following:	*All* of the following:	*Any* of the following:
T1-Gad + lesions	None	≥50% ↓	<50% ↓ to <25% ↑	≥25% ↑
T2/FLAIR lesions	Stable or ↓	Stable or ↓	Stable or ↓	↑
New lesions	None	None	None	Present
Corticosteroids	None[a]	Stable or ↓	Stable or ↓	NA
Clinical status	Stable or ↑	Stable or ↑	Stable or ↑	↓[b]

Abbreviations: FLAIR, fluid attenuated inversion recovery; Gad +, gadolinium contract enhancement; NA, not applicable; T1, T1-weighted MRI; T2, T2-weighted MRI.

Note: Patient should be assessed more than 12 weeks following cessation of chemoradiotherapy. Imaging features should be sustained for at least 4 weeks.

[a]Physiological replacement doses permitted.

[b]Not attributable to nontumor causes or steroid dose reduction.

1.4 Selected Papers on the Treatment Outcomes of Recurrent Glioblastoma

- Park C-K, Kim JH, Nam D-H, et al. A practical scoring system to determine whether to proceed with surgical resection in recurrent glioblastoma. Neurooncol 2013;15(8):1096–1101.
- Tully PA, Gogos AJ, Love C, Liew D, Drummond KJ, Morokoff AP. Reoperation for recurrent glioblastoma and its association with survival benefit. Neurosurgery 2016;79(5):678–689.
- Lu VM, Jue TR, McDonald KL, Rovin RA. The survival effect of repeat surgery at glioblastoma recurrence and its trend: a systematic review and meta-analysis. World Neurosurg 2018;115:453–459.e3.

1.5 Treatment Options for Recurrent Glioblastoma

Following recurrence of GBM, no available salvage treatment has clearly achieved improved survival (▶ Fig. 1.3). At present, treatment choices should be individualized, and clinical trials strongly considered. In patients with good performance status, more active treatment options can be considered; patients who are nonambulatory or heavily dependent on others at the time of recurrence are best managed with supportive care alone. Conventional treatment of recurrent GBM is predominantly palliative, with the patient's quality of life the primary concern.

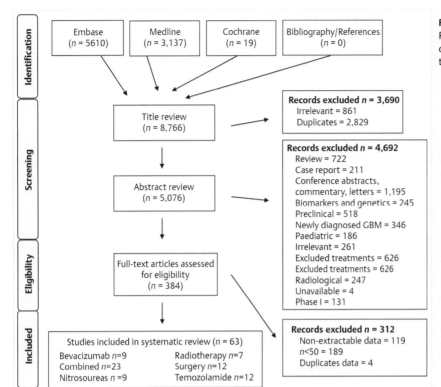

Fig. 1.3 Preferred Reporting Items for Systematic Reviews and Meta-Analyses (PRISMA) chart demonstrating the systematic search process for the treatment outcomes of recurrent glioblastoma.

1.5.1 Repeat Surgery

The role of repeat resection as a cytoreductive measure to prolong survival following tumor recurrence is unclear. Tumor location and size determine whether reoperation is feasible. The objective may be to alleviate mass effect, to improve tolerance of further adjuvant therapy, or, increasingly, to provide further tissue samples that may discern eligibility to a clinical trial. A recent meta-analysis by Lu et al of 1906 recurrent GBM patients has demonstrated that repeat resection is associated with a 28% improvement in survival.[43] However, prospective randomized data to support this strategy are lacking. Available evidence are retrospective and subject to inherent selection bias, where surgery is performed in younger patients, with higher performance status and better general health.[37,38,44] Additionally, patients who undergo repeat surgery may be more likely to also receive more aggressive adjuvant treatment. To address these limitations, Tully et al omitted patients who would be unlikely to be considered for repeat GBM surgery (patients older than 80 years and those with a poor performance status and brainstem or posterior fossa tumors) from an analysis comparing the survival of patients who did and did not undergo repeat surgery; this demonstrated no benefit of repeat surgery.[37] In contrast, a case control study conducted by Wann et al suggested instead that repeat operation may improve survival.[45]

To simplify surgical decision-making for recurrent GBM, the National Institutes of Health (NIH) Recurrent Glioblastoma Scale has been proposed (▶ Table 1.3).[46,47] Although these scales are based on retrospective data, and essentially repeat the same factors that promote survival in all patients, they provide some clinical guidance and facilitate discussions with patients.

Table 1.3 Simplified WHO Recurrent Glioblastoma Scale for survival after repeat resection

Calculating score		
Patient factor	**Threshold**	**Score**
KPS	≤ 70	1 point
Ependymal enhancement	Present	1 point
Interpreting score		
Score	**Survival (mo)**	**Operative prospects**
0	18	Good
1	10	Intermediate
2	4	Poor

Abbreviation: KPS, Karnofsky's Performance Score.

Retrospective analyses have demonstrated that gross total resection of recurrent GBM is associated with an improved outcome; Oppenlander et al have proposed that a threshold of 80% resection is associated with a survival benefit.[48] In contrast to primary resection of GBM, carmustine wafers do not show any evidence of benefit in recurrent GBM. Experimental surgical therapies may also be considered for treatment of recurrent GBM. An example is provided by Desjardins et al, who have shown a 36-month survival rate of 21% in patients treated with recombinant poliovirus therapeutic vector, compared with 4% survival in historical controls, with obvious concern regarding the use of historical controls given the history of poor translation of such promising phase II trials to meaningful therapies in phase III studies.[49]

1.5.2 Further Radiotherapy

Similarly, the role of re-irradiation for recurrent GBM is unclear, with most studies subjected to the limitation of retrospective data bias. Available evidence suggests some utility of repeat irradiation in selected patients with a reasonable performance status and small recurrent tumors.[50] Consensus expert opinion suggests that benefit of re-irradiation is higher when there has been a prolonged time since the first course of radiotherapy, and GBM recurrence is in a noneloquent location.[51] Stereotactic radiosurgery (SRS) may also be deployed to treat very localized recurrent GBM. Several groups have demonstrated improved survival and reduced complication rates from SRS when compared to repeat resection, raising SRS as a possible alternative to reoperation.[52,48]

1.5.3 Further Chemotherapy

In contrast, the role of additional chemotherapy for recurrent GBM has been well studied in more than 100 clinical trials since 1995. However, no clear evidence has emerged to support use of any specific drugs, alone or in combination. The most commonly used treatments are bevacizumab, rechallenge with temozolomide (generally after a significant interval from last course), or other nitrosoureas.

A significant research effort has been spent examining the efficacy of bevacizumab, a monoclonal antibody that binds vascular endothelial growth factor. Phase I and II trials that examined the role of bevacizumab for recurrent GBM did not find consistent evidence to support its use as a standard. More recently, a phase III trial (EORTC 26101) demonstrated a benefit of bevacizumab in combination with lomustine in prolonging progression-free survival, but not overall survival.[49] A previous trial found no evidence of benefit for bevacizumab monotherapy.[50]

In the largest trial examining repeat temozolomide for recurrent GBM, the RESCUE study, 120 patients were administered continuous temozolomide for up to 1 year. RESCUE demonstrated 27% 1-year survival in patients who had recurred early in their initial chemoradiotherapy course, 15% survival in patients who stayed on temozolomide following their initial course, and 29% survival in patients who returned to temozolomide following a different drug.[51]

In the pre-temozolomide era, nitrosourea-based chemotherapy was standard treatment for GBM. Nitrosureas such as carmustine or fotemustine, either alone or in combinations such as procarbazine, lomustine (CCNU), and vincristine (PCV), have shown some evidence of activity. PCV was compared to temozolomide following recurrence of high-grade glioma in patients initially treated with radiotherapy alone; a 447 patient phase III trial (including 277 with recurrent GBM) showed no difference in survival between groups.[52]

1.6 Authors' Recommendations

- Delineating true tumor recurrence from "pseudoprogression" due to treatment is important. The RANO criteria may be used to assist diagnosis.
- GBM invariably recurs; there are no treatments with a sound evidence base.

- Resection of recurrent GBM may be performed to relieve mass effect, or to gain tissue for further investigations.
- Surgery to prolong survival should be performed rarely, in younger patients with good performance status and tumors in favorable, resectable locations.
- Treatment of recurrent GBM has a poor evidence base with little to commend any specific treatment; clinical trials are strongly encouraged for patients with this condition.

References

[1] Ostrom QT, Gittleman H, Truitt G, Boscia A, Kruchko C, Barnholtz-Sloan JS. CBTRUS statistical report: primary brain and other central nervous system tumors diagnosed in the United States in 2011–2015. Neuro-oncol. 2018; 20 (4) suppl_4:iv1–iv86

[2] Ohgaki H, Dessen P, Jourde B, et al. Genetic pathways to glioblastoma: a population-based study. Cancer Res. 2004; 64(19):6892–6899

[3] Ohgaki H, Kleihues P. The definition of primary and secondary glioblastoma. Clin Cancer Res. 2013; 19(4):764–772

[4] Bleeker FE, Atai NA, Lamba S, et al. The prognostic IDH1(R132) mutation is associated with reduced NADP +-dependent IDH activity in glioblastoma. Acta Neuropathol. 2010; 119(4):487–494

[5] Yan H, Parsons DW, Jin G, et al. IDH1 and IDH2 mutations in gliomas. N Engl J Med. 2009; 360(8):765–773

[6] Ichimura K, Pearson DM, Kocialkowski S, et al. IDH1 mutations are present in the majority of common adult gliomas but rare in primary glioblastomas. Neuro-oncol. 2009; 11(4):341–347

[7] Dobes M, Khurana VG, Shadbolt B, et al. Increasing incidence of glioblastoma multiforme and meningioma, and decreasing incidence of Schwannoma (2000–2008): Findings of a multicenter Australian study. Surg Neurol Int. 2011; 2(1):176

[8] Hochberg FH, Pruitt A. Assumptions in the radiotherapy of glioblastoma. Neurology. 1980; 30(9):907–911

[9] Louis DN, Perry A, Reifenberger G, et al. The 2016 World Health Organization Classification of Tumors of the Central Nervous System: a summary. Acta Neuropathol. 2016; 131(6):803–820

[10] Verhaak RGW, Hoadley KA, Purdom E, et al. Cancer Genome Atlas Research Network. Integrated genomic analysis identifies clinically relevant subtypes of glioblastoma characterized by abnormalities in PDGFRA, IDH1, EGFR, and NF1. Cancer Cell. 2010; 17(1):98–110

[11] Watanabe K, Tachibana O, Sata K, Yonekawa Y, Kleihues P, Ohgaki H. Overexpression of the EGF receptor and p53 mutations are mutually exclusive in the evolution of primary and secondary glioblastomas. Brain Pathol. 1996; 6(3):217–223, discussion 23–24

[12] Stupp R, Hegi ME, Mason WP, et al. European Organisation for Research and Treatment of Cancer Brain, Tumour and Radiation Oncology Groups, National Cancer Institute of Canada Clinical Trials Group. Effects of radiotherapy with concomitant and adjuvant temozolomide versus radiotherapy alone on survival in glioblastoma in a randomised phase III study: 5-year analysis of the EORTC-NCIC trial. Lancet Oncol. 2009; 10(5):459–466

[13] Dandy WE. Removal of right cerebral hemisphere for certain tumors with hemiplegia: Preliminary report. JAMA. 1928; 90(11):823–825

[14] Stummer W, Pichlmeier U, Meinel T, Wiestler OD, Zanella F, Reulen HJ, ALA-Glioma Study Group. Fluorescence-guided surgery with 5-aminolevulinic acid for resection of malignant glioma: a randomised controlled multicentre phase III trial. Lancet Oncol. 2006; 7(5):392–401

[15] Brown TJ, Brennan MC, Li M, et al. Association of the extent of resection with survival in glioblastoma: a systematic review and meta-analysis. JAMA Oncol. 2016; 2(11):1460–1469

[16] Sanai N, Polley M-Y, McDermott MW, Parsa AT, Berger MS. An extent of resection threshold for newly diagnosed glioblastomas. J Neurosurg. 2011; 115(1):3–8

[17] Chaichana KL, Jusue-Torres I, Navarro-Ramirez R, et al. Establishing percent resection and residual volume thresholds affecting survival and recurrence for patients with newly diagnosed intracranial glioblastoma. Neuro-oncol. 2014; 16(1):113–122

[18] Laperriere N, Zuraw L, Cairncross G, Cancer Care Ontario Practice Guidelines Initiative Neuro-Oncology Disease Site Group. Radiotherapy for newly diagnosed malignant glioma in adults: a systematic review. Radiother Oncol. 2002; 64(3):259–273

[19] Stupp R, Mason WP, van den Bent MJ, et al. European Organisation for Research and Treatment of Cancer Brain Tumor and Radiotherapy Groups, National Cancer Institute of Canada Clinical Trials Group. Radiotherapy plus concomitant and adjuvant temozolomide for glioblastoma. N Engl J Med. 2005; 352(10):987–996

[20] Taal W, Brandsma D, de Bruin HG, et al. Incidence of early pseudo-progression in a cohort of malignant glioma patients treated with chemoirradiation with temozolomide. Cancer. 2008; 113(2):405–410

[21] Chamberlain MC, Glantz MJ, Chalmers L, Van Horn A, Sloan AE. Early necrosis following concurrent Temodar and radiotherapy in patients with glioblastoma. J Neurooncol. 2007; 82(1):81–83

[22] Young RJ, Gupta A, Shah AD, et al. Potential utility of conventional MRI signs in diagnosing pseudoprogression in glioblastoma. Neurology. 2011; 76(22): 1918–1924

[23] O'Brien BJ, Colen RR. Post-treatment imaging changes in primary brain tumors. Curr Oncol Rep. 2014; 16(8):397

[24] Wen PY, Macdonald DR, Reardon DA, et al. Updated response assessment criteria for high-grade gliomas: response assessment in neuro-oncology working group. J Clin Oncol. 2010; 28(11):1963–1972

[25] Okada H, Weller M, Huang R, et al. Immunotherapy response assessment in neuro-oncology: a report of the RANO working group. Lancet Oncol. 2015; 16(15):e534–e542

[26] Amini A, Altoos B, Karam SD, et al. Outcomes of symptomatic compared to asymptomatic recurrences in patients with glioblastoma multiforme (GBM). J Radiat Oncol. 2015; 5(1):33–39

[27] Azoulay M, Santos F, Shenouda G, et al. Benefit of re-operation and salvage therapies for recurrent glioblastoma multiforme: results from a single institution. J Neurooncol. 2017; 132(3):419–426

[28] Ciammella P, Podgornii A, Galeandro M, et al. Hypofractionated stereotactic radiation therapy for recurrent glioblastoma: single institutional experience. Radiat Oncol. 2013; 8(1):222

[29] De Bonis P, Fiorentino A, Anile C, et al. The impact of repeated surgery and adjuvant therapy on survival for patients with recurrent glioblastoma. Clin Neurol Neurosurg. 2013; 115(7):883–886

[30] Hau P, Baumgart U, Pfeifer K, et al. Salvage therapy in patients with glioblastoma: is there any benefit? Cancer. 2003; 98(12):2678–2686

[31] Kappelle AC, Postma TJ, Taphoorn MJ, et al. PCV chemotherapy for recurrent glioblastoma multiforme. Neurology. 2001; 56(1):118–120

[32] McNamara MG, Lwin Z, Jiang H, et al. Factors impacting survival following second surgery in patients with glioblastoma in the temozolomide treatment era, incorporating neutrophil/lymphocyte ratio and time to first progression. J Neurooncol. 2014; 117(1):147–152

[33] Michaelsen SR, Christensen IJ, Grunnet K, et al. Clinical variables serve as prognostic factors in a model for survival from glioblastoma multiforme: an observational study of a cohort of consecutive non-selected patients from a single institution. BMC Cancer. 2013; 13(1):402

[34] Parakh S, Thursfield V, Cher L, et al. Recurrent glioblastoma: current patterns of care in an Australian population. J Clin Neurosci. 2016; 24:78–82

[35] Socha J, Kepka L, Ghosh S, et al. Outcome of treatment of recurrent glioblastoma multiforme in elderly and/or frail patients. J Neurooncol. 2016; 126(3):493–498

[36] van Linde ME, Brahm CG, de Witt Hamer PC, et al. Treatment outcome of patients with recurrent glioblastoma multiforme: a retrospective multicenter analysis. J Neurooncol. 2017; 135(1):183–192

[37] Tully PA, Gogos AJ, Love C, Liew D, Drummond KJ, Morokoff AP. Reoperation for recurrent glioblastoma and its association with survival benefit. Neurosurgery. 2016; 79(5):678–689

[38] Ringel F, Pape H, Sabel M, et al. SN1 study group. Clinical benefit from resection of recurrent glioblastomas: results of a multicenter study including 503 patients with recurrent glioblastomas undergoing surgical resection. Neurooncol. 2016; 18(1):96–104

[39] Bette S, Barz M, Huber T, et al. Retrospective analysis of radiological recurrence patterns in glioblastoma, their prognostic value and association to postoperative infarct volume. Sci Rep. 2018; 8(1):4561

[40] Helseth R, Helseth E, Johannesen TB, et al. Overall survival, prognostic factors, and repeated surgery in a consecutive series of 516 patients with glioblastoma multiforme. Acta Neurol Scand. 2010; 122(3):159–167

[41] da Fonseca CO, Simão M, Lins IR, Caetano RO, Futuro D, Quirico-Santos T. Efficacy of monoterpene perillyl alcohol upon survival rate of patients with recurrent glioblastoma. J Cancer Res Clin Oncol. 2011; 137(2):287–293

[42] Mandel JJ, Cachia D, Liu D, et al. Impact of IDH1 mutation status on outcome in clinical trials for recurrent glioblastoma. J Neurooncol. 2016; 129(1):147–154

[43] Lu VM, Jue TR, McDonald KL, Rovin RA. The survival effect of repeat surgery at glioblastoma recurrence and its trend: a systematic review and meta-analysis. World Neurosurg. 2018; 115:453–459.e3

[44] Chen MW, Morsy AA, Liang S, Ng WH. Re-do craniotomy for recurrent grade IV glioblastomas: impact and outcomes from the National Neuroscience Institute Singapore. World Neurosurg. 2016; 87:439–445

[45] Wann A, Tully PA, Barnes EH, et al. Outcomes after second surgery for recurrent glioblastoma: a retrospective case-control study. J Neurooncol. 2018; 137(2):409–415

[46] Park JK, Hodges T, Arko L, et al. Scale to predict survival after surgery for recurrent glioblastoma multiforme. J Clin Oncol. 2010; 28(24):3838–3843

[47] Park C-K, Kim JH, Nam D-H, et al. A practical scoring system to determine whether to proceed with surgical resection in recurrent glioblastoma. Neuro-oncol. 2013; 15(8):1096–1101

[48] Oppenlander ME, Wolf AB, Snyder LA, et al. An extent of resection threshold for recurrent glioblastoma and its risk for neurological morbidity. J Neurosurg. 2014; 120(4):846–853

[49] Desjardins A, Gromeier M, Herndon JE, II, et al. Recurrent glioblastoma treated with recombinant poliovirus. N Engl J Med. 2018; 379(2):150–161

[50] Kazmi F, Soon YY, Leong YH, Koh WY, Vellayappan B. Re-irradiation for recurrent glioblastoma (GBM): a systematic review and meta-analysis. J Neurooncol. 2019; 142(1):79–90

[51] Krauze AV, Attia A, Braunstein S, et al. Expert consensus on re-irradiation for recurrent glioma. Radiat Oncol. 2017; 12(1):194

[52] Skeie BS, Enger PØ, Brøgger J, et al. γ knife surgery versus reoperation for recurrent glioblastoma multiforme. World Neurosurg. 2012; 78(6):658–669

[53] Kim HR, Kim KH, Kong D-S, et al. Outcome of salvage treatment for recurrent glioblastoma. J Clin Neurosci. 2015; 22(3):468–473

[54] Wick W, Gorlia T, Bendszus M, et al. Lomustine and bevacizumab in progressive glioblastoma. N Engl J Med. 2017; 377(20):1954–1963

[55] Taal W, Oosterkamp HM, Walenkamp AME, et al. Single-agent bevacizumab or lomustine versus a combination of bevacizumab plus lomustine in patients with recurrent glioblastoma (BELOB trial): a randomised controlled phase 2 trial. Lancet Oncol. 2014; 15(9):943–953

[56] Perry JR, Bélanger K, Mason WP, et al. Phase II trial of continuous dose-intense temozolomide in recurrent malignant glioma: RESCUE study. J Clin Oncol. 2010; 28(12):2051–2057

[57] Brada M, Stenning S, Gabe R, et al. Temozolomide versus procarbazine, lomustine, and vincristine in recurrent high-grade glioma. J Clin Oncol. 2010; 28(30):4601–4608

2 Natural History and Management Options of Unruptured Brain Arteriovenous Malformation

Michael Kerin Morgan

Abstract

The annual risk of intracranial hemorrhage (ICH) from an unruptured brain arteriovenous malformation (bAVM) is likely to be 1.8% with a 20-year risk of 29%. There is a strong case for venous outflow stenosis (VOS) associated proximal intracranial aneurysms (APIA), and increasing age to be included as risk factors for bAVM ICH. The risk associated with ICH during pregnancy is inconsistent and confusing, although it is reasonable to state that pregnancy provides no protection against ICH. The consequence of ICH in association with bAVM very much depends upon the context. For patients who cannot be treated and therefore may sustain multiple ICH, the risks of cumulative morbidity and mortality is 70% (95% confidence interval [95% CI]: 63–76) including a 42% (95% CI: 36–49) risk of death. For an initially conservatively treated patient with an unruptured bAVM who will be treated if an ICH occurs (i.e., they will have a single ICH), there is a 42% (95% CI: 33–51) risk of morbidity and mortality, including a 9% (95% CI: 6–15) risk of death. The grading systems that should be utilized to assist decision-making in the management of bAVM include the Spetzler–Martin Grade (SMG) and its simplification into the three-tier Spetzler–Ponce Classification class (SPC classes A, B, or C), the Lawton–Young Supplementary (LYS) score, and the Virginia Radiosurgery AVM Scale (VRAS). Familiarity with cohort data allows guidance for the best recommendation of treatment for the individual patient. Unfavorable outcomes (unFOs; persistent bAVM, permanent complication of treatment or posttreatment hemorrhage) following surgery are expected to occur in 1 to 11% of cases for SPC class A (complication increasing with increasing size within class) and 10 to 38% for SPC class B (complication increasing with increasing size within class). Unruptured SPC class C bAVMs normally have such a high complication rate that they do not warrant consideration for surgery. Following radiosurgery, unFO is predicted to occur in 19, 25, 34, 52, and 59% for VRAS scores of 0, 1, 2, 3, and 4, respectively. It is important to remember that the proportion of permanent neurological deficit contributing to the unFO is greater for surgery than that for radiosurgery and the proportion of persisting bAVM contributing to the unFO is greater for radiosurgery than that for surgery. Embolization may be appropriate in some centers that have results comparable to those achieved by other treatments. However, as yet, embolization has not achieved the same level of evidence warranting its general support as an intent-to-cure treatment option for unruptured bAVM.

Keywords: brain, arteriovenous malformation, natural history, risk of hemorrhage, laminar wall shear stress, surgery, radiosurgery, embolization

2.1 Introduction

A brain arteriovenous malformation (bAVM) may cause no problems (an unknown proportion of the population with bAVM) or cause intracranial hemorrhage (ICH; presentation in ~50% of cases), seizures (presentation in ~25% of cases), headaches (presentation in ~16% of cases), neurological deficits not associated with ICH (presentation in ~8% of cases), or a combination of these events.[1,2] Therefore, defining the natural history to be studied can be very complex given the variety of event types and variations in the risk factors for differing events. As an example, posterior fossa bAVMs are very unlikely to present with seizures, neurological deficits without ICH are most likely to occur in large bAVMs near critical brain, and headaches are not likely to be associated with small bAVMs unless associated with venous obstruction. Furthermore, consequences of these events may be highly variable and may produce cumulative problems.

There is no study that could claim to be a study of the true natural history, that is, a study that captures a sufficiently large number of representative cases from the overall population at the inception of the disease and follows these cases without intervention until death. This is not to say that a good estimate of the risk of ICH cannot be made. A number of studies do shed some light on the future risk of ICH. However, the limitations of these studies need to be understood so that, as far as possible, the inevitable biases that distort the results may be taken into consideration and discrepancies between studies explained.

Prevention of ICH is the most important management goal in bAVMs and is the reason for preemptive treatment. Although the various other ways that bAVM can cause symptoms are of importance, for the most part, these on their own do not warrant treatment. Therefore, knowing the risk of ICH is important for bAVM management. The purpose of this chapter is to provide reasonable estimates of the future risk of ICH in unruptured bAVMs and to discuss how this is best prevented.

2.2 Selected Papers on the Natural History of Unruptured bAVM

- Gross BA, Du R. Natural history of cerebral arteriovenous malformations: a meta-analysis. J Neurosurg 2013;118(2):437–443
- Kim H, Al-Shahi Salman R, McCulloch CE, Stapf C, Young WL; MARS Coinvestigators. Untreated brain arteriovenous malformation: patient-level meta-analysis of hemorrhage predictors. Neurology 2014;83(7):590–597
- Hernesniemi JA, Dashti R, Juvela S, Väärt K, Niemelä M, Laakso A. Natural history of brain arteriovenous malformations: a long-term follow-up study of risk of hemorrhage in 238 patients. Neurosurgery 2008;63(5):823–829, discussion 829–831
- Al-Shahi Salman R, White PM, Counsell CE, et al; Scottish Audit of Intracranial Vascular Malformations Collaborators. Outcome after conservative management or intervention for unruptured brain arteriovenous malformations. JAMA 2014;311(16):1661–1669

2.2.1 Comparing Future Risk of ICH for Unruptured bAVM

From two recent pooled data analyses, the annual risk of ICH following diagnosis of an unruptured bAVM is reported to be 1.3% (95% CI: 1.0–1.7) for the "Multicenter AVM Research Study" (MARS) and 2.2% (95% CI: 0.9–5.5) for the Gross and Du study.[2,3] The Gross and Du study was a meta-analysis of a number of cohorts. The MARS was formulated from a combination of two large cohort studies (UCSF AVM database and Columbia AVM database) and two population-based studies ("Scottish Intracranial Vascular Malformation Study" [SIVMS] and the Kaiser Permanente of Northern California) with analysis of individual patient data.[3] Utilizing the decay equation ($e^{-1.\text{annual risk as proportion.years}}$),[4] the projected cumulative incidence of a patient experiencing a first intraventricular hemorrhage (IVH) for the Gross and Du study was 11% at 5 years, 20% at 10 years, and 35% at 10 years. For the Mars, these results were 6% at 5 years, 12% at 10 years,

and 23% at 10 years (▶ Fig. 2.1). The methodological differences of these two pooled data studies do not entirely explain the different outcomes. Because the risk of ICH may not be constant with respect to time, these projected data from annualized risks need to be tested against large series with long-term follow-up. Results of short-term follow-up for unruptured bAVMs suggest a higher rate of ICH in the first 12 months compared with longer periods (▶ Fig. 2.1).[1,4] Therefore, the use of cohorts with long-term results is more appropriate to test the projected results from which to compare the projected annualized long-term risks from MARS and Gross and Du.[2,3] When confining our search to cohort studies with a minimum of 90 cases and at least 10% of the initial cohort remaining assessable at 10 years of follow-up (this provides reliable data for a minimum of 10 years), four studies are of interest (▶ Fig. 2.1).[5,6,7,8] These cohort studies provide moderation to the risks calculated from the projected annualized ICH rates derived from the two pooled data studies of MARS and that of Gross and Du. The longer-term studies lay between the projected

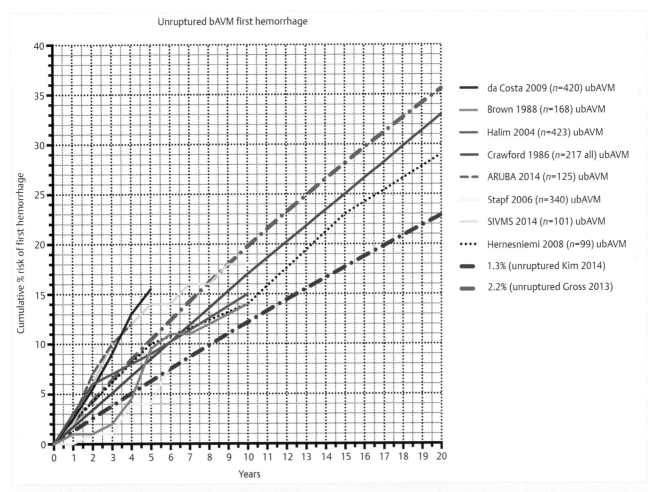

Fig. 2.1 The percentage free of first intracranial hemorrhage (ICH) with respect to time following diagnosis of an unruptured brain arteriovenous malformation (ubAVM). This graph represents data provided by series with greater than 90 cases followed with a reliable number of patients at risk (10% of the initial patient cohort): *orange* (Brown et al[6])—168 cases; *black* (Hernesniemi et al[7])—99 cases; *green* (Crawford et al[5])—217 cases; *blue* (Al-Shahi Salman et al[8])—101 cases; *red thin* (Mohr et al[40])—125 cases; *yellow* (Stapf et al[19])—340 cases; *brown* (Halim et al[9])—423 cases; *purple* (da Costa et al[15])—420 cases. Studies with short-term data (Mohr et al,[40] Stapf et al,[19] Halim et al,[9] and da Costa et al[15]) have also been included to demonstrate their inclusion would suggest a higher risk of first hemorrhage as compared with longer-term studies. The meta-analyses (*blue*—Gross and Du[2]; *red*—Kim et al[3]), represented by the *broken dashed* and *dotted lines*, are extrapolated from the annualized 2.2%[2] and 1.3%[3] calculated by the decay equation ($e^{-1.\text{annual risk as proportion.years}}$).[4]

annualized rates of MARS and Gross and Du.[5,6,7,8] Therefore, it is reasonable to assume (apart from the very early period after diagnosis when some studies report a higher rate of ICH) that fitting the curve of a projected constant ICH rate in the decay equation over 10 to 20 years is a good fit in long-term studies and that MARS underestimates the risk of ICH and the Gross and Du meta-analysis overestimates the risk.[2,3] Underestimating the risk of ICH may be explained partly by event identification (a lower capture rate for patients experiencing ICH as compared with those returning for routine follow-up) and censoring patients to treatment with a higher risk of future ICH.[4] Overestimating the risk may be partly explained by event identification (a higher capture rate for patients experiencing ICH as compared with those returning for routine follow-up) and studies weighted for short-term follow-up (see ▶ Fig. 2.1). The study by Hernesniemi et al,[7] from a time when most unruptured bAVMs were untreated, in which there was a 9.3-year median follow-up and only 1% of cases were lost to follow-up, is worthy of special attention.[7] This cohort found an almost exact intermediate result between the two pooled data studies with cumulative incidence of a patient experiencing a first IVH of 8, 16, and 29% at 5, 10, and 20 years from diagnosis, respectively (▶ Fig. 2.1).[7] Applying the decay function to Hernesniemi et al's results approximates an annualized ICH rate for patients with unruptured bAVM to be 1.8%.[4] This would seem to be a reasonable intermediate rate between the annualized rates of 1.3% from MARS and 2.2% from the Gross and Du meta-analysis.[2,3] Therefore, we believe a reasonable estimation of annual risk of ICH for unruptured bAVM is 1.8% and the 20-year risk is 29%.

2.2.2 Factors that Impact on the Risk of First ICH

There are a number of factors that have been proposed to increase the risk of subsequent ICH in unruptured bAVMs. These include venous outflow stenosis (VOS) an associated proximal intracranial aneurysm (APIA), older age, and pregnancy (see below).

- *VOS*: VOS may be associated with venous ectasia and may be more common with bAVMs associated with deep venous drainage (DVD).[2,3] Although acute venous thrombosis may be a cause for VOS, the most common cause is an acquired intimal hyperplasia.[10,11,12] There is considerable evidence implicating VOS as a risk factor of ICH as well as a reasonable underlying physiological basis for the association (reduced laminar wall shear stress [LWSS]). However, there are no prospective data following untreated patients with VOS compared with those without VOS. Such studies may not be feasible given the widespread acceptance of this condition as a risk factor suggesting the likelihood of a selection bias (due to the preference for intervening when VOS is identified) and the small proportion of cases with VOS in a rare disease making statistical significance difficult to achieve. A consequence of VOS is its effect on the upstream bAVM vasculature. The impact is twofold. There will develop an increased pressure arising once the progression of stenosis is significant and there is a reduction in LWSS with the consequent vascular degeneration. Both of these physiological perturbations, either on their own or in combination, may be a reason for ultimate vascular integrity failure and ICH.

- *APIA*: Aneurysms may be intranidal, APIAs, or coincidental (occurring in an artery not contributing to the bAVM). The association of aneurysms with an increased risk of ICH was first reported prior to 1991.[13,14] The source of an ICH may be either the APIA or aneurysm. The predominant source of ICH when APIAs are present is the bAVM.[13] More recent cohorts have observed this association inconsistently.[15,16,17] An identified association reported in an earlier study of a cohort was not confirmed in later analysis of a larger cohort from the same database.[18,19] This association was identified in the Gross and Du meta-analysis (hazard ratio: 1.8; 95% CI: 1.6–2.0) but was studied in only two of the nine series incorporated in the study. For one of the studies that identified the association of aneurysms with ICH, the mean follow-up was only 2.8 years.[2] In MARS, the association was significant for the first 12 months but was not significant beyond this period.[3] Therefore, the association of an increased risk with APIA is complex and may be present for only a short period after diagnosis, disappearing beyond the initial 12 months.[4] APIAs are acquired.[20] As with intracranial aneurysm formation in the absence of bAVM, high LWSS is likely to be responsible for aneurysm formation (although low LWSS may be associated with aneurysm rupture).[21] LWSS may only be elevated at the time of bAVM formation and early growth and may be normal or low at other times. Therefore, there may be only a limited period of time for the development of APIA after which the conditions favor vascular stability. Following treatment by radiosurgery, prior to bAVM occlusion, there is an increased risk of bAVM rupture in the presence of APIAs.[22] This may be considered support for the proposition that APIA increases the risk of bAVM ICH because the period between treatment and obliteration is considered to follow the natural history of untreated bAVMs. However, the alternate explanation is that during progressive thrombosis of the bAVM as a consequence of treatment, LWSS is reduced, leading to degeneration and disruption of the bAVM. It may be argued that those bAVMs with an APIA are, overall, more likely to have had periods of high LWSS in their past as compared with bAVMs without APIA. If so, they have the vascular angioarchitecture that may lead to a greater reduction in LWSS and greater increase in pressure arising as the consequence of the progressive obliteration by radiosurgery. The reduction of LWSS may increase the inflammation of the vascular wall and the increase in pressure may challenge the integrity of the vascular wall. Therefore, the data from postradiosurgery ICH cannot be legitimately extrapolated to an untreated bAVM with APIA. In summary, with regard to APIAs, it is reasonable to suggest that there may be an association with the risk of bAVM ICH. However, this may be transient. Furthermore, APIA may be a surrogate marker for age, and it may prove to be that increasing age is the factor associated with increasing the risk of bAVM ICH rather than the APIA.

- *Older age*: Age was found to be a factor associated with an increased risk of bAVM ICH in the combined cohort and population series of MARS.[3] However, this was not found in the Gross and Du meta-analysis. This suggests that this association, if true, is likely to be weak.[2] The importance of bias is significant as younger patients are more likely to be offered treatment because of their lower chance of complications of treatment and the longer time they have to live with a threat of ICH. Therefore, there is an age-related selection bias. In order to reduce this bias, evidence from a time when conservative management was more prevalent is important. Two such studies supported the effect of increasing age being associated with an increasing risk of bAVM ICH,[5,13] but a third failed to demonstrate this association.[7] Overall, it would seem reasonable to accept there is an association between increasing age and bAVM ICH, but suggest that such additional risk, in comparison with that of presentation with ICH, is small. Furthermore, increasing age has been reported to be associated with both the development of VOS and the diagnosis of APIA.[11,12] Therefore, there may well be a complex interaction of these factors. This is perhaps best illustrated by contrasting a study from Toronto that found APIA, but not age, was associated with increased risk of bAVM ICH,[15] in comparison with a study from Columbia that found the converse result.[18,19] Furthermore, the Columbia database reported an association with APIA and presentation with bAVM ICH,[24] but subsequently failed to confirm this association.[19]

- *Pregnancy*: Few areas related to bAVM have resulted in such confusing results and consequentially inconsistent management recommendations (including pregnancy termination, avoidance of pregnancy, and no change in management).[25,26,27,28,29] Studying the risk of pregnancy in patients with bAVM presents many challenges. This is highlighted by the variation in annualized risk of first ICH during pregnancy for cohorts ranging from 3.0% (95% CI: 1.7–5.2) to 30% (95% CI: 18–49).[27,28] Even in a study in which the same methodology was employed for two different cohorts, the results vary widely with one cohort having 8.6% (95% CI: 1.8–25) annualized risk of first ICH during pregnancy and the second 30% (95% CI: 18–49).[27] Furthermore, no reasonable explanation for why a normal pregnancy would increase the risk for hemorrhage has been provided. The argument that a hormonal or increased blood volume has an influence on the predisposition to ICH from a bAVM is still speculative. The issue of the risk of bAVM ICH during pregnancy remains to be determined. However, it is reasonable to state that pregnancy does not offer any reduction in risk of bAVM ICH.

2.2.3 The Expected Outcome from bAVM ICH

The outcomes of bAVM ICH are more complex to determine than other causes of spontaneous ICH. This is because there is an increased likelihood of multiple ICHs if the bAVM remains untreated with the risk of recurrent hemorrhage greater than that for the first ICH. Furthermore, the risks of complications from treatment can be significant and may be difficult to separate from those of the ICH itself. For all cases, the reported range of combined morbidity and mortality is 40 to 90% and the range for mortality alone is 0 to 60%.[4] However, the specific situation is an important consideration. Patients presenting with an acute ICH have a 40% (95% CI: 32–48) risk of new permanent neurological deficit or death including a 15% (95% CI: 12–19) risk of death as a consequence of this single ICH.[4] Untreated patients followed until ICH have a 42% (95% CI: 33–51)

risk of morbidity and mortality including a 9% (95% CI: 6–15) risk of death after the next single ICH.[4] Untreated patients followed long term who may be subject to multiple ICHs have a cumulative 70% (95% CI: 63–76) morbidity and mortality including a 42% (95% CI: 36–49) risk of death.[4] Patients treated by radiosurgery followed until the next ICH or subsequent ICH have a 41% (95% CI: 33–50) risk of new permanent neurological deficit or death and a 27% (95% CI: 22–33) risk of death.[4] These various situations need to be understood as the clinical pathway will vary between those patients who cannot reasonably be treated and those who will be treated when diagnosed. For example, it may be reasonable to assume that the risk of morbidity and mortality for a patient with an SPC class A unruptured bAVM would be about 40% if an ICH were to occur and that for a patient with an SPC class C case would be about 70% (because of multiple ICH or subsequent treatment following ICH). In order to simplify these data, an estimated risk of permanent neurological deficit or death from a first ICH of 40% is reasonable if the bAVM would be otherwise suitable to treat if it had presented with ICH rather than unruptured. This is because it is possible to change management pathways if ICH should occur.

2.2.4 Understanding the Cause for ICH Associated with bAVM

In order to better understand the natural history ICH associated with bAVM, the cause for vascular integrity failure needs to be understood. The associated risk factors of bAVM ICH discussed earlier do not directly explain why blood vessels break to cause ICH. VOS, APIA, and age are not independent of each other. Both the identification of VOS and occurrence of APIA are associated with increasing age. A unifying underlying physiological association of these factors is deviation of LWSS from normal. APIA is associated with high LWSS, VOS associated with a point of low LWSS, and age (if VOS progresses) may be associated with a reduction in LWSS. There is a reasonable basis to suspect that a reduction in LWSS explains the ICH. Although this is yet to be verified prospectively (in part because of the difficulties until recently in calculating LWSS), the hypothetical basis is compelling.

LWSS is tightly controlled within a normal range by the endothelial mechanoreceptor-vascular wall response and is likely to remain intact in patients with bAVM.[30] LWSS in the feeding vessels of bAVM may vary with the life cycle of a bAVM (▶ Fig. 2.2). After the initiation of the fistulas, the increased velocity of the involved vasculature leads to increased LWSS resulting in vasodilation, angiogenesis, and arterial recruitment.[31] These responses have the effect of returning the LWSS toward normal (although with persisting increased velocity of blood flow) within the dilated bAVM vasculature. The initial high LWSS may also explain the presence of APIA formation.[20] Studies of LWSS in the proximal arteries of bAVM confirm that values do not vary widely from normal.[32,33] High or normal LWSS is associated with normal healthy endothelium.[34] As with arteriovenous shunts from any cause, points of low LWSS may be present to produce VOS.[35] Low LWSS is responsible for an inflammatory-degenerative process resulting in most of the histopathological degenerative process evident in bAVM and intimal hyperplasia

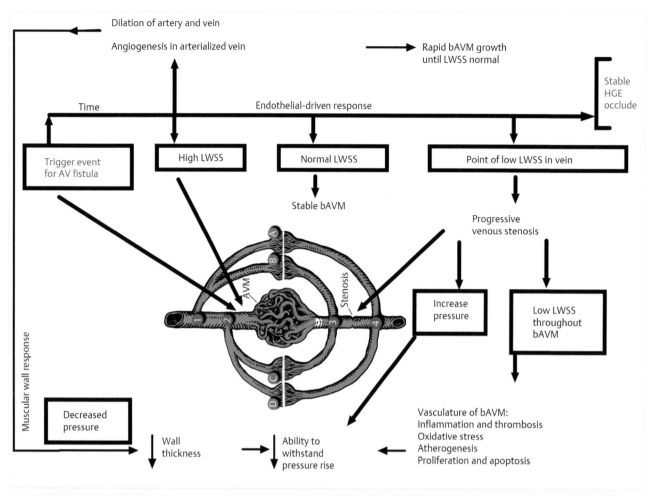

Fig. 2.2 The hypothetical progression over time of a brain arteriovenous malformation (bAVM) commencing with a trigger event and ending in a stable bAVM, intracranial hemorrhage (ICH), or bAVM occlusion. The progress from high laminar wall shear stress (LWSS) through to normal LWSS (after dilatation, recruitment, and angiogenesis) and a stable bAVM. With the development of venous intimal hyperplasia resulting in venous outflow obstruction that results in a reduction in LWSS and an increase in pressure upstream (within the abnormal vasculature). This will lead to endothelial oxidative stress and the changes that can lead to vascular wall degeneration challenged by the increase in pressure within these vessels. Measuring LWSS may prove to be an opportunity to more accurately predict the risk for an individual with a bAVM of ICH.

in the VOS.[34] A vicious cycle may ensue to progress the degenerative process with ultimate rupture resulting from the combination of the vascular degeneration and the rise in pressure if the VOS is significant. This explanation is given in detail in ▶ Fig. 2.2.

2.3 Selected Papers on the Treatment Options for Unruptured Brain AVM

- Spetzler RF, Ponce FA. A 3-tier classification of cerebral arteriovenous malformations. Clinical article. J Neurosurg 2011;114(3):842–849
- Patel NJ, Bervini D, Eftekhar B, et al. Results of surgery for low-grade brain arteriovenous malformation resection by early career neurosurgeons: an observational study. Neurosurgery 2019;84(3):655–661

2.4 Treatment Options for Unruptured Brain AVM

Cushing and Bailey described the first resection of an unruptured bAVM (a probable Spetzler–Martin Grade [SMG] III).[36] The patient was treated by radiotherapy through a bone window created for surgery on a 5-cm dominant central sulcus convexity bAVM in 1924. At the time of surgery, Cushing judged that it was "inconceivable that [the bAVM] could be attacked without fatal hemorrhage" and had the patient treated with radiotherapy. Surgery on this patient was repeated by Cushing in 1927, following which the patient developed progressive dysphasia. At this second surgery, Cushing and Bailey[36] reported:

"The lesion proved to be of stony hardness. The tangle of pulsating vessels previously encountered was largely thrombosed and transformed into a multitude of small bloodless shreds… On finally tilting the growth out from its deep pocket, there passed …

a large thick-walled, partly calcified vessel almost the size of a lead pencil…there was nothing to do but to ligate the vessel and to remove the lesion…. As a result of this operation the patient was rendered aphasic and hemiplegic."

Cushing's management decisions, surgical performance, and consequent outcome remain current. The decision to treat a 64-year-old patient with unruptured SMG III bAVM with combined therapy with an adverse outcome from each treatment would be controversial today. While treatment at this time may be considered controversial, it was based on a misunderstanding of the natural history of bAVM. Norlen asserted, in 1949, that "probably most, if not all, patients die of hemorrhage or are completely incapacitated."[37] Despite the sinister view of the natural history, the opinion of the role of surgery was equally dire. Walter Dandy's review in 1928 of his clinical experience concluded that "the radical attempt at cure is attended by such supreme difficulties and is so exceedingly dangerous as to be contraindicated except in certain selected cases."[38] Radiotherapy outcomes were also initially considered fruitless. Olivecrona and Riives concluded that there is no "proof that Roentgen treatment…in any way alters the spontaneous course (of bAVM ICH)."[39] What progress has been made in our understanding of various management pathways over the last nearly 100 years of attempted treatments?

The highest level of evidence upon which to base management recommendations is the randomized controlled trial (RCT). Such a trial for unruptured bAVM, the "A Randomized trial of Unruptured Brain Arteriovenous malformations" (ARUBA) found in favor of medical management in comparison to intervention with intent to cure.[40] However, lumping the three intent-to-cure methods together fails to acknowledge that there is in fact multiple treatment pathways rather than a dichotomy of pathways to consider for unruptured bAVM: conservative treatment, endovascular treatment, radiosurgery, surgery (with or without planned preoperative embolization), and a combination of the aforementioned treatments. Because of the likelihood of heterogeneity with regard to adverse outcomes among the treatment methods, it is reasonable to conclude that ARUBA has not resolved the question of management despite the expertise of the ARUBA researchers.[41] The failure to identify the best management pathway is largely related to the small number of patients, which reflects the rarity of the disease (unruptured bAVMs are diagnosed in < 1 per 100,000 per year)[42,43]; the ethical dilemma in denying treatment to patients whose risk of treatment was perceived to be low; and randomizing patients with immediate high-stakes outcomes. By contrast, many pharmaceutical trials allow a crossover in management after the end of the trial period once the best course is known.[41]

In the absence of an RCT, what is the best evidence upon which management decisions can be made? Case-controlled series can be a good basis upon which to make decisions providing patients included in the analysis can be seen to be a reasonable representation of all similar cases both treated and untreated (i.e., there is an explanation of how selection bias may have impacted the results); can be reliably divided into risk categories that can be reliably reproduced by others (e.g., grading systems); have sufficient numbers that there is a great deal of confidence in the reported outcomes; and results can be reliably demonstrated to be reproduced by others. In order to compare different treatments from such case series, there must be an acceptable categorization of cases by grade of risk, as well as outcomes, that when applied across different treatments is reliable. Fortunately, such conditions can be met for some of the treatments.

The Spetzler–Martin grading system, developed for risk assessment of surgery, has gained the widest acceptance and has been validated independently by a number of authors for surgery, radiosurgery, and embolization.[44,45,46,47,48,49,50] SMG was established by allocating points for size (1 for maximum diameter < 3 cm, 2 for maximum diameter between 3 and 6 cm, and 3 for maximum diameter > 6 cm), the presence of DVD (adding 1 point if present), and location in eloquent brain (adding 1 point as defined earlier).[44] The SPC categories for bAVM are derived from combining SMG 1 and 2 into SPC class A, SMG 3 into SPC class B, and SMG 4 and 5 into SPC class C.[45] The inter- and intraobserver reliability of the SMG evaluation of the score is generally reasonable.[44,51,52] Unoperated cases have been incorporated into a sensitivity analysis to confirm that maximum diameter, eloquent location, DVD, and presentation in the absence of hemorrhage remain as risk factors, confirming that these factors are valid for use in risk assessment classification scales.[1,46] The relative impact of these factors is high, with an odds ratio of 1.8 per cm (95% CI: 1.5–2.2) for maximum bAVM diameter as a continuous variable, 5.4 (95% CI: 2.5–11.5) for DVD, and 4.4 (95% CI: 2.1–9.2) for eloquent location.[1] Taking into consideration the size grouping in the SMG, the relative risk as depicted by the odds ratio of each of these variables is well represented by their weighting of the SMG points. Therefore, there should be a high degree of confidence as to their reliability and validity of SMG and SPC to predict risk of surgery.

The SMG is useful in a number of ways. These include audit, comparing cohorts, and informing recommendation of treatment. For the first two of these uses, it is common to report outcomes in a binary fashion (e.g., modified Rankin scale [mRS] > 1 or < 2) in order to allow for statistical analysis. However, with regard to its use in the recommendation of treatment, it is only a good first step of many. Adverse outcomes are diverse in both what is affected and how profound is the effect. For one patient, any permanent neurological impairment that may follow immediately from surgery would be considered unacceptable, but for another, avoidance of early death from subsequent bAVM ICH may be given greater priority.

Despite these considerations, the SMG is a useful first step in estimating the risk of surgical treatment and they can reliably predict the risk of new permanent neurological deficits.[44,45] However, for the purpose of comparing treatments, new permanent neurological deficits are only one aspect of the sum of unFOs. Other considerations that need to be incorporated in the assessment of an unFO include failure to occlude along with delayed ICH following treatment. Furthermore, because of the latency period until occlusion, time needs to elapse for the results of radiosurgery to report unFOs. Large cohort series that have incorporated selection bias for surgery, and multicenter for radiosurgery, facilitate such comparison by having a common definition of unFO and have divided cases by SMG.[47,53,54]

There are two assessment instruments specifically developed with the intent of predicting unFOs:

- The modified Pollock–Flickinger (mPF) score[54]:

mPF score = 0.1 × Volume (mL) + 0.02 × age (years) + 0.5

(if located in basal ganglia, thalamus, or brainstem).

- The VRAS[47]:
  VRAS score = the sum of points awarded to bAVM volume ($2–4 cm^3$ = 1 point; smaller = 0 points and larger =2 points) with additional 1 point awarded for each if there was a history of hemorrhage or the hemorrhage occurred in eloquent brain (as defined by the SMG defined below).

Both these scores correlate well with predicting unFOs after radiosurgery. For patients followed for more than 12 months (patients with a complication or hemorrhage occurring in the first year were also included) for a mean of 7 years, these are excellent methods of communicating expectations of radiosurgery.[47] In addition, the SMG also correlated well with unFOs for radiosurgery.[47,48,55] Therefore, the SMG and the outcomes reported with respect to unFOs are a good basis upon which to commence with decision-making for the individual patient as it allows some comparison between the radiosurgery and surgery.

2.4.1 Embolization

Embolization continues to evolve rapidly. These changes can be explained by an increased experience with ethylene vinyl acetyl copolymer, innovation in catheter technology, and the introduction of the promising role of venous approaches.[49,50,56,57] There is some support for selected cases to be treated by embolization with an intent to cure.[49,50] However, because of the results from ARUBA, caution needs to be exercised with its widespread adoption outside those few highly specialized centers that are achieving outstanding results and are exploring the place of embolization as an intent-to-cure treatment.[40,56] In the treatment arm of ARUBA, the breakdown of the adverse outcomes by treatment modality was not published. However, 62% of the intention-to-treat arm included cases for embolization (32% as the only treatment).[40] There was only a small number of surgical cases (5% surgery alone and 14% embolization followed by surgery) and a low likelihood that a significant number of complications would have occurred in those undergoing focused irradiation during a mean follow-up of 33 months. Therefore, it is reasonable to speculate that embolization was a major cause of adverse outcomes (occurring in 36 cases, i.e., 37% of all treated patients) in the treatment arm. A conclusion that may be drawn is that the role of embolization in unruptured bAVM is questionable if alternate management options are reasonable.[56]

Despite the above note of caution, there are two case series of more than 100 treated patients that report (for those completing treatment) obliteration for SPC class A bAVM of 92 and 98% with a decline in neurological condition of 6 and 2.5%.[49,50] However, not all cases in these series have completed treatment (reported as 19% for one of the series and an exclusion criterion from any form of analysis in the other). This allows for the possibility that the overall results may be worse than those reported for the completed treatment group.

Barring advances in technique, the role for embolization with intent to cure for SPC classes greater than A remains limited. The best results from a center that attempts maximum treatment with

embolization reported an 11% new permanent neurological deficit rate with a minority of cases cured by embolization.[49] This is a deceptive figure given there will be a tradeoff between complications of embolization with effectiveness of treatment as well as the exclusion of cases not considered treatable by embolization.[50,56]

The role for embolization as a preoperative treatment is discussed in the section "Radiosurgery."

2.4.2 Radiosurgery

The predictability of the physics and radiobiology of radiosurgery makes risk prediction for radiosurgery reliable.[47,54] A consideration of radiosurgery needs to include the risks of radiation-related complications, time delay between treatment and cure (with a continuing risk of hemorrhage during this latency period), and the likelihood of cure. Because of the interplay between these variables (e.g., a higher marginal dose reduces the time to obliteration but may be at the expense of increasing radiation-induced complications), an overall assessment of unFO is a good method of looking at the overall expected outcome.[54] With the more consistent and reliable principles of the physics of radiosurgery than the much more operator-dependent approaches of surgery or embolization, it is not surprising that there has been only modest improvement in obliteration rate among experts and experienced radiosurgical centers with time.[55]

The mPF score, at a mean follow-up of 70 months, predicts an unFO in approximately 10% for scores ≤ 1, 30% for scores higher than 1 and ≤ 1.5, 40% for scores higher than 1.5 and ≤ 2, and more than 50% for scores higher than 2.[54] In order to roughly calculate volume, the three orthogonal axes (that include the largest diameter) can be estimated by the following equation:

$$\text{Volume (mL)} = \frac{\text{Diameter X (cm)} \times \text{Diameter Y (cm)} \times \text{Diameter Z (cm)}}{2}.$$

Although this equation does not have the accuracy of that involved in the radiosurgery planning protocols, for the purpose of decision-making, it is judged to be reasonable.[58]

Because of the reliable prediction of outcomes from both surgery and radiosurgery by categorizing bAVMs into SPC classes, it is appropriate to specifically look for reports of these outcomes for radiosurgery. Considering all bAVMs treated by radiosurgery (i.e., both ruptured and unruptured), unFO was observed in 25, 31, 39, and 63% for SMG I, II, III, and IV, respectively.[47] Because of the delay to obliteration and the potential for hemorrhage during this period, it is not surprising that unruptured, in comparison to ruptured, bAVMs are less likely to have an unFO after adjustment for the marginal dose, presence of aneurysms, and bAVM volume.[55] Therefore, it is likely that the above-stated unFO rates are lower when considering only unruptured cases. When utilizing the VRAS score, the author's extrapolation for unFO from data provided by a large multicenter study was 19% (95% CI: 13.7–25.8), 25% (95% CI: 21.6–28.8), 34% (95% CI: 30.1–38.1), 52% (95% CI: 47.9–56.0), and 59% (95% CI: 53.8–63.8) for VRAS scores of 0, 1, 2, 3, and 4, respectively (▶ Fig. 2.3).[48]

Larger bAVMs may be unsuitable for treatment by a single radiosurgery session. For such patients, there has been a case

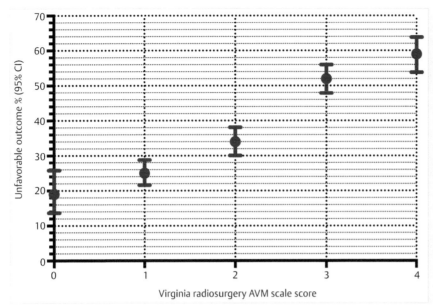

Fig. 2.3 The results of radiosurgery for Virginia Radiosurgery Arteriovenous Malformation Scale (VRAS) scores of 0 to 4 from a large multicenter study of more than 2,000 patients.[48] VRAS score = the sum of points awarded to brain arteriovenous malformation (bAVM) volume (2–4 cm³ = 1 point; smaller = 0 points and larger = 2 points) with additional 1 point awarded for each if there was a history of hemorrhage or location occurred in eloquent brain (as defined by the Spetzler–Martin grade). The point estimates have been made from a graph from the publication and the 95% confidence interval (95% CI) calculated by the author.

series on a small number of bAVM treated by planned staged volumetric reduction (with repeat focused irradiation for residual bAVM). For these, the obliteration rate was no better than 20% at 4 years with a similar percentage of patients dying of hemorrhage.[59] Therefore, treatment for large unruptured bAVMs by radiosurgery should be recommended only after alternative management pathways (including conservative management) have been considered.

2.4.3 Surgery with or without Planned Preoperative Embolization

Important Principles of Surgery

The important principles of surgery that must be followed include the following:

- Awareness and appropriate action related to changes in physiology that occur during anesthesia. This includes anticipating the increase in feeding arterial pressure during and after arteriovenous shunt elimination. Anesthesia with significant blood pressure control to levels lower than normal (but avoiding ischemia) may require both the use of vasodilation and cardiac output suppression (e.g., beta-blockade and barbiturates). Cerebral protection needs to be ensured at low pressures. A reduction in cerebral metabolic activity of the brain will assist brain relaxation. This reduces the need for retraction during surgery. This is particularly pertinent at low pressures, during which retraction may result in ischemia.
- Craniotomies need to be executed to optimize exposure, minimize retraction (by maximizing the range of angles from which the bAVM can be approached), and facilitate access to feeding arteries. Distinguishing arteries from arterialized veins may be difficult but is possible with sufficient proximal and distal exposure of the vasculature. Intraoperative indocyanine green (ICG) may assist with distinguishing arteries from arterialized veins. Accessing arteries from normal to abnormal provides confidence that arteries can be distinguished from arterialized veins. When appropriate, a craniotomy should consider exposure crossing the dural boundaries. As an example, a bAVM presenting on the medial surface may be accessed from both the ipsilateral interhemispheric approach and a contralateral approach through a wide opening in the falx cerebri. This may improve the angle at which the most lateral component of the bAVM may be reached. Therefore, consideration as to positioning must, when appropriate, include free access across dural boundaries (falx cerebri or tentorium cerebelli).
- Feeding arteries need to be dissected proximal to all terminal tributaries of the bAVM (to ensure that arteries can be distinguished from arterialized veins) as well as ensuring the preservation of distal arterial supply to normal brain. This is often best achieved by commencing the dissection distally, beyond the bAVM, and progressing proximally. This allows correct identification of the arteries supplying critical brain. These distal arteries may be much smaller than those branching to the bAVM and therefore may be confused with small terminal bAVM arteries if not sufficiently exposed distally. This requires extensive opening of the relevant sulci by sharp dissection.
- Regional hypotension within the bAVM can be achieved by temporary arterial clips applied to as many feeding arteries as possible. Even when it is thought by the surgeon that all feeding arteries are controlled by this technique, in the author's experience, this can never be assumed until the bAVM is delivered on its venous umbilicus. Irrespective of how well controlled the arterial feeders are believed to be prior to bAVM delivery, venous drainage should not be impeded. Embolization can be used to assist with regional hypotension but may be unnecessary depending upon surgical technique.[1,46,60]
- Retraction of the brain may exacerbate ischemia as perfusion pressure to the brain may be low. Retraction of the bAVM itself is safe providing that the venous drainage is not impaired. Impeding the venous outflow may result from coagulation of the surface vessels of the bAVM (that are most likely venous) coupled with the effects of bAVM retraction.

- Division of the feeding arteries requires competence in a number of techniques. The use of bipolar forceps is more difficult than usual because of the thinness of the walls of the arteries relative to the vessel radius. This can make coagulation difficult with rupture of the vessels if not performed appropriately. Very clean bipolar tips and a coagulation setting lower than one might normally use in other situations are important. Assistance can be gained by the use of microclips to arrest flow. Microclips can also be employed permanently to ligate the smallest vessel and miniclips for larger vessels. The smallest clip that can affect hemostasis is appropriate as these have smaller clip handles, which reduce the chance of accidental dislodgement by the sucker. Some surgeons prefer irrigating bipolar forceps or disposable bipolar forceps exclusively for hemostasis. An additional technique suitable for some vessels includes incorporating adjacent brain with broader blades to spread the current and incorporate more proteinaceous material. This is particularly useful when following vessels into the white matter to swoop them back to the plane of the bAVM.
- Because of the importance of securing all arterial input before compromising venous drainage, a useful strategy is to first secure all the accessible superficial feeding arteries followed by a partial and very limited bAVM marginal dissection on a small arc and white matter dissection directly to the deepest component of the bAVM (including entry into the ventricles if the bAVM juxtaposes the ventricle) to secure arteries to the deep nose cone. This differs from the normal circumferential corkscrew spiral dissection employed for brain tumors. Such a corkscrew circumferential dissection is not initiated until after the deep feeders have been controlled and the deep nosecone is dissected (▶ Fig. 2.4).
- It is necessary to follow small arterialized vessels into the white matter during the dissection. This is because small feeding arteries (few in number) need to be distinguished from the more frequently occurring arterialized venous loops that leave the imagined surface plane of the bAVM and loop in and out of the white matter and are distended and elongated because of the forces associated with high flow in small vessels. The cumulative ligation of venous loops,

mistaken for arteries, will impede venous drainage from the depth of the bAVM. This may produce a problem for the resection of the final nose cone as it will become very tense when the nose cone continues to have arterial feeders. The venous loops should be left unligated and only the infrequent arterial input ligated and divided.
- Before ligation and division of the main draining vein is attempted, the resected bAVM should be deliverable from the resection bed on its venous umbilical attachment in order to be sure that there are no underlying feeding arteries often found in the axilla of the draining vein.
- A satisfactory resection bed has no arterialized bleeding. Bleeding suggests the possibility of retained bAVM and needs to be further explored. Even when this bleeding is not due to retained bAVM, the small vessels responsible for persistent bleeding do not have the capacity to constrict due to the thinness of their muscular wall component and require surgical intervention. Bleeding needs to be specifically surgically arrested rather than allow time to pass for the possibility of arterial vasoconstriction response for hemostasis control. It is important not to stress test the security of hemostasis by raising the blood pressure during the surgery.
- Transdural arterial recruitment (from meningeal arteries) to the bAVM is occasionally significant. When transdural arterial recruitment occurs, the dura and the brain must not be retracted apart because of the risk of tearing the vascular connection. Creating an island of dura and leaving this on the brain over the bAVM is an effective strategy to prevent catastrophic hemorrhage in these cases. The tentorium or the falx can be incised at a considerable distance from the bAVM facilitating blood supply security. Techniques such as division of the tentorium from lateral to medial (to secure the meningeal arterial supply from the carotid artery) or opening of the falx from a contralateral approach at a distance from the bAVM can eliminate feeders entering from the dura.
- Multiple transosseous arterial supply may be present and can lead to catastrophic bleeding on elevation of the craniotomy flap if the craniotomy is performed in the normal way. When present, it is safer to do narrow strip craniotomies, removing

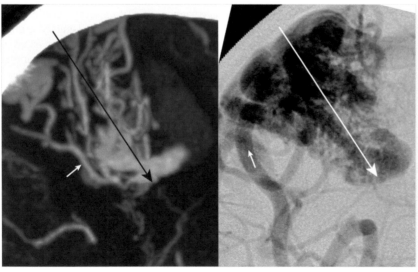

Fig. 2.4 This convexity-based brain arteriovenous malformation (bAVM) illustrates the reason for reaching the deep nose cone early in surgery. The computed tomography angiography (CTA) scan on the left demonstrates the pattern of arterial contribution. Although this is supplied by a middle cerebral M4 branch on the surface of the brain, there is a significant proportion of small arteries (e.g., *white small arrow*) that can be seen diving into the deep sulci to enter the bAVM at the deep nose cone. The digital subtraction angiography (DSA) on the right demonstrates that the veins envelope the body of the abnormal vasculature, making it difficult to gain access to individual arteries. However, taking a trajectory on the lateral side of the bAVM directly to the nose cone by following the *long arrows* facilitates the isolation of the arterial contribution.

multiple narrow strips one at a time and securing bleeding at each stage. Preoperative embolization may seem appealing in such cases; however, the result may interfere with wound healing, given the targeting of the extracranial supply, and is ill advised.

Technical Execution of Microsurgery

Advances in technology (such as ICG) are useful but should not be seen as a substitute for principles or practices of surgery. The most important instruments are the scalpel, microscissors, sucker, bipolar forceps, and microscope. These must be appropriate and used competently for the situation. The following description is by necessity a personal approach. Unlike the principles mentioned above (that must always be followed), there are undoubtedly many ways to effect surgery. This is, therefore, a personal recommendation.

Arachnoid Dissection

A no. 11 blade that is changed often (to ensure that it remains sharp) is used for dissecting within the sulci and for releasing vessels from ensnaring arachnoid. For the efficiency of surgery, it is important that a no. 11 blade can act as both a knife and a retractor. For this, a no. 11 blade that has the spine (or blade flat) beveled as it approaches the tip with the distal half of the tip incorporated in the grind of the cutting edge (or grind) can achieve this dual purpose. This no. 11 blade can serve both as a knife that divides the arachnoid (the arachnoid is placed under slight tension with appropriate positioning of the sucker) and a retractor-dissector. The use of the blade as a retractor-dissector can be achieved by using the back (spine) of the blade (ensuring the tip or blade does not contact either vessels under tension or brain, facilitated by the beveled angle of the tip of the spine) after release of arachnoid tension provided by the sucker. For the smaller sulci as well as in the depths of sulci, an eye knife (that is considerably smaller than the no. 11 blade) is used. These blades lack the distal bevel so that the dual-purpose use of incision and retractor-dissector becomes more difficult.

The selection of suckers is critical for the retraction role during dissection. Because of the fragility of the vessels and the need to use the terminal part of the barrel of the sucker in retraction, a fine-tipped (although rounded to avoid sharp edges) sucker of the smallest sizes (nos. 3 and 4) should be used with low-pressure suction. Pressure should be sufficient to clear the field of cerebrospinal fluid (CSF) and blood, but insufficient to disrupt the small vessels. Sucker tips should be free of burs at the tip to ensure that they do not catch the arachnoid or vessels. Because small suckers may more easily block, a number of spare suckers should be available on the setup to prevent delays during surgery. In addition, as hemorrhage may be dramatic when it occurs, a variety of larger suckers on a separate suction line at higher pressure allows for immediate action if required. By the interplay between the suckers as a retractor and keeping the field clear, and the no. 11 blade as a knife dividing the arachnoid and the dissector, efficiency in minimizing instrument changes can be achieved. Tension to the arachnoid is provided by the sucker, allowing the caress of the no. 11 blade to divide the arachnoid; when tension is released, the no. 11 blade's spine can be used as a dissector.

Controlling Blood Vessels in the Sulci

Controlling every single artery is imperative. This can commence by applying temporary clips on arteries at a distance from the bAVM. As the sulci and fissure are gradually opened, the temporary clips can be advanced closer to the bAVM. Once an artery is judged to be terminating in the bAVM (without supply to critical brain), it can be ligated and divided. By dividing the artery, this point of bAVM anchoring is removed, thus reducing the tension when the bAVM needs to be manipulated. Ligation can be achieved by microclips or by bipolar coagulation. The bipolar tips and current are both important considerations. For the small vessels in the sulci, a very fine-tipped bipolar applied with a low current is appropriate. Avoiding charring is critical as charring may cause uneven concentration of current, resulting in vessel rupture. Having very clean mirror tips of the bipolar is essential. This is assisted, as with the scalpel, by having more than one bipolar available on the setup. By applying the bipolar to a length of artery (much longer than the width of the tips of the bipolar) and taking time to ensure that coagulation is complete, the artery can be divided. This process may require a change of bipolar during the diathermy application of each individual artery. Remember that it is the state of the vessel and the bipolar that determines the exchange, not the impatience of the surgeon to complete the job. For the arteries with walls that are too thin to perform bipolar coagulation without rupture, arresting the flow within the artery by microclips before bipolar coagulation is reasonable. Using a broader-tipped bipolar may assist with distribution of current along a greater length of artery, reducing the risk of premature vessel rupture. However, broader-tipped bipolar forceps take up more room in this often very highly magnified field before the corticotomy is performed. The author favors the use of broader-tipped bipolar forceps when traversing the white matter when a far more agricultural (harvesting the adjacent brain) approach to dissection is practical and appropriate, swooping the white matter into the plane of the bAVM.

Corticotomy

There are two corticotomy strategies to be considered. The first is through a normal cortex. The second occurs when a large number of small arterial feeders need to be divided on the surface of the cortex. For the first scenario, the corticotomy should be in the deepest part of the sulcus to make best use of the sulcal opening. This often affords a shorter course to the deep nose cone. In the second technique, with a number of arterialized vessels crossing the cortical surface, the broadest bipolar can be used to coagulate a broad width of vessels and cortex as one, followed by division of both with microscissors. In the second scenario, the fine-tipped bipolar forceps are less helpful than the broader-tipped insulated bipolar forceps.

White Matter Dissection

Dissection of the adjacent white matter can be performed quickly but needs to be performed in a way that allows arterialized vessels on the surface of the bAVM that loop out into the white matter (for the most part, these are venous loops) to be swept back onto the bAVM. The arterialized venous loops sweep out into the white matter because of the forces involved in the higher-velocity flow within the bAVM causing elongation and straightening of vessels to minimize the flow (▶ Fig. 2.5). For this phase, the suction and the bipolar are used as dissectors and retractors. The suction used at this point is often a little larger (no. 4) together with a broad insulated bipolar forceps. As the suction retracts and removes the peripheral white matter, the bipolar sweeps the immediate margin of the bAVM by lightly closing the bipolar blades upon immediately adjacent white matter while coagulating. This allows arterialized loops to be brought back to the bAVM surface without placing them under undue tension. By using this sweeping motion, many of

the arterialized vessels crossing the dissection void will not require coagulation.

The first goal of the white matter dissection should be to access the deep nose cone and then dissect around the nose cone. The deepest target maybe within the ventricle itself, and entry into the ventricle should be anticipated and encouraged. Identifying the choroidal feeders within the ventricle rather than through the white matter is preferred as the vessels are thicker and more readily controlled by bipolar diathermy (or microclip) within the ventricle and the circumferential dissection around the deep nose cone is easier when incorporating the ventricular ependyma.

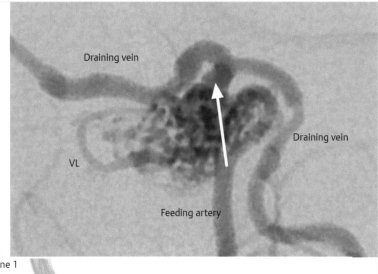

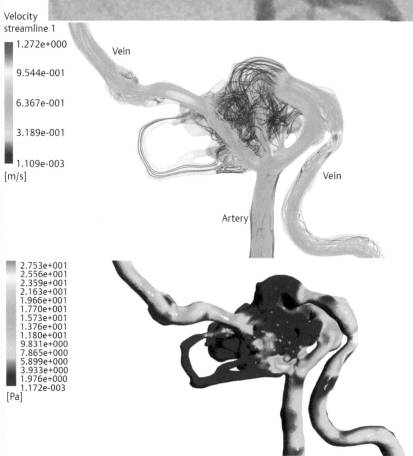

Fig. 2.5 The digital subtraction angiography (DSA) and the computational fluid dynamic models created highlight the forces of flow and the straightening of the venous loop (VL) projecting into the white matter. As one exposes this VL close to the brain arteriovenous malformation (bAVM), each arm of the loop may be mistaken for an arterial feeder. The general arrangement of at least some of the venous drainage being opposite the feeding artery (following the *arrow*) is likely a response to the forces involved in the high-velocity (although normal laminar wall shear stress) flow. It is necessary to use a sweeping motion of the broad bipolar toward the bAVM to bring the loop back to the plane of the bAVM and avoid its disruption. This prevents the need to divide each of the arms of the loops as well as preserving the venous drainage.

Final Surgical Hemostasis

For those familiar with the crystal clear rock pools by the sea at Manly, this appearance is what needs to be achieved in the bed of the bAVM after resection with irrigation fluid in the bAVM cavity. Neither the bleeding should be concealed by cottonoid or covering material nor should there be compression of bleeding points. Both these techniques, appropriate in other neurosurgical contexts, can be catastrophic with bAVM surgery. The small arteries do not have the muscular wall to constrict, and attempted packing may merely conceal a significant hemorrhage. If a point in the cavity wall is bleeding, by using the smallest sucker placed immediately over the point of bleeding, and a second small sucker to dissect around the point of bleeding, it can be ascertained if this is a solitary vessel or belongs to a nest of vessels under tension that need to be resected. In the case of a solitary vessel, the sucker holds the bleeding vessel tip while applying a microclip to control the bleeding. It is very difficult to perform bipolar coagulation on these vessels at this point in the operation. A small square of surgicel over the clip handles will cage the microclip to the brain, preventing accidental dislodgement later by inadvertent contact between the microclip and the sucker. If a nest of vessels is the source of bleeding, it should be assumed that there is "retained nidus" and that further dissection at a slight margin from this nest is appropriate to regain control and allow completion of the resection.

2.4.4 Results of Surgery

A number of factors associated with an increased risk of adverse outcome from bAVM surgery have been identified. These include the following: maximum diameter; eloquent location (defined as motor cortex, primary sensory cortex, visual cortex, language cortex, internal capsule, diencephalon, brainstem, deep cerebellar nuclei, and cerebellar peduncle)[44]; DVD; nonhemorrhagic presentation; diffuse type; older age; and lenticulostriate arterial supply.[1,44,61,62,63,64] There is a strong evidence that these factors have an influence on the outcome of surgery, with the exception of lenticulostriate supply.[61] Of these factors, maximum diameter, eloquent location, DVD, presentation in the absence of hemorrhage, age, and diffuse bAVM have been validated from large surgical cohorts other than those from which the factors were proposed and first identified.[1,45,62]

To understand the impact of selection bias, unoperated cases have been incorporated into a sensitivity analysis and have confirmed that maximum diameter, eloquent location, DVD, and presentation in the absence of hemorrhage are valid for use in risk assessment classification scales.[1,46] The relative impact of some of these factors has been discussed earlier. These risk factors are both generalizable and useful and, as a consequence, there should be a high degree of confidence as to their validity to predict risk of surgery when incorporated into grading schemes. The SMG and the simplified SPC stratifications provide a good basis to estimate the risk of complications leading to a new permanent disabling neurological deficit from surgery. The points allocated for the SMG to the variables are close to their relative weighting as determined by a logistic regression model.[46]

A meta-analysis reported the incidence of adverse outcome following surgery for bAVM to be 8% (95% CI: 6–10), 18% (95% CI: 15–22), and 32% (95% CI: 27–38) for SPC A, B, and C, respectively,

with good concordance between the included studies.[45] Furthermore, four of the studies included in this meta-analysis, comprising more than 1,200 patients, have reported the incidence of late adverse outcomes (complication with new permanent neurological deficit leading to an mRS score >1) to be 2.3% (95% CI: 1.4–3.5), 14% (95% CI: 11–19), and 38% (95% CI: 30–48) for SPC A, B, and C, respectively.[46,65,66,67] These results are not only consistent between reporting expert groups but also, for SPC class A, achievable for young, inexperienced cerebrovascular neurosurgeons.[68]

To have an accurate and useful system for estimating the risk of surgery, selection bias should be corrected by including both the incidence of reported adverse outcomes from patients treated by surgery and cases not recommended for surgery because of perceived greater risk of surgery. Following an adjustment for unoperated cases deemed to have a greater risk of adverse outcome, the risk of adverse outcome is more likely to be closer to 21% (95% CI: 16–27) for SPC B and 57% (95% CI: 48–66) for SPC C.[46] Because of the small number of SPC A patients recommended for nonsurgical management, the incidence of adverse outcomes for SPC A is not significantly different to the risk obtained by analyzing just the surgically treated cases (2.3% [95% CI: 1.4–3.5%]).[46]

Additional variables of age, diffusion, and hemorrhagic presentation in LYS allows for nuancing the SMG.[63] In this grading system, 1 point is added to the SMG score for age less than 20 years, 2 points for age between 20 and 40 years, and 3 points for age greater than 40 years.[63] In addition, a point is added if the patient does not present with hemorrhage and a point if the bAVM is judged to be diffuse.[63] This results in a score of between 3 and 10 for unruptured bAVMs. A validation study on more than 1,000 surgical patients from four cohorts demonstrated that the LYS improves the accuracy of SMG following surgery. The incidence of adverse outcomes from surgery for the combined cohort was no greater than 10% for LYS scores less than 5, approximately 20% for a score of 5, approximately 25% for a score of 6, and approximately ≥40% for scores greater than 6 (▶ Fig. 2.6).[62]

Utilizing the LYS system adds nuance to predicting complication surgery. For instance, an SPC class A patient with an LYS score greater than 6 (e.g., 50 years of age with an unruptured diffuse SMG 2 bAVM) should raise a flag that the complications from surgery may be significantly greater than would normally be expected for an SPC class A bAVM. Therefore, the LYS system can add to the personalized assessment of the risk of surgery.

In addition to adverse outcome from treatment, in order to facilitate comparison between treatments (at least between surgery and radiosurgery), surgical outcomes should utilize the unFO as defined by radiosurgery. Although most bAVMs are immediately effectively obliterated by surgery, those that are not need to be accounted for in the unFO assessment to allow comparison with radiosurgery. A systematic review of the literature has shown that surgical resection results in cure in 96% of patients.[69] At 9 years after surgery, the cumulative incidence of recurrence or residual is 3% for SPC A and 8% for SPC B or C.[53,70] The likelihood of recurrence is greatest in childhood, and in bAVM with DVD.[70] This allows the ascertainment of unFO following surgery for SPC classes A and B bAVM (at 8 years following surgery) to be within the range (depending upon size) of 1 and 11% for SPC class A bAVM and 10 to 38% for SPC class B bAVM (▶ Fig. 2.7).[53]

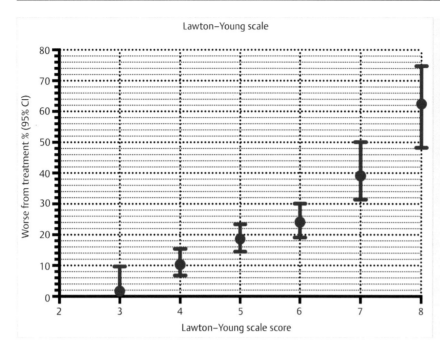

Fig. 2.6 The Lawton–Young supplementary (LYS) score allows for nuancing the Spetzler–Martin Grade (SMG).[63] In this grading system, 1 point is added to the SMG score for age less than 20 years, 2 points for age between 20 and 40 years, and 3 points for age greater than 40 years. In addition, a point is added if the patient does not present with hemorrhage and 1 point if the brain arteriovenous malformation (bAVM) is judged to be diffuse. These data are from the validation study with the 95% confidence intervals (95% CI) calculated by me.[62]

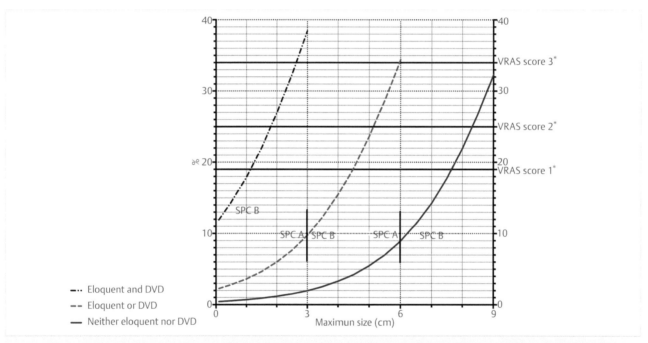

Fig. 2.7 The risk of developing an unfavorable outcome (unFO; complication from surgery or preoperative embolization leading to a permanent neurological deficit with a modified Rankin scale [mRS] >1 or failing to obliterate an arteriovenous malformation) 8 years following treatment from surgery for Spetzler–Ponce Classification class A (SPC A) and SPC B. This is derived from the Morgan et al equation: $\frac{e^{exponent}}{1+e^{exponent}}$, where $exponent$ = 5.076 – (0.473 × maximum diameter) – 1.488 (if located in eloquent brain) and – 1.679 (if deep venous drainage [DVD] is present).[53] The *blue line* is the risk of unFO following surgery for brain arteriovenous malformation (bAVM) with neither DVD nor eloquent location, and the *red line* is the risk of unFO following surgery when either eloquent or DVD (but not both) is present. The *black line* is the risk of unFO following surgery when both DVD and eloquent location are present. For reference, the boundary between SPC A and SPC B bAVM is present. Because of the nongeneralizable results of SPC class and the irrelevance of surgery in the case of SPC C unruptured bAVM, this is not included. For reference, the Virginia Radiosurgery AVM Scale (VRAS) scores of 1 to 3 are also placed on the figure, derived from a large multicenter study.[62] It should be remembered that a higher proportion of unFO for surgery is permanent disability in comparison with radiosurgery. Therefore, this figure should act as a guide but with thought as to what the individual patient concerns may be.

Range of Adverse Outcomes as a Consequence of Surgical Complications

Although the focus is often initially upon whether or not a permanent neurological deficit will arise as a consequence of surgery, it is important to consider the degree and nature of the disability as well in addition to changes in the quality of life (QOL). When a new permanent adverse outcome occurs as a consequence of surgery, with increasing SPC, there is an increasing likelihood of this deficit resulting in death or major disability (mRS >2).[46] Focusing on SPC class B and C bAVMs (as too few SPC class A patients have a deficit to be statistically examined), the number of patients who develop a permanent new neurological deficit (mRS >1) with an mRS score of greater than 2 is reported to be 29% for SPC class B and 49% for SPC class C.[46] A significant proportion of patients undergo change in at least one domain of QOL after surgery.[70] However, QOL changes happen in conservatively managed patients as well. Despite a prospective hospital-based study and a population-based study looking at this question, there is no clear evidence of a worse QOL outcome 12 months after surgery in comparison to conservatively managed patients followed for 12 months.[70]

Time to Likely Benefit from Surgery

The time that it takes for a proportion of untreated patients to develop a hemorrhage or deficit, if untreated, compared to the proportion of patients with that level of deficit arising as a complication of surgery (time to benefit from surgery) for an unruptured bAVM (using mRS >1 as the prespecified level of deficit), is less than 5 years for SPC class A bAVM, more than 8 years for SPC class B bAVM, and will never occur for SPC class C bAVM (▶ Fig. 2.8).[1] If this outcome were to be an mRS >2 for unruptured bAVMs, the time to benefit from surgery for SPC class B would likely be less than 8 years (but no benefit can be found for SPC class C).[1]

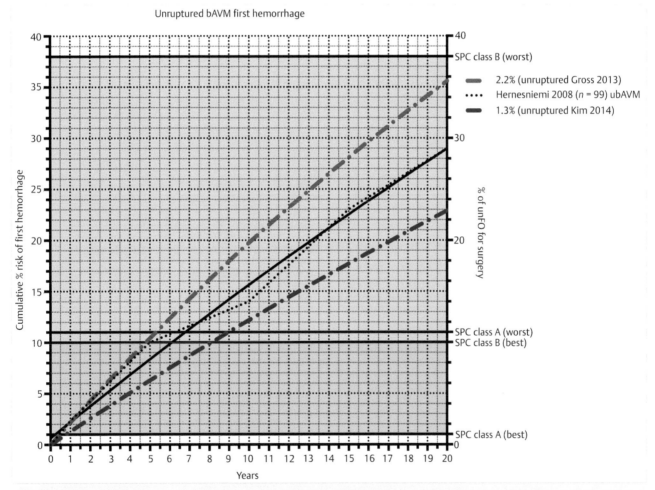

Fig. 2.8 The band of unfavorable outcome (unFO) for Spetzler–Ponce Classification (SPC) class A brain arteriovenous malformation (bAVM; 1–11% depending on size) from ▶ Fig. 2.7 is colored *blue* with the band of unFO for SPC class B bAVM (10–38%) at 8 years following surgery overlaying the risk of intracranial hemorrhage (ICH) as extrapolated from the annualized 2.2% (*red*—Gross and Du[2]) and 1.3% (*blue*—Kim et al[3]) calculated by the decay equation ($e^{-1.annual\ risk\ as\ proportion.years}$) along with the curve fit for Hernesniemi et al[7] (*black*) with the annualized risk of ICH of 1.8%.[4] Whereas it is apparent that surgery for SPC class A bAVM is generally associated with a lower risk than the risk of CH) from bAVM, this cannot be said for SPC class B in the first 5 years following diagnosis. SPC class C would be extremely unlikely to be best treated by surgery.

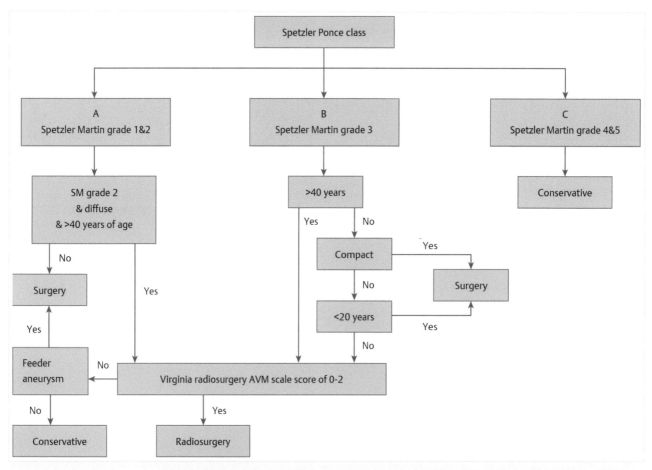

Fig. 2.9 The treatment protocol followed by the author. Commencing at the Spetzler–Ponce Classification and then utilizing the Lawton–Young supplementary score (LYS) to nuancing the Spetzler–Martin grade (SMG) (AVM, arteriovenous malformation).

2.4.5 Combined Treatment

For unruptured bAVMs, combined treatment (with the probable exception of planned embolization followed by surgery) is unlikely to be superior to a single-modality treatment because of the summation of risks. This is supported by the ARUBA study.[40]

2.4.6 Conclusion Regarding Treatment

Selecting a treatment paradigm to assist the decision-making with regard to unruptured AVMs needs to be shaped by both the evidence from the literature and the audit results from treatments that are available to the individual patient. The author's recommended protocol for treatment of unruptured bAVMs, based on the different treatments discussed, is illustrated in ► Fig. 2.9.

References

[1] Bervini D, Morgan MK, Ritson EA, Heller G. Surgery for unruptured arteriovenous malformations of the brain is better than conservative management for selected cases: a prospective cohort study. J Neurosurg. 2014; 121(4):878–890

[2] Gross BA, Du R. Natural history of cerebral arteriovenous malformations: a meta-analysis. J Neurosurg. 2013; 118(2):437–443

[3] Kim H, Al-Shahi Salman R, McCulloch CE, Stapf C, Young WL, MARS Coinvestigators. Untreated brain arteriovenous malformation: patient-level meta-analysis of hemorrhage predictors. Neurology. 2014; 83(7):590–597

[4] Morgan MK, Davidson AS, Assaad NNA, Stoodley MA. Critical review of brain AVM surgery, surgical results and natural history in 2017. Acta Neurochir (Wien). 2017; 159(8):1457–1478

[5] Crawford PM, West CR, Chadwick DW, Shaw MDM. Arteriovenous malformations of the brain: natural history in unoperated patients. J Neurol Neurosurg Psychiatry. 1986; 49(1):1–10

[6] Brown RD, Jr, Wiebers DO, Forbes G, et al. The natural history of unruptured intracranial arteriovenous malformations. J Neurosurg. 1988; 68(3):352–357

[7] Hernesniemi JA, Dashti R, Juvela S, Väärt K, Niemelä M, Laakso A. Natural history of brain arteriovenous malformations: a long-term follow-up study of risk of hemorrhage in 238 patients. Neurosurgery. 2008; 63(5):823–829, discussion 829–831

[8] Al-Shahi Salman R, White PM, Counsell CE, et al. Scottish Audit of Intracranial Vascular Malformations Collaborators. Outcome after conservative management or intervention for unruptured brain arteriovenous malformations. JAMA. 2014; 311(16):1661–1669

[9] Halim AX, Johnston SC, Singh V, et al. Longitudinal risk of intracranial hemorrhage in patients with arteriovenous malformation of the brain within a defined population. Stroke. 2004; 35(7):1697–1702

[10] Shakur SF, Hussein AE, Amin-Hanjani S, Valyi-Nagy T, Charbel FT, Alaraj A. Cerebral arteriovenous malformation flow is associated with venous intimal hyperplasia. Stroke. 2017; 48(4):1088–1091

[11] Shakur SF, Brunozzi D, Ismail R, Pandey D, Charbel FT, Alaraj A. Effect of age on cerebral arteriovenous malformation draining vein stenosis. World Neurosurg. 2018; 113:e654–e658

[12] Mendoza-Elias N, Shakur SF, Charbel FT, Alaraj A. Cerebral arteriovenous malformation draining vein stenosis is associated with atherosclerotic risk factors. J Neuro Intervent Surg. 2018; 10(8):788–790

[13] Brown RD, Jr, Wiebers DO, Forbes GS. Unruptured intracranial aneurysms and arteriovenous malformations: frequency of intracranial hemorrhage and relationship of lesions. J Neurosurg. 1990; 73(6):859–863

[14] Willinsky R, Lasjaunias P, Terbrugge K, Pruvost P. Brain arteriovenous malformations: analysis of the angio-architecture in relationship to hemorrhage (based on 152 patients explored and/or treated at the hopital de Bicêtre between 1981 and 1986). J Neuroradiol. 1988; 15(3):225–237

[15] da Costa L, Wallace MC, Ter Brugge KG, O'Kelly C, Willinsky RA, Tymianski M. The natural history and predictive features of hemorrhage from brain arteriovenous malformations. Stroke. 2009; 40(1):100–105

[16] Redekop G, TerBrugge K, Montanera W, Willinsky R. Arterial aneurysms associated with cerebral arteriovenous malformations: classification, incidence, and risk of hemorrhage. J Neurosurg. 1998; 89(4):539–546

[17] Marks MP, Lane B, Steinberg GK, Chang PJ. Hemorrhage in intracerebral arteriovenous malformations: angiographic determinants. Radiology. 1990; 176(3):807–813

[18] Stapf C, Khaw AV, Sciacca RR, et al. Effect of age on clinical and morphological characteristics in patients with brain arteriovenous malformation. Stroke. 2003; 34(11):2664–2669

[19] Stapf C, Mast H, Sciacca RR, et al. Predictors of hemorrhage in patients with untreated brain arteriovenous malformation. Neurology. 2006; 66(9):1350–1355

[20] Morgan MK, Alsahli K, Wiedmann M, Assaad NN, Heller GZ. Factors associated with proximal intracranial aneurysms to brain arteriovenous malformations: a prospective cohort study. Neurosurgery. 2016; 78(6):787–792

[21] Can A, Du R. Association of hemodynamic factors with intracranial aneurysm formation and rupture: systematic review and meta-analysis. Neurosurgery. 2016; 78(4):510–520

[22] Kano H, Kondziolka D, Flickinger JC, et al. Aneurysms increase the risk of rebleeding after stereotactic radiosurgery for hemorrhagic arteriovenous malformations. Stroke. 2012; 43(10):2586–2591

[23] Graf CJ, Perret GE, Torner JC. Bleeding from cerebral arteriovenous malformations as part of their natural history. J Neurosurg. 1983; 58(3):331–337

[24] Stapf C, Mohr JP, Pile-Spellman J, et al. Concurrent arterial aneurysms in brain arteriovenous malformations with haemorrhagic presentation. J Neurol Neurosurg Psychiatry. 2002; 73(3):294–298

[25] Robinson JL, Hall CS, Sedzimir CB. Arteriovenous malformations, aneurysms, and pregnancy. J Neurosurg. 1974; 41(1):63–70

[26] Forster DMC, Kunkler IH, Hartland P. Risk of cerebral bleeding from arteriovenous malformations in pregnancy: the Sheffield experience. Stereotact Funct Neurosurg. 1993; 61 Suppl 1:20–22

[27] van Beijnum J, Wilkinson T, Whitaker HJ, et al. Scottish Audit of Intracranial Vascular Malformations collaborators. Relative risk of hemorrhage during pregnancy in patients with brain arteriovenous malformations. Int J Stroke. 2017; 12(7):741–747

[28] Horton JC, Chambers WA, Lyons SL, Adams RD, Kjellberg RN. Pregnancy and the risk of hemorrhage from cerebral arteriovenous malformations. Neurosurgery. 1990; 27(6):867–871, discussion 871–872

[29] Liu XJ, Wang S, Zhao YL, et al. Risk of cerebral arteriovenous malformation rupture during pregnancy and puerperium. Neurology. 2014; 82(20):1798–1803

[30] Morgan MK, Guilfoyle M, Kirollos R, Heller GZ. Remodeling of the feeding arterial system after surgery for resection of brain arteriovenous malformations: an observational study. Neurosurgery. 2019; 84(1):84–94

[31] Bervini D, Morgan MK, Stoodley MA, Heller GZ. Transdural arterial recruitment to brain arteriovenous malformation: clinical and management implications in a prospective cohort series. J Neurosurg. 2017; 127(1):51–58

[32] Alaraj A, Shakur SF, Amin-Hanjani S, et al. Changes in wall shear stress of cerebral arteriovenous malformation feeder arteries after embolization and surgery. Stroke. 2015; 46(5):1216–1220

[33] Chang W, Loecher MW, Wu Y, et al. Hemodynamic changes in patients with arteriovenous malformations assessed using high-resolution 3D radial phase-contrast MR angiography. AJNR Am J Neuroradiol. 2012; 33(8):1565–1572

[34] Chiu J-J, Chien S. Effects of disturbed flow on vascular endothelium: pathophysiological basis and clinical perspectives. Physiol Rev. 2011; 91(1):327–387

[35] Jia L, Wang L, Wei F, et al. Effects of wall shear stress in venous neointimal hyperplasia of arteriovenous fistulae. Nephrology (Carlton). 2015; 20(5):335–342

[36] Cushing H, Bailey P. Tumors Arising from the Blood-Vessels of the Brain: Angiomatous Malformations and Hemangioblastomas. Baltimore, MD: Charles C Thomas; 1928:40–48

[37] Norlen G. Arteriovenous aneurysms of the brain; report of ten cases of total removal of the lesion. J Neurosurg. 1949; 6(6):475–494

[38] Dandy WE. Venous abnormalities and angiomas of the brain. Arch Surg. 1928; 17(5):715–793

[39] Olivecrona H, Riives J. Arteriovenous aneurysms of the brain, their diagnosis and treatment. Arch Neurol Psychiatry. 1948; 59(5):567–602

[40] Mohr JP, Parides MK, Stapf C, et al. International ARUBA investigators. Medical management with or without interventional therapy for unruptured brain arteriovenous malformations (ARUBA): a multicentre, non-blinded, randomised trial. Lancet. 2014; 383:614–621

[41] Korja M, Hernesniemi J, Lawton MT, Spetzler RF, Morgan MK. Is cerebrovascular neurosurgery sacrificed on the altar of RCTs? Lancet. 2014; 384(9937):27–28

[42] Al-Shahi R, Bhattacharya JJ, Currie DG, et al. Scottish Intracranial Vascular Malformation Study Collaborators. Prospective, population-based detection of intracranial vascular malformations in adults: the Scottish Intracranial Vascular Malformation Study (SIVMS). Stroke. 2003; 34(5):1163–1169

[43] Stapf C, Mast H, Sciacca RR, et al. New York Islands AVM Study Collaborators. The New York Islands AVM Study: design, study progress, and initial results. Stroke. 2003; 34(5):e29–e33

[44] Spetzler RF, Martin NA. A proposed grading system for arteriovenous malformations. J Neurosurg. 1986; 65(4):476–483

[45] Spetzler RF, Ponce FA. A 3-tier classification of cerebral arteriovenous malformations. Clinical article. J Neurosurg. 2011; 114(3):842–849

[46] Korja M, Bervini D, Assaad N, Morgan MK. Role of surgery in the management of brain arteriovenous malformations: prospective cohort study. Stroke. 2014; 45(12):3549–3555

[47] Starke RM, Yen C-P, Ding D, Sheehan JP. A practical grading scale for predicting outcome after radiosurgery for arteriovenous malformations: analysis of 1012 treated patients. J Neurosurg. 2013; 119(4):981–987

[48] Starke RM, Kano H, Ding D, et al. Stereotactic radiosurgery for cerebral arteriovenous malformations: evaluation of long-term outcomes in a multicenter cohort. J Neurosurg. 2017; 126(1):36–44

[49] Saatci I, Geyik S, Yavuz K, Cekirge HS. Endovascular treatment of brain arteriovenous malformations with prolonged intranidal Onyx injection technique: long-term results in 350 consecutive patients with completed endovascular treatment course. J Neurosurg. 2011; 115(1):78–88

[50] Bahavahdat H, Blanc R, Fahed R, et al. Endovascular treatment for low-grade (Spetzler-Martin I–II) brain arteriovenous · malformations. AJNR Am J Neuroradiol. 2019; 40(4):668–672

[51] Griessenauer CJ, Miller JH, Agee BS, et al. Observer reliability of arteriovenous malformations grading scales using current imaging modalities. J Neurosurg. 2014; 120(5):1179–1187

[52] Iancu-Gontard D, Weill A, Guilbert F, Nguyen T, Raymond J, Roy D. Inter- and intraobserver variability in the assessment of brain arteriovenous malformation angioarchitecture and endovascular treatment results. AJNR Am J Neuroradiol. 2007; 28(3):524–527

[53] Morgan MK, Hermann Wiedmann MK, Stoodley MA, Heller GZ. Microsurgery for Spetzler-Ponce Class A and B arteriovenous malformations utilizing an outcome score adopted from Gamma Knife radiosurgery: a prospective cohort study. J Neurosurg. 2017; 127(5):1105–1116

[54] Pollock BE, Flickinger JC. Modification of the radiosurgery-based arteriovenous malformation grading system. Neurosurgery. 2008; 63(2):239–243, discussion 243

[55] Patibandla MR, Ding D, Kano H, et al. Effect of treatment period on outcomes after stereotactic radiosurgery for brain arteriovenous malformations: an international multicenter study. J Neurosurg. 2018; 130:1–10

[56] Wu EM, El Ahmadieh TY, McDougall CM, et al. Embolization of brain arteriovenous malformations with intent to cure: a systematic review. J Neurosurg. 2019; 132(2):388–399

[57] Fahed R, Darsaut TE, Mounayer C, et al. Transvenous approach for the treatment of cerebral arteriovenous malformations (TATAM): study protocol of a randomised controlled trial. Interv Neuroradiol. 2019; 25(3):305–309

[58] Kashanian A, Sparks H, Kaprealian T, Pouratian N. Assessing the volume of large cerebral arteriovenous malformations: can the ABC/2 formula reliably predict true volume? J Clin Neurosci. 2019; 65:1–5

[59] Kano H, Kondziolka D, Flickinger JC, et al. Stereotactic radiosurgery for arteriovenous malformations, part 6: multistaged volumetric management of large arteriovenous malformations. J Neurosurg. 2012; 116(1):54–65

[60] Morgan MK, Davidson AS, Koustais S, Simons M, Ritson EA. The failure of ethylene-vinyl alcohol copolymer embolization to improve outcomes in

arteriovenous malformation management: case series. J Neurosurg. 2013; 118(5):969–977

[61] Du R, Keyoung HM, Dowd CF, Young WL, Lawton MT. The effects of diffuseness and deep perforating artery supply on outcomes after microsurgical resection of brain arteriovenous malformations. Neurosurgery. 2007; 60(4):638–646, discussion 646–648

[62] Kim H, Abla AA, Nelson J, et al. Validation of the supplemented Spetzler-Martin grading system for brain arteriovenous malformations in a multicenter cohort of 1009 surgical patients. Neurosurgery. 2015; 76(1):25–31, discussion 31–32, quiz 32–33

[63] Lawton MT, Kim H, McCulloch CE, Mikhak B, Young WL. A supplementary grading scale for selecting patients with brain arteriovenous malformations for surgery. Neurosurgery. 2010; 66(4):702–713, discussion 713

[64] Morgan MK, Drummond KJ, Grinnell V, Sorby W. Surgery for cerebral arteriovenous malformation: risks related to lenticulostriate arterial supply. J Neurosurg. 1997; 86(5):801–805

[65] Moon K, Levitt MR, Almefty RO, et al. Safety and efficacy of surgical resection of unruptured low-grade arteriovenous malformations from the modern decade. Neurosurgery. 2015; 77(6):948–952, discussion 952–953

[66] Potts MB, Lau D, Abla AA, Kim H, Young WL, Lawton MT, UCSF Brain AVM Study Project. Current surgical results with low-grade brain arteriovenous malformations. J Neurosurg. 2015; 122(4):912–920

[67] Schramm J, Schaller K, Esche J, Boström A. Microsurgery for cerebral arteriovenous malformations: subgroup outcomes in a consecutive series of 288 cases. J Neurosurg. 2017; 126(4):1056–1063

[68] Patel NJ, Bervini D, Eftekhar B, et al. Results of surgery for low-grade brain arteriovenous malformation resection by early career neurosurgeons: an observational study. Neurosurgery. 2019; 84(3):655–661

[69] van Beijnum J, van der Worp HB, Buis DR, et al. Treatment of brain arteriovenous malformations: a systematic review and meta-analysis. JAMA. 2011; 306(18):2011–2019

[70] Morgan MK, Patel NJ, Simons M, Ritson EA, Heller GZ. Influence of the combination of patient age and deep venous drainage on brain arteriovenous malformation recurrence after surgery. J Neurosurg. 2012; 117(5):934–941

[71] O'Donnell JM, Al-Shahi Salman R, Manuguerra M, Assaad N, Morgan MK. Quality of life and disability 12 months after surgery vs. conservative management for unruptured brain arteriovenous malformations: Scottish population-based and Australian hospital-based studies. Acta Neurochir (Wien). 2018; 160(3):559–566

3 Natural History and Surgical Management of Spontaneous Intracerebral Hemorrhage

Jonathan Rychen and David Bervini

Abstract

The following chapter provides a literature review on the natural history and management options of spontaneous intracerebral hemorrhage (ICH). ICH is associated with high morbidity/mortality risks and requires evidence-based management. Tremendous efforts have been made to produce high-level evidence studies. The most important trials are discussed in this chapter. For many ICH cases, the presented reviewed literature allows to define surgical and conservative candidates. However, there are still some ICH cases "in between," where management remains controversial. The different surgical and medical management options are reviewed.

Keywords: spontaneous intracerebral hemorrhage, stroke, natural history, conservative therapy, surgical therapy, neurosurgery, outcome

3.1 Introduction

Spontaneous intracerebral hemorrhage (ICH) is a devastating form of stroke (the second most common form of stroke, accounting for 9–27% of all strokes) and is associated with high mortality and morbidity risks (the most deadly form of stroke).[1,2,3] The term *spontaneous* is meant to specify ICH in the absence of trauma or underlying structural lesions. The overall incidence of spontaneous ICH is 24.6 per 100,000 person-years and increases with age, with a slight male preponderance.[3]

The clinical presentation of acute ICH includes focal neurological deficits, headache, vomiting, impaired consciousness, and epilepsy. Neuroimaging with computed tomography (CT; ▶ Fig. 3.1) or magnetic resonance imaging (MRI) is necessary to confirm the diagnosis. Contrast-enhanced CT or MR and CT or MR angiography/venography as well as catheter angiography are useful to look at underlying structural lesions. Possible underlying structural lesions causing ICH include cerebral aneurysms, arteriovenous malformations and fistulas, cavernous angiomas, venous thrombosis, and tumors (primary or metastatic neoplasia). It is important to distinguish spontaneous ICH from hemorrhages due to an underlying vascular etiology such as cerebral aneurysm or arteriovenous malformation rupture because these different entities develop at a different bleeding pressure and have different natural histories.

This chapter focuses on the natural history and management options for spontaneous ICH without underlying structural lesions. This subgroup of spontaneous ICH is mainly caused by the following:

- Hypertension.
- Amyloid angiopathy.
- Clotting disorders.
- Recreational drugs (e.g., cocaine).
- Hemorrhagic conversion of an ischemic stroke.

In the cases where no underlying cause is identified with currently available diagnostic tools, spontaneous ICH may be considered cryptogenic or *sine materia*.

3.2 Selected Papers on the Natural History of Spontaneous ICHs

- van Asch CJ, Luitse MJ, Rinkel GJ, van der Tweel I, Algra A, Klijn CJ. Incidence, case fatality, and functional outcome of intracerebral haemorrhage over time, according to age, sex, and ethnic origin: a systematic review and meta-analysis. Lancet Neurol 2010;9(2):167–176

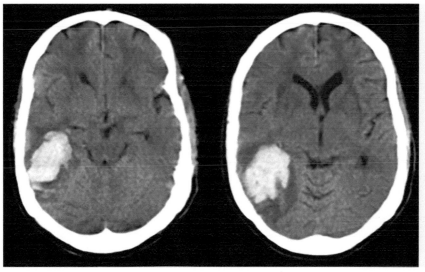

Fig. 3.1 Intracerebral hemorrhage. Axial native computed tomography (CT) scan demonstrating a hyperdense lesion in the right temporal lobe, corresponding to an acute spontaneous intracerebral hemorrhage.

- Mendelow AD, Gregson BA, Fernandes HM, et al; STICH investigators. Early surgery versus initial conservative treatment in patients with spontaneous supratentorial intracerebral haematomas in the International Surgical Trial in Intracerebral Haemorrhage (STICH): a randomised trial. Lancet 2005;365(9457):387–397
- Mendelow AD, Gregson BA, Rowan EN, Murray GD, Gholkar A, Mitchell PM; STICH II Investigators. Early surgery versus initial conservative treatment in patients with spontaneous supratentorial lobar intracerebral haematomas (STICH II): a randomised trial. Lancet 2013;382(9890):397–408

3.3 Natural History of Spontaneous ICHs

A total of 24 studies[4,5,6,7,8,9,10,11,12,13,14,15,16,17,18,19,20,21,22,23,24,25,26,27] related to the natural history and 64 studies[4,5,6,7,8,9,10,11,12,13,14,16,17,18,19,20,21,22,23,24,26,28,29,30,31,32,33,34,35,36,37,38,39,40,41,42,43,44,45,46,47,48,49,50,51,52,53,54,55,56,57,58,59,60,61,62,63,64,65,66,67,68,70] related to surgical management of spontaneous ICH are summarized in ▶ Table 3.1. In all, 13,026 cases (conservatively and surgically treated ICH,

supra- and infratentorial ICH) in 66 studies eligible for the systematic review were included in the analysis. The mean age at presentation of ICH was 59 years (range: 12–94 years) with a slight male preponderance (56%). ▶ Fig. 3.2 demonstrates the common locations of ICH. Spontaneous hemorrhage was most commonly located in the basal ganglia and/or the thalamus (64.8%). ICH was associated with intraventricular hematoma in 21.6% of cases. This was usually related to deep-seated ICH in the basal ganglia and/or the thalamus. In 46% of cases, the hematoma was in the left hemisphere. Considerable hematoma expansion after initial CT scan occurred in 7% of the patients.

From an overall cohort of 13,026 patients, 46% were treated conservatively (i.e., without surgery) with best medical management. The mean age of the conservatively treated cohort was 63 years (range: 12–94 years). The mean Glasgow Coma Scale (GCS) at presentation was 11 (range: 3–15) and the mean ICH volume was 25 mL (range: not reported [NR]). As in the overall cohort, the most common ICH location was the basal ganglia and/or the thalamus with 68.0% of cases. Mortality reached 20% (95% confidence interval [CI]: 14–26) at a mean follow-up time of 7 months (range: 0.5–12 months).

Table 3.1 Pooled literature analysis on the natural history and surgical outcomes following spontaneous intracerebral hemorrhages

Study	Study type	Treatment	No. of patients	Type of surgical treatment (n)	Death (n)	Favorable outcome (n)
Liliang et al[15]	RCS	Conservative	36		3	24[a]
Yildiz et al[25]	RCS	Conservative	153		NR	NR
Auer et al[4]	RCT	Conservative	50		35	NR
		Surgical	50	End (50)	21	NR
Batjer et al[5]	RCT	Conservative	13		11	2[b]
		Surgical	8	Cra (8)	4	2[b]
Bilbao et al[6]	PNRS	Conservative	276		115	NR
		Surgical	80	Cra (58), StA (1), BH (1), Oth (20)	42	NR
Cho et al[7]	RCS	Conservative	201		NR	NR
		Surgical	199	Cra (101), End (74), StA (24)	NR	NR
Fujitsu et al[8]	PNRS	Conservative	111		NR	NR
		Surgical	69	Cra (69)	NR	NR
Guo et al[9]	RCS	Conservative	3,007		321	NR
		Surgical	226	NR	61	NR
Jang et al[10]	RCS	Conservative	195		94	18[c]
		Surgical	86	StA (35), DCraHE (16), Cra (2), Oth (33)	16	9[c]
Juvela et al[11]	RCT	Conservative	26		10	5[a]
		Surgical	26	NR	12	1[a]
Kanno et al[12]	RCS	Conservative	305		NR	NR
		Surgical	154	NR	NR	NR
Kaya et al[13]	RCS	Conservative	19		12	0[a]
		Surgical	47	Cra (47)	16	0[a]
Kobayashi et al[14]	RCS	Conservative	65		NR	NR
		Surgical	36	DCraHE (36)	NR	NR
Liu et al[16]	RCS	Conservative	181		31	NR
		Surgical	129	Cra (129)	18	NR
Lo et al[17]	RCS	Conservative	72		31	5[a]; 10[b]
		Surgical	54	DCraHE (49), DCra (5)	16	0[a]; 13[b]

(Continued)

Table 3.1 (*Continued*) Pooled literature analysis on the natural history and surgical outcomes following spontaneous intracerebral hemorrhages

Study	Study type	Treatment	No. of patients	Type of surgical treatment (n)	Death (n)	Favorable outcome (n)
Melamed et al[18]	RCS	Conservative	15		7	8[a]
		Surgical	2	DCraHE (2)	1	1[a]
Mendelow et al[19]	RCT	Conservative	530		189	118[a]
		Surgical	503	Cra (346), BH (37), End (31), StA (34), Oth (55)	173	122[a]
Mendelow et al[20]	RCT	Conservative	292		69	108[a]
		Surgical	305	Cra (284), Oth (21)	54	123[a]
Sumer et al[21]	PNRS	Conservative	46		5	30[a]
		Surgical	1	DCraHE (1)	1	0[a]
Tan et al[22]	PNRS	Conservative	17		6	NR
		Surgical	17	Cra (17)	8	NR
Wang et al[23]	RCT	Conservative	234		45	29[a]
		Surgical	266	NR	31	21[a]
Xu and Hai[24]	RCT	Conservative	50		NR	NR
		Surgical	50	StA (50)	NR	NR
Zuccarello et al[26]	RCT	Conservative	11		3	4[b]
		Surgical	9		2	5[b]
Hanley et al[28]	RCT	Conservative	42		4	6[c]
		Surgical	54	StA (54)	8	8[c]
Barrett et al[29]	RCS	Surgical	15	StA (15)	2	NR
Bauer et al[30]	PNRS	Surgical	18	Oth (18)	1	NR
Chen and Feng[31]	RCS	Surgical	322	NR	NR	NR
Chi et al[32]	RCS	Surgical	1,310	Cra (312), BH (298), End (144), StA (475), Oth (81)	241	NR
Esquenazi et al[33]	PNRS	Surgical	73	DCraHE (63), DCra (10)	20	11[a]
Fu et al[34]	RCS	Surgical	267	IVF (267)	NR	NR
Gao et al[35]	RCS	Surgical	106	Cra (106)	7	NR
Goedemans et al[36]	RCS	Surgical	29	DCra (15), DCraHE (14)	NR	9[b]
Hayes et al[37]	RCS	Surgical	51	Cra (33), DCraHE (18)	15	15[c]
Hinson et al[38]	RCS	Surgical	14	IVF (8), Oth (6)	6	NR
Jianwei et al[39]	RCS	Surgical	28	Cra (28)	NR	NR
Kim et al[40]	RCS	Surgical	24	DCraHE (24)	6	12[b]
Kwon et al[41]	RCS	Surgical	47	StA (47)	2	16[b]
Labib et al[42]	PNRS	Surgical	39	Oth (39)	0	22[c]
Ma et al[43]	RCS	Surgical	84	DCraHE (46), Cra (38)	32	1[a]
Marquardt et al[44]	PNRS	Surgical	64	StA (64)	2	NR
Matsumoto and Hondo[45]	RCS	Surgical	51	StA (51)	7	12[a]
Moussa and Khedr[46]	RCT	Surgical	40	DCraHE (20), Cra (20)	7	18[a]
Murthy et al[47]	RCS	Surgical	12	DCraHE (12)	1	5[d]
Naff et al[48]	RCT	Surgical	48	IVF (26), Other (22)	10	NR
Niizuma et al[49]	RCS	Surgical	190	StA (175), Cra (15)	NR	NR
Piotrowski and Rochowanski[50]	RCS	Surgical	275	Cra (275)	NR	NR
Rehman et al[51]	RCS	Surgical	27	Cra (27)	6	NR
Sadahiro et al[52]	PNRS	Surgical	10	End (10)	0	0[a]
Takeda et al[53]	RCS	Surgical	25	Cra (20), DCraHE (5)	NR	NR
Shin et al[54]	RCS	Surgical	45	Cra (45)	14	0[a]
Singh et al[55]	RCS	Surgical	28	DCraHE (28)	10	NR
Spiotta et al[56]	RCS	Surgical	29	End (29)	4	NR
Staykov et al[57]	PNRS	Surgical	32	IVF (32)	5	13[d]

(*Continued*)

Table 3.1 (*Continued*) Pooled literature analysis on the natural history and surgical outcomes following spontaneous intracerebral hemorrhages

Study	Study type	Treatment	No. of patients	Type of surgical treatment (*n*)	Death (*n*)	Favorable outcome (*n*)
Takeuchi et al[58]	RCS	Surgical	21	DCraHE (21)	4	6[b]
Vespa et al[59]	RCT	Surgical	14	End (14)	1	6[c]
Wang et al[60]	PNRS	Surgical	104	StA (70), End (34)	32	48[b]
Wang et al[61]	RCS	Surgical	309	StA (309)	44	NR
Wu et al[62]	RCS	Surgical	126	StA (126)	NR	NR
Yadav et al[63]	PNRS	Surgical	25	End (25)	6	13[a]
Yang et al[64]	RCS	Surgical	21	StA (21)	0	20[a]
Yang and Shao[65]	RCT	Surgical	156	StA (78), Cra (78)	NR	NR
Fei et al[66]	RCS	Surgical	112	NR	NR	NR
Zhang et al[67]	RCS	Surgical	33	DCraHE (33)	8	5[a]
Zhao et al[68]	PNRS	Surgical	296	DCraHE (127), Cra (116), StA (53)	63	151[b]
Ziai et al[69]	RCS	Surgical	12	IVF (12)	1	NR
Zuo et al[70]	RCS	Surgical	176	End (176)	NR	NR
Total (*n*; %)	RCS (40; 60%) PNRS (13; 20%) RCT (13; 20%)	Conservative (5,947; 46%) Surgical (7,079; 54%)		Cra (2,211; 38%), StA (1,682; 29%), End (553; 9.5%), DCraHE (515; 9%), IVF (345; 6%), BH (336; 6%), DCra (30; 0.5%), Oth (101; 2%)	Conservative (991; 20% [95% CI: 14–26]) Surgical (1,041; 21% [95% CI: 15–27])	Conservative (362; 24% [95% CI: 14–34]) Surgical (688; 29% [95% CI: 21–37])

Abbreviations: BH, burr hole or keyhole craniotomy; CI, confidence interval; Cra, craniotomy; DCra, decompressive craniectomy alone; DCraHE, decompressive craniectomy and hematoma evacuation; End, endoscopy; IVF, intraventricular fibrinolysis with EVD; NR, not reported; Oth, other; PNRS, prospective nonrandomized study; RCS, retrospective case series; RCT, randomized controlled trial; StA, stereotactic or CT-guided aspiration.
[a]Favorable outcome defined as Glasgow Outcome Scale (GOS) ≥ 5.
[b]Favorable outcome defined as GOS ≥ 4.
[c]Favorable outcome defined as modified Rankin scale (mRS) ≤ 3.
[d]Favorable outcome defined as mRS ≤ 2.

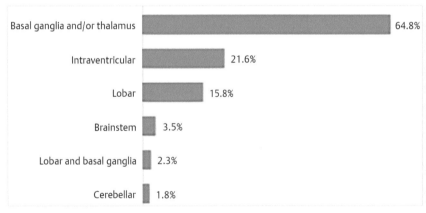

Fig. 3.2 Location of intracerebral hemorrhage (ICH): basal ganglia and/or thalamus (*n* = 6,417), intraventricular (*n* = 2,134), lobar (*n* = 1,569), brainstem (*n* = 349), lobar and basal ganglia (*n* = 228), and cerebellar (*n* = 176). The sum of percentages is not equal to 100% because patients can be classified to more than one location category.

A favorable functional outcome was seen in 24% (95% CI: 14–34) of patients at a mean follow-up time of 6 months (range: 0.5–12 months; the definition of favorable outcome varied among the different studies; for details, see ▶ Table 3.1).

3.4 Natural History of Spontaneous Supratentorial ICH

There are high morbidity and mortality risks following spontaneous ICH. The presence of intraventricular hemorrhage (IVH) or hydrocephalus is associated with a significantly poorer outcome.

A subgroup analysis from the International Surgical Trials in Intracerebral Hemorrhage (STICH) data showed that only 15% of patients with ICH and IVH had a favorable outcome, compared to 31% of patients without IVH.[71] The most important risk factor for development of ICH is patient's age. However, the most important modifiable risk factor is hypertension.[72] The ICH score has been developed as a grading scale for spontaneous ICH. It can be calculated based on the clinical features depicted in ▶ Table 3.2 and has been validated to estimate 30-day mortality[73,74,75] (▶ Table 3.3) and 12-month functional outcome (conservative and surgical treatment combined).[76] Factors associated with 30-day mortality and worse functional

Table 3.2 Intracerebral hemorrhage score[73]

Feature	Finding	Points
GCS score	3–4	2
	5–12	1
	13–15	0
Age	≥80 y	1
	<80 y	0
Location	Infratentorial	1
	Supratentorial	0
ICH volume	≥30 mL	1
	<30 mL	0
Intraventricular blood	Yes	1
	No	0
Total points (ICH score)		0–6

Abbreviations: GCS, Glasgow Coma Scale; ICH, intracerebral hemorrhage.

Table 3.3 Thirty-day mortality based on ICH score[73]

ICH score	30-d mortality
0	0%
1	13%
2	26%
3	72%
4	97%
5	100%
6	100%[a]

Abbreviation: ICH, intracerebral hemorrhage.
[a]No patients in the study had a score of 6, but it is expected that a score of 6 has a high mortality rate.

outcome are lower GCS, age ≥80 years, infratentorial origin of ICH, higher ICH volume, and presence of IVH. Thirty-day mortality increases steadily with ICH score.[73] If patients survive the acute stage after spontaneous ICH, about one-third of them continue to improve neurologically across the first year post ictus.[76]

3.5 Natural History of Spontaneous Infratentorial ICH

In the cohort presented earlier, cerebellar hemorrhages represent around 2% of all spontaneous ICH. Heros reported rates ranging between 5 and 10%.[77] Because of the narrow confines of the posterior fossa, infratentorial ICH is associated with a higher mortality than supratentorial ICH. Indeed, cerebellar hemorrhage can quickly lead to obstructive hydrocephalus, compression of the brainstem, and eventually to death. Mortality at 12 months was reported to range from 28 to 43% and good outcomes (modified Rankin scale [mRS]: 0–3) at 3 months from 31 to 36%, regardless of treatment modality.[78] Neurological condition at presentation based on GCS has been significantly associated with outcome, with GCS ≥13 being a significant predictor of good outcome.[79]

3.6 Selected Papers on Surgical Management of Spontaneous ICHs

- Prasad K, Mendelow AD, Gregson B. Surgery for primary supratentorial intracerebral haemorrhage. Cochrane Database Syst Rev 2008; (4):CD000200
- Hemphill JC III, Greenberg SM, Anderson CS, et al; American Heart Association Stroke Council; Council on Cardiovascular and Stroke Nursing; Council on Clinical Cardiology. Guidelines for the management of spontaneous intracerebral hemorrhage: a guideline for healthcare professionals from the American Heart Association/American Stroke Association. Stroke 2015;46(7):2032–2060
- Mendelow AD, Gregson BA, Fernandes HM, et al; STICH investigators. Early surgery versus initial conservative

treatment in patients with spontaneous supratentorial intracerebral haematomas in the International Surgical Trial in Intracerebral Haemorrhage (STICH): a randomised trial. Lancet 2005;365(9457):387–397
- Mendelow AD, Gregson BA, Rowan EN, Murray GD, Gholkar A, Mitchell PM; STICH II Investigators. Early surgery versus initial conservative treatment in patients with spontaneous supratentorial lobar intracerebral haematomas (STICH II): a randomised trial. Lancet 2013;382(9890):397–408

3.7 Surgical Management Options for Spontaneous ICHs

Among the 13,026 patients, 54% of cases were treated surgically. The mean age of the surgical cohort was 58 years (range: 12–94 years). The mean GCS at presentation was 8 (range: 3–15) and the mean ICH volume was 62 mL (range: 8.2–140 mL). The most common ICH location in the surgically treated cohort was the basal ganglia and/or the thalamus with 64.0% of cases.

Craniotomy and hematoma evacuation were performed in 38% of the cases, followed by stereotactic or CT-guided aspiration of the hematoma (29%; ▶ Fig. 3.3). The need for an external ventricular drain (EVD) and ventriculoperitoneal shunting (VPS) was 19 and 12%, respectively. The overall surgical complication rate (i.e., rebleedings, wound healing disturbances, infections, etc.) reached 11% (95% CI: 0–25), including 9% (95% CI: 0–25) of postoperative rebleedings.

In the surgically treated cohort, mortality reached 21% (95% CI: 15–27) at a mean follow-up time of 6 months (range: 0.5–39). A favorable functional outcome was noted in 29% (95% CI: 21–37) of patients at a mean follow-up period of 6 months (range: 0.5–39).

When analyzing mortality for each surgical subgroup, we found that the decompressive craniectomy subgroup (with or without hematoma evacuation) is associated with a mortality of 24% (95% CI: 6–42), compared to 21% (95% CI: 9–33) in the craniotomy subgroup, 17% (95% CI: 0–47) in the endoscopic subgroup, 14% (95% CI: 0–39) in the keyhole craniotomy subgroup, and 13% (95% CI: 0–31) in the stereotactic or CT-guided aspiration subgroup. Functional outcome was inconsistently reported for the different subgroups, so that a meaningful analysis was not possible. Notwithstanding these findings, these pooled data are subjected to inherent selection bias and need to be interpreted with consideration.

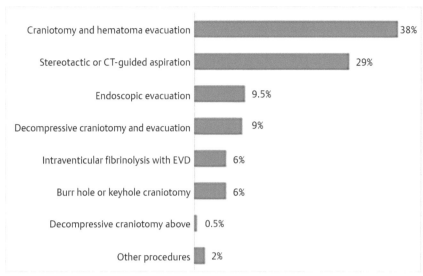

Fig. 3.3 Different surgical managements for spontaneous intracerebral hemorrhage (ICH): craniotomy and hematoma evacuation (*n* = 2,211), stereotactic or computed tomography (CT) guided aspiration (*n* = 1,682), endoscopic evacuation (*n* = 553), decompressive craniectomy and hematoma evacuation (*n* = 515), intraventricular fibrinolysis with external ventricular drain (EVD; *n* = 345), burr hole or keyhole craniotomy (*n* = 336), decompressive craniectomy alone (*n* = 30), and other procedures (*n* = 101).

Table 3.4 Major randomized controlled trials on surgical therapy for ICH

RCT	Type of bleeding	Type of treatment	Results
STICH[19]	ICH, supratentorial, any location	Early surgery (conventional and MI) vs. medical treatment	No difference in clinical outcome (positive trend for surgery in ICH within 1 cm of the cortical surface)
STICH II[20]	ICH, supratentorial, lobar (without intraventricular hematoma)	Early surgery (conventional and MI) vs. medical treatment	Surgery is safe, but no difference in clinical outcome
MISTIE III[81]	ICH, supratentorial, any location	MI catheter aspiration and alteplase irrigation vs. medical treatment	Surgery is safe but no difference in clinical outcome
ICES[59]	ICH, supratentorial, any location	MI image-guided endoscopic surgery vs. medical therapy	Surgery is safe and effective in reducing ICH volume, but data on clinical outcome are missing (no phase 3 trial to date)
Wang et al[88]	ICH in basal ganglia	MI puncture vs. medical therapy	Functional outcome better with surgery; no difference in mortality
CLEAR III[27]	IVH obstructing the third and fourth ventricles	Alteplase through EVD	Alteplase is safe but no difference in functional outcome

Abbreviations: EVD, external ventricular drain; ICH, intracerebral hemorrhage; IVH, intraventricular hemorrhage; MI, minimally invasive; RCT, randomized controlled trial.

3.8 Surgical Management of Spontaneous Supratentorial ICH

Despite efforts in conducting prospective randomized trials comparing surgical management with the best medical care, surgical evacuation of spontaneous ICH remains controversial. The major randomized controlled trials on surgical therapy for supratentorial ICH are summarized in ▶ Table 3.4. STICH I and II compared early surgical hematoma evacuation with the best medical treatment in patients with supratentorial ICH (any location in STICH I and lobar ICH without intraventricular hematoma in STICH II) and found that early surgery did not show an overall benefit compared with the best medical management.[19,20] However, a subgroup analysis in the STICH I trial revealed a positive trend for surgery in those patients with hemorrhages within 1 cm of the cortical surface.[19] In a meta-analysis of 10 randomized trials of surgical outcomes for supratentorial ICH, early surgery was superior to medical treatment, but there was significant heterogeneity between the trials, which mandates cautious interpretation of these results.[80]

Decompressive hemicraniectomy with or without hematoma evacuation reduces mortality for patients with large ICH, significant midline shift, and comatose status in comparison to medical management.[83,84,85]

When analyzing each surgical subgroup of the above-presented literature review, minimally invasive surgical techniques such as stereotactic or CT-guided hematoma aspiration, keyhole craniotomy, and endoscopic evacuation seem to have lower mortality rates (13, 14, and 17%, respectively) than conventional craniotomy or decompressive craniectomy (21 and 24%, respectively). This is in line with several studies suggesting the beneficial role of minimally invasive surgical evacuation of ICH.[4,86,87,88] However, cautious interpretation of these results is necessary due to potential selection bias (decompressive craniectomy may be used more frequently as salvage surgery for patients with a bad clinical condition). A prospective randomized trial from China analyzed the results of needle aspiration of ICH in the basal ganglia compared to medical management. At 3 months, functional outcome was significantly better in the surgical arm, without any differences regarding mortality in comparison to the medical treatment arm.[88] The Minimally Invasive Surgery Plus Recombinant Tissue-Type Plasminogen Activator for ICH Evacuation (MISTIE, phase II) trial reported that minimally invasive catheter aspiration of ICH followed by alteplase clot irrigation seems to be safe, and hematoma removal significantly reduces perihematomal edema.[28,87] The recent results of MISTIE III, a randomized phase III clinical trial with 500 patients, confirmed that the method can be used safely, but failed to show a significant improvement of the functional outcome in comparison to medical therapy.[89] Finally, the Intraoperative Stereotactic Computed Tomography-Guided Endoscopic Surgery (ICES) study is a randomized trial comparing image-guided endoscopic removal of ICH versus medical management. The results showed that the ICH volume can be reduced safely and effectively.[59] However, the impact on mortality and functional outcome needs to be analyzed in an appropriate phase III clinical trial.

As it is widely accepted that surgical intervention for patients older than 80 years is associated with significantly higher morbidity and mortality,[73,76,90] conservative management of supratentorial ICH in this cohort is generally recommended. On balance, the decision to operate must be individualized, based on the neurological condition, size, and localization of the hematoma, patient's age, and the possible existence of a "living will."

3.9 Surgical Management of Spontaneous Infratentorial ICH

Randomized controlled trials comparing surgical versus conservative management of infratentorial ICH have not been performed and are probably ethically not feasible, due to the multiple retrospective series reporting more favorable outcome with surgery in patients with neurological deterioration (GCS <13), brainstem compression, hydrocephalus, or large hematomas.[78,91,92,93,94,95,96] Different studies have examined varying hematoma size thresholds for surgical therapy; a hematoma size larger than 3 cm is considered a meaningful threshold for surgical therapy.[91,92,93,97] A recent meta-analysis by Kuramatsu et al showed that surgical hematoma evacuation was associated with a significant greater probability of survival (78.3 vs. 61.2%) compared with conservative management for cerebellar hemorrhage. However, there was no significant difference in the functional outcome.[78] In this meta-analysis, the hematoma size threshold hypothesis of more than 3 cm was reinforced. Indeed, a threshold hematoma volume ranging between 12 and 15 cm^3 was identified (a hematoma with 3-cm diameter corresponds approximately to 13.5 cm^3); below this level, surgical hematoma evacuation was associated with lower likelihood of favorable functional outcome, whereas above, it was associated with greater likelihood of survival.[78]

Hydrocephalus in the presence of an infratentorial ICH can be due to a "packed posterior fossa" with effacement of the cisterns and compression of the fourth ventricle and/or due to a cerebellar hemorrhage with an intraventricular obstructive component. In the presence of an obstructive clot in the fourth ventricle without "packed posterior fossa," there is some evidence that placement of a ventricular drain as a sole therapy can be considered to treat hydrocephalus[93]; however, it is not recommended by the American Heart Association (AHA)/American Stroke Association (ASA) ICH guidelines.[82] Cerebellar upward

herniation after sole treatment with a ventricular drain occurred in 2 of 30 patients (6.7%) in the series of van Loon et al.[93] In the presence of hydrocephalus and a "packed posterior fossa," sole placement of an EVD is clearly not sufficient due to the compression of the brainstem. In this scenario, additional surgical decompression of the posterior fossa is necessary.[93,98,99,100]

Due to the highly eloquent location, surgical evacuation of brainstem ICH is associated with a high morbidity and in those ICH, a conservative treatment should be preferred.[82,101,102] Although there are reports that suggest that surgical treatment of brainstem hemorrhages is safe and effective,[103,104,105] the invasive treatment of spontaneous ICH in these location remains controversial.

3.10 Surgical Management for Spontaneous ICH Associated with Intraventricular Hemorrhage

When a spontaneous ICH results in intraventricular hemorrhagic extension with hydrocephalus, placement of an EVD helps drain blood and cerebrospinal fluid from the ventricles. However, difficulty to maintain catheter patency and the slow removal of intraventricular blood are some of the limitations of EVD. The adjunctive use of thrombolytic agents has shown to be helpful in minimizing these limitations.[82] The largest trials of intraventricular fibrinolysis to date are the Clot lysis: Evaluating Accelerated Resolution of IVH (CLEAR-IVH) trials.[27,48] The CLEAR-IVH (phase II) study concluded that intraventricular injection of low-dose recombinant tissue-type plasminogen activator enhances clot resolution in IVH with an acceptable safety profile.[48] The phase III clinical trial (CLEAR III) randomized a total of 500 patients to intraventricular fibrinolysis and placebo injection. The safety of intraventricular fibrinolysis has been confirmed, but no improvement in functional outcome could be confirmed. The mortality rate was lower, but at the cost of a greater proportion of patients with bad neurological outcome. There was no difference in ventriculoperitoneal shunt dependency.[27]

3.11 Medical Management of Spontaneous ICH

Patients with ICH frequently have elevated blood pressure. High blood pressure has been shown to increase hematoma volume and to worsen outcome following spontaneous ICH.[73] The Intensive Blood Pressure Reduction in Acute Cerebral Hemorrhage Trial 1 (INTERACT-1) study demonstrated that intensive blood pressure control (systolic blood pressure [SBP] < 140 mm Hg) resulted in significantly less hematoma growth on follow-up CT.[106] The INTERACT-2 study showed that intensive blood pressure lowering (<140 mm Hg) results in a moderate improvement of the functional outcome.[107] However, a second trial (Antihypertensive Treatment of Acute Cerebral Hemorrhage 2 [ATACH-2]) did not show any benefits of an intensive blood pressure lowering regimen and raised concerns over an increase in renal adverse events of such treatment.[108] Despite those discordant results, the actual recommendation is still to lower the SBP to 140 mm Hg.[81,82]

Patients with a severe coagulation factor deficiency or severe thrombocytopenia should receive appropriate factor replacement therapy or platelets, respectively. Patients with ICH whose international normalized ratio (INR) is elevated because of vitamin K antagonists should receive prothrombin complex concentrates (PCCs) and intravenous vitamin K. High-dose PCCs have been suggested as possible treatments for newer oral anticoagulants; specific antidots are under investigations. Protamine sulfate is the best agent to reverse unfractionated heparin. The use of platelet transfusions in ICH patients with a history of antiplatelet medication is not recommended (PATCH-study).[109]

3.12 Authors' Recommendations

3.12.1 Medical Management of Spontaneous ICH

- Blood pressure should be monitored and lowered to a systolic target of 140 mm Hg.
- Patients with ICH whose INR is elevated because of vitamin K antagonists should receive PCCs and intravenous vitamin K.
- High-dose PCCs should be administered to reverse newer oral anticoagulants.
- Protamine sulfate reverses unfractionated heparin.

3.12.2 Management of Supratentorial Hemorrhage

- Neurologically stable patients (GCS score ≥ 13) can be treated conservatively.
- Early surgical evacuation of supratentorial hematoma can be considered in patients with superficial lobar hematoma and mass effect.
- Decompressive craniectomy with or without hematoma evacuation might reduce mortality in those patients with deep-seated ICH who are comatose, have large hematomas, and have a significant midline shift.

3.12.3 Management of Infratentorial Hemorrhage

- Patients with infratentorial hemorrhage who deteriorate neurologically (GCS < 13) or have brainstem compression and/or hydrocephalus should undergo emergent surgical removal of the hematoma.
- Initial management with an EVD as a stand-alone procedure (i.e., without surgical removal of the hematoma) is generally not sufficient/recommended.
- A cerebellar hematoma less than 3 cm without hydrocephalus or brainstem compression and a GCS score ≥ 13 can be managed medically with close neurological observation.
- Brainstem hemorrhages are usually managed conservatively due to the highly eloquent location.

3.12.4 Management of Intraventricular Hemorrhage

- Ventricular drainage should be placed in patients with IVH and hydrocephalus, especially in patients with decreased level of consciousness.

References

[1] Zhu XL, Chan MS, Poon WS. Spontaneous intracranial hemorrhage: which patients need diagnostic cerebral angiography? A prospective study of 206 cases and review of the literature. Stroke. 1997; 28(7):1406–1409

[2] Feigin VL, Lawes CM, Bennett DA, Barker-Collo SL, Parag V. Worldwide stroke incidence and early case fatality reported in 56 population-based studies: a systematic review. Lancet Neurol. 2009; 8(4):355–369

[3] van Asch CJ, Luitse MJ, Rinkel GJ, van der Tweel I, Algra A, Klijn CJ. Incidence, case fatality, and functional outcome of intracerebral haemorrhage over time, according to age, sex, and ethnic origin: a systematic review and meta-analysis. Lancet Neurol. 2010; 9(2):167–176

[4] Auer LM, Deinsberger W, Niederkorn K, et al. Endoscopic surgery versus medical treatment for spontaneous intracerebral hematoma: a randomized study. J Neurosurg. 1989; 70(4):530–535

[5] Batjer HH, Reisch JS, Allen BC, Plaizier LJ, Su CJ. Failure of surgery to improve outcome in hypertensive putaminal hemorrhage. A prospective randomized trial. Arch Neurol. 1990; 47(10):1103–1106

[6] Bilbao G, Garibi J, Pomposo I, et al. A prospective study of a series of 356 patients with supratentorial spontaneous intracerebral haematomas treated in a neurosurgical department. Acta Neurochir (Wien). 2005; 147(8):823–829

[7] Cho DY, Chen CC, Lee HC, Lee WY, Lin HL. Glasgow Coma Scale and hematoma volume as criteria for treatment of putaminal and thalamic intracerebral hemorrhage. Surg Neurol. 2008; 70(6):628–633

[8] Fujitsu K, Muramoto M, Ikeda Y, Inada Y, Kim I, Kuwabara T. Indications for surgical treatment of putaminal hemorrhage. Comparative study based on serial CT and time-course analysis. J Neurosurg. 1990; 73(4):518–525

[9] Guo R, Blacker DJ, Wang X, et al. INTERACT Investigators. Practice patterns for neurosurgical utilization and outcome in acute intracerebral hemorrhage: intensive blood pressure reduction in acute cerebral hemorrhage trials 1 and 2 studies. Neurosurgery. 2017; 81(6):980–985

[10] Jang JH, Song YG, Kim YZ. Predictors of 30-day mortality and 90-day functional recovery after primary pontine hemorrhage. J Korean Med Sci. 2011; 26(1):100–107

[11] Juvela S, Heiskanen O, Poranen A, et al. The treatment of spontaneous intracerebral hemorrhage. A prospective randomized trial of surgical and conservative treatment. J Neurosurg. 1989; 70(5):755–758

[12] Kanno T, Sano H, Shinomiya Y, et al. Role of surgery in hypertensive intracerebral hematoma. A comparative study of 305 nonsurgical and 154 surgical cases. J Neurosurg. 1984; 61(6):1091–1099

[13] Kaya RA, Türkmenoğlu O, Ziyal IM, Dalkiliç T, Sahin Y, Aydin Y. The effects on prognosis of surgical treatment of hypertensive putaminal hematomas through transsylvian transinsular approach. Surg Neurol. 2003; 59(3):176–183, discussion 183

[14] Kobayashi S, Sato A, Kageyama Y, Nakamura H, Watanabe Y, Yamaura A. Treatment of hypertensive cerebellar hemorrhage–surgical or conservative management? Neurosurgery. 1994; 34(2):246–250, discussion 250–251

[15] Liliang PC, Liang CL, Lu CH, et al. Hypertensive caudate hemorrhage prognostic predictor, outcome, and role of external ventricular drainage. Stroke. 2001; 32(5):1195–1200

[16] Liu H, Zen Y, Li J, et al. Optimal treatment determination on the basis of haematoma volume and intra-cerebral haemorrhage score in patients with hypertensive putaminal haemorrhages: a retrospective analysis of 310 patients. BMC Neurol. 2014; 14:141

[17] Lo YT, See AAQ, King NKK. Decompressive craniectomy in spontaneous intracerebral hemorrhage: a case-control study. World Neurosurg. 2017; 103:815–820.e2

[18] Melamed N, Satya-Murti S. Cerebellar hemorrhage. A review and reappraisal of benign cases. Arch Neurol. 1984; 41(4):425–428

[19] Mendelow AD, Gregson BA, Fernandes HM, et al. STICH investigators. Early surgery versus initial conservative treatment in patients with spontaneous supratentorial intracerebral haematomas in the International Surgical Trial in Intracerebral Haemorrhage (STICH): a randomised trial. Lancet. 2005; 365 (9457):387–397

[20] Mendelow AD, Gregson BA, Rowan EN, Murray GD, Gholkar A, Mitchell PM, STICH II Investigators. Early surgery versus initial conservative treatment in patients with spontaneous supratentorial lobar intracerebral haematomas (STICH II): a randomised trial. Lancet. 2013; 382(9890):397–408

[21] Sumer MM, Açikgöz B, Akpinar G. External ventricular drainage for acute obstructive hydrocephalus developing following spontaneous intracerebral haemorrhages. Neurol Sci. 2002; 23(1):29–33

[22] Tan SH, Ng PY, Yeo TT, Wong SH, Ong PL, Venketasubramanian N. Hypertensive basal ganglia hemorrhage: a prospective study comparing surgical and nonsurgical management. Surg Neurol. 2001; 56(5):287–292, discussion 292–293

[23] Wang YF, Wu JS, Mao Y, Chen XC, Zhou LF, Zhang Y. The optimal time-window for surgical treatment of spontaneous intracerebral hemorrhage: result of prospective randomized controlled trial of 500 cases. Acta Neurochir Suppl (Wien). 2008; 105:141–145

[24] Xu K, Hai J. The clinical study of stereotactic microsurgery. Cell Biochem Biophys. 2014; 69(2):259–263

[25] Yildiz OK, Arsava EM, Akpinar E, Topcuoglu MA. Previous antiplatelet use is associated with hematoma expansion in patients with spontaneous intracerebral hemorrhage. J Stroke Cerebrovasc Dis. 2012; 21(8):760–766

[26] Zuccarello M, Brott T, Derex L, et al. Early surgical treatment for supratentorial intracerebral hemorrhage: a randomized feasibility study. Stroke. 1999; 30(9):1833–1839

[27] Hanley DF, Lane K, McBee N, et al. CLEAR III Investigators. Thrombolytic removal of intraventricular haemorrhage in treatment of severe stroke: results of the randomised, multicentre, multiregion, placebo-controlled CLEAR III trial. Lancet. 2017; 389(10069):603–611

[28] Hanley DF, Thompson RE, Muschelli J, et al. MISTIE Investigators. Safety and efficacy of minimally invasive surgery plus alteplase in intracerebral haemorrhage evacuation (MISTIE): a randomised, controlled, open-label, phase 2 trial. Lancet Neurol. 2016; 15(12):1228–1237

[29] Barrett RJ, Hussain R, Coplin WM, et al. Frameless stereotactic aspiration and thrombolysis of spontaneous intracerebral hemorrhage. Neurocrit Care. 2005; 3(3):237–245

[30] Bauer AM, Rasmussen PA, Bain MD. Initial single-center technical experience with the BrainPath system for acute intracerebral hemorrhage evacuation. Oper Neurosurg (Hagerstown). 2017; 13(1):69–76

[31] Chen SC, Feng G. Clinic investigation and logistic analysis of risk factors of recurrent hemorrhage after operation in the earlier period of cerebral hemorrhage. Acta Neurochir Suppl (Wien). 2005; 95:119–121

[32] Chi FL, Lang TC, Sun SJ, et al. Relationship between different surgical methods, hemorrhage position, hemorrhage volume, surgical timing, and treatment outcome of hypertensive intracerebral hemorrhage. World J Emerg Med. 2014; 5(3):203–208

[33] Esquenazi Y, Savitz SI, El Khoury R, McIntosh MA, Grotta JC, Tandon N. Decompressive hemicraniectomy with or without clot evacuation for large spontaneous supratentorial intracerebral hemorrhages. Clin Neurol Neurosurg. 2015; 128:117–122

[34] Fu C, Liu L, Chen B, et al. Risk factors for poor outcome in hypertensive intraventricular hemorrhage treated by external ventricular drainage with intraventricular fibrinolysis. World Neurosurg. 2017; 102:240–245

[35] Gao Z, Qian L, Niu C, et al. Evacuating hypertensive intracerebral hematoma with a cortical sulcus approach. World Neurosurg. 2016; 95:341–347

[36] Goedemans T, Verbaan D, Coert BA, et al. Neurologic outcome after decompressive craniectomy: predictors of outcome in different pathologic conditions. World Neurosurg. 2017; 105:765–774

[37] Hayes SB, Benveniste RJ, Morcos JJ, Aziz-Sultan MA, Elhammady MS. Retrospective comparison of craniotomy and decompressive craniectomy for surgical evacuation of nontraumatic, supratentorial intracerebral hemorrhage. Neurosurg Focus. 2013; 34(5):E3

[38] Hinson HE, Melnychuk E, Muschelli J, Hanley DF, Awad IA, Ziai WC. Drainage efficiency with dual versus single catheters in severe intraventricular hemorrhage. Neurocrit Care. 2012; 16(3):399–405

[39] Jianwei G, Weiqiao Z, Xiaohua Z, Qizhong L, Jiyao J, Yongming Q. Our experience of transsylvian-transinsular microsurgical approach to hypertensive putaminal hematomas. J Craniofac Surg. 2009; 20(4):1097–1099

[40] Kim KT, Park JK, Kang SG, et al. Comparison of the effect of decompressive craniectomy on different neurosurgical diseases. Acta Neurochir (Wien). 2009; 151(1):21–30

[41] Kwon WK, Park DH, Park KJ, et al. Prognostic factors of clinical outcome after neuronavigation-assisted hematoma drainage in patients with spontaneous intracerebral hemorrhage. Clin Neurol Neurosurg. 2014; 123:83–89

[42] Labib MA, Shah M, Kassam AB, et al. the safety and feasibility of image-guided BrainPath-mediated transsulcul hematoma evacuation: a multicenter study. Neurosurgery. 2017; 80(4):515–524

[43] Ma L, Liu WG, Sheng HS, Fan J, Hu WW, Chen JS. Decompressive craniectomy in addition to hematoma evacuation improves mortality of patients with spontaneous basal ganglia hemorrhage. J Stroke Cerebrovasc Dis. 2010; 19(4):294–298

[44] Marquardt G, Wolff R, Seifert V. Multiple target aspiration technique for subacute stereotactic aspiration of hematomas within the basal ganglia. Surg Neurol. 2003; 60(1):8–13, discussion 13–14

[45] Matsumoto K, Hondo H. CT-guided stereotaxic evacuation of hypertensive intracerebral hematomas. J Neurosurg. 1984; 61(3):440–448

[46] Moussa WM, Khedr W. Decompressive craniectomy and expansive duraplasty with evacuation of hypertensive intracerebral hematoma, a randomized controlled trial. Neurosurg Rev. 2017; 40(1):115–127

[47] Murthy JM, Chowdary GV, Murthy TV, Bhasha PS, Naryanan TJ. Decompressive craniectomy with clot evacuation in large hemispheric hypertensive intracerebral hemorrhage. Neurocrit Care. 2005; 2(3):258–262

[48] Naff N, Williams MA, Keyl PM, et al. Low-dose recombinant tissue-type plasminogen activator enhances clot resolution in brain hemorrhage: the intraventricular hemorrhage thrombolysis trial. Stroke. 2011; 42(11):3009–3016

[49] Niizuma H, Shimizu Y, Yonemitsu T, Nakasato N, Suzuki J. Results of stereotactic aspiration in 175 cases of putaminal hemorrhage. Neurosurgery. 1989; 24(6):814–819

[50] Piotrowski WP, Rochowanski E. Operative results in hypertensive intracerebral hematomas in patients over 60. Gerontology. 1996; 42(6):339–347

[51] Rehman WA, Anwar MS. Surgical outcome of spontaneous supra tentorial intracerebral hemorrhage. Pak J Med Sci. 2017; 33(4):804–807

[52] Sadahiro H, Nomura S, Goto H, et al. Real-time ultrasound-guided endoscopic surgery for putaminal hemorrhage. J Neurosurg. 2015; 123(5):1151–1155

[53] Takeda T, Nakano T, Asano K, Shimamura N, Ohkuma H. Usefulness of thallium-201 SPECT in the evaluation of tumor natures in intracranial meningiomas. Neuroradiology. 2011; 53(11):867–873

[54] Shin DS, Yoon SM, Kim SH, Shim JJ, Bae HG, Yun IG. Open surgical evacuation of spontaneous putaminal hematomas: prognostic factors and comparison of outcomes between transsylvian and transcortical approaches. J Korean Neurosurg Soc. 2008; 44(1):1–7

[55] Singh TG, Ghalige HS, Karthik K, et al. Primary supratentorial haemorrhage: surgery or no surgery in an Indian setup. J Clin Diagn Res. 2014; 8(9):NC01–NC03

[56] Spiotta AM, Fiorella D, Vargas J, et al. Initial multicenter technical experience with the Apollo device for minimally invasive intracerebral hematoma evacuation. Neurosurgery. 2015; 11 Suppl 2:243–251, discussion 251

[57] Staykov D, Huttner HB, Struffert T, et al. Intraventricular fibrinolysis and lumbar drainage for ventricular hemorrhage. Stroke. 2009; 40(10):3275–3280

[58] Takeuchi S, Nawashiro H, Wada K, et al. Ventriculomegaly after decompressive craniectomy with hematoma evacuation for large hemispheric hypertensive intracerebral hemorrhage. Clin Neurol Neurosurg. 2013; 115(3):317–322

[59] Vespa P, Hanley D, Betz J, et al. ICES Investigators. ICES (Intraoperative Stereotactic Computed Tomography-Guided Endoscopic Surgery) for brain hemorrhage: a multicenter randomized controlled trial. Stroke. 2016; 47(11):2749–2755

[60] Wang W, Zhou N, Wang C. minimally invasive surgery for patients with hypertensive intracerebral hemorrhage with large hematoma volume: a retrospective study. World Neurosurg. 2017; 105:348–358

[61] Wang T, Guan Y, Du J, Liu G, Gao F, Zhao X. Factors affecting the evacuation rate of intracerebral hemorrhage in basal ganglia treated by minimally invasive craniopuncture. Clin Neurol Neurosurg. 2015; 134:104–109

[62] Wu G, Shen Z, Wang L, Sun S, Luo J, Mao Y. Post-operative re-bleeding in patients with hypertensive ICH is closely associated with the CT blend sign. BMC Neurol. 2017; 17(1):131

[63] Yadav YR, Mukerji G, Shenoy R, Basoor A, Jain G, Nelson A. Endoscopic management of hypertensive intraventricular haemorrhage with obstructive hydrocephalus. BMC Neurol. 2007; 7:1

[64] Yang Z, Hong B, Jia Z, et al. Treatment of supratentorial spontaneous intracerebral hemorrhage using image-guided minimally invasive surgery: initial experiences of a flat detector CT-based puncture planning and navigation system in the angiographic suite. AJNR Am J Neuroradiol. 2014; 35(11):2170–2175

[65] Yang G, Shao G. Clinical effect of minimally invasive intracranial hematoma in treating hypertensive cerebral hemorrhage. Pak J Med Sci. 2016; 32(3):677–681

[66] Fei Z, Zhang X, Song SJ. Secondary insults and outcomes in patients with hypertensive basal ganglia hemorrhage. Acta Neurochir Suppl (Wien). 2005; 95:265–267

[67] Zhang HT, Xue S, Li PJ, Fu YB, Xu RX. Treatment of huge hypertensive putaminal hemorrhage by surgery and cerebrospinal fluid drainage. Clin Neurol Neurosurg. 2013; 115(9):1602–1608

[68] Zhao Z, Wang H, Li Z, et al. Assessment of the effect of short-term factors on surgical treatments for hypertensive intracerebral haemorrhage. Clin Neurol Neurosurg. 2016; 150:67–71

[69] Ziai W, Moullaali T, Nekoovaght-Tak S, et al. No exacerbation of perihematomal edema with intraventricular tissue plasminogen activator in patients with spontaneous intraventricular hemorrhage. Neurocrit Care. 2013;18(3):354–361

[70] Zuo Y, Cheng G, Gao DK, et al. Gross-total hematoma removal of hypertensive basal ganglia hemorrhages: a long-term follow-up. J Neurol Sci. 2009; 287(1–2):100–104

[71] Bhattathiri PS, Gregson B, Prasad KS, Mendelow AD, STICH Investigators. Intraventricular hemorrhage and hydrocephalus after spontaneous intracerebral hemorrhage: results from the STICH trial. Acta Neurochir Suppl (Wien). 2006; 96:65–68

[72] Hypertension Detection and Follow-up Program Cooperative Group. Five-year findings of the hypertension detection and follow-up program. III. Reduction in stroke incidence among persons with high blood pressure. JAMA. 1982; 247(5):633–638

[73] Hemphill JC, III, Bonovich DC, Besmertis L, Manley GT, Johnston SC. The ICH score: a simple, reliable grading scale for intracerebral hemorrhage. Stroke. 2001; 32(4):891–897

[74] Clarke JL, Johnston SC, Farrant M, Bernstein R, Tong D, Hemphill JC, III. External validation of the ICH score. Neurocrit Care. 2004; 1(1):53–60

[75] Schmidt FA, Liotta EM, Prabhakaran S, Naidech AM, Maas MB. Assessment and comparison of the max-ICH score and ICH score by external validation. Neurology. 2018; 91(10):e939–e946

[76] Hemphill JC, III, Farrant M, Neill TA, Jr. Prospective validation of the ICH score for 12-month functional outcome. Neurology. 2009; 73(14):1088–1094

[77] Heros RC. Cerebellar hemorrhage and infarction. Stroke. 1982; 13(1):106–109

[78] Kuramatsu JB, Biffi A, Gerner ST, et al. Association of surgical hematoma evacuation vs conservative treatment with functional outcome in patients with cerebellar intracerebral hemorrhage. JAMA. 2019; 322(14):1392–1403

[79] Dammann P, Asgari S, Bassiouni H, et al. Spontaneous cerebellar hemorrhage: experience with 57 surgically treated patients and review of the literature. Neurosurg Rev. 2011; 34(1):77–86

[80] Prasad K, Mendelow AD, Gregson B. Surgery for primary supratentorial intracerebral haemorrhage. Cochrane Database Syst Rev. 2008(4):CD000200

[81] Cordonnier C, Demchuk A, Ziai W, Anderson CS. Intracerebral haemorrhage: current approaches to acute management. Lancet. 2018; 392(10154):1257–1268

[82] Hemphill JC, III, Greenberg SM, Anderson CS, et al. American Heart Association Stroke Council, Council on Cardiovascular and Stroke Nursing, Council on Clinical Cardiology. Guidelines for the management of spontaneous intracerebral hemorrhage: a guideline for healthcare professionals from the American Heart Association/American Stroke Association. Stroke. 2015; 46(7):2032–2060

[83] Fung C, Murek M, Z'Graggen WJ, et al. Decompressive hemicraniectomy in patients with supratentorial intracerebral hemorrhage. Stroke. 2012; 43 (12):3207–3211

[84] Takeuchi S, Wada K, Nagatani K, Otani N, Mori K. Decompressive hemicraniectomy for spontaneous intracerebral hemorrhage. Neurosurg Focus. 2013; 34(5):E5

[85] Heuts SG, Bruce SS, Zacharia BE, et al. Decompressive hemicraniectomy without clot evacuation in dominant-sided intracerebral hemorrhage with ICP crisis. Neurosurg Focus. 2013; 34(5):E4

[86] Morgan T, Zuccarello M, Narayan R, Keyl P, Lane K, Hanley D. Preliminary findings of the minimally-invasive surgery plus rtPA for intracerebral hemorrhage evacuation (MISTIE) clinical trial. Acta Neurochir Suppl (Wien). 2008; 105:147–151

[87] Mould WA, Carhuapoma JR, Muschelli J, et al. MISTIE Investigators. Minimally invasive surgery plus recombinant tissue-type plasminogen activator for intracerebral hemorrhage evacuation decreases perihematomal edema. Stroke. 2013; 44(3):627–634

[88] Wang WZ, Jiang B, Liu HM, et al. Minimally invasive craniopuncture therapy vs. conservative treatment for spontaneous intracerebral hemorrhage: results from a randomized clinical trial in China. Int J Stroke. 2009; 4(1):11–16

[89] Hanley DF, Thompson RE, Rosenblum M, et al. MISTIE III Investigators. Efficacy and safety of minimally invasive surgery with thrombolysis in intracerebral haemorrhage evacuation (MISTIE III): a randomised, controlled, open-label, blinded endpoint phase 3 trial. Lancet. 2019; 393(10175):1021–1032

[90] Stein M, Misselwitz B, Hamann GF, Scharbrodt W, Schummer DI, Oertel MF. Intracerebral hemorrhage in the very old: future demographic trends of an aging population. Stroke. 2012; 43(4):1126–1128

[91] Da Pian R, Bazzan A, Pasqualin A. Surgical versus medical treatment of spontaneous posterior fossa haematomas: a cooperative study on 205 cases. Neurol Res. 1984; 6(3):145–151

[92] Firsching R, Huber M, Frowein RA. Cerebellar haemorrhage: management and prognosis. Neurosurg Rev. 1991; 14(3):191–194

[93] van Loon J, Van Calenbergh F, Goffin J, Plets C. Controversies in the management of spontaneous cerebellar haemorrhage. A consecutive series of 49 cases and review of the literature. Acta Neurochir (Wien). 1993; 122 (3–4):187–193

[94] Waidhauser E, Hamburger C, Marguth F. Neurosurgical management of cerebellar hemorrhage. Neurosurg Rev. 1990; 13(3):211–217

[95] Yanaka K, Meguro K, Fujita K, Narushima K, Nose T. Immediate surgery reduces mortality in deeply comatose patients with spontaneous cerebellar hemorrhage. Neurol Med Chir (Tokyo). 2000; 40(6):295–299, discussion 299–300

[96] Dahdaleh NS, Dlouhy BJ, Viljoen SV, et al. Clinical and radiographic predictors of neurological outcome following posterior fossa decompression for spontaneous cerebellar hemorrhage. J Clin Neurosci. 2012; 19(9):1236–1241

[97] Salvati M, Cervoni L, Raco A, Delfini R. Spontaneous cerebellar hemorrhage: clinical remarks on 50 cases. Surg Neurol. 2001; 55(3):156–161, discussion 161

[98] Greenberg J, Skubick D, Shenkin H. Acute hydrocephalus in cerebellar infarct and hemorrhage. Neurology. 1979; 29(3):409–413

[99] Amar AP. Controversies in the neurosurgical management of cerebellar hemorrhage and infarction. Neurosurg Focus. 2012; 32(4):E1

[100] Mathew P, Teasdale G, Bannan A, Oluoch-Olunya D. Neurosurgical management of cerebellar haematoma and infarct. J Neurol Neurosurg Psychiatry. 1995; 59(3):287–292

[101] Komiyama M, Boo YE, Yagura H, et al. A clinical analysis of 32 brainstem haemorrhages; with special reference to surviving but severely disabled cases. Acta Neurochir (Wien). 1989; 101(1–2):46–51

[102] Manno EM, Atkinson JL, Fulgham JR, Wijdicks EF. Emerging medical and surgical management strategies in the evaluation and treatment of intracerebral hemorrhage. Mayo Clin Proc. 2005; 80(3):420–433

[103] Hara T, Nagata K, Kawamoto S, et al. Functional outcome of primary pontine hemorrhage: conservative treatment or stereotaxic surgery. No Shinkei Geka. 2001; 29(9):823–829

[104] Mangiardi JR, Epstein FJ. Brainstem haematomas: review of the literature and presentation of five new cases. J Neurol Neurosurg Psychiatry. 1988; 51 (7):966–976

[105] Takahama H, Morii K, Sato M, Sekiguchi K, Sato S. Stereotactic aspiration in hypertensive pontine hemorrhage: comparative study with conservative therapy. No Shinkei Geka. 1989; 17(8):733–739

[106] Anderson CS, Huang Y, Arima H, et al. INTERACT Investigators. Effects of early intensive blood pressure-lowering treatment on the growth of hematoma and perihematomal edema in acute intracerebral hemorrhage: the Intensive Blood Pressure Reduction in Acute Cerebral Haemorrhage Trial (INTERACT). Stroke. 2010; 41(2):307–312

[107] Anderson CS, Heeley E, Huang Y, et al. INTERACT2 Investigators. Rapid blood-pressure lowering in patients with acute intracerebral hemorrhage. N Engl J Med. 2013; 368(25):2355–2365

[108] Qureshi AI, Palesch YY, Barsan WG, et al. ATACH-2 Trial Investigators and the Neurological Emergency Treatment Trials Network. Intensive blood-pressure lowering in patients with acute cerebral hemorrhage. N Engl J Med. 2016; 375(11):1033–1043

[109] Baharoglu MI, Cordonnier C, Al-Shahi Salman R, de Gans K, Koopman MM, Brand A, et al. Platelet transfusion versus standard care after acute stroke due to spontaneous cerebral haemorrhage associated with antiplatelet therapy (PATCH): a randomised, open-label, phase 3 trial. Lancet. 2016 Jun 25;387(10038):2605–2613. PubMed PMID: 27178479. Epub 2016/05/15

4 Natural History and Management Options of Pineal Cyst

Michael J. Mulcahy and Behzad Eftekhar

Abstract

A thorough understanding of the natural history and treatment options of pineal cysts is required for the neurosurgeon managing these patients, as the cysts are usually incidental, yet their critical location affords them catastrophic potential.

The results of a pooled literature analysis suggest that most pineal cysts remain stable in size. There are case reports of sudden death attributed to pineal cysts; however, no patient who was under clinical or radiological surveillance died.

Direct treatment of a symptomatic pineal cyst (causing CSF circulation disturbance or neurological deficit) should be considered. When direct intervention is deemed appropriate, microsurgical resection (or at least wide opening of the cyst) is the preferred method of treatment.

Keywords: pineal cyst, natural history, pineal gland, sudden death

4.1 Introduction

Pineal cysts are common incidental findings with contemporary neuroimaging. They are typically found in young adults (20–30 years of age) with a predilection for female (3:1 female-to-male ratio). Their reported prevalence varies from 1.3% (95% confidence interval [CI]: 1.0–1.6) to 23% (95% CI: 15.8–32.2) conditional to the methodology, sample size, and the quality of the magnetic resonance imaging (MRI) used.[1,2] The rate is much higher (20–40%) among autopsy studies[3] and in children where size threshold among studies can be variable (2% prevalence for cysts > 5 mm and up to 57% for cysts of any size).[4,5]

Pineal cysts are thought to arise from exaggeration of the microcysts that occur in the normal pineal gland.[12] Their importance arises from the difficulty in differentiating benign cyst from cystic tumors in the pineal region, especially when large or when there are atypical features. The classic histopathologic appearance describes a thin wall composed of three layers: a delicate fibrous external layer, a middle layer of pineal parenchyma, and an inner layer of glial tissue, often containing Rosenthal fibers.[7,13,14]

On computed tomography (CT), pineal cysts appear as well-circumscribed fluid density lesions. The typical MRI appearance is of a thin-walled cyst with homogeneous contents that are isointense or slightly hyperintense to cerebrospinal fluid (CSF) on T1- and T2-weighted imaging, and slightly hyperintense to CSF on fluid-attenuated inversion recovery (FLAIR) weighted sequence.[15] Septations are frequently present within the cyst. The thin, smooth wall can display contrast enhancement, thought to be due to the involvement of pineal tissue, which is outside the blood–brain barrier.[16,17] The cyst should be bereft of nodules (▶ Fig. 4.1).

Most pineal cysts are small (< 1 cm) and asymptomatic. Larger cysts can cause a spectrum of clinical presentation secondary to hydrocephalus, Parinaud's syndrome, or gaze paresis.[6,7,8] Almost all published cases of symptomatic cysts have been greater than 1 cm in size. Headache, especially in the absence of hydrocephalus, is a controversial topic. Proposed mechanisms include intermittent obstruction of the aqueduct of Sylvius, abnormalities in melatonin secretion, or venous congestion from compression of the internal cerebral veins or the vein of Galen.[9,10,11]

A thorough understanding of the natural history and treatment options is required of the surgeon managing patients with pineal cysts, as they are usually incidental and common, but they have a catastrophic potential because of their critical location.

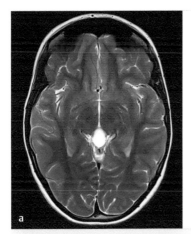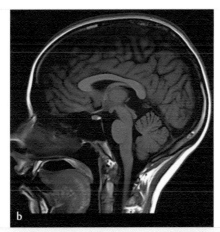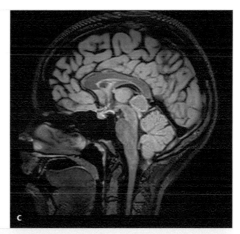

Fig. 4.1 Pineal cyst. The cyst is isointense to cerebrospinal fluid (CSF) on **(a)** the axial T2 magnetic resonance imaging (MRI) and **(b)** the midsagittal T1 MRI, with a thin smooth wall. The cyst contents are homogeneous. **(c)** The cyst contents are hyperintense compared to CSF on the T2 fluid-attenuated inversion recovery (FLAIR).

4.2 Selected Papers on the Natural History of Pineal Cyst

- Nevins EJ, Das K, Bhojak M, et al. Incidental pineal cysts: is surveillance necessary? World Neurosurg 2016;90:96–102
- Al-Holou WN, Terman SW, Kilburg C, et al. Prevalence and natural history of pineal cysts in adults. J Neurosurg 2011;115(6):1106–1114
- Al-Holou WN, Maher CO, Muraszko KM, Garton HJ. The natural history of pineal cysts in children and young adults. J Neurosurg Pediatr 2010;5(2):162–166

4.3 Natural History

The natural history of pineal cysts is not well understood. Many cysts are identified incidentally on MRI or at autopsy. However, there are cases of sudden death attributed to pineal cysts in the literature. In the first mortality attributed to a pineal cyst, a microscopic vascular malformation was found in the wall of a hemorrhagic pineal cyst; the term "pineal apoplexy" was thus coined.[18] In addition, there are rare reports of sudden death attributed to compressive effects of the pineal cyst.[19,20,21] Possible mechanisms could be transient obstruction of the aqueduct of Sylvius, or compression of the midbrain affecting the function of the reticular formation.

Pooled literature analysis on the natural history included nine retrospective studies (▶ Table 4.1), encompassing a total of 735 patients with pineal cysts. Across a highly variable follow-up period ranging from 1 month to 16 years, 633 of the 735 (86.1%) cysts remained stable in size. Of the remainder, 36 (4.9%) increased in size, 40 (5.4%) decreased in size, and 4 (0.5%) cysts spontaneously resolved. No case of traumatic hemorrhage in a pineal cyst was found. Even cysts that increased in size often remained asymptomatic and did not require surgery. No patient

Table 4.1 Natural history studies of pineal cysts

Study	Patients	Age (y)	Size (mm)	Indication for magnetic resonance imaging (MRI)	Follow-up (mo)	Increased, n (%)	Stable, n (%)	Decreased, n (%)	Resolved, n (%)	Surgery performed, n (%)
Májovský et al[23]	110	Mean: 32.6 ± 12.6 (range: 7–62)	Mean: 14.2 ± 5.4 (range: 7–35)	Symptoms and incidental	Mean: 71.2 (range: 12–192)	6	74	9	0	21
Jussila et al[15]	79	Mean: 8.6 ± 4.6 (range: 1–16)	Minimum: 10	Incidental cysts	Median: 10 (range: 3–145)	9	70	0	0	0
Nevins et al[35]	181	Range: 16–84	Median: 10 (range: 2–28)	Incidental cysts	Median: 6 (1–68)	7	170	4	0	0
Al-holou et al[28]	151	Mean: 40.1 ± 14.5 (all >18)	Mean: 9.7 ± 3.8	Incidental cysts	Mean 3.4 ± 2.9 y (6 mo–13 y)	4	124	23	0	0
Al-holou et al[27]	106	Mean: 11.7 ± 7.2 (all <25)	Mean: 9.9 ± 4.5	Incidental cysts	Mean: 3 ± 2.8 y (minimum: 6)	6	99	1	0	1
Cauley et al[26]	20	Range: 10–57	Range: 6–26	Incidental cysts	Range: 7–97	0	20	0	0	0
Mandera et al[22]	24	Range: 4–18	Range: 8 to >20	Symptoms	Range: 24–60	1	23	0	0	6
Barboriak et al[17]	32	Range: 0–67	Range: 5–22	Incidental cysts	Range: 6–54	3	24	3	2	0
Tamaki et al[36]	32	Range: 8–69	Unknown	Incidental cysts	Range: 3–48	0	29	0	2	1
Total	735					36 (4.9)	633 (86.1)	40 (5.4)	4 (0.5)	29 (3.9)

who was being observed had an acute clinical deterioration or died secondary to the cyst.

Most of the cysts were incidental findings. A point of controversy is whether pineal cysts can cause headache in the absence of hydrocephalus or tectal plate compression. Indeed, this controversy existed across these series, with most studies reporting pineal cysts to be incidental, even if the indication for MRI was headache.

Some authors, however, attributed headache to the pineal cyst and this may be reflected by the higher rates of surgery performed in these studies.[22,23] Of the 735 patients observed, 29 (3.9%) underwent surgery. Most were performed by series that attributed headache to the pineal cyst. This is a controversial indication. It has been postulated that a pineal cyst, in the absence of ventriculomegaly, could cause headache; indeed, there is anecdotal evidence of resolution of headache postsurgery.[24] However, the arguments against this unproven viewpoint are robust.[25]

Cases of acute hydrocephalus and sudden death secondary to a pineal cyst have been reported, but death is rare and has not been recorded in a patient with a pineal cyst that is being clinically or radiologically observed.

Recommendations for surveillance of pineal cysts varied between the studies. Based on the observed natural history, however, most authors suggested that radiologic follow-up was not mandatory, and clinical follow-up is sufficient.[15,17,26,27,28]

4.4 Selected Papers on the Treatment Options for Pineal Cyst

- Májovský M, Netuka D, Beneš V. Conservative and surgical treatment of patients with pineal cysts: prospective case series of 110 patients. World Neurosurg 2017;105:199–205
- Fain JS, Tomlinson FH, Scheithauer BW, et al. Symptomatic glial cysts of the pineal gland. J Neurosurg 1994;80(3):454–460

4.5 Treatment Options for Pineal Cysts

Management strategies for pineal cysts include observation or surgery. Incidental pineal cysts do not require intervention. Symptomatic patients with chronic progressive obstructive hydrocephalus should be treated. In the rare circumstances of obtundation due to acute hydrocephalus, an external ventricular drain (EVD) should be placed. Restoration of CSF circulation can then be achieved later by cyst resection.

Surgical approaches for pineal cysts are variable (▶ Table 4.2) and include craniotomy (supracerebellar infratentorial, suboccipital transtentorial, or transcallosal interforniceal); endoscopy (intraventricular or supracerebellar); stereotactic aspiration; or

CSF diversion (ventricular shunt or endoscopic third ventriculostomy). Of the 199 cases performed across the eight studies, 74% (134/181) were treated by resection via a supracerebellar infratentorial approach.

Some surgeons advocate resection of the cyst and others fenestration. There is little evidence to advocate one method over the other; however, in the series by Eide and Ringstad, there was greater improvement in symptoms if the cyst was resected rather than fenestrated.[29] There were no recurrences in cysts that were resected or fenestrated; there was one recurrence in a patient who underwent a stereotactic biopsy.[13]

Nonobstructive headache (along with other nonspecific symptoms) is a controversial indication for surgery. Eide et al[30] and Eide and Ringstad[31] have attempted to look at preoperative indicators that headache may be due to a pineal cyst, including tectum-splenium-cyst ratio, raised thalamic-to-periventricular apparent diffusion coefficient (ADC) ratios, and elevated pulsatile intracranial pressure (ICP) measurements. These criteria are currently not widely accepted and need to be evaluated and replicated in larger patient series before surgical recommendations can be deduced.

Most studies report symptomatic improvement for nonspecific symptoms (▶ Table 4.2). It is important to note that there may be an element of reporting bias considering the retrospective nature of the studies and the small numbers of patients included. The placebo effect must also be considered.

There were inconsistencies among the reported complications, with some studies reporting transient neurologic deficits and some not. Overall, there were 26 (13%) reported complications, including one perioperative death (from an acute cardiovascular event). An analysis of the complications according to surgical approach was not possible due to imprecise reporting across the series. The uncertainty appertaining to the surgical outcomes and complications is indicative of the common limitations encountered when reviewing small retrospective series.

4.6 Authors' Recommendations

- The diagnosis of pineal cysts can be made radiologically.
- Incidental pineal cysts (with typical MRI appearance) do not require intervention. One-year follow-up with neuroimaging is suggested. Should there be no significant change in size or configuration of the cyst, no further investigations are recommended.
- Direct treatment of a symptomatic pineal cyst (causing CSF circulation disturbance or neurological deficit) should be considered.
- When direct intervention is deemed appropriate, microsurgical resection (or at least wide opening of the cyst) via a supracerebellar infratentorial approach is the preferred method for those cysts located predominantly infratentorially.

Table 4.2 Surgical treatment of pineal cysts

Study	Patients	Age, mean (y)	Surgical approaches					Clinical outcomes				FU mean (mo)	Complications
			SOT	SCI	EIV/ETV	STA/B	VPS	Improved	Unchanged	Worse	Cyst recurrence		
Berhouma et al[32]	24	23.5 (7.0–49.0)	20	0	4	0	0	NR	NR	6	0	144	6 (25%): 4 hemianopias and 2 pseudomeningoceles
Eide et al[29]	27	3 groups: 36.6, 27.0, and 30.2	0	21	0	0	6	20	NR	NR	0	34.8	Nil
Fain et al[7]	24	28.7 (15.0–46.0)	0	23	0	1	0	NR	NR	2	0	Range: 3–120	2 (8%): 1 ocular palsy and 1 venous infarct
Hajnsek et al[33]	56	30.0	0	56	0	0	0	56 (100%)	0	0	NR	NR	Nil
Kalani et al[24]	18	24.0	SCI or SOT cyst resections		0	0	0	17 (94%)	1	0	0	19.1	14 (78%): transient neurologic symptoms
Kreth et al[34]	14	30.0	0	0	0	14	0	6 (43%)	8	0	0	Median: 48	NR
Májovský et al[23]	21	39.7 (20.0–63.0)	0	21	0	0	0	20 (95%)	0	1	0	201.7 (12.0–228.0)	2 (10%): 1 IVH requiring EVD and 1 wound infection
Mena et al[13]	15	33 (7.0–69.0)	1	13	0	1	0	13 (87%)	0	2	1	Range: 26.0–144.0	2 (13%): 1 death and 1 epilepsy
Total	199		21	134	4	16	6						

Abbreviations: EIV, endoscopic intraventricular; ETV, endoscopic third ventriculostomy; EVD, external ventricular drain; FU, follow-up; NR, not reported; SCI, supracerebellar infratentorial; SOT, suboccipital transtentorial; STA, stereotactic aspiration/biopsy; VPS, ventriculoperitoneal shunt.

References

[1] Sawamura Y, Ikeda J, Ozawa M, Minoshima Y, Saito H, Abe H. Magnetic resonance images reveal a high incidence of asymptomatic pineal cysts in young women. Neurosurgery. 1995; 37(1):11–15, discussion 15–16

[2] Pu Y, Mahankali S, Hou J, et al. High prevalence of pineal cysts in healthy adults demonstrated by high-resolution, noncontrast brain MR imaging. AJNR Am J Neuroradiol. 2007; 28(9):1706–1709

[3] Hasegawa A, Ohtsubo K, Mori W. Pineal gland in old age; quantitative and qualitative morphological study of 168 human autopsy cases. Brain Res. 1987; 409(2):343–349

[4] Al-Holou WN, Garton HJ, Muraszko KM, Ibrahim M, Maher CO. Prevalence of pineal cysts in children and young adults. Clinical article. J Neurosurg Pediatr. 2009; 4(3):230–236

[5] Whitehead MT, Oh CC, Choudhri AF. Incidental pineal cysts in children who undergo 3-T MRI. Pediatr Radiol. 2013; 43(12):1577–1583

[6] Wisoff JH, Epstein F. Surgical management of symptomatic pineal cysts. J Neurosurg. 1992; 77(6):896–900

[7] Fain JS, Tomlinson FH, Scheithauer BW, et al. Symptomatic glial cysts of the pineal gland. J Neurosurg. 1994; 80(3):454–460

[8] Michielsen G, Benoit Y, Baert E, Meire F, Caemaert J. Symptomatic pineal cysts: clinical manifestations and management. Acta Neurochir (Wien). 2002; 144(3):233–242, discussion 242

[9] Miyatake S, Kikuchi H, Yamasaki T, et al. Glial cyst of the pineal gland with characteristic computed tomography, magnetic resonance imaging, and pathological findings: report of two cases. Surg Neurol. 1992; 37(4):293–299

[10] Peres MF, Zukerman E, Porto PP, Brandt RA. Headaches and pineal cyst: a (more than) coincidental relationship? Headache. 2004; 44(9):929–930

[11] Seifert CL, Woeller A, Valet M, et al. Headaches and pineal cyst: a case-control study. Headache. 2008; 48(3):448–452

[12] Cooper ER. The human pineal gland and pineal cysts. J Anat. 1932; 67(Pt 1):28–46

[13] Mena H, Armonda RA, Ribas JL, Ondra SL, Rushing EJ. Nonneoplastic pineal cysts: a clinicopathologic study of twenty-one cases. Ann Diagn Pathol. 1997; 1(1):11–18

[14] Engel U, Gottschalk S, Niehaus L, et al. Cystic lesions of the pineal region: MRI and pathology. Neuroradiology. 2000; 42(6):399–402

[15] Jussila MP, Olsén P, Salokorpi N, Suo-Palosaari M. Follow-up of pineal cysts in children: is it necessary? Neuroradiology. 2017; 59(12):1265–1273

[16] Mamourian AC, Yarnell T. Enhancement of pineal cysts on MR images. AJNR Am J Neuroradiol. 1991; 12(4):773–774

[17] Barboriak DP, Lee L, Provenzale JM. Serial MR imaging of pineal cysts: implications for natural history and follow-up. AJR Am J Roentgenol. 2001; 176(3):737–743

[18] Richardson JK, Hirsch CS. Sudden, unexpected death due to "pineal apoplexy.". Am J Forensic Med Pathol. 1986; 7(1):64–68

[19] Milroy CM, Smith CL. Sudden death due to a glial cyst of the pineal gland. J Clin Pathol. 1996; 49(3):267–269

[20] Na JY, Lee KH, Kim HS, Park JT. An autopsy case of sudden unexpected death due to a glial cyst of the pineal gland. Am J Forensic Med Pathol. 2014; 35(3):186–188

[21] Barranco R, Lo Pinto S, Cuccì M, et al. Sudden and unexpected death during sexual activity, due to a glial cyst of the pineal gland. Am J Forensic Med Pathol. 2018; 39(2):157–160

[22] Mandera M, Marcol W, Bierzyńska-Macyszyn G, Kluczewska E. Pineal cysts in childhood. Childs Nerv Syst. 2003; 19(10–11):750–755

[23] Májovský M, Netuka D, Beneš V. Conservative and surgical treatment of patients with pineal cysts: prospective case series of 110 patients. World Neurosurg. 2017; 105:199–205

[24] Kalani MY, Wilson DA, Koechlin NO, et al. Pineal cyst resection in the absence of ventriculomegaly or Parinaud's syndrome: clinical outcomes and implications for patient selection. J Neurosurg. 2015; 123(2):352–356

[25] Kulkarni AV. Pineal cyst resection. J Neurosurg. 2015; 123(2):350

[26] Cauley KA, Linnell GJ, Braff SP, Filippi CG. Serial follow-up MRI of indeterminate cystic lesions of the pineal region: experience at a rural tertiary care referral center. AJR Am J Roentgenol. 2009; 193(2):533–537

[27] Al-Holou WN, Maher CO, Muraszko KM, Garton HJ. The natural history of pineal cysts in children and young adults. J Neurosurg Pediatr. 2010; 5(2):162–166

[28] Al-Holou WN, Terman SW, Kilburg C, et al. Prevalence and natural history of pineal cysts in adults. J Neurosurg. 2011; 115(6):1106–1114

[29] Eide PK, Ringstad G. Results of surgery in symptomatic non-hydrocephalic pineal cysts: role of magnetic resonance imaging biomarkers indicative of central venous hypertension. Acta Neurochir (Wien). 2017; 159(2):349–361

[30] Eide PK, Pripp AH, Ringstad GA. Magnetic resonance imaging biomarkers indicate a central venous hypertension syndrome in patients with symptomatic pineal cysts. J Neurol Sci. 2016; 363:207–216

[31] Eide PK, Ringstad G. Increased pulsatile intracranial pressure in patients with symptomatic pineal cysts and magnetic resonance imaging biomarkers indicative of central venous hypertension. J Neurol Sci. 2016; 367:247–255

[32] Berhouma M, Ni H, Delabar V, et al. Update on the management of pineal cysts: case series and a review of the literature. Neurochirurgie. 2015; 61(2–3):201–207

[33] Hajnsek S, Paladino J, Gadze ZP, Nanković S, Mrak G, Lupret V. Clinical and neurophysiological changes in patients with pineal region expansions. Coll Antropol. 2013; 37(1):35–40

[34] Kreth FW, Schätz CR, Pagenstecher A, Faist M, Volk B, Ostertag CB. Stereotactic management of lesions of the pineal region. Neurosurgery. 1996; 39(2):280–289, discussion 289–291

[35] Nevins EJ, Das K, Bhojak M, et al. Incidental pineal cysts: is surveillance necessary? World Neurosurg. 2016; 90:96–102

[36] Tamaki N, Shirataki K, Lin TK, Masumura M, Katayama S, Matsumoto S. Cysts of the pineal gland. A new clinical entity to be distinguished from tumors of the pineal region. Childs Nerv Syst. 1989; 5(3):172–176

5 Natural History and Management Options of Colloid Cysts

Anthea H. O'Neill, Cristian Gragnaniello, and Leon T. Lai

Abstract

Colloid cysts are benign epithelial lined cysts and are generally located in the anterior third ventricle, in the region of the foramen of Monroe. Understanding the natural history of colloid cysts has been challenging, given their low incidence and the small number of cases in most reported series. Published data suggest that while the majority of colloid cysts will remain stable over time, and a small percentage will regress, there is a significant risk of progression necessitating operative intervention. The risk of acute deterioration and cyst-related mortality is low. The literature supports the need for surveillance of asymptomatic colloid cysts. Operative intervention is recommended for symptomatic patients, or those with cysts ≥ 10 mm, or those with hydrocephalus. When intervention is deemed appropriate, microsurgical resection via a transcallosal or transcortical approach should be considered.

Keywords: colloid cyst, natural history, intraventricular tumor, microsurgery, endoscopic surgery, stereotactic aspiration

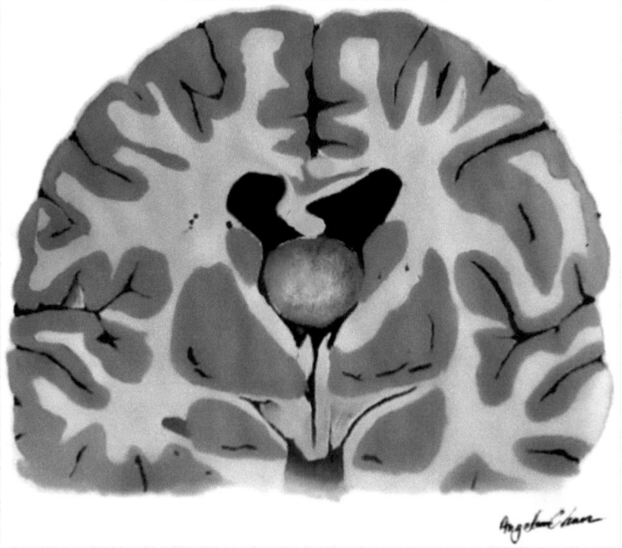

Fig. 5.1 Coronal section demonstrating a large colloid cyst in the roof of the third ventricle.

5.1 Introduction

Colloid cysts are benign epithelial lined cysts, and are generally located in the anterior third ventricle, in the region of the foramen of Monroe.[1] They account for 0.5 to 2% of intracranial tumors[1,2] correlating to an incidence of 3.2 per million population per year.[2,3] The true prevalence is unknown but has been estimated at approximately 1 in 8,500 people.[4] Typical age of presentation is between 20 and 50 years, with a possible familial predisposition,[1,5,6] and a slight male preponderance.[7]

Prior to the availability of modern neuroimaging, most colloid cysts encountered in the clinical setting were symptomatic. With increased use of neuroradiology, asymptomatic colloid cysts are readily discovered following cranial imaging for unrelated indications. Symptomatic colloid cysts present with headache, which may be postural, associated with nausea and vomiting, blurred vision, gait ataxia, and altered cognition.[2,8,9] Incontinence, tinnitus, seizures, syncope, psychological manifestations, and dizziness have also been reported.[1,2] Because of their location (▶ Fig. 5.1), an enlarging cyst may cause obstructive hydrocephalus, resulting in acute rapid neurological deterioration and sudden death.

5.2 Selected Papers on the Natural History of Colloid Cysts

- Beaumont TL, Limbrick DD Jr, Rich KM, Wippold FJ II, Dacey RG Jr. Natural history of colloid cysts of the third ventricle. J Neurosurg 2016;125(6):1420–1430
- Pollock BE, Huston J III. Natural history of asymptomatic colloid cysts of the third ventricle. J Neurosurg 1999;91(3):364–369

5.3 Natural History of Colloid Cysts

Understanding the natural history of colloid cysts has been challenging given their low incidence and the small number of cases in most reported series. An overview of currently published case series regarding presenting clinical features and the natural history of colloid cysts is presented in ▶ Table 5.1.[2,7,10,11,12,13]

In general, colloid cysts may remain stable (88.3%), progress (9.9%), or regress in size (1.8%) during a median follow-up of 33.0 months (range: 1.0–276.0) from the time of diagnosis. Acute clinical deterioration occurred in 0.6% of cases. The risk of cyst-related mortality for asymptomatic colloid is estimated at 0.2% per year.

Most cysts less than 10 mm in diameter size do not cause hydrocephalus and are asymptomatic.[1] However, data indicate that most cysts will progress to some extent over time, as many patients with incidental colloid cysts nevertheless have some degree of hydrocephalus, indicating gradually enlarging cysts causing compromise of cerebrospinal fluid (CSF) flow during the patient's lifetime.[12,14] One-third of asymptomatic patients will have hydrocephalus at diagnosis. The rate of cyst progression necessitating surgical intervention was 6.7% (95% confidence interval [CI]: 3.6–11.7) during a median follow-up interval of 3 years following diagnosis. Approximately half of these patients required surgery due to development of symptoms related to their colloid cyst, and the other half due to growth of the cyst on follow-up radiological imaging. It is believed that younger patients with incidentally diagnosed colloid cysts are more likely to become symptomatic in the future than older patients with equivalent lesions.[7,15]

Table 5.1 General demographics and clinical features of asymptomatic colloid cysts of the third ventricle

Studies	No. of patients	Mean age (y) (range)	Mean size (mm) (range)	Mean follow-up (mo) (range)	Radiologically stable, n (%, 95% CI)	Radiological progression, n (%, 95% CI)	Radiological regression, n (%, 95% CI)	Surgical intervention required, n (%; 95% CI)	Acute neurological deterioration, n (%; 95% CI)	Sudden death (%)	Cyst-related mortality, n (%; 95% CI)
Camacho et al[10]	24	52.0 (NR)	NR	19.3 (1.0–89.0)	NR	NR	NR	0	0	0	0
Kondziolka and Lunsford[11]	6	NR	<7.0[a]	NR (36.0–84.0)	NR	NR	NR	0	0	0	0
Mathiesen et al[7]	7	47.9 (9.0–78.0)	15.9 (3.0–16.0)	22.0 (6.0–37.0)	3	4	0	4	0	0	0
Pollock and Huston[12]	58	57.0 (7.0–88.0)	8.0 (4.0–18.0)	79.0 (7.0–268.0)	32	2	0	2	1	0	1
Beaumont et al[2]	57	54.2 (NR)	7.0 (NR)	61.2 (6.0–276.0)	50	5	2	5	0	0	0
Roth et al[13]	13	35.0 (27.0–58.5)	6.9 (6.0–9.1)	33.0 (12.6–67.0)	13	0	0	0	0	0	0
	213	52.0[b] (7.0–88.0)	7.0[b] (3.0–18.0)	33.0[b] (1.0–276.0)	98 (88.3; 95% CI 80.9–93.2)	11 (9.9; 95% CI 5.5–17.0)	2 (1.8; 95% CI 0.1–6.7)	11 (6.7, 95% CI 3.6–11.7)	1 (0.6, 95% CI −0.2–3.7)	0	1 (0.6, 95% CI −0.2–3.7)

Abbreviations: CI, confidence interval; mo, months; NR, not reported; y, years.
[a]Size reported as less than the cutoff value.
[b]Median.

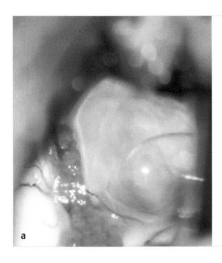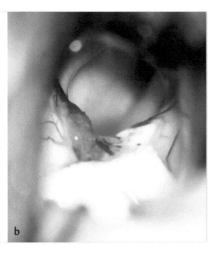

Fig. 5.2 An intraoperative image of a colloid cyst, **(a)** occluding the foramen of Monro and **(b)** following cyst removal.

The most concerning presentation of a colloid cyst is an acute neurological deterioration, which has been reported in between 3 and 45% of patients, with an associated 5 to 38% risk of death.[1,2,4,9,16,17] In most cases, it is thought to be caused by rapid cyst enlargement leading to acute obstruction of the foramen of Monroe, and subsequent acute hydrocephalus and cerebral herniation (▶ Fig. 5.2).[4,12,14] However, alternative proposed mechanisms include disturbance of hypothalamic-mediated cardiovascular reflex control, venous infarction, spinal cord infarction, neurogenic pulmonary edema, and intracystic haemorrhage.[1,2,7,16,18,19,20,21,22] Finally, several deaths have been precipitated by performing lumbar punctures in patients with colloid cysts.[3,9]

In rare cases, colloid cysts have also been reported to spontaneously regress in size.[2,6,23] The mechanism by which the regression occurred is unclear; however, it has been postulated to be the result of asymptomatic cyst rupture.[5,24]

5.4 Predicting the Risk of Sudden Death

There is considerable variation in the literature regarding the prognostic features of patients with colloid cysts who are at risk of sudden death. Acute hydrocephalus, with neurological deterioration and death, has been reported to be more likely in patients who are young, with ventriculomegaly, with cysts greater than 10 mm in diameter size, or T2 hyperintense lesions.[2,7,12,14,16] It has been variably reported that both long-standing and acute onset of symptoms increase the likelihood of an acute deterioration.[2,4,12,14] However, multiple studies have concluded that neither clinical nor neuroimaging features can be reliably used to estimate the risk of acute deterioration.[4,16,25]

5.5 Selected Papers on the Treatment Outcomes of Colloid Cysts

- Mathiesen T, Grane P, Lindquist C, von Holst H. High recurrence rate following aspiration of colloid cysts in the third ventricle. J Neurosurg 1993;78(5):748–752

- Konovalov AN, Pitskhelauri DI, Shkarubo M, Buklina SB, Poddubskaya AA, Kolycheva M. Microsurgical treatment of colloid cysts of the third ventricle. World Neurosurg 2017;105:678–688
- Samadian M, Ebrahimzadeh K, Maloumeh EN, et al. Colloid cyst of the third ventricle: long-term results of endoscopic management in a series of 112 cases. World Neurosurg 2018;111:e440–e448

5.6 Treatment Options

Management options for colloid cysts include observation or surgery. Asymptomatic colloid cysts can be conservatively managed with serial neuroimaging to assess for radiological progression.[2,5,12,17] However, prompt neurosurgical intervention is indicated should the patient develop symptoms, when the cyst enlarges, or when CSF flow is compromised. Prevention of sudden death is not a surgical indication in asymptomatic patients with small cysts and no hydrocephalus. Lumbar puncture should be avoided in patients with colloid cysts prior to definitive management or ventriculoperitoneal shunt (VPS) insertion due to the risk of herniation.

In patients with acute hydrocephalus, immediate CSF diversion strategies with bilateral external ventricular drains or a VPS may be considered. The rationale for definitive surgery is to restore CSF drainage. In general, the entire cyst capsule should be removed to prevent recurrence.[26] Direct operative options include stereotactic cyst aspiration, endoscopic cyst removal, and microsurgical resection (transcallosal or transcortical). An overview of the outcomes of the available operative treatment options published between 1974 and 2020 is presented in ▶ Table 5.2.[7,9,10,11,13,22,26,27,28,29,30,31,32,33,34,35,36,37,38,39,40,41,42,43,44,45,46,47,48,49,50,51,52,53,54,55,56,57,58,59,60,61,62,63,64,65,66,67,68,69,70,71,72,73,74,75,76,77,78,79,80,81,82,83,84,85,86,87,88,89,90,91,92,93,94,95,96,97,98,99,100,101,102,103,104]

Endoscopic and microsurgical resections are the most common surgical treatment strategies for colloid cysts. Microsurgical resection of colloid cysts has a higher rate of complete resection than endoscopic removal (95.9 vs. 69.2%) and corresponding lower rates of recurrence (0.9 vs. 5.2%) and the need for reoperation (0.8 vs. 2.5%). Clinical outcomes are equivalent between the two techniques, with 96.0% of microsurgical patients and 96.3% of endoscopic patients independent

Table 5.2 Summary of the literature regarding surgical management of colloid cysts

	Microsurgical series (1,263 patients in 36 studies)	Endoscopic series (1,374 patients in 53 studies)	Stereotactic aspiration series (113 patients in 9 studies)
Study period	1929–2017	1981–2017	1969–1995
Patient age, median (range)	41.0 (1.0–78.0)	41.0 (0.5–87.0)	39.4 (12.0–70.0)
Colloid cyst size, median (range) (mm)	14.0 (4.0–52.0)	14.4 (3.0–50.0)	18.9 (10.0–50.0)
Degree of resection			
Complete (%)	95.9	69.2	0.0
Residual (%)	4.1	30.8	100.0
Perioperative complications (%)	20.6	18.9	26.3
Length of operation, min (range)	208.0 (83.0–257.0)	104.0 (20.0–300.0)	120.0 (NR)
ICU stay, d (range)	3.4 (1.0–7.0)	1.5 (1.0–7.0)	NR
LOS, d (range)	6.0 (2.0–24.0)	3.8 (1.0–63.0)	3.5 (NR)
Clinical outcomes			
Independence (%)	96.0	96.3	96.5
Morbidity (%)	4.0	3.7	3.5
Mortality (%)	1.3	0.5	0.9
Shunt dependency (%)	4.1	3.7	8.1
Radiological outcomes			
Recurrence (%)	0.9	5.2	27.6
Reoperation (%)	0.8	2.5	61.9
Conversion to open (%)	NA	3.1	NA
Median time to follow-up, mo (range)	24.5 (1.0–300.0)	37.0 (1.0–275.0)	45.5 (0.0–108.0)

Abbreviations: d, day; ICU, intensive care unit; LOS, length of stay; mo, month; NA, not applicable; NR, not reported.

following treatment. Both groups also had similar rates of perioperative mortality (1.3 vs. 0.5%) and shunt dependency (4.1 vs. 3.7%). Current literature reports that the transcallosal approach has a lower morbidity rate compared to the transcortical approach, notwithstanding reporting biases of these case series.[17]

Stereotactic aspiration involves insertion of a stereotactic needle anterior to the right coronal suture, and application of negative pressure using a syringe to remove the cyst contents.[1] Complete removal of the cyst is precluded, and recurrence and reoperation are common at 27.6 and 61.9%, respectively.

5.7 Authors' Recommendations

- Asymptomatic patients, and patients with cysts less than 10 mm in diameter size, can be safely managed conservatively with serial neuroimaging: initially every 3 months, then every 6 months, and then annually.
- Symptomatic patients, or those with cysts ≥ 10 mm in diameter, or those with hydrocephalus, should be managed surgically as the risk of acute deterioration is high.
- Prevention of sudden death is not a surgical indication in asymptomatic patients with small cysts and no hydrocephalus. However, prompt neurosurgical intervention is indicated should the patient develop symptoms, when the cyst enlarges, or hydrocephalus develops.
- When intervention is deemed appropriate, microsurgical resection via a transcallosal or transcortical approach should be considered.

- The use of VPS or stereotactic aspiration of the cyst as definitive form of treatment is not recommended.
- In patients with acute deterioration in conscious state and hydrocephalus, bilateral external ventricular drains (EVDs) or VPS should be inserted prior to consideration of further surgical management.

References

[1] Greenberg MS, Arredondo N. Handbook of neurosurgery. 2006
[2] Beaumont TL, Limbrick DD, Jr, Rich KM, Wippold FJ, II, Dacey RG, Jr. Natural history of colloid cysts of the third ventricle. J Neurosurg. 2016; 125(6): 1420–1430
[3] Hernesniemi J, Leivo S. Management outcome in third ventricular colloid cysts in a defined population: a series of 40 patients treated mainly by transcallosal microsurgery. Surg Neurol. 1996; 45(1):2–14
[4] de Witt Hamer PC, Verstegen MJT, De Haan RJ, et al. High risk of acute deterioration in patients harboring symptomatic colloid cysts of the third ventricle. J Neurosurg. 2002; 96(6):1041–1045
[5] Peeters SM, Daou B, Jabbour P, Ladoux A, Abi Lahoud G. Spontaneous regression of a third ventricle colloid cyst. World Neurosurg. 2016; 90: 704.e19–704.e22
[6] Gbejuade H, Plaha P, Porter D. Spontaneous regression of a third ventricle colloid cyst. Br J Neurosurg. 2011; 25(5):655–657
[7] Mathiesen T, Grane P, Lindgren L, Lindquist C. Third ventricle colloid cysts: a consecutive 12-year series. J Neurosurg. 1997; 86(1):5–12
[8] Kaye AH. Essential neurosurgery. Chicester, UK: John Wiley & Sons; 2009
[9] Little JR, MacCarty CS. Colloid cysts of the third ventricle. J Neurosurg. 1974; 40(2):230–235
[10] Camacho A, Abernathey CD, Kelly PJ, Laws ER, Jr. Colloid cysts: experience with the management of 84 cases since the introduction of computed tomography. Neurosurgery. 1989; 24(5):693–700

[11] Kondziolka D, Lunsford LD. Microsurgical resection of colloid cysts using a stereotactic transventricular approach. Surg Neurol. 1996; 46(5):485–490, discussion 490–492

[12] Pollock BE, Huston J, III. Natural history of asymptomatic colloid cysts of the third ventricle. J Neurosurg. 1999; 91(3):364–369

[13] Roth J, Sela G, Andelman F, Nossek E, Elran H, Ram Z. The impact of colloid cyst treatment on neurocognition. World Neurosurg. 2019; 125:e372–e377

[14] Pollock BE, Schreiner SA, Huston J, III. A theory on the natural history of colloid cysts of the third ventricle. Neurosurgery. 2000; 46(5):1077–1081, discussion 1081–1083

[15] Macdonald RL, Humphreys RP, Rutka JT, Kestle JRW. Colloid cysts in children. Pediatr Neurosurg. 1994; 20(3):169–177

[16] Ryder JW, Kleinschmidt-DeMasters BK, Keller TS. Sudden deterioration and death in patients with benign tumors of the third ventricle area. J Neurosurg. 1986; 64(2):216–223

[17] Sheikh AB, Mendelson ZS, Liu JK. Endoscopic versus microsurgical resection of colloid cysts: a systematic review and meta-analysis of 1,278 patients. World Neurosurg. 2014; 82(6):1187–1197

[18] Turillazzi E, Bello S, Neri M, Riezzo I, Fineschi V. Colloid cyst of the third ventricle, hypothalamus, and heart: a dangerous link for sudden death. Diagn Pathol. 2012; 7:144

[19] Findler G, Cotev S. Neurogenic pulmonary edema associated with a colloid cyst in the third ventricle. Case report. J Neurosurg. 1980; 52(3):395–398

[20] Siu TL, Bannan P, Stokes BA. Spinal cord infarction complicating acute hydrocephalus secondary to a colloid cyst of the third ventricle. Case report. J Neurosurg Spine. 2005; 3(1):64–67

[21] Godano U, Ferrai R, Meleddu V, Bellinzona M. Hemorrhagic colloid cyst with sudden coma. Minim Invasive Neurosurg. 2010; 53(5–6):273–274

[22] Jeffree RL, Besser M. Colloid cyst of the third ventricle: a clinical review of 39 cases. J Clin Neurosci. 2001; 8(4):328–331

[23] Annamalai G, Lindsay KW, Bhattacharya JJ. Spontaneous resolution of a colloid cyst of the third ventricle. Br J Radiol. 2008; 81(961):e20–e22

[24] Motoyama Y, Hashimoto H, Ishida Y, Iida J. Spontaneous rupture of a presumed colloid cyst of the third ventricle: case report. Neurol Med Chir (Tokyo). 2002; 42(5):228–231

[25] Büttner A, Winkler PA, Eisenmenger W, Weis S. Colloid cysts of the third ventricle with fatal outcome: a report of two cases and review of the literature. Int J Legal Med. 1997; 110(5):260–266

[26] Decq P, Le Guerinel C, Brugières P, et al. Endoscopic management of colloid cysts. Neurosurgery. 1998; 42(6):1288–1294, discussion 1294–1296

[27] Kumar K, Kelly M, Toth C. Stereotactic cyst wall disruption and aspiration of colloid cysts of the third ventricle. Stereotact Funct Neurosurg. 1998; 71(3): 145–152

[28] Mohadjer M, Teshmar E, Mundinger F. CT-stereotaxic drainage of colloid cysts in the foramen of Monro and the third ventricle. J Neurosurg. 1987; 67 (2):220–223

[29] Musolino A, Fosse S, Munari C, Daumas-Duport C, Chodkiewicz JP. Diagnosis and treatment of colloid cysts of the third ventricle by stereotactic drainage. Report on eleven cases. Surg Neurol. 1989; 32(4):294–299

[30] Rajshekhar V. Rate of recurrence following stereotactic aspiration of colloid cysts of the third ventricle. Stereotact Funct Neurosurg. 2012; 90(1):37–44

[31] Acerbi F, Rampini P, Egidi M, Locatelli M, Borsa S, Gaini SM. Endoscopic treatment of colloid cysts of the third ventricle: long-term results in a series of 6 consecutive cases. J Neurosurg Sci. 2007; 51(2):53–60

[32] Bergsneider M. Complete microsurgical resection of colloid cysts with a dual-port endoscopic technique. Neurosurgery. 2007; 60(2) Suppl 1:ONS33–ONS42, discussion ONS42–ONS43

[33] Birski M, Birska J, Paczkowski D, et al. Combination of neuroendoscopic and stereotactic procedures for total resection of colloid cysts with favorable neurological and cognitive outcomes. World Neurosurg. 2016; 85:205–214

[34] Boogaarts HD, Decq P, Grotenhuis JA, et al. Long-term results of the neuroendoscopic management of colloid cysts of the third ventricle: a series of 90 cases. Neurosurgery. 2011; 68(1):179–187

[35] Charalampaki P, Filippi R, Welschehold S, Perneczky A. Endoscope-assisted removal of colloid cysts of the third ventricle. Neurosurg Rev. 2006; 29(1): 72–79

[36] Chibbaro S, Champeaux C, Poczos P, et al. Anterior trans-frontal endoscopic management of colloid cyst: an effective, safe, and elegant way of treatment. Case series and technical note from a multicenter prospective study. Neurosurg Rev. 2014; 37(2):235–241, discussion 241

[37] Delitala A, Brunori A, Russo N. Supraorbital endoscopic approach to colloid cysts. Neurosurgery. 2011; 69(2) Suppl Operative:ons176–ons182, discussion ons182–ons183

[38] Doron O, Feldman Z, Zauberman J. MRI features have a role in pre-surgical planning of colloid cyst removal. Acta Neurochir (Wien). 2016; 158(4):671–676

[39] El-Ghandour NM. Endoscopic treatment of third ventricular colloid cysts: a review including ten personal cases. Neurosurg Rev. 2009; 32(4):395–402

[40] Engh JA, Lunsford LD, Amin DV, et al. Stereotactically guided endoscopic port surgery for intraventricular tumor and colloid cyst resection. Neurosurgery. 2010; 67(3) Suppl Operative:ons198–ons204, discussion ons204–ons205

[41] Girgis F, Diaz R, Hader W, Hamilton M. Comparison of intracranial neuroendoscopic procedures in children versus adults. Can J Neurol Sci. 2015; 42(6):427–435

[42] Gonzalez-Martinez JA, Zamorano L, Li QH, Diaz FG. Interactive image-guided management of colloid cysts of the third ventricle. Minim Invasive Neurosurg. 2003; 46(4):193–197

[43] Greenlee JD, Teo C, Ghahreman A, Kwok B. Purely endoscopic resection of colloid cysts. Neurosurgery. 2008; 62(3) Suppl 1:51–55, discussion 55–56

[44] Hellwig D, Bauer BL, Schulte M, Gatscher S, Riegel T, Bertalanffy H. Neuroendoscopic treatment for colloid cysts of the third ventricle: the experience of a decade. Neurosurgery. 2003; 52(3):525–533, discussion 532–533

[45] Hoffman CE, Savage NJ, Souweidane MM. The significance of cyst remnants after endoscopic colloid cyst resection: a retrospective clinical case series. Neurosurgery. 2013; 73(2):233–237, discussion 237–239

[46] Iacoangeli M, di Somma LG, Di Rienzo A, Alvaro L, Nasi D, Scerrati M. Combined endoscopic transforaminal-transchoroidal approach for the treatment of third ventricle colloid cysts. J Neurosurg. 2014; 120(6):1471–1476

[47] Ibáñez-Botella G, Domínguez M, Ros B, De Miguel L, Márquez B, Arráez MA. Endoscopic transchoroidal and transforaminal approaches for resection of third ventricular colloid cysts. Neurosurg Rev. 2014; 37(2):227–234, discussion 234

[48] Kwiek S, Kocur D, Doleżych H, et al. Endoscopic technique in the treatment of patients with colloid cysts of the third ventricle. Report based on over a decade of experience. Neurol Neurochir Pol. 2012; 46(3):216–223

[49] Levine NB, Miller MN, Crone KR. Endoscopic resection of colloid cysts: indications, technique, and results during a 13-year period. Minim Invasive Neurosurg. 2007; 50(6):313–317

[50] Longatti P, Godano U, Gangemi M, et al. Italian neuroendoscopy group. Cooperative study by the Italian neuroendoscopy group on the treatment of 61 colloid cysts. Childs Nerv Syst. 2006; 22(10):1263–1267

[51] Longatti P, Martinuzzi A, Moro M, Fiorindi A, Carteri A. Endoscopic treatment of colloid cysts of the third ventricle: 9 consecutive cases. Minim Invasive Neurosurg. 2000; 43(3):118–123

[52] Margetis K, Christos PJ, Souweidane M. Endoscopic resection of incidental colloid cysts. J Neurosurg. 2014; 120(6):1259–1267

[53] Mishra S, Chandra PS, Suri A, Rajender K, Sharma BS, Mahapatra AK. Endoscopic management of third ventricular colloid cysts: eight years' institutional experience and description of a new technique. Neurol India. 2010; 58(3):412–417

[54] Pinto FC, Chavantes MC, Fonoff ET, Teixeira MJ. Treatment of colloid cysts of the third ventricle through neuroendoscopic Nd: YAG laser stereotaxis. Arq Neuropsiquiatr. 2009; 67(4):1082–1087

[55] Raouf A, Zidan I. Endoscopic removal of third ventricular colloid cyst: experience of 90 cases. Neurosurg Q. 2015; 25(1):46–50

[56] Rodziewicz GS, Smith MV, Hodge CJ, Jr. Endoscopic colloid cyst surgery. Neurosurgery. 2000; 46(3):655–660, discussion 660–662

[57] Schroeder HWS, Oertel J, Gaab MR. Incidence of complications in neuroendoscopic surgery. Childs Nerv Syst. 2004; 20(11–12):878–883

[58] Sharifi G, Bakhtevari MH, Samadian M, Alavi E, Rezaei O. Endoscopic surgery in nonhydrocephalous third ventricular colloid cysts: a feasibility study. World Neurosurg. 2015; 84(2):398–404

[59] Sribnick EA, Dadashev VY, Miller BA, Hawkins S, Hadjipanayis CG. Neuroendoscopic colloid cyst resection: a case cohort with follow-up and patient satisfaction. World Neurosurg. 2014; 81(3–4):584–593

[60] Stachura K, Grzywna E. Neuronavigation-guided endoscopy for intraventricular tumors in adult patients without hydrocephalus. Wideochir Inne Tech Malo Inwazyjne. 2016; 11(3):200–207

[61] Tirakotai W, Schulte DM, Bauer BL, Bertalanffy H, Hellwig D. Neuroendoscopic surgery of intracranial cysts in adults. Childs Nerv Syst. 2004; 20(11–12):842–851

[62] Vandertop WP, Verdaasdonk RM, van Swol CF. Laser-assisted neuroendoscopy using a neodymium-yttrium aluminum garnet or diode contact laser with pretreated fiber tips. J Neurosurg. 1998; 88(1):82–92

[63] Wait SD, Gazzeri R, Wilson DA, Abla AA, Nakaji P, Teo C. Endoscopic colloid cyst resection in the absence of ventriculomegaly. Neurosurgery. 2013; 73 (1) Suppl Operative:ons39–ons46, ons46–ons47

[64] Wilson DA, Fusco DJ, Wait SD, Nakaji P. Endoscopic resection of colloid cysts: use of a dual-instrument technique and an anterolateral approach. World Neurosurg. 2013; 80(5):576–583

[65] Yadav YR, Parihar V, Pande S, Namdev H. Endoscopic management of colloid cysts. J Neurol Surg A Cent Eur Neurosurg. 2014; 75(5):376–380

[66] Zohdi A, El Kheshin S. Endoscopic approach to colloid cysts. Minim Invasive Neurosurg. 2006; 49(5):263–268

[67] Abernathey CD, Davis DH, Kelly PJ. Treatment of colloid cysts of the third ventricle by stereotaxic microsurgical laser craniotomy. J Neurosurg. 1989; 70(4):525–529

[68] Barlas O, Karadereler S. Stereotactically guided microsurgical removal of colloid cysts. Acta Neurochir (Wien). 2004; 146(11):1199–1204

[69] Brostigen CS, Meling TR, Marthinsen PB, Scheie D, Aarhus M, Helseth E. Surgical management of colloid cyst of the third ventricle. Acta Neurol Scand. 2017; 135(4):484–487

[70] Cabbell KL, Ross DA. Stereotactic microsurgical craniotomy for the treatment of third ventricular colloid cysts. Neurosurgery. 1996; 38(2):301–307

[71] Carmel PW. Tumours of the third ventricle. Acta Neurochir (Wien). 1985; 75 (1–4):136–146

[72] Cohen-Gadol AA. Minitubular transcortical microsurgical approach for gross total resection of third ventricular colloid cysts: technique and assessment. World Neurosurg. 2013; 79(1):207.e7–207.e10

[73] Desai KI, Nadkarni TD, Muzumdar DP, Goel AH. Surgical management of colloid cyst of the third ventricle: a study of 105 cases. Surg Neurol. 2002; 57(5):295–302, discussion 302–304

[74] Easwer HV, Bhattacharya RN, Nair S, et al. Pre-coronal, paramedian minicraniotomy: a minimal access approach for microsurgical, transcallosal, transforaminal removal of colloid cysts of the third ventricle. Minim Invasive Neurosurg. 2008; 51(5):253–257

[75] Eliyas JK, Glynn R, Kulwin CG, et al. Minimally invasive transsulcal resection of intraventricular and periventricular lesions through a tubular retractor system: multicentric experience and results. World Neurosurg. 2016; 90: 556–564

[76] Gökalp HZ, Yüceer N, Arasil E, Erdogan A, Dincer C, Baskaya M. Colloid cyst of the third ventricle. Evaluation of 28 cases of colloid cyst of the third ventricle operated on by transcortical transventricular (25 cases) and transcallosal/transventricular (3 cases) approaches. Acta Neurochir (Wien). 1996; 138(1):45–49

[77] Haciyakupoglu E, Yilmaz DM, Kinali B, Arpac T, Akbas T, Haciyakupoglu S. Colloid cyst of third ventricle: report of 11 cases with transcallosal transforaminal and transcolumna fornicis approach and clinical, radiological features. Int J Clin Exp Med. 2017; 10(6):8819–8828

[78] Hernesniemi J, Romani R, Dashti R, et al. Microsurgical treatment of third ventricular colloid cysts by interhemispheric far lateral transcallosal approach: experience of 134 patients. Surg Neurol. 2008; 69(5):447–453, discussion 453–456

[79] Konovalov AN, Pitskhelauri DI, Shkarubo M, Buklina SB, Poddubskaya AA, Kolycheva M. Microsurgical treatment of colloid cysts of the third ventricle. World Neurosurg. 2017; 105:678–688

[80] Mathiesen T, Grane P, Lindquist C, von Holst H. High recurrence rate following aspiration of colloid cysts in the third ventricle. J Neurosurg. 1993; 78(5):748–752

[81] Mazher S, Imran M, Ashraf J, Ahmed A, Shah IU, Zulfiqar F. Outcome of open transcortical approach in the management of intraventricular lesions. J Coll Physicians Surg Pak. 2013; 23(12):857–861

[82] Milligan BD, Meyer FB. Morbidity of transcallosal and transcortical approaches to lesions in and around the lateral and third ventricles: a single-institution experience. Neurosurgery. 2010; 67(6):1483–1496, discussion 1496

[83] Morita A, Kelly PJ. Resection of intraventricular tumors via a computer-assisted volumetric stereotactic approach. Neurosurgery. 1993; 32(6):920–926, discussion 926–927

[84] Pamir MN, Peker S, Ozgen S, Kiliç T, Türe U, Ozek MM. Anterior transcallosal approach to the colloid cysts of the third ventricle: case series and review of the literature. Zentralbl Neurochir. 2004; 65(3):108–115, discussion 116

[85] Sampath R, Vannemreddy P, Nanda A. Microsurgical excision of colloid cyst with favorable cognitive outcomes and short operative time and hospital stay: operative techniques and analyses of outcomes with review of previous studies. Neurosurgery. 2010; 66(2):368–374, discussion 374–375

[86] Shapiro S, Rodgers R, Shah M, Fulkerson D, Campbell RL. Interhemispheric transcallosal subchoroidal fornix-sparing craniotomy for total resection of colloid cysts of the third ventricle. J Neurosurg. 2009; 110(1):112–115

[87] Solaroglu I, Beskonakli E, Kaptanoglu E, Okutan O, Ak F, Taskin Y. Transcortical-transventricular approach in colloid cysts of the third ventricle: surgical experience with 26 cases. Neurosurg Rev. 2004; 27(2):89–92

[88] Symss NP, Ramamurthi R, Rao SM, Vasudevan MC, Jain PK, Pande A. Management outcome of the transcallosal, transforaminal approach to colloid cysts of the anterior third ventricle: an analysis of 78 cases. Neurol India. 2011; 59(4):542–547

[89] Wild AM, Xuereb JH, Marks PV, Gleave JR. Computerized tomographic stereotaxy in the management of 200 consecutive intracranial mass lesions. Analysis of indications, benefits and outcome. Br J Neurosurg. 1990; 4(5): 407–415

[90] Azzazi A, Almekawi S. Colloid cysts of the third ventricle: endoscopic versus microsurgical removal. Neurosurg Q. 2010; 20(3):142–145

[91] Grondin RT, Hader W, MacRae ME, Hamilton MG. Endoscopic versus microsurgical resection of third ventricle colloid cysts. Can J Neurol Sci. 2007; 34(2):197–207

[92] Horn EM, Feiz-Erfan I, Bristol RE, et al. Treatment options for third ventricular colloid cysts: comparison of open microsurgical versus endoscopic resection. Neurosurgery. 2007; 60(4):613–618, discussion 618–620

[93] Kehler U, Brunori A, Gliemroth J, et al. Twenty colloid cysts: comparison of endoscopic and microsurgical management. Minim Invasive Neurosurg. 2001; 44(3):121–127

[94] King WA, Ullman JS, Frazee JG, Post KD, Bergsneider M. Endoscopic resection of colloid cysts: surgical considerations using the rigid endoscope. Neurosurgery. 1999; 44(5):1103–1109, discussion 1109–1111

[95] Kondziolka D, Lunsford LD. Stereotactic techniques for colloid cysts: roles of aspiration, endoscopy, and microsurgery. Acta Neurochir Suppl (Wien). 1994; 61:76–78

[96] Lewis AI, Crone KR, Taha J, van Loveren HR, Yeh HS, Tew JM, Jr. Surgical resection of third ventricle colloid cysts. Preliminary results comparing transcallosal microsurgery with endoscopy. J Neurosurg. 1994; 81(2):174–178

[97] Stachura K, Libionka W, Moskała M, Krupa M, Polak J. Colloid cysts of the third ventricle. Endoscopic and open microsurgical management. Neurol Neurochir Pol. 2009; 43(3):251–257

[98] Vorbau C, Baldauf J, Oertel J, Gaab MR, Schroeder HWS. Long-term results after endoscopic resection of colloid cysts. World Neurosurg. 2019; 122: e176–e185

[99] Eshra MA. Endoscopic management of third ventricular colloid cysts in mildly dilated lateral ventricles. Neurosurg Rev. 2019; 42(1):127–132

[100] Azab WA, Abdelnabi EA, Mostafa KH. Efficacy and safety of the rotational technique for endoscopic transforaminal excision of colloid cysts of the third ventricle. World Neurosurg. 2019; 125:e602–e611

[101] Samadian M, Ebrahimzadeh K, Maloumeh EN, et al. Colloid cyst of the third ventricle: long-term results of endoscopic management in a series of 112 cases. World Neurosurg. 2018; 111:e440–e448

[102] Brunori A, de Falco R, Delitala A, Schaller K, Schonauer C. Tailoring endoscopic approach to colloid cysts of the third ventricle: a multicenter experience. World Neurosurg. 2018; 117:e457–e464

[103] Husain M, Jha D, Vatsal DK, et al. Neuro-endoscopic surgery: experience and outcome analysis of 102 consecutive procedures in a busy neurosurgical centre of India. Acta Neurochir (Wien). 2003; 145(5):369–375, discussion 375–376

[104] Lin M, Bakhsheshian J, Strickland B, et al. Navigable channel-based trans-sulcal resection of third ventricular colloid cysts: a multicenter retrospective case series and review of the literature. World Neurosurg. 2020; 133:e702–e710

6 Natural History and Management Options of Vestibular Schwannomas

Jordan Jones, Andrew H. Kaye, and Andrew Morokoff

Abstract

An understanding of the natural history as well as the effectiveness of treatment modalities is essential when managing patients diagnosed with vestibular schwannomas. In this chapter, we review the literature pertaining to the rate and predictive features of growth in both sporadic and neurofibromatosis type 2 associated vestibular schwannomas. We then summarize the outcomes following surgery, stereotactic radiosurgery, and a combination of subtotal resection and adjuvant radiosurgery.

Keywords: vestibular schwannoma, natural history, growth, predictors, microsurgery, stereotactic radiosurgery, tumor control, facial nerve outcomes

6.1 Introduction

Vestibular schwannomas (VS; acoustic neurinomas) are benign tumors that typically arise from the vestibular division of the vestibulocochlear nerve.[1] They account for approximately 6 to 8% of all primary intracranial tumors and are responsible for between 78 and 85% of tumors that arise within the cerebellopontine angle.[2,3] The incidence of VS is best estimated by the Danish epidemiology study by Tos et al at 9.4 tumors per year per million inhabitants.[4] A more recent review of their database in 2004 indicated that this was increasing to a peak of 23 tumors per year per million, likely reflecting the improved diagnostic capabilities of modern magnetic resonance imaging (MRI).[5] Post mortem studies have found a higher incidence of VS from 1.7 to 2.4%, suggesting a substantial number remain asymptomatic or undiagnosed and follow a benign course.[6,7]

VS are sporadic and unilateral in 96% of cases (▶ Fig. 6.1a). Bilateral VS (▶ Fig. 6.1b) are far less common and are associated with the inherited condition neurofibromatosis type 2 (NF2). NF2, first described by the Scottish surgeon Wishart in 1822, results from a mutation in the tumor suppressor *nf2* gene located on chromosome 22q12.2 that encodes for the Merlin protein. Merlin exerts its tumor suppressor effects primarily through maintaining membrane stability and by promoting cell contact inhibition.[1]

Unilateral sensorineural hearing loss, tinnitus, and disequilibrium are the most common presenting symptoms in VS; however, only 10% of patients with these symptoms will be found to have a VS.[8] Unilateral hearing loss that is present for a median of 1 to 3 years is the most common symptom (94–96%), followed by disequilibrium (77%), tinnitus (71%), headache (20–85%), otalgia (28%), facial numbness (7%), and diplopia (7%), with cerebellar dysfunction and facial hypoesthesia more common in larger tumors.[9,10,11] Recently, there has been an increase in the detection of asymptomatic tumors (5–12%) found incidentally on neuroimaging.[12]

Prior to management decisions, all patients should have appropriate neuroimaging with MRI and computed tomography (CT), baseline audiometry assessment, and evaluation of facial nerve function.

6.2 Selected Papers on Natural History

- Paldor I, Chen AS, Kaye AH. Growth rate of vestibular schwannoma. J Clin Neurosci 2016;32:1–8
- Stangerup SE, Caye-Thomasen P, Tos M, Thomsen J. The natural history of vestibular schwannoma. Otol Neurotol 2006;27(4):547–552
- Hunter JB, Francis DO, O'Connell BP, et al. Single institutional experience with observing 564 vestibular schwannomas: factors associated with tumor growth. Otol Neurotol 2016;37(10):1630–1636
- Moffat DA, Kasbekar A, Axon PR, Lloyd SK. Growth characteristics of vestibular schwannomas. Otol Neurotol 2012;33(6):1053–1058

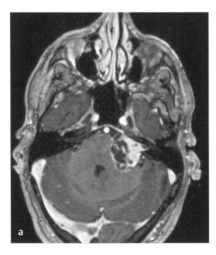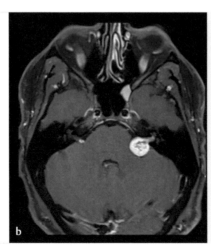

Fig. 6.1 (a) Axial T1 postgadolinium contrast magnetic resonance imaging (MRI) demonstrating large cystic left vestibular schwannoma with brainstem compression and **(b)** bilateral vestibular schwannoma as seen in neurofibromatosis type 2 with larger left- and smaller right-sided tumors.

6.3 Natural History

There is wide variability in the reported natural history of untreated VS (▶ Table 6.1). In sporadic tumors, the incidence of tumor growth during follow-up has been reported to be between 12 and 85% of cases. A total of 7,581 tumors were reported in the 50 series of non-NF2 VS; of these, 2,816 (37%) were reported as growing, during a median follow-up of 39 months. The duration of follow-up affects the incidence of growth as suggested by Paldor et al in their systematic review, in which approximately one-third of patients demonstrated growth in a follow-up period of 1 to 3 years; however, that increased to 50% when follow-up extended beyond 5 years.[13]

6.3.1 Rate of Growth

The reported rate of growth is also highly variable, typically less than 2 mm/y with an average of 1.48 mm/y in reports on non-NF2 VS. A small subset of patients though will demonstrate more rapid growth as reported by Charabi et al who found that 8% will grow greater than 10 mm/y,[14] similar to that reported by Modugno et al, where 12% grew by greater than 9 mm/y.[15] The pattern of growth is also not always constant with up to 40% showing exponential growth compared to linear enlargement.[16] Growth in the first few years of follow-up tended to be more rapid and suggestive of continued enlargement, whereas several reports have suggested a slow or absent pattern of growth for 3 years indicates that future growth is unlikely to be of significance.

6.3.2 Risk Factors for Growth

Forty-one of the 56 reports attempted to identify predictive features of growth. Both patient and tumor factors were identified and included the following:

- *Age*: Younger patients are more likely to grow at an increased rate.
- *Tumor size*: Larger tumors demonstrated greater tendency for growth, but not at a faster rate.
- *Tumor location*: VS with extension into the cerebellopontine angle reported to more likely grow and at a faster rate compared to purely intracanalicular VS.
- *Tumor features*: Cystic tumors and those that have demonstrated hemorrhage show increased rate and tendency to grow.
- *Presenting symptoms*: Disequilibrium and tinnitus were reported in a small number of studies to be predictive of tumor growth. Hearing loss and vertigo as presenting symptoms were not found to be risk factors. Tumors found incidentally were reported either to have no effect on natural history[17] or to behave more indolently.[18]
- *Previous growth*: VS growth within the first year was reported in five studies to be a significant predictor of further tumor growth. Similarly, the longer a tumor remains stable, the likelihood of subsequent growth also reduces; Sethi et al recently demonstrated the risk of growth after 4 years of stability to be less than 2%.[19] On the other hand, a separate report by Macielak et al found that 3.9% of all observed tumors and 8.1% of previously reported growing tumors have delayed growth beyond 5 years arguing for lifelong surveillance of all untreated VS.[20]

Table 6.1 Selective series reporting on the natural history of vestibular schwannomas

Studies	No. of patients	Median follow-up (mo)	Mean age (y)	Tumor size	Tumor growth (%)	Growth rate (mm/y)	Predictors of growth
Stangerup et al[24]	552	43.2	59.0	IM: 42% EM: 1–10 mm, 33% EM: >10 mm, 25%	132 (23.9)	5.0	Tumor location (CPA >IAC) Early growth
Bakkouri et al[21]	325	54	58.0	IM: 54% EM: 1–10 mm, 43% EM: 10–20 mm, 3%	130 (40.0)	1.2	Delay in diagnosis
Moffat et al[23]	381	50.4	61.0	Mean: 9.9 mm IM: 62.4%	124 (32.5)	2.3	Nil
Peyre et al[26]	92	58	25.0	Mean: 13 mm IM: 56%	79 (85.9)	1.8	Early age of diagnosis Unpredictable
Plotkin et al[25]	166	31.3	26.0	Median volume: 0.4 cm^3	105 (63.2)	–	Nil
Hunter et al[22]	564	22.9	59.0	Median: 10 mm	230 (40.8)	>2.0	Disequilibrium Larger tumor size
Lees et al[18]	361	49	62.0	Median volume: 0.161 cm^3 IM: 64%	249 (69.0)	0.054 cm^3/y	Aural fullness Facial numbness Nonincidental
Sethi et al[19]	341	60	67.0	IM: 49% Small: 39% Medium: 17% Large: 1%	139 (40.8)	>2.0	Previous growth

Abbreviations: CPA, cerebellopontine angle; EM, extrameatal; IAC, internal acoustic canal; IM, intrameatal; VS, vestibular schwannoma.

Although a number of risk factors for tumor growth were identified, the results were not consistent across all studies and 10 series found no features that were predictive of growth during follow-up. The clinical significance of tumor growth was also mixed with symptom progression or need for retreatment ranging from 23 to 42% when reported.[18,21,22,23,24] Nevertheless, the majority of these studies were limited by selection bias whereby tumors deemed high risk for growth, including larger tumors, or tumors with symptom progression, were excluded from surveillance.

6.3.3 Growth in Neurofibromatosis Type 2 Vestibular Schwannomas

The growth of VS in patients with NF2 differs to that of non-NF2 patients due to underlying differences in tumor biology and the fact that they occur in a younger population. In six studies, the rate of growing tumors ranged from 32 to 100% of cases. Overall in 468 VS in NF2 patients, 263 (56%) were reported to grow during a median follow-up of 53 months. Growth rates were variable, with three series reporting younger age of onset as a risk factor for tumor growth and the median time to tumor progression was significantly shorter than the median time to hearing decline when reported.[25,26]

6.4 Selected Papers on Treatment

- Goldbrunner R, Weller M, Regis J, et al. EANO guideline on the diagnosis and treatment of vestibular schwannoma. Neuro-Oncol 2020;22(1):31–45[27]
- Ben Ammar M, Piccirillo E, Topsakal V, Taibah A, Sanna M. Surgical results and technical refinements in translabyrinthine excision of vestibular schwannomas: the Gruppo Otologico experience. Neurosurgery 2012;70(6):1481–1491, discussion 1491
- Johnson S, Kano H, Faramand A, et al. Long term results of primary radiosurgery for vestibular schwannomas. J Neurooncol 2019;145(2):247–255
- Golfinos JG, Hill TC, Rokosh R, et al. A matched cohort comparison of clinical outcomes following microsurgical resection or stereotactic radiosurgery for patients with small- and medium-sized vestibular schwannomas. J Neurosurg 2016;125(6):1472–1482

- Chung L, Nguyen T, Sheppard J, Lagman C. A systematic review of radiosurgery versus surgery for neurofibromatosis type 2 vestibular schwannomas. World Neurosurg 2018;109:47–58

6.5 Treatment

There are four main treatment strategies in patients with VS: conservative management with tumor monitoring, microsurgical resection, stereotactic radiosurgery (SRS) or a planned combination of subtotal resection and adjuvant SRS. Treatment decisions must consider tumor morphology and size, patient symptoms and comorbidities, as well as the experience of the treating team.

6.5.1 Microsurgery

The first reported successful operation on a cerebellopontine angle tumor was by Sir Charles Ballance in 1894 and early series were complicated by high morbidity and mortality.[1] Current advances in anesthesia, facial nerve electromyographic (EMG) monitoring, and microsurgical techniques, as described by House in 1964 and others, have resulted in significant reductions in mortality rates and high rates of anatomical facial nerve preservation. In general, there are retrosigmoid and presigmoid approaches with the choice dependent on tumor characteristics, hearing status, bony and venous sinus anatomy, and expertise of treating surgeons.

In the last 26 years, 114 studies have reported on outcomes following surgical resection of sporadic non-NF2 VS (▶ Table 6.2). The total number of patients included was 28,470 patients with median follow-up of 37 months. A gross macroscopic resection was reported in 42 to 100% of cohorts with Ahmad et al reporting 93.8% gross total resection in a large cohort of 2,400 VS.[28] Larger tumors and cystic characteristics were associated with lower rates of GTR[29,30]; however, several series reported high rates of GTR despite these features.[31] Along with the good chance of complete resection, tumor control was high and the need for retreatment was low in most reported series. Ben Ammar et al in a series of 1,865 patients reported 99.5% tumor control during a median follow-up of 68 months.[32] Subtotal resection was associated with higher rates of retreatment (▶ Fig. 6.2) as

Table 6.2 Summary of the literature regarding treatment of vestibular schwannoma

	Microsurgery	Stereotactic radiosurgery	STR and SRS
No. of studies	114	92	11
No. of patients	28,740	13,347	439
Median age (y)	49.0	56.0	52.0
Study period	1994–2020	1995–2020	2003–2018
Median follow-up (mo)	37.0	57.0	51.0
GTR or NTR (%)	87.8	–	–
Tumor control (%)	95.7	85.7	89.0
Retreatment rate (%)	3.3	6.0	8.8
Facial nerve outcome	75.5% HB I or II	94.8% stable	94% HB I or II
Functional hearing (%)	47.7	57.0	62.0

Abbreviations: GTR, gross total resection; HB, House–Brackmann, NTR, near-total resection; STR, subtotal resection.

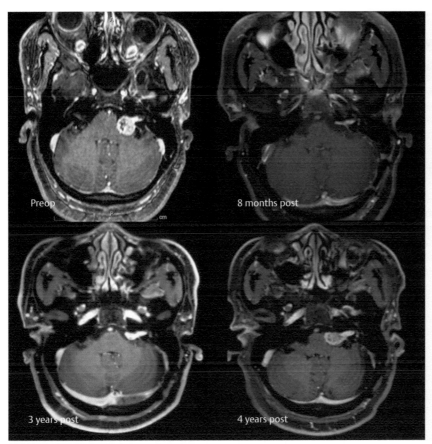

Fig. 6.2 Recurrent vestibular schwannoma. A 40-year-old man underwent a retrosigmoid craniotomy and near-complete macroscopic resection of tumor, with the aim of hearing preservation. At 8 months postsurgery, magnetic resonance imaging (MRI) showed a small enhancing residual. However, at 3 and 4 years, there was progressive regrowth of the residual tumor. Progressive recurrence is unusual in vestibular schwannoma and underlines the importance of postresection follow-up imaging. This recurrent tumor was treated with second surgery via a translabyrinthine approach.

was cystic tumors,[30,33,34] although in a series of 131 solid versus 131 matched cystic tumors there was minimal differences between the two groups.[35]

Reported good facial nerve outcomes, defined as either House–Brackmann (HB) grade I or II at last follow-up, were variable across historical series ranging from 42 to 100%. In 23,956 patients with reported facial nerve outcomes, HB grade I or II was found in 75.5%. Series reporting larger tumors[31,36,37] were associated with lower rates of good facial nerve outcomes, as were two early series.[38,39] Sinha and Sharma reported lower rates of good facial nerve outcomes in 58 cystic tumors when compared to 226 solid tumors[30]; however, this finding was not found by Tang et al.[35] Functional hearing preservation was more variable ranging from 2 to 87%. In 58 studies with a total 11,198 patients in which hearing preservation surgery was attempted, serviceable hearing was reported in 47.7% at last follow-up. The reporting of hearing outcomes was more heterogenous than the facial nerve outcome with the American Academy of Otolaryngology–Head and Neck Surgery (AAO-HNS) and Gardner–Robertson hearing classifications most commonly used. Surgery was complicated by cerebrospinal fluid (CSF) leak in 1 to 12.5% of reported studies. Ansari et al found the retrosigmoid approach (10.3%) had higher rates of CSF leak compared to the translabyrinthine (7.1%) and middle fossa approaches (5.3%).[40] Sughrue et al reported that most CSF leaks (68%) required some form of intervention including lumbar drainage, CSF diversion procedure, or open surgical repair.[41] Overall mortality from microsurgery, however, was very low at 0.2%.

6.5.2 Stereotactic Radiosurgery

The first VS treated with SRS was in 1967 by Lars Leksell.[42] Delivery of gamma radiation was targeted to the tumor from a cobalt-60 source and termed Gamma Knife. Since that time, there have been several alterations to delivery including reduction of the marginal tumor dose to reduce the incidence of cranial nerve neuropathy.[43,44] Other methods of delivering radiation treatment include the linear particle accelerator (LINAC) that accelerated charged particles (electrons) to velocities near the speed of light using oscillating electric fields,[45] Cyber Knife, which utilizes a robotic arm to allow radiation to be delivered from any desired angle,[46] and proton beam therapy that allows reduction of integral dose, reducing surrounding radiation toxicity.[47] Additionally, treatment can be delivered in fractions, reducing the potential side effects when compared to single-dose SRS.[48]

Ninety-two studies in the last 25 years have reported on outcomes following SRS. The total number of patients was 13,347 with a median follow-up of 57 months (▶ Table 6.2). Tumor control in the follow-up was 85.7%, with 6% of the 7,315 patients requiring retreatment either with surgery or further SRS. Patients with smaller tumors had improved tumor control as opposed to larger tumors.[49,50,51] This finding, however, is influenced by the natural history of VS as discussed previously, with larger tumors more likely to demonstrate growth with or without treatment. The majority of treatment failures occurred early after SRS as reported by Hasegawa et al with almost all growths occurring within the first 5 years of follow-up.[52]

The incidence of facial nerve injury from SRS has improved in recent years and reported rates are low. Lunsford et al, in a series of 829 patients, described 21% new facial palsies following treatment in 2005,[53] with modern large series demonstrating less than 5% of new facial palsies.[49,52,54,55] Similar to microsurgery, preservation of functional hearing is variable ranging from 18 to 100% with an average of 57% in 10,980 patients who reported hearing outcomes with hearing status at the time of SRS and cochlear dose predictors of hearing preservation.[56,57] The incidence of permanent trigeminal neuropathy following SRS is low, ranging from 0 to 5.8% in modern large series[49,52,53,55,58,59,60] with post-SRS hydrocephalus occurring in 3.2% of patients.[61] Malignant transformation has been raised as a concern following radiosurgery; however, there is little evidence to suggest a significant risk.[62,63] Carlson et al reviewed the Surveillance, Epidemiology, and End Results (SEER) database and found that the 5-year risk of developing a malignancy after treatment of a unilateral VS to be 0.1% with no differences between radiotherapy, microsurgery, and observation.[64]

Four nonrandomized studies compared microsurgery to SRS and found lower rates of facial nerve palsies and hearing loss with SRS in tumors less than 3 cm in size.[65,66,67,68] However, the cohort with the longest follow-up reported slightly higher rates of retreatment with SRS,[66] whereas the largest study with 85 patients in each treatment arm had significantly longer follow-up in the surgery group (36 vs. 19 months).[65] Due to the lack of randomized trials, a Cochrane review in 2014 concluded that treatment needs to be selected on an individual basis, taking into account patient preference, clinical experience, and the availability of radiotherapeutic equipment.[69]

6.5.3 Microsurgery and Stereotactic Radiosurgery

A combination of planned subtotal resection followed by SRS has been considered an option to reduce morbidity in treatment of large VS.[70] Eleven studies have reported this approach with tumor control in 89% in 439 patients with a median follow-up of 51 months (▶ Table 6.2). Good facial nerve outcome was reported in 94% of patients with 62% of patients with serviceable hearing preoperatively reporting preserved function at last follow-up.

6.5.4 Neurofibromatosis Type 2

Ten studies with 629 patients and 792 VS reported outcomes following microsurgery in NF2 patients. Gross total resection was reported in 86% of VS and recurrence was seen in 6% of 486 VS who reported retreatment rates. Good facial nerve outcomes were seen in 67% and hearing preservation in 46% of patients following surgery with significantly lower rates for both functional outcomes in larger tumors.[71,72,73,74] Nineteen studies with 643 patients and 803 VS reported outcomes following SRS. Tumor control was 79% with a median follow-up of 65 months, with good facial nerve outcomes in 92% and hearing preservation in 40%. Only one study reported on 12 NF2 patients with combined microsurgery followed by SRS.[75] These 12 patients reported a control rate of 83% at a median follow-up of 73 months with good facial nerve outcome in 92% and hearing

preservation in 3 patients. Management of VS in NF2 patients is particularly challenging and the goal of treatment is to preserve functional hearing for as long as possible. Tumors occur in younger patients and although variable tend to grow more rapidly than sporadic VS. Additionally, audiological symptoms tend to occur late in the disease and the chance of preserving hearing following treatment is low leading to difficulties in decisions regarding timing of treatment.[1]

6.6 Authors' Recommendations

- The growth rate of VS is generally slow, around 1 to 2 mm/y, but some tumors can exhibit rapid growth. Monitoring small asymptomatic tumors is appropriate, but follow-up should continue in the long term as there is a small incidence of delayed growth.
- The decision to treat depends on patient age, tumor size and appearance, symptoms, and patient preference. In general, the younger the patient and the larger the tumor, the more reason to recommend treatment, in order to avoid the complications of growth in the long term.
- Microsurgery with modern techniques has a very high rate of complete tumor resection, good chance of facial nerve function preservation, and low rates of recurrence and retreatment. It is suitable for most patients, especially those with larger tumors.
- We use the retrosigmoid approach in cases of smaller tumors where preoperative hearing is good and hearing preservation is attempted. In large tumors or those patients with nonfunctional hearing, a translabyrinthine approach is preferred. More rarely, for small intracanalicular tumors requiring resection, a middle fossa approach is appropriate.
- We recommend treatment of purely intracanalicular VS in cases of documented growth or progressive symptoms, usually deafness or disequilibrium, in young patients or those without significant medical comorbidities.
- SRS (or fractionated radiotherapy) has shown high rates of tumor control over 20 years or more with low morbidity and is the recommended technique in small to medium tumors (< 3 cm) and older patients or those with significant surgical risks.
- VS in NF2 patients grow more aggressively and often present difficult management decisions. The aim is to preserve hearing for as long as possible and a combination of timed subtotal resection and SRS is used. Brainstem implants provide a way to restore some hearing in cases of bilateral acoustic nerve loss.

References

[1] Kaye AH, Laws ER. Brain Tumors: An Encyclopedic Approach. New York, NY: Saunders/Elsevier; 2012

[2] House WF. Transtemporal bone microsurgical removal of acoustic neuromas. Evolution of transtemporal bone removal of acoustic tumors. Arch Otolaryngol. 1964; 80:731–742

[3] Moffat DA, Ballagh RH. Rare tumours of the cerebellopontine angle. Clin Oncol (R Coll Radiol). 1995; 7(1):28–41

[4] Tos M, Thomsen J, Charabi S. Incidence of acoustic neuromas. Ear Nose Throat J. 1992; 71(9):391–393

[5] Stangerup SE, Tos M, Thomsen J, Caye-Thomasen P. True incidence of vestibular schwannoma? Neurosurgery. 2010; 67(5):1335–1340, discussion 1340

[6] Hardy M, Crowe SJ. Early asymptomatic acoustic tumor: report of six cases. Arch Surg. 1936; 32:292–301

[7] Leonard JR, Talbot ML. Asymptomatic acoustic neurilemoma. Arch Otolaryngol. 1970; 91(2):117–124

[8] Valvassori GE, Mafee MF, Dobben GD. Computerized tomography of the temporal bone. Laryngoscope. 1982; 92(5):562–565

[9] Hardy DG, Macfarlane R, Baguley D, Moffat DA. Surgery for acoustic neurinoma. An analysis of 100 translabyrinthine operations. J Neurosurg. 1989; 71(6):799–804

[10] Tos M, Thomsen J. Epidemiology of acoustic neuromas. J Laryngol Otol. 1984; 98(7):685–692

[11] Kentala E, Pyykkö I. Clinical picture of vestibular schwannoma. Auris Nasus Larynx. 2001; 28(1):15–22

[12] Selesnick SH, Deora M, Drotman MB, Heier LA. Incidental discovery of acoustic neuromas. Otolaryngol Head Neck Surg. 1999; 120(6):815–818

[13] Paldor I, Chen AS, Kaye AH. Growth rate of vestibular schwannoma. J Clin Neurosci. 2016; 32:1 8

[14] Charabi S, Thomsen J, Tos M, Charabi B, Mantoni M, Børgesen SE. Acoustic neuroma/vestibular schwannoma growth: past, present and future. Acta Otolaryngol. 1998; 118(3):327–332

[15] Modugno GC, Pirodda A, Ferri GG, et al. Small acoustic neuromas: monitoring the growth rate by MRI. Acta Neurochir (Wien). 1999; 141(10):1063–1067

[16] Dirks MS, Butman JA, Kim HJ, et al. Long-term natural history of neurofibromatosis type 2-associated intracranial tumors. J Neurosurg. 2012; 117(1):109–117

[17] Carlson ML, Lees KA, Patel NS, et al. The clinical behavior of asymptomatic incidental vestibular schwannomas is similar to that of symptomatic tumors. Otol Neurotol. 2016; 37(9):1435–1441

[18] Lees KA, Tombers NM, Link MJ, et al. Natural history of sporadic vestibular schwannoma: a volumetric study of tumor growth. Otolaryngol Head Neck Surg. 2018; 159(3):535–542

[19] Sethi M, Borsetto D, Cho Y, et al. The conditional probability of vestibular schwannoma growth at different time points after initial stability on an observational protocol. Otol Neurotol. 2020; 41(2):250–257

[20] Macielak RJ, Patel NS, Lees KA, et al. Delayed tumor growth in vestibular schwannoma: an argument for lifelong surveillance. Otol Neurotol. 2019; 40 (9):1224–1229

[21] Bakkouri WE, Kania RE, Guichard JP, Lot G, Herman P, Huy PT. Conservative management of 386 cases of unilateral vestibular schwannoma: tumor growth and consequences for treatment. J Neurosurg. 2009; 110(4):662–669

[22] Hunter JB, Francis DO, O'Connell BP, et al. Single institutional experience with observing 564 vestibular schwannomas: factors associated with tumor growth. Otol Neurotol. 2016; 37(10):1630–1636

[23] Moffat DA, Kasbekar A, Axon PR, Lloyd SK. Growth characteristics of vestibular schwannomas. Otol Neurotol. 2012; 33(6):1053–1058

[24] Stangerup SE, Caye-Thomasen P, Tos M, Thomsen J. The natural history of vestibular schwannoma. Otol Neurotol. 2006; 27(4):547–552

[25] Plotkin SR, Merker VL, Muzikansky A, Barker FG, II, Slattery W, III. Natural history of vestibular schwannoma growth and hearing decline in newly diagnosed neurofibromatosis type 2 patients. Otol Neurotol. 2014; 35(1): e50–e56

[26] Peyre M, Goutagny S, Bah A, et al. Conservative management of bilateral vestibular schwannomas in neurofibromatosis type 2 patients: hearing and tumor growth results. Neurosurgery. 2013; 72(6):907–913, discussion 914, quiz 914

[27] Goldbrunner R, Weller M, Regis J, et al. EANO guideline on the diagnosis and treatment of vestibular schwannoma. Neuro-oncol. 2020; 22(1):31–45

[28] Ahmad RA, Sivalingam S, Topsakal V, Russo A, Taibah A, Sanna M. Rate of recurrent vestibular schwannoma after total removal via different surgical approaches. Ann Otol Rhinol Laryngol. 2012; 121(3):156–161

[29] Wanibuchi M, Fukushima T, McElveen JT, Jr, Friedman AH. Hearing preservation in surgery for large vestibular schwannomas. J Neurosurg. 2009; 111(4):845–854

[30] Sinha S, Sharma BS. Cystic acoustic neuromas: surgical outcome in a series of 58 patients. J Clin Neurosci. 2008; 15(5):511–515

[31] Sluyter S, Graamans K, Tulleken CA, Van Veelen CW. Analysis of the results obtained in 120 patients with large acoustic neuromas surgically treated via the translabyrinthine-transtentorial approach. J Neurosurg. 2001; 94 (1):61–66

[32] Ben Ammar M, Piccirillo E, Topsakal V, Taibah A, Sanna M. Surgical results and technical refinements in translabyrinthine excision of vestibular schwannomas: the Gruppo Otologico experience. Neurosurgery. 2012; 70(6): 1481–1491, discussion 1491

[33] Monfared A, Corrales CE, Theodosopoulos PV, et al. Facial nerve outcome and tumor control rate as a function of degree of resection in treatment of large acoustic neuromas: preliminary report of the Acoustic Neuroma Subtotal Resection Study (ANSRS). Neurosurgery. 2016; 79(2):194–203

[34] Arlt F, Trantakis C, Seifert V, Bootz F, Strauss G, Meixensberger J. Recurrence rate, time to progression and facial nerve function in microsurgery of vestibular schwannoma. Neurol Res. 2011; 33(10):1032–1037

[35] Tang IP, Freeman SR, Rutherford SA, King AT, Ramsden RT, Lloyd SK. Surgical outcomes in cystic vestibular schwannoma versus solid vestibular schwannoma. Otol Neurotol. 2014; 35(7):1266–1270

[36] Silva J, Cerejo A, Duarte F, Silveira F, Vaz R. Surgical removal of giant acoustic neuromas. World Neurosurg. 2012; 77(5–6):731–735

[37] Samii M, Gerganov VM, Samii A. Functional outcome after complete surgical removal of giant vestibular schwannomas. J Neurosurg. 2010; 112(4):860–867

[38] Briggs RJ, Luxford WM, Atkins JS, Jr, Hitselberger WE. Translabyrinthine removal of large acoustic neuromas. Neurosurgery. 1994; 34(5):785–790, discussion 790–791

[39] Elsmore AJ, Mendoza ND. The operative learning curve for vestibular schwannoma excision via the retrosigmoid approach. Br J Neurosurg. 2002; 16(5):448–455

[40] Ansari SF, Terry C, Cohen-Gadol AA. Surgery for vestibular schwannomas: a systematic review of complications by approach. Neurosurg Focus. 2012; 33 (3):E14

[41] Sughrue ME, Yang I, Aranda D, et al. Beyond audiofacial morbidity after vestibular schwannoma surgery. J Neurosurg. 2011; 114(2):367–374

[42] Leksell L. A note on the treatment of acoustic tumours. Acta Chir Scand. 1971; 137(8):763–765

[43] Flickinger JC, Kondziolka D, Pollock BE, Lunsford LD. Evolution in technique for vestibular schwannoma radiosurgery and effect on outcome. Int J Radiat Oncol Biol Phys. 1996; 36(2):275–280

[44] Miller RC, Foote RL, Coffey RJ, et al. Decrease in cranial nerve complications after radiosurgery for acoustic neuromas: a prospective study of dose and volume. Int J Radiat Oncol Biol Phys. 1999; 43(2):305–311

[45] Zeman EM. The biological basis of radiation oncology. In: Gunderson LL, Tepper JE, eds. Clinical Radiation Oncology. 4th ed. Philadelphia, PA: Elsevier; 2016:2–40.e5

[46] Kurup G. CyberKnife: a new paradigm in radiotherapy. J Med Phys. 2010; 35 (2):63–64

[47] DeLaney TF. Proton therapy in the clinic. Front Radiat Ther Oncol. 2011; 43: 465–485

[48] Lederman G, Lowry J, Wertheim S, et al. Acoustic neuroma: potential benefits of fractionated stereotactic radiosurgery. Stereotact Funct Neurosurg. 1997; 69(1–4, Pt 2):175–182

[49] Johnson S, Kano H, Faramand A, et al. Long term results of primary radiosurgery for vestibular schwannomas. J Neurooncol. 2019; 145(2): 247–255

[50] Mezey G, Cahill J, Rowe JG, et al. A retrospective analysis of the role of single-session gamma knife stereotactic radiosurgery in sporadic vestibular schwannomas with tumor volumes greater than 10 cm³: is it worth stretching the boundaries? Stereotact Funct Neurosurg. 2020; 98(2):85–94

[51] Yang HC, Kano H, Awan NR, et al. Gamma Knife radiosurgery for larger-volume vestibular schwannomas. Clinical article. J Neurosurg. 2011; 114(3): 801–807

[52] Hasegawa T, Kida Y, Kato T, Iizuka H, Kuramitsu S, Yamamoto T. Long-term safety and efficacy of stereotactic radiosurgery for vestibular schwannomas: evaluation of 440 patients more than 10 years after treatment with Gamma Knife surgery. J Neurosurg. 2013; 118(3):557–565

[53] Lunsford LD, Niranjan A, Flickinger JC, Maitz A, Kondziolka D. Radiosurgery of vestibular schwannomas: summary of experience in 829 cases. J Neurosurg. 2005; 102 Suppl:195–199

[54] Rueß D, Pöhlmann L, Hellerbach A, et al. Acoustic neuroma treated with stereotactic radiosurgery: follow-up of 335 patients. World Neurosurg. 2018; 116:e194–e202

[55] Klijn S, Verheul JB, Beute GN, et al. Gamma Knife radiosurgery for vestibular schwannomas: evaluation of tumor control and its predictors in a large patient cohort in The Netherlands. J Neurosurg. 2016; 124(6):1619–1626

[56] Jacob JT, Carlson ML, Schiefer TK, Pollock BE, Driscoll CL, Link MJ. Significance of cochlear dose in the radiosurgical treatment of vestibular schwannoma: controversies and unanswered questions. Neurosurgery. 2014; 74(5):466–474, discussion 474

[57] Mousavi SH, Niranjan A, Akpinar B, et al. Hearing subclassification may predict long-term auditory outcomes after radiosurgery for vestibular schwannoma patients with good hearing. J Neurosurg. 2016; 125(4):845–852

[58] Watanabe S, Yamamoto M, Kawabe T, et al. Stereotactic radiosurgery for vestibular schwannomas: average 10-year follow-up results focusing on long-term hearing preservation. J Neurosurg. 2016; 125 Suppl 1:64–72

[59] Sun S, Liu A. Long-term follow-up studies of Gamma Knife surgery with a low margin dose for vestibular schwannoma. J Neurosurg. 2012; 117 Suppl:57–62

[60] Boari N, Bailo M, Gagliardi F, et al. Gamma Knife radiosurgery for vestibular schwannoma: clinical results at long-term follow-up in a series of 379 patients. J Neurosurg. 2014; 121 Suppl:123–142

[61] De Sanctis P, Green S, Germano I. Communicating hydrocephalus after radiosurgery for vestibular schwannomas: does technique matter? A systematic review and meta-analysis. J Neurooncol. 2019; 145(2):365–373

[62] Pollock BE, Link MJ, Stafford SL, Parney IF, Garces YI, Foote RL. The risk of radiation-induced tumors or malignant transformation after single-fraction intracranial radiosurgery: results based on a 25-year experience. Int J Radiat Oncol Biol Phys. 2017; 97(5):919–923

[63] Maducdoc MM, Ghavami Y, Linskey ME, Djalilian HR. Evaluation of reported malignant transformation of vestibular schwannoma: de novo and after stereotactic radiosurgery or surgery. Otol Neurotol. 2015; 36(8):1301–1308

[64] Carlson ML, Glasgow AE, Jacob JT, Habermann EB, Link MJ. The short-term and intermediate-term risk of second neoplasms after diagnosis and treatment of unilateral vestibular schwannoma: analysis of 9460 cases. Int J Radiat Oncol Biol Phys. 2016; 95(4):1149–1157

[65] Golfinos JG, Hill TC, Rokosh R, et al. A matched cohort comparison of clinical outcomes following microsurgical resection or stereotactic radiosurgery for patients with small- and medium-sized vestibular schwannomas. J Neurosurg. 2016; 125(6):1472–1482

[66] Pollock BE, Driscoll CL, Foote RL, et al. Patient outcomes after vestibular schwannoma management: a prospective comparison of microsurgical resection and stereotactic radiosurgery. Neurosurgery. 2006; 59(1):77–85, discussion 77–85

[67] Myrseth E, Møller P, Pedersen PH, Lund-Johansen M. Vestibular schwannoma: surgery or gamma knife radiosurgery? A prospective, nonrandomized study. Neurosurgery. 2009; 64(4):654–661, discussion 661–663

[68] Régis J, Pellet W, Delsanti C, et al. Functional outcome after gamma knife surgery or microsurgery for vestibular schwannomas. J Neurosurg. 2002; 97(5):1091–1100

[69] Muzevic D, Legcevic J, Splavski B, Cayé-Thomasen P. Stereotactic radiotherapy for vestibular schwannoma. Cochrane Database Syst Rev. 2014(12):CD009897

[70] Starnoni D, Daniel RT, Tuleasca C, George M, Levivier M, Messerer M. Systematic review and meta-analysis of the technique of subtotal resection and stereotactic radiosurgery for large vestibular schwannomas: a "nerve-centered" approach. Neurosurg Focus. 2018; 44(3):E4

[71] Zhao F, Wang B, Yang Z, et al. Surgical treatment of large vestibular schwannomas in patients with neurofibromatosis type 2: outcomes on facial nerve function and hearing preservation. J Neurooncol. 2018; 138(2):417–424

[72] Moffat DA, Lloyd SK, Macfarlane R, et al. Outcome of translabyrinthine surgery for vestibular schwannoma in neurofibromatosis type 2. Br J Neurosurg. 2013; 27(4):446–453

[73] Odat HA, Piccirillo E, Sequino G, Taibah A, Sanna M. Management strategy of vestibular schwannoma in neurofibromatosis type 2. Otol Neurotol. 2011; 32(7):1163–1170

[74] Nowak A, Dziedzic T, Czernicki T, et al. Strategy for the surgical treatment of vestibular schwannomas in patients with neurofibromatosis type 2. Neurol Neurochir Pol. 2015; 49(5):295–301

[75] Troude L, Boucekine M, Montava M, et al. Does NF2 status impact the results of combined surgery and adjunctive Gamma Knife surgery for large vestibular schwannomas? Neurosurg Rev. 2020; 43(4):1191–1199

7 Natural History and Management Options of Acromegaly

Mendel Castle-Kirszbaum and Tony Goldschlager

Abstract

Acromegaly is a clinical syndrome related to growth hormone excess from a somatotroph adenoma. It is a highly morbid disease, significantly reducing quality of life and is associated with increased risk of cardiovascular disease, cancer, and death. Screening for acromegaly is performed by measuring serum IGF-1, and the diagnosis is confirmed by measuring the GH response to a glucose load. Treatment requires an experienced multidisciplinary team of surgeons, endocrinologists, radiologists, and radiation oncologists. Surgical resection of the adenoma is first-line therapy, with reoperation, stereotactic radiosurgery, and medical therapy all options for residual or recurrent disease. Hormonal control is an essential aim for all patients to reduce mortality and improve quality of life.

Keywords: acromegaly, transsphenoidal surgery, pegvisomant, octreotide, sterotactic radiosurgery

7.1 Introduction

Acromegaly describes the clinical syndrome resulting from excess of growth hormone (GH) and insulin-like growth factor 1 (IGF-1) caused, almost always, by a somatotroph adenoma.[1] Acromegaly is a disease of adulthood, as identical pathology in a child with unfused epiphyses leads to gigantism. Symptoms of acromegaly may be due to local sellar mass effect in addition to the effects of excess circulating GH and its downstream mediators, particularly IGF-1. Acromegaly is an important disease to recognize, as untreated acromegaly is associated with higher all-cause mortality,[2] which can be normalized by adequate treatment.[3] As a hormone-driven tumor, it may be responsive to endocrine therapy, although transsphenoidal resection remains the first-line treatment for most cases.

An overview of population studies evaluating the epidemiology and presentation of acromegaly is shown in ▶ Table 7.1.[4,5,6,7,8,9,10,11,12,13] Somatotroph adenomas are typically a disease of middle age, with diagnosis averaging in the fifth decade,[14] and affect men and women in roughly equal numbers.[14,15,16] In general, there is a significant delay, a median interval of 5 years,[4,5] between symptom onset and diagnosis, demonstrating the often-cryptic nature of the disease. The prevalence of acromegaly ranges between 2.8 and 13.7 cases per 100,000 in the general population, whereas its incidence ranges from 0.2 to 1.1 cases per 100,000.[14] Familial clustering has been noted in kindreds with multiple endocrine neoplasia type 1, McCune–Albright syndrome, Carney complex, familial acromegaly, and familial isolated pituitary adenoma (FIPA).[9,10,17,18,19,20,21,22,23,24]

7.2 Pathology

Somatotrophs lie in the anterolateral aspect of the adenohypophysis and derive, along with lactotrophs, from somatomammotrophs (▶ Fig. 7.1). Most acromegaly cases are due to pure GH hypersecreting adenomas. A further one-third of cases are mixed somatotroph–lactotroph adenomas, whereas somatomammotroph and acidophil stem cell tumors comprise the remaining 10%; each of these cosecrete GH and prolactin. Somatomammotroph tumors tend to appear in the young, and thus are more associated with gigantism than acromegaly,[25] whereas acidophil stem cell tumors are rapidly growing, invasive adenomas where symptoms relating to hyperprolactinemia, rather than acromegaly, are the harbinger to diagnosis.[26,27,28] Additionally, it is not uncommon to detect modest hyperprolactinemia in pure somatotroph adenomas as a result of stalk compression, permitting uninhibited lactotroph secretion due to interruption of the inhibitory infundibulo-hypophyseal dopaminergic pathway.[16,21]

Table 7.1 Summary of large epidemiological studies of acromegaly

Studies	*n*	Prevalence (per 100,000 population)	Incidence (per 100,000 population)	M:F ratio	Age at diagnosis, mean, y (range)	Macroadenoma (%)
Mestron et al[10]	41,035,271	3.4	0.2	1:1.5	45.0	73.0
Daly et al[5]	71,972	12.5	NR	3:1	43.7 (17.0–65.0)	100.0
Bex et al[9]	10,850,000	4.0	0.2	1:1	NR	79.0
Fernandez et al[4]	81,449	8.6	NR	1.3:1	47.0[a] (30.0–63.0)	86.0
Raappana et al[7]	722,000–733,000	NR	0.3	1.6:1	40.5[a] (12.0–69.0)	78.0
Gruppetta et al[11]	417,608	12.4	0.3	1:1.3	44.0[a] (19.0–69.0)	73.0
Kwon et al[13]	48,456,369	2.8	0.4	1:1.2	44.1	83.0
Hoskuldsdottir et al[6]	316,075	13.3	0.8	1.6:1	44.5 (24.0–49.0)	71.0
Dal et al[8]	7,200,000	8.5 (in 2010)	0.4	1.1:1	48.7	69.0
Burton et al[12]	50,170,946	7.8	1.1	1.1:1	41.0	Not reported

Abbreviation: NR, not reported.
[a]Median age (mean not given or able to be calculated).
Population of Iceland between 1955 and 2013.
Population of Denmark between 1991 and 2010.

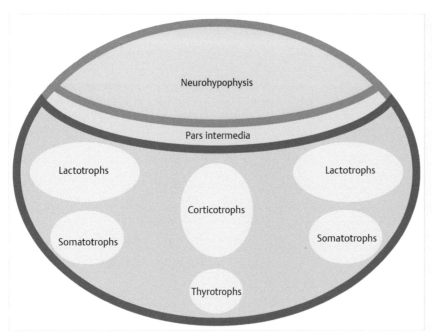

Fig. 7.1 Schematic diagram of an axial slice of the pituitary, demonstrating an idealized distribution of pituicytes.

At the time of diagnosis, greater than two-thirds of cases are macroadenomas[14] and may be classified into two histological subtypes based on the distribution of cytoplasmic cytokeratin: densely granulated or sparsely granulated. The latter is more common in younger patients and tends to be more invasive, larger, and less likely to respond to endocrine therapy.[29] The *AIP* gene is commonly mutated in FIPA, although 3% of sporadic somatotroph adenomas harbor spontaneous mutations, and AIP mutations are associated with younger presentation, larger, and more invasive tumors.[30,31] It is important to mention the extra-pituitary causes of acromegaly; although exceedingly rare, they include growth hormone–releasing hormone (GHRH) hypersecretion from the hypothalamus[32] and systemic neuroendocrine tumors, particularly carcinoid and pancreatic tumors[33,34,35,36,37,38]; ectopic GH hypersecretion from ectopic pituitary remnants, and rarely pancreatic tumors, and lymphoma[39,40,41,42]; and *acromegaloidism*, caused by apparent excess of downstream growth factors.[43,44,45]

7.3 Clinical Signs and Presentation

The clinical presentation of acromegaly may be due to the endocrinopathy or mass effect on the fragile structures in and around the sella, the latter being particularly relevant as greater than two-thirds of cases are macroadenomas.[14]

The hypophyseal fossa is encircled by eloquent anatomy and the symptoms of an expanding somatotroph adenoma are common to any sellar mass. The optic pathway runs in the roof of the suprasellar cistern, and superior extension may compress the optic chiasm, nerves, or tracts in normal, post-, and prefixed chiasmata, respectively. As a result, visual disturbance has been quoted to occur in 26 to 35% of cases[6,46] and is the primary presenting complaint in 3%.[47] The classical visual presentation is a bitemporal hemianopsia due to chiasmal compression. Lateral extension into the cavernous sinus is particularly relevant as it reduces the surgical cure rate. Tumor may compress the oculomotor nerve onto the interclinoid and petroclinoid ligaments, whereas the trochlear, ophthalmic, maxillary, and abducens nerves are similarly vulnerable in the cavernous sinus; however, presentation with diplopia or ophthalmoplegia is rare.[47]

As macroadenomas grow, they may compress the surrounding adenohypophysis and the infundibulum, which may lead to dysfunction in vital hormonal axes, as hypothalamic factors that modulate the release of pituitary hormones pass through the infundibulum and its portal venous system. Biochemical hyperprolactinemia is seen in almost a third of patients, whereas overt galactorrhea is seen in 9%.[46] Hypogonadism has been documented in 38% of patients,[46] whereas disturbance of menses and decreased libido are the primary presenting complaint in 13 and 3% of cases, respectively.[47]

Headache is a common symptom of pituitary mass lesions, due to stretching of the richly innervated diaphragma and related structures. Headache is present in 55% of acromegalic patients and is the primary presenting complaint in 8%.[21,47] The headache of somatotroph adenomas appears particularly disabling, generating higher Migraine Disability Assessment scores (MIDAS) than any other adenoma type.[48] The headache approximates migraines most commonly but sometimes mimics a trigeminal autonomic cephalalgia.[48]

The systemic features of acromegaly are due to high circulating levels of GH and IGF-1 and their resultant stimulation of peripheral tissues to grow. A selection of the typical signs and symptoms of acromegaly is shown in ▶ Fig. 7.2.[10,15,21,49,50,51,52] Some signs are highly sensitive such as somatic changes (prognathism, frontal bossing, and acral enlargement), and some are specific, such as secondary diabetes (odds ratio [OR]: 3.7), hyperhidrosis (OR: 6.1), colorectal polyps (OR: 10.4), spaced teeth (OR: 25.4), carpal tunnel syndrome (OR: 4.3), and finger widening (OR: 131.2).[53]

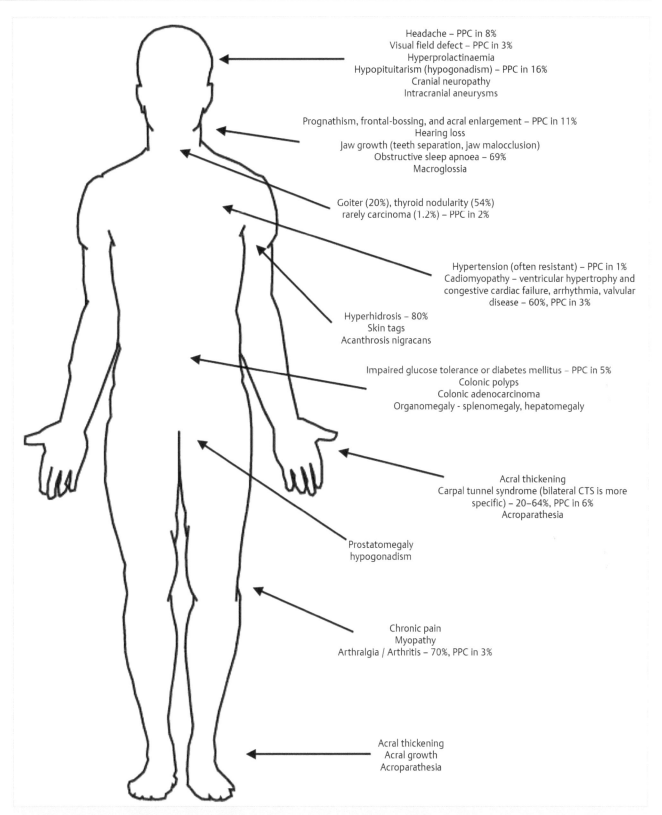

Headache – PPC in 8%
Visual field defect – PPC in 3%
Hyperprolactinaemia
Hypopituitarism (hypogonadism) – PPC in 16%
Cranial neuropathy
Intracranial aneurysms

Prognathism, frontal-bossing, and acral enlargement – PPC in 11%
Hearing loss
Jaw growth (teeth separation, jaw malocclusion)
Obstructive sleep apnoea – 69%
Macroglossia

Goiter (20%), thyroid nodularity (54%)
rarely carcinoma (1.2%) – PPC in 2%

Hypertension (often resistant) – PPC in 1%
Cadiomyopathy – ventricular hypertrophy and
congestive cardiac failure, arrhythmia, valvular
disease – 60%, PPC in 3%

Hyperhidrosis – 80%
Skin tags
Acanthrosis nigracans

Impaired glucose tolerance or diabetes mellitus – PPC in 5%
Colonic polyps
Colonic adenocarcinoma
Organomegaly - splenomegaly, hepatomegaly

Acral thickening
Carpal tunnel syndrome (bilateral CTS is more
specific) – 20–64%, PPC in 6%
Acroparathesia

Prostatomegaly
hypogonadism

Chronic pain
Myopathy
Arthralgia / Arthritis – 70%, PPC in 3%

Acral thickening
Acral growth
Acroparathesia

Fig. 7.2 Clinical signs and symptoms of acromegaly. Percentages denote the incidence of symptoms (PPC, primary presenting complaint).

7.4 Imaging

Magnetic resonance imaging (MRI) is the imaging modality of choice for evaluation of pituitary adenomas and is mandatory for a complete evaluation of the disease. Macroadenomas are usually isointense to cortex and may cause the physiological "bright spot" of the neurohypophysis to be absent (20%) or displaced (80%).[69] Hyperintensity of the optic apparatus on T2/fluid-attenuated inversion recovery (FLAIR) is a sign of compression. Heterogeneous, strong enhancement is the norm; however, in 5 to 10% of cases, adjacent dural thickening may be noted, which may be misinterpreted as the "dural tail" of a meningioma.[69] Microadenomas may be elusive on non-contrast-enhanced imaging, and generally are hypointense to the surrounding gland when contrast is given. Some microadenomas enhance to a similar degree to normal pituitary parenchyma; however, their rate of gadolinium uptake is slower. This may be exploited in dynamic scanning where time lapsed images can demonstrate the delayed enhancement of the 10 to 30% of microadenomas not visible on standard contrast-enhanced imaging.[69] On T2-weighted imaging, GH adenomas are hypointense in 52.9%, hyperintense in 25.9%, and isointense in 21.2% of cases, with T2 hypointensity associated with smaller tumors, lower likelihood of optic nerve compression, and higher IGF-1 levels.[70]

7.5 Diagnosis and Follow-up

Acromegaly should be suspected in those with typical acral or facial features, or those who have multiple of the associated conditions including sleep apnea, type 2 diabetes mellitus, carpal tunnel syndrome, hyperhidrosis, and severe or treatment-resistant hypertension.[54] The accepted screening test is measurement of serum IGF-1.[54] IGF-1 has a half-life of 15 hours (unlike 20 minutes for GH), is not pulsatile (unlike GH), and correlates well with overall GH load.[55] As such, a normal IGF-1 level effectively rules out acromegaly.[54] Importantly, elevated "false-positive" IGF-1 levels may occur in pregnancy, and late adolescence; lowered "false-negative" levels may be seen with oral estrogens, malnutrition, hepatic and renal failure, hypothyroidism, severe infection, and impaired glucose metabolism (i.e., uncontrolled diabetes mellitus).[54,55] Furthermore, IGF-1 levels decrease with age after peaking in adolescence, and there is significant variation between IGF-1 assays[56]; thus, levels must be compared to age-matched and assay-specific normal values.

For those with positive or equivocal serum IGF-1 levels, an oral glucose tolerance test (OGTT) should be performed, whereupon an inappropriately normal (nonsuppressed) GH level after a glucose load is diagnostic of acromegaly. Newer "ultrasensitive" assays use a cutoff of > 0.4 µg/L; however, reference levels for the IDS-iSYS GH assay, which account for BMI, sex, and oestrogen therapy, should be used wherever possible.[57] Elevated IGF-1 with normal GH suppression may indicate early-stage disease.[58] Although GHRH hypersecretion is responsible for only 0.5% of acromegaly, when a nonpituitary etiology is suspected or imaging is negative, measurement of GHRH should be performed.[59]

A positive diagnosis of acromegaly necessitates further work-up to examine the extent of disease. Evaluation of metabolic derangements should be performed including fasting blood sugar and fasting lipids. Cardiovascular and cerebrovascular complications are the major cause of death in acromegaly, and echocardiography and ambulatory electrocardiography should be arranged; early intervention is particularly important as these changes appear nonreversible.[60] A thyroid ultrasound should be performed if there is palpable thyroid nodularity, and patients should be questioned about symptoms of sleep apnea.[54] If not already performed, a complete pituitary screen should be arranged, as well as a colonoscopy, as the ORs for colonic adenomas (OR = 2.49) and colonic carcinomas (OR = 4.35) are significant.[61]

7.6 Selected Papers on the Natural History of Acromegaly

- Wright AD, McLachlan MS, Doyle FH, Fraser TR. Serum growth hormone levels and size of pituitary tumour in untreated acromegaly. BMJ 1969;4(5683):582–584
- Wright AD, Hill DM, Lowy C, Fraser TR. Mortality in acromegaly. Q J Med 1970;39(153):1–16

7.7 Natural History of Acromegaly

Although the literature is scant, the natural history of acromegaly appears one of progressive adenoma growth and symptom progression. Tumor size, as estimated by sella area, correlates with disease duration.[62] GH concentration after OGTT did not escalate during 13 months of observation of 22 patients,[62] suggesting disease progression is often slow, and systemic manifestations may correlate more with the chronicity of elevated GH and IGF-1 rather than their absolute value. Untreated patients have a much higher mortality than those who are successfully treated.[63]

Acromegaly is a life-limiting condition, with a standardized mortality ratio (SMR) of 1.72 (95%CI: 1.62–1.83) compared to the general population.[2] With active treatment, those who achieve normal IGF-1 levels restore their elevated mortality to normal levels (SMR = 1.1; 95%CI: 0.9–1.4), whereas those with persistently elevated IGF-1 maintain a significantly greater risk of death (SMR = 2.5; 95%CI: 1.6–4.0).[3] Given these findings, disease control should be the goal in every patient and should be defined as a normal aged-matched IGF-1 or a nadir GH < 0.4 µg/L on ultrasensitive assay, following OGTT.[64]

Biochemical monitoring should include measurement of both GH and IGF-1, with normalization of the latter being the chief goal[65]; the exception to this is patients receiving pegvisomant, where only IGF-1 levels are of value. After biochemical control, regular follow-up every 6 months is the norm. Many of the sequelae of untreated disease are irreversible, and thus aggressive management of acromegaly-related comorbidities including insulin resistance, obstructive sleep apnea, hypertension, cardiomyopathy, and joint pathology is strongly recommended.[65] Recently, two tools for monitoring disease have been developed and validated, which are the SAGIT (*S*igns and symptoms, *A*ssociated comorbidities, *G*H levels, *I*GF-1, and *T*umor profile) and ACRODAT (ACROmegaly

Disease Activity Tool).[66,67] These combine symptomatologic and biochemical outcomes to objectively measure disease control and are useful indicators of disease burden.

7.8 Selected Papers on the Management Options for Acromegaly

- Melmed S, Bronstein MD, Chanson P, Klibanski A, Casanueva FF, Wass JAH, et al. A Consensus Statement on acromegaly therapeutic outcomes. Nat Rev Endocrinol 2018;14(9):552–561
- Katznelson L, Laws ER Jr, Melmed S, et al; Endocrine Society. Acromegaly: an endocrine society clinical practice guideline. J Clin Endocrinol Metab 2014;99(11):3933–3951
- Abu Dabrh AM, Mohammed K, Asi N, et al. Surgical interventions and medical treatments in treatment-naïve patients with acromegaly: systematic review and meta-analysis. J Clin Endocrinol Metab 2014;99(11):4003–4014[68]

7.9 Management Options

The management of acromegaly is complex and requires a multidisciplinary team including a primary care physician, an endocrinologist, and the neurosurgeon. ▶ Fig. 7.3 demonstrates our recommended management pathway.[54,65,64,71]

7.9.1 Surgery

Acromegaly is best treated in centers with significant experience with the disease, where patients can be managed by a multidisciplinary team including a neurosurgeon well trained in transsphenoidal resection and operating with sufficient case volume. It requires a team of endocrinologists up-to-date with the latest medical therapies, neuroradiologists well versed in sellar imaging, neuropathologists with expertise in molecular analysis, and radiation oncologists trained in pituitary irradiation.[65] Endoscopic transsphenoidal resection is the treatment of choice for all surgical candidates.[54] In expert centers, surgery can offer biochemical cure in 75 to 90% of microadenomas and 45 to 70% of macroadenomas. ▶ Table 7.2 summarizes the surgical remission rates in large trials using modern criteria for cure.

Surgical remission appears to correlate with cavernous sinus invasion, quantified by the Knosp grade, preoperative GH and IGF-1 levels, postoperative GH level, and tumor size,[84] as well as parasellar invasion,[72] male gender,[85] and the experience of the surgical center.[86] The postoperative decline in IGF-1 is often delayed in comparison to GH levels; thus, a period of at least 12 weeks should elapse before assessing the success of surgery with IGF-1 levels.[65]

Given larger and more invasive tumors have a poorer chance of surgical cure, presurgical "neoadjuvant" somatostatin receptor ligand (SRL) therapy has been advocated as a method of shrinking the adenoma and facilitating complete resection. Pretreatment with SRL increases the chance of IGF-1 normalization at 3 months postsurgery (relative risk [RR] = 2.47) but does not affect the rate of surgical complications.[87] However, long-term follow-up after 1 and 5 years fails to demonstrate any benefit,

suggesting that early biochemical changes may be due to carry-over effect of the SRL itself.[88] Preoperative SRL is recommended in those with severe pharyngeal thickness and sleep apnea, or high-output heart failure, as it reduces anesthetic risk.[54,89] It may also be used, at the discretion of the surgeon, preoperatively in patients with large, invasive tumors, in which case a 3-month course is standard[90]; however, there is little quality evidence supporting this practice.

When complete surgical excision is not possible, maximal safe debulking of the tumor enhances the efficacy of subsequent medical therapy. In a small prospective series (n = 26), control of IGF-1 levels with SRL significantly improved (from 42 to 89%) after surgical debulking, demonstrating that a poor prospect of surgical cure should not prohibit surgery.[91]

In the hands of an experienced surgeon, endoscopic transsphenoidal resection is a safe and effective treatment. Complications of transsphenoidal surgery (TSS) for acromegaly are generally minor and commonly include nasal congestion (42%), sinusitis (30%), epistaxis (7%), and disturbances of smell (30%), though these are almost always transient.[84] Cerebrospinal fluid (CSF) leaks occur in about 1% of cases,[72] and thus for CSF leaks in macroadenoma surgery, we advocate for graded repair, guided by the grade of intraoperative CSF leak.[92] Major complications including meningitis and damage to cranial nerves or carotid arteries occur in less than 1% of cases in experienced pituitary centers.[21]

Reoperation after TSS is recommended if the tumor remnant is readily identifiable on imaging and surgically accessible.[54] In a small series (n = 14) where initial surgery did not achieve biochemical remission, repeat surgery was able to achieve disease control in 57%, and was more likely to be successful in those with random GH < 10 μg/L preoperatively.[93] Recurrence after surgical biochemical cure is rare, with only 2 of 668 patients over 10 years of follow-up presenting with recurrent disease.[72]

7.9.2 Stereotactic Radiosurgery

Stereotactic radiosurgery (SRS) is emerging as an adjuvant therapy for medically resistant acromegaly; indeed, most studies of SRS are in postsurgical patients, refractory to medical therapy. Occasionally SRS may be chosen as the primary treatment modality, particularly in patients not fit for surgery or patients who wish to avoid surgery. ▶ Table 7.3 and ▶ Table 7.4 summarize the data for primary and postoperative SRS, respectively. Predictors of a durable response from SRS include prior surgery (p = 0.02), only mildly elevated GH and IGF1 (p = 0.0004), cessation of medical therapy prior to SRS (p = 0.04), and higher marginal and maximal dosages (p = 0.0007).[106] Unfortunately, the latter factor as well as a tumor volume >2.5 cm^3 predicted a more than twofold risk developing a new hormone deficiency.[108,109]

The temporality of the response to SRS is varied and may take years to take full effect. Thus, medical therapy is required while awaiting the response to SRS and should be annually withdrawn to assess the response[54]; SRLs need to be discontinued for 2 months and GH receptor antagonists (GHRAs) and dopamine agonists (DAs) for 2 to 3 weeks before assessment.[109] Importantly, SRLs and DAs decrease the efficacy of SRS and thus medical therapy should be temporarily interrupted prior to SRS,[110] as this practice increases the chances of durable

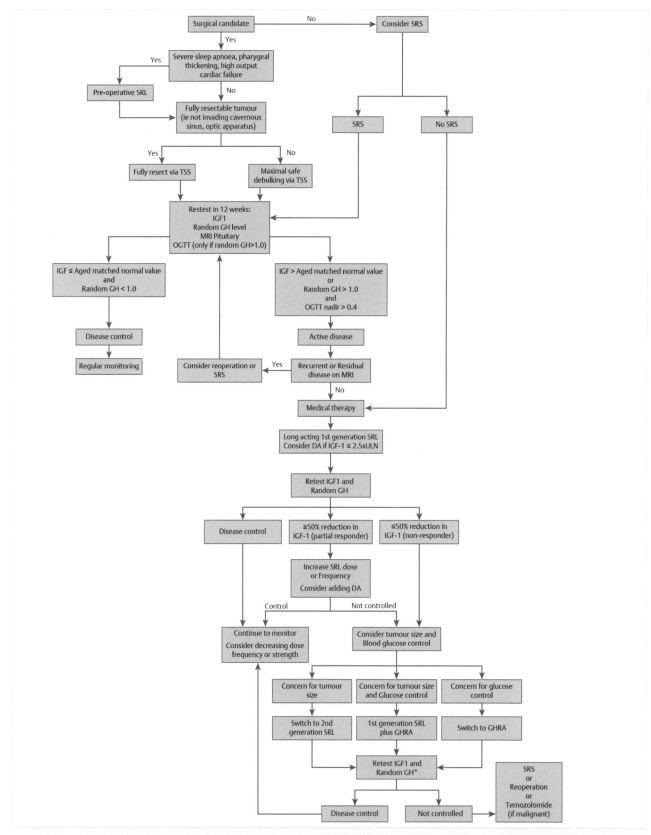

Fig. 7.3 Our recommended management pathway (SRS, stereotactic radiosurgery; SRL, somatostatin receptor ligand; GHRA, growth hormone receptor antagonist; DA, dopamine agonist; OGTT, oral glucose tolerance test; TSS, transsphenoidal surgery). All units are in µg/L. *Do not measure GH if using GHRA.

Table 7.2 Studies of transsphenoidal surgery with ≥ 100 patients in the cohort where modern definitions of cure are used (i.e., OGTT and IGF1)

Studies	*n*	Remission, total (%)	Remission, microadenoma (%)	Remission, macroadenoma (%)	Remission criteria
Davis et al[77]	174	51.7	NR	NR	Normal IGF-1, OGTT <2 ng/mL, and postoperative GH <5 ng/mL
Tindall et al[78]	103	76.2	87	56.7	IGF-1 <2.2 U/mL, and postoperative GH <5 ng/mL
Freda et al[80]	115	61	88	53	Normal IGF-1, or OGTT <2 ng/mL
Beauregard et al[73]	103	52	82	39	Normal IGF-1, and OGTT <1 ng/mL
Mortini et al[76]	320	59.1	83.1	53.6	Normal IGF-1, and OGTT <1 ng/mL
Nomikos et al[72]	506	57.3	75.3	50.3	Normal GH and IGF-1, and OGTT <1 ng/mL
Hazer et al[74]	214	62.6	62.8	62.6	Normal IGF-1, tumor-free MRI, and OGTT <1 ng/mL
Shirvani et al[75]	130	56.9	66.7	52.9	Normal IGF-1, resolution of symptoms, first postoperative GH <2.5 ng/mL
Zhou et al[79]	133	66.2	NR	NR	Normal IGF-1, and OGTT <1 ng/mL
Anik et al[82]	401	68.1	81.3	63.3	Normal IGF-1, OGTT <0.4 ng/mL, or postoperative GH <1 ng/mL
Fernández Mateos et al[83]	548	61.7	91.5	53.4	Normal IGF-1, OGTT <0.4 ng/mL, and postoperative GH <2 ng/mL
Kim et al[81]	134	73.1	86.7	72.3	Normal IGF-1, and OGTT <1 ng/mL

Abbreviations: GH, growth hormone; IGF-1, insulin-like growth factor 1; NR, not reported; OGTT, oral glucose tolerance test.

Table 7.3 Studies of primary stereotactic radiosurgery for acromegaly

Author (y)	*n*	Median marginal dose (Gy)	Cure at last F/U	Hormonal control ± medical Rx at last F/U	Hypopituitarism
Mohammed (2019)[93]	26	23.7	19.2 (5/26)	69.2 (18/26)	15.3 (4/26)
Sims-Williams (2019)[94]	20	27.5	25 (3/12)	100 (12/12)	52.9 (9/17)
Total	46		21.1 (8/38)	78.9 (30/38)	30.2 (13/43)

Abbreviations: F/U, follow-up; GH, growth hormone; OGTT, oral glucose tolerance test.

Notes: Cure is defined as IGF-1 normalization and normal GH OGTT off any medical therapy. Hormonal control is defined as IGF-1 normalization with or without medical therapy. Cured patients are included in the hormonal control group. Results are given as percentage (*n* event/*n* total)

Table 7.4 Studies of postoperative stereotactic radiosurgery for acromegaly

Author (y)	*n*	Median marginal dose (Gy)	Cure at last F/U	Hormonal control ± medical Rx at last F/U	Hypopituitarism	Visual deficit attributed to SRS
Castinetti (2005)[95]	82	30	17.1 (14/82)	40.2 (33/82)	17.1 (14/82)	0 (0/82)
Ding (2019)[96]	371	24.2	38.5 (143/371)	NR	26.1 (97/371)	3.5 (13/371)
Iwata (2016)[97]	52	NR	17.3 (9/52)	NR	1.9 (1/52)	0 (0/52)
Ježková (2006)[98]	96	35	44.2 (19/43)	NR	27.1 (26/96)	0 (0/96)
Knappe (2020)[99]	119	NR	52.1 (62/119	NR	63 (56/89)	NR
Kong (2018)[100]	138	25	34.1 (47/138)	58.0 (80/138)	8.7 (12/138)	NR
Lee (2014)[101]	136	25	66.7 (18/27)	NR	31.6 (43/136)	2.9 (4/136)
Pai (2018)[102]	76	15.8	28.9 (22/76)	NR	11.8 (9/76)	0 (0/76)
Vik-Mo (2007)[103]	61	26.5	50.8 (31/61)	NR	52.9 (9/17)	5.0 (1/20)
Wilson (2013)[104]	86	20	14.0 (12/86)	NR	19.8 (17/86)	1.2 (1/86)
Total	1217		35.7 (377/1055)	51.4 (113/220)	24.8 (284/1143)	2.1 (19/919)

Abbreviations: F/U, follow-up; GH, growth hormone; OGTT, oral glucose tolerance test; SRS, stereotactic radiosurgery.

Notes: Cure is defined as IGF-1 normalization and normal GH OGTT off any medical therapy. Hormonal control is defined as IGF-1 normalization with or without medical therapy. Cured patients are included in the hormonal control group. Results are given as percentage (*n* event/*n* total).

remission 2.5-fold.[106] Specifically, SRLs and DAs should be withheld for 6 to 8 weeks prior to SRS, whereas GHRA do not need to be withheld; medical therapy may restart 4 to 8 weeks after SRS.[106]

The most common complication of SRS is hypopituitarism in one or more axes, occurring in 26 to 32% of patients, with hypothyroidism (64%), hypogonadism (51%), and hypocortisolism (40%) being the most common.[106,108] Endocrine follow-up following SRS is critical. Apart from the previously discussed association with higher marginal and maximal dosages, hypopituitarism is also associated with SRS targeting the whole sella (p = 0.02).[106] Therefore, whole sella SRS should only be used when no residual or recurrent tumor can be distinguished on MRI. Cranial neuropathies are uncommon, seen in 4.3% of patients, and generally involve the optic apparatus; not surprisingly, extension into the suprasellar region is a risk factor (p = 0.02).[106] These complications, like the benefits of SRS, may only occur many years after administration.

7.9.3 Medical Therapy

When biochemical remission has not been achieved from surgery, medical therapy is recommended. The armamentarium of therapies includes SRLs and DAs, both of which are directed at the somatotroph adenoma, and GHRAs, which peripherally block the action of GH. SRLs are the preferred "first-line" agent, with DAs reserved for select patients with mild disease; GHRAs may augment or replace SRL therapy when there is a suboptimal response.[54,71] Rarely, in patients with unusually aggressive or proven malignant tumors, temozolomide may be given in cooperation with a neuro-oncologist.[65] Medical therapies are summarized in ▶ Table 7.5.

SRLs possess a longer half-life than the natural ligand of the somatostatin receptor and exert their antisecretory and antiproliferative effects by binding to somatostatin receptor (commonly type 2) which are frequently expressed by somatotroph adenomas.[111] Newer, long-acting SRL formulations are the treatment of choice, with long-acting octreotide able to induce normalization of IGF-1 levels in 67% of cases; success rates are even greater in those with only mildly elevated pretreatment GH levels.[112] In treatment-naïve patients (no previous medical or surgical intervention), long-acting octreotide normalized IGF-1 levels in 34% of patients after 48 weeks of treatment, with likelihood of remission correlating inversely with tumor size.[113]

When followed over a period of many years, 69% of patients are able to achieve biochemical control on SRLs.[21] Predictors of response to SRLs include female gender, older age, lower IGH-1 and GH levels,[114] densely granulated histology,[29] robust somatostatin receptor expression,[115] and previous surgical or SRS treatment.[116] Apart from biochemical respite, SRLs also decrease tumor size in 53% of patients by an average of 37%, which may provide relief from mass effect symptoms.[117] Side effects from SRLs are generally mild and include diarrhea (36%), abdominal discomfort (29%), cholelithiasis (22%), and bradycardia (25%).[118] Additionally, despite theoretical risks, the effect of first-generation SRLs on glucose control is minimal.[119] A newer, second-generation SRL Pasireotide has been shown to confer greater rates of biochemical control than long-acting octreotide; however, it is highly diabetogenic, with nearly 70% of patients experiencing hyperglycemia.[65] Thus, Pasireotide is reserved for first-generation SRL-resistant disease, and blood glucose should be strictly monitored. In patients who have demonstrated biochemical response to injectable SRL, novel oral octreotide can be considered.[107]

DAs are effective in patients with mild disease, defined as GH levels and IGF-1 levels less than twice the upper limit of normal.[120] When pretreatment IGF-1 levels are greater than 2.5 times the upper limit of normal, the likelihood of successful DA monotherapy is low.[71] DAs may have a role in augmenting SRL or GHRA therapy, with the addition of DA allowing biochemical control in 52 and 28% of cases suboptimally controlled on SRLs and GHRAs, respectively.[120,121] Despite the theoretical advantage, DAs are no more effective in cases of acromegaly with hyperprolactinemia.[122,123]

The GHRA pegvisomant blocks postreceptor GH signal transduction and thus peripheral synthesis of IGF-1. GHRA therapy normalizes IGF-1 in 73% of the cases at 10-year follow-up, with efficacy improving with both time and dose.[125,126] Because of its mechanism of action, response can only be measured using IGF-1. Serial imaging of the sella is required to rule out tumor growth, especially in macroadenomas, although only 6.8% demonstrated radiological progression in 10-year follow-up.[124] GHRAs are well tolerated, with adverse reactions including transaminitis, injection site reactions (lipodystrophy), and headache occurring in less than 10%.[21] When added to SRL therapy, GHRA may induce remission in up to 95% of cases; however, this combination is potentially hepatotoxic, and vigilant monitoring of liver function is required.[127]

Table 7.5 Overview of the medications used in the treatment of acromegaly and their side effects

Drug	Route	Initial dose	Side effects
Somatostatin receptor ligand			
Octreotide	SC	50–100 µg; every 8–12 h	Common: nausea/vomiting, cholelithiasis/cholestasis, bradycardia, alopecia, hyperglycemia, altered bowel habits, abdominal pain, fatigue
Octreotide XR	IM	20–40 mg; monthly	Rarely: hypothyroidism, pancreatitis, hepatopathy
Pasireotide	IM	20–60 mg; monthly	
Dopamine agonist			
Cabergoline	PO	1–4 mg; twice weekly or daily	Nausea/vomiting, orthostatic hypotension, systemic fibrosis (cardiac, retroperitoneal, pleuropulmonary), abdominal pain, constipation, headache, psychiatric disorders
Growth hormone receptor antagonist			
Pegvisomant	IM	20–60 mg; monthly	Transaminitis, injection site lipodystrophy, arthralgias, headache, ongoing adenoma growth

Abbreviations: IM, intramuscular; PO, per os; SC, subcutaneous.

7.10 Authors' Recommendations

- Our recommended management plan is summarized in ▶ Fig. 7.3.
- Surgical resection should be considered the first-line treatment, through an endoscopic transsphenoidal approach, where possible. This should be performed by an experienced surgical team working in a multidisciplinary setting. Complete resection is the goal.
- Patients who are not surgical candidates should be considered for SRS.
- Those who do not achieve remission 12 weeks after surgery, where remission is defined by normalized IGF-1 and either random GH < 1 ng/mL or OGTT < 0.4 ng/mL, should be considered for reoperation or SRS if there is macroscopic remnant on MRI, or medical therapy if there is no macroscopic remnant.
- Medical therapy should be initiated in conjunction with an endocrinologist, but generally begins with a long-acting first-generation SRL.
- Depending on the response to first-line medical therapy, the dose can be maintained, uptitrated, or a GHRA may be added.
- Patients should be regularly monitored for the sequelae of acromegaly, including regular colonoscopy, hemoglobin A1c, and blood pressure checks.

References

[1] Marie P. Sur deux cas d'acromégalie; hypertrophie singuliére non congénitale des extrémités supérieures, inférieures et céphalique. Rev Med Liege. 1886; 6:297–333

[2] Dekkers OM, Biermasz NR, Pereira AM, Romijn JA, Vandenbroucke JP. Mortality in acromegaly: a metaanalysis. J Clin Endocrinol Metab. 2008; 93(1):61–67

[3] Holdaway IM, Bolland MJ, Gamble GD. A meta-analysis of the effect of lowering serum levels of GH and IGF-I on mortality in acromegaly. Eur J Endocrinol. 2008; 159(2):89–95

[4] Fernandez A, Karavitaki N, Wass JAH. Prevalence of pituitary adenomas: a community-based, cross-sectional study in Banbury (Oxfordshire, UK). Clin Endocrinol (Oxf). 2010; 72(3):377–382

[5] Daly AF, Rixhon M, Adam C, Dempegioti A, Tichomirowa MA, Beckers A. High prevalence of pituitary adenomas: a cross-sectional study in the province of Liege, Belgium. J Clin Endocrinol Metab. 2006; 91(12):4769–4775

[6] Hoskuldsdottir GT, Fjalldal SB, Sigurjonsdottir HA. The incidence and prevalence of acromegaly, a nationwide study from 1955 through 2013. Pituitary. 2015; 18(6):803–807

[7] Raappana A, Koivukangas J, Ebeling T, Pirilä T. Incidence of pituitary adenomas in Northern Finland in 1992–2007. J Clin Endocrinol Metab. 2010; 95(9):4268–4275

[8] Dal J, Feldt-Rasmussen U, Andersen M, et al. Acromegaly incidence, prevalence, complications and long-term prognosis: a nationwide cohort study. Eur J Endocrinol. 2016; 175(3):181–190

[9] Bex M, Abs R, T'Sjoen G, et al. AcroBel: the Belgian registry on acromegaly—a survey of the "real-life" outcome in 418 acromegalic subjects. Eur J Endocrinol. 2007; 157(4):399–409

[10] Mestron A, Webb SM, Astorga R, et al. Epidemiology, clinical characteristics, outcome, morbidity and mortality in acromegaly based on the Spanish Acromegaly Registry (Registro Espanol de Acromegalia, REA). Eur J Endocrinol. 2004; 151(4):439–446

[11] Gruppetta M, Mercieca C, Vassallo J. Prevalence and incidence of pituitary adenomas: a population based study in Malta. Pituitary. 2013; 16(4):545–553

[12] Burton T, Le Nestour E, Neary M, Ludlam WH. Incidence and prevalence of acromegaly in a large US health plan database. Pituitary. 2016; 19(3):262–267

[13] Kwon O, Song YD, Kim SY, Lee EJ, Rare Disease Study Group, Science and Research Committee, Korean Endocrine, Society. Nationwide survey of acromegaly in South Korea. Clin Endocrinol (Oxf). 2013; 78(4):577–585

[14] Lavrentaki A, Paluzzi A, Wass JAH, Karavitaki N. Epidemiology of acromegaly: review of population studies. Pituitary. 2016; 20(1):4–9

[15] Ezzat S, Forster MJ, Berchtold P, Redelmeier DA, Boerlin V, Harris AG. Acromegaly. Clinical and biochemical features in 500 patients. Medicine (Baltimore). 1994; 73(5):233–240

[16] Kaye AH, Laws ER Jr. Brain Tumors. Philadelphia, PA: Elsevier Health Sciences; 2011:1

[17] Katznelson L, Atkinson JL, Cook DM, Ezzat SZ, Hamrahian AH, Miller KK, AACE Acromegaly Task Force. American Association of Clinical Endocrinologists Medical Guidelines for Clinical Practice for the Diagnosis and Treatment of Acromegaly: 2011 update: executive summary. Endocr Pract. 2011; 17(4):636–646

[18] Weinstein LS, Yu S, Warner DR, Liu J. Endocrine manifestations of stimulatory G protein alpha-subunit mutations and the role of genomic imprinting. Endocr Rev. 2001; 22(5):675–705

[19] Boikos SA, Stratakis CA. Carney complex: the first 20 years. Curr Opin Oncol. 2007; 19(1):24–29

[20] Correa R, Salpea P, Stratakis CA. Carney complex: an update. Eur J Endocrinol. 2015; 173(4):M85–M97

[21] Capatina C, Wass JAH. 60 years of neuroendocrinology: acromegaly. J Endocrinol. 2015; 226(2):T141–T160

[22] Pellegata NS, Quintanilla-Martinez L, Siggelkow H, et al. Germ-line mutations in p27Kip1 cause a multiple endocrine neoplasia syndrome in rats and humans. Proceedings of the National Academy of Sciences. National Academy of Sciences. 2006; 103(42):15558–15563

[23] Georgitsi M, Raitila A, Karhu A, et al. Germline CDKN1B/p27Kip1 mutation in multiple endocrine neoplasia. J Clin Endocrinol Metab. 2007; 92(8):3321–3325

[24] Agarwal SK, Ozawa A, Mateo CM, Marx SJ. The MEN1 gene and pituitary tumours. Horm Res. 2009; 71(2) Suppl 2:131–138

[25] Jameson JL, De Groot LJ. Endocrinology: Adult and Pediatric. Philadelphia, PA: Elsevier Health Sciences; 2015:1

[26] Lloyd RV, Cano M, Chandler WF, Barkan AL, Horvath E, Kovacs K. Human growth hormone and prolactin secreting pituitary adenomas analyzed by in situ hybridization. Am J Pathol. 1989; 134(3):605–613

[27] Halmi NS. Occurrence of both growth hormone- and prolactin-immunoreactive material in the cells of human somatotropic pituitary adenomas containing mammotropic elements. Virchows Arch A Pathol Anat Histopathol. 1982; 398(1):19–31

[28] Horvath E, Kovacs K, Singer W, Ezrin C, Kerenyi NA. Acidophil stem cell adenoma of the human pituitary. Arch Pathol Lab Med. 1977; 101(11):594–599

[29] Larkin S, Reddy R, Karavitaki N, Cudlip S, Wass J, Ansorge O. Granulation pattern, but not GSP or GHR mutation, is associated with clinical characteristics in somatostatin-naive patients with somatotroph adenomas. Eur J Endocrinol. 2013; 168(4):491–499

[30] Cazabat L, Bouligand J, Salenave S, et al. Germline AIP mutations in apparently sporadic pituitary adenomas: prevalence in a prospective single-center cohort of 443 patients. J Clin Endocrinol Metab. 2012; 97(4):E663–E670

[31] Cazabat L, Libè R, Perlemoine K, et al. Germline inactivating mutations of the aryl hydrocarbon receptor-interacting protein gene in a large cohort of sporadic acromegaly: mutations are found in a subset of young patients with macroadenomas. Eur J Endocrinol. 2007; 157(1):1–8

[32] Asa SL, Scheithauer BW, Bilbao JM, et al. A case for hypothalamic acromegaly: a clinicopathological study of six patients with hypothalamic gangliocytomas producing growth hormone-releasing factor. J Clin Endocrinol Metab. 1984; 58(5):796–803

[33] Thorner MO, Perryman RL, Cronin MJ, et al. Somatotroph hyperplasia. Successful treatment of acromegaly by removal of a pancreatic islet tumor secreting a growth hormone-releasing factor. J Clin Invest. 1982; 70(5):965–977

[34] Guillemin R, Brazeau P, Böhlen P, Esch F, Ling N, Wehrenberg WB. Growth hormone-releasing factor from a human pancreatic tumor that caused acromegaly. Science. 1982; 218(4572):585–587

[35] Rivier J, Spiess J, Thorner M, Vale W. Characterization of a growth hormone-releasing factor from a human pancreatic islet tumour. Nature. 1982; 300(5889):276–278

[36] Barkan AL, Shenker Y, Grekin RJ, Vale WW. Acromegaly from ectopic growth hormone-releasing hormone secretion by a malignant carcinoid tumor.

Successful treatment with long-acting somatostatin analogue SMS 201–995. Cancer. 1988; 61(2):221–226

[37] Melmed S, Ziel FH, Braunstein GD, Downs T, Frohman LA. Medical management of acromegaly due to ectopic production of growth hormone-releasing hormone by a carcinoid tumor. J Clin Endocrinol Metab. 1988; 67 (2):395–399

[38] Drange MR, Melmed S. Long-acting lanreotide induces clinical and biochemical remission of acromegaly caused by disseminated growth hormone-releasing hormone-secreting carcinoid. J Clin Endocrinol Metab. 1998; 83(9):3104–3109

[39] Lloyd RV, Chandler WF, Kovacs K, Ryan N. Ectopic pituitary adenomas with normal anterior pituitary glands. Am J Surg Pathol. 1986; 10(8):546–552

[40] Corenblum B, LeBlanc FE, Watanabe M. Acromegaly with an adenomatous pharyngeal pituitary. JAMA. 1980; 243(14):1456–1457

[41] Beuschlein F, Strasburger CJ, Siegerstetter V, et al. Acromegaly caused by secretion of growth hormone by a non-Hodgkin's lymphoma. N Engl J Med. 2000; 342(25):1871–1876

[42] Melmed S, Ezrin C, Kovacs K, Goodman RS, Frohman LA. Acromegaly due to secretion of growth hormone by an ectopic pancreatic islet-cell tumor. N Engl J Med. 1985; 312(1):9–17

[43] Low L, Chernausek SD, Sperling MA. Acromegaloid patients with type A insulin resistance: parallel defects in insulin and insulin-like growth factor-I receptors and biological responses in cultured fibroblasts. J Clin Endocrinol Metab. 1989; 69(2):329–337

[44] Ashcraft MW, Hartzband PI, Van Herle AJ, Bersch N, Golde DW. A unique growth factor in patients with acromegaloidism. J Clin Endocrinol Metab. 1983; 57(2):272–276

[45] Dahlqvist P, Spencer R, Marques P, et al. Pseudoacromegaly: a differential diagnostic problem for acromegaly with a genetic solution. J Endocr Soc. 2017; 1(8):1104–1109

[46] Drange MR, Fram NR, Herman-Bonert V, Melmed S. Pituitary tumor registry: a novel clinical resource. J Clin Endocrinol Metab. 2000; 85(1): 168–174

[47] Melmed S. The Pituitary. London, UK: Academic Press; 2016:1

[48] Levy MJ, Matharu MS, Meeran K, Powell M, Goadsby PJ. The clinical characteristics of headache in patients with pituitary tumours. Brain. 2005; 128(Pt 8):1921–1930

[49] Molitch ME. Clinical manifestations of acromegaly. Endocrinol Metab Clin North Am. 1992; 21(3):597–614

[50] Reid TJ, Post KD, Bruce JN, Nabi Kanibir M, Reyes-Vidal CM, Freda PU. Features at diagnosis of 324 patients with acromegaly did not change from 1981 to 2006: acromegaly remains under-recognized and under-diagnosed. Clin Endocrinol (Oxf). 2010; 72(2):203–208

[51] Lugo G, Pena L, Cordido F. Clinical manifestations and diagnosis of acromegaly. Int J Endocrinol. 2012; 2012:540398

[52] Melmed S. Medical progress: acromegaly. N Engl J Med. 2006; 355(24): 2558–2573

[53] Prencipe N, Floriani I, Guaraldi F, et al. ACROSCORE: a new and simple tool for the diagnosis of acromegaly, a rare and underdiagnosed disease. Clin Endocrinol (Oxf). 2016; 84(3):380–385

[54] Katznelson L, Laws ER, Jr, Melmed S, et al. Endocrine Society. Acromegaly: an endocrine society clinical practice guideline. J Clin Endocrinol Metab. 2014; 99(11):3933–3951

[55] Brooke AM, Drake WM. Serum IGF-I levels in the diagnosis and monitoring of acromegaly. Pituitary. 2007; 10(2):173–179

[56] Pokrajac A, Wark G, Ellis AR, Wear J, Wieringa GE, Trainer PJ. Variation in GH and IGF-I assays limits the applicability of international consensus criteria to local practice. Clin Endocrinol (Oxf). 2007; 67(1):65–70

[57] Schilbach K, Gar C, Lechner A, Nicolay SS, Schwerdt L, Haenelt M et al (2019) Determinants of the growth hormone nadir during oral glucose tolerance test in adults. Eur J Endocrinol 181(1):55–67. https://doi.org/10.1530/EJE-19-0139

[58] Dimaraki EV, Jaffe CA, DeMott-Friberg R, Chandler WF, Barkan AL. Acromegaly with apparently normal GH secretion: implications for diagnosis and follow-up. J Clin Endocrinol Metab. 2002; 87(8):3537–3542

[59] Losa M, von Werder K. Pathophysiology and clinical aspects of the ectopic GH-releasing hormone syndrome. Clin Endocrinol (Oxf). 1997; 47(2):123–135

[60] Colao A, Ferone D, Marzullo P, Lombardi G. Systemic complications of acromegaly: epidemiology, pathogenesis, and management. Endocr Rev. 2004; 25(1):102–152

[61] Rokkas T, Pistiolas D, Sechopoulos P, Margantinis G, Koukoulis G. Risk of colorectal neoplasm in patients with acromegaly: a meta-analysis. World J Gastroenterol. 2008; 14(22):3484–3489

[62] Wright AD, McLachlan MS, Doyle FH, Fraser TR. Serum growth hormone levels and size of pituitary tumour in untreated acromegaly. BMJ. 1969; 4 (5683):582–584

[63] Wright AD, Hill DM, Lowy C, Fraser TR. Mortality in acromegaly. Q J Med. 1970; 39(153):1–16

[64] Giustina A, Chanson P, Bronstein MD, et al. Acromegaly Consensus Group. A consensus on criteria for cure of acromegaly. J Clin Endocrinol Metab. 2010; 95(7):3141–3148

[65] Melmed S, Bronstein MD, Chanson P, Klibanski A, Casanueva FF, Wass JAH, et al. A Consensus Statement on acromegaly therapeutic outcomes. Nat Rev Endocrinol. 2018; 14(9):552–561

[66] van der Lely AJ, Gomez R, Pleil A, et al. Development of ACRODAT®, a new software medical device to assess disease activity in patients with acromegaly. Pituitary. 2017; 20(6):692–701

[67] Giustina A, Bevan JS, Bronstein MD, et al. SAGIT Investigator Group. SAGIT®: clinician-reported outcome instrument for managing acromegaly in clinical practice—development and results from a pilot study. Pituitary. 2016; 19(1): 39–49

[68] Abu Dabrh AM, Mohammed K, Asi N, et al. Surgical interventions and medical treatments in treatment-naïve patients with acromegaly: systematic review and meta-analysis. J Clin Endocrinol Metab. 2014; 99(11): 4003–4014

[69] Osborn AG, Hedlund GL, Salzman KL. Osborn's Brain. Philadelphia, PA: Elsevier Health Sciences; 2017:1

[70] Potorac I, Petrossians P, Daly AF, et al. Pituitary MRI characteristics in 297 acromegaly patients based on T2-weighted sequences. Endocr Relat Cancer. 2015; 22(2):169–177

[71] Giustina A, Chanson P, Kleinberg D, et al. Acromegaly Consensus Group. Expert consensus document: a consensus on the medical treatment of acromegaly. Nat Rev Endocrinol. 2014; 10(4):243–248

[72] Nomikos P, Buchfelder M, Fahlbusch R. The outcome of surgery in 668 patients with acromegaly using current criteria of biochemical 'cure'. Eur J Endocrinol. 2005; 152(3):379–387

[73] Beauregard C, Truong U, Hardy J, Serri O. Long-term outcome and mortality after transsphenoidal adenomectomy for acromegaly. Clin Endocrinol (Oxf). 2003; 58(1):86–91

[74] Hazer DB, Işık S, Berker D, et al. Treatment of acromegaly by endoscopic transsphenoidal surgery: surgical experience in 214 cases and cure rates according to current consensus criteria. J Neurosurg. 2013; 119(6):1467–1477

[75] Shirvani M, Motiei-Langroudi R. Transsphenoidal surgery for growth hormone-secreting pituitary adenomas in 130 patients. World Neurosurg. 2014; 81(1):125–130

[76] Mortini P, Losa M, Barzaghi R, Boari N, Giovanelli M. Results of transsphenoidal surgery in a large series of patients with pituitary adenoma. Neurosurgery. 2005; 56(6):1222–1233, discussion 1233

[77] Davis DH, Laws ERJ, Jr, Ilstrup DM, et al. Results of surgical treatment for growth hormone-secreting pituitary adenomas. J Neurosurg. 1993; 79(1): 70–75

[78] Tindall GT, Oyesiku NM, Watts NB, Clark RV, Christy JH, Adams DA. Transsphenoidal adenomectomy for growth hormone-secreting pituitary adenomas in acromegaly: outcome analysis and determinants of failure. J Neurosurg. 1993; 78(2):205–215

[79] Zhou T, Wang F, Meng X, Ba J, Wei S, Xu B. Outcome of endoscopic transsphenoidal surgery in combination with somatostatin analogues in patients with growth hormone producing pituitary adenoma. J Korean Neurosurg Soc. 2014; 56(5):405–409

[80] Freda PU, Wardlaw SL, Post KD. Long-term endocrinological follow-up evaluation in 115 patients who underwent transsphenoidal surgery for acromegaly. J Neurosurg. 1998; 89(3):353–358

[81] Kim JH, Hur KY, Lee JH, et al. Outcome of endoscopic transsphenoidal surgery for acromegaly. World Neurosurg. 2017; 104:272–278

[82] Anik I, Cabuk B, Gokbel A, et al. Endoscopic transsphenoidal approach for acromegaly with remission rates in 401 patients: 2010 consensus criteria. World Neurosurg. 2017; 108:278–290

[83] Fernández Mateos C, García-Uria M, Morante TL, García-Uría J. Acromegaly: surgical results in 548 patients. Pituitary. 2017; 20(5):522–528

[84] Jane JA, Jr, Starke RM, Elzoghby MA, et al. Endoscopic transsphenoidal surgery for acromegaly: remission using modern criteria, complications, and predictors of outcome. J Clin Endocrinol Metab. 2011; 96(9):2732–2740

[85] van Bunderen CC, van Varsseveld NC, Baayen JC, et al. Predictors of endoscopic transsphenoidal surgery outcome in acromegaly: patient and tumor characteristics evaluated by magnetic resonance imaging. Pituitary. 2013; 16(2):158–167

[86] Schöfl C, Franz H, Grussendorf M, et al. participants of the German Acromegaly Register. Long-term outcome in patients with acromegaly: analysis of 1344 patients from the German Acromegaly Register. Eur J Endocrinol. 2012; 168(1):39–47

[87] Nunes VS, Correa JMS, Puga MES, Silva EMK, Boguszewski CL. Preoperative somatostatin analogues versus direct transsphenoidal surgery for newly-diagnosed acromegaly patients: a systematic review and meta-analysis using the GRADE system. Pituitary. 2015; 18(4):500–508

[88] Fougner SL, Bollerslev J, Svartberg J, Øksnes M, Cooper J, Carlsen SM. Preoperative octreotide treatment of acromegaly: long-term results of a randomised controlled trial. Eur J Endocrinol. 2014; 171(2):229–235

[89] Friedel ME, Johnston DR, Singhal S, et al. Airway management and perioperative concerns in acromegaly patients undergoing endoscopic transsphenoidal surgery for pituitary tumors. Otolaryngol Head Neck Surg. 2013; 149(6):840–844

[90] Jacob JJ, Bevan JS. Should all patients with acromegaly receive somatostatin analogue therapy before surgery and, if so, for how long? Clin Endocrinol (Oxf). 2014; 81(6):812–817

[91] Karavitaki N, Turner HE, Adams CBT, et al. Surgical debulking of pituitary macroadenomas causing acromegaly improves control by lanreotide. Clin Endocrinol (Oxf). 2008; 68(6):970–975

[92] Patel KS, Komotar RJ, Szentirmai O, et al. Case-specific protocol to reduce cerebrospinal fluid leakage after endonasal endoscopic surgery. J Neurosurg. 2013; 119(3):661–668

[93] Wilson TJ, McKean EL, Barkan AL, Chandler WF, Sullivan SE. Repeat endoscopic transsphenoidal surgery for acromegaly: remission and complications. Pituitary. 2013; 16(4):459–464

[94] Mohammed N, Ding D, Hung Y-C, Xu Z, Lee C-C, Kano H, et al. Primary versus postoperative stereotactic radiosurgery for acromegaly: a multicenter matched cohort study. J Neurosurg. 2019 Apr 26;1–10

[95] Sims-Williams HP, Rajapaksa K, Sinha S, Radatz M, Walton L, Yianni J, et al. Radiosurgery as primary management for acromegaly. Clinical Endocrinology. 2019;90(1):114–121

[96] Castinetti F, Taieb D, Kuhn J-M, Chanson P, Tamura M, Jaquet P, et al. Outcome of Gamma Knife Radiosurgery in 82 Patients with Acromegaly: Correlation with Initial Hypersecretion. The Journal of Clinical Endocrinology & Metabolism. 2005 Aug 1;90(8):4483–4488.

[97] Ding D, Mehta GU, Patibandla MR, Lee C-C, Liscak R, Kano H, et al. Stereotactic Radiosurgery for Acromegaly: An International Multicenter Retrospective Cohort Study. Neurosurgery. 2018;355(24):2558

[98] Iwata H, Sato K, Nomura R, Tabei Y, Suzuki I, Yokota N, et al. Long-term results of hypofractionated stereotactic radiotherapy with CyberKnife for growth hormone-secreting pituitary adenoma: evaluation by the Cortina consensus. J Neurooncol. 2016 Jun;128(2):267–275

[99] Ježková J, Marek J, Hána V, Kršek M, Weiss V, Vladyka V, et al. Gamma knife radiosurgery for acromegaly – long-term experience. Clinical Endocrinology. 2006;64(5):588–595

[100] Knappe UJ, Petroff D, Quinkler M, Schmid SM, Schöfl C, Schopohl J, et al. Fractionated radiotherapy and radiosurgery in acromegaly: analysis of 352 patients from the German Acromegaly Registry. European Journal of Endocrinology. 2020 Mar 1;182(3):275–284

[101] Kong D-S, Kim Y-H, Kim YH, Hur KY, Kim JH, Kim M-S, et al. Long-Term Efficacy and Tolerability of Gamma Knife Radiosurgery for Growth Hormone-Secreting Adenoma: A Retrospective Multicenter Study (MERGE-001). World Neurosurgery. 2019 Feb 1;122:e1291–e1299

[102] Lee C-C, Vance ML, Xu Z, Yen C-P, Schlesinger D, Dodson B, et al. Stereotactic Radiosurgery for Acromegaly. The Journal of clinical endocrinology and metabolism. 2014;99(4):1273–1281

[103] Pai F-Y, Chen C-J, Wang W-H, Yang H-C, Lin CJ, Wu H-M, et al. Low-Dose Gamma Knife Radiosurgery for Acromegaly. Neurosurgery. 2019 Jul 1;85(1):E20–E30

[104] Vik-Mo EO, Øksnes M, Pedersen P-H, Wentzel-Larsen T, Rødahl E, Thorsen F, et al. Gamma knife stereotactic radiosurgery for acromegaly. European Journal of Endocrinology. 2007 Sep 1;157(3):255–263

[105] Wilson PJ, De-loyde KJ, Williams JR, Smee RI. Acromegaly: A single centre's experience of stereotactic radiosurgery and radiotherapy for growth hormone secreting pituitary tumours with the linear accelerator. Journal of Clinical Neuroscience. 2013 Nov 1;20(11):1506–1513

[106] Ding D, Mehta GU, Patibandla MR, et al. Stereotactic radiosurgery for acromegaly: an international multicenter retrospective cohort study. Neurosurgery. 2019; 84(3):717–725

[107] Fleseriu M, Biller BMK, Freda PU, et al. A Pituitary Society update to acromegaly management guidelines. Pituitary. 2021 Feb;24(1):1-13. doi: 10.1007/s11102-020-01091-7. Epub 2020 Oct 20. PMID: 33079318; PMCID: PMC7864830.

[108] Lee C-C, Vance ML, Xu Z, et al. Stereotactic radiosurgery for acromegaly. J Clin Endocrinol Metab. 2014; 99(4):1273–1281

[109] Lee C-C, Vance ML, Lopes MB, Xu Z, Chen C-J, Sheehan J. Stereotactic radiosurgery for acromegaly: outcomes by adenoma subtype. Pituitary. 2015; 18(3):326–334

[110] Pollock BE, Nippoldt TB, Stafford SL, Foote RL, Abboud CF. Results of stereotactic radiosurgery in patients with hormone-producing pituitary adenomas: factors associated with endocrine normalization. J Neurosurg. 2002; 97(3):525–530

[111] Hofland LJ, Lamberts SW. Somatostatin receptor subtype expression in human tumors. Ann Oncol. 2001; 12 Suppl 2:S31–S36

[112] Freda PU, Katznelson L, van der Lely AJ, Reyes CM, Zhao S, Rabinowitz D. Long-acting somatostatin analog therapy of acromegaly: a meta-analysis. J Clin Endocrinol Metab. 2005; 90(8):4465–4473

[113] Mercado M, Borges F, Bouterfa H, et al. SMS995B2401 Study Group. A prospective, multicentre study to investigate the efficacy, safety and tolerability of octreotide LAR (long-acting repeatable octreotide) in the primary therapy of patients with acromegaly. Clin Endocrinol (Oxf). 2007; 66(6):859–868. Wiley/Blackwell (10.1111)

[114] Cuevas-Ramos D, Fleseriu M. Somatostatin receptor ligands and resistance to treatment in pituitary adenomas. J Mol Endocrinol. 2014; 52 (3):R223–R240

[115] Espinosa de los Monteros AL, Carrasco CA, Albarrán AAR, Gadelha M, Abreu A, Mercado M. The role of primary pharmacological therapy in acromegaly. Pituitary. 2014; 17 Suppl 1:S4–S10

[116] Howlett TA, Willis D, Walker G, Wass JAH, Trainer PJ, UK Acromegaly Register Study Group (UKAR-3). Control of growth hormone and IGF1 in patients with acromegaly in the UK: responses to medical treatment with somatostatin analogues and dopamine agonists. Clin Endocrinol (Oxf). 2013; 79(5):689–699

[117] Giustina A, Mazziotti G, Torri V, Spinello M, Floriani I, Melmed S. Meta-analysis on the effects of octreotide on tumor mass in acromegaly. PLoS One. 2012; 7(5):e36411. Luque RM, editor

[118] Ben-Shlomo A, Melmed S. Somatostatin agonists for treatment of acromegaly. Mol Cell Endocrinol. 2008; 286(1–2):192–198

[119] Mazziotti G, Floriani I, Bonadonna S, Torri V, Chanson P, Giustina A. Effects of somatostatin analogs on glucose homeostasis: a metaanalysis of acromegaly studies. J Clin Endocrinol Metab. 2009; 94(5):1500–1508

[120] Sandret L, Maison P, Chanson P. Place of cabergoline in acromegaly: a meta-analysis. J Clin Endocrinol Metab. 2011; 96(5):1327–1335

[121] Bernabeu I, Alvarez-Escolá C, Paniagua AE, et al. Pegvisomant and cabergoline combination therapy in acromegaly. Pituitary. 2013; 16(1):101–108

[122] Cozzi R, Attanasio R, Lodrini S, Lasio G. Cabergoline addition to depot somatostatin analogues in resistant acromegalic patients: efficacy and lack of predictive value of prolactin status. Clin Endocrinol (Oxf). 2004; 61(2): 209–215

[123] Sherlock M, Fernandez-Rodriguez E, Alonso AA, et al. Medical therapy in patients with acromegaly: predictors of response and comparison of efficacy of dopamine agonists and somatostatin analogues. J Clin Endocrinol Metab. 2009; 94(4):1255–1263

[124] Buchfelder M, van der Lely AJ, Biller BMK, Webb SM, Brue T, Strasburger CJ et al (2018) Long-term treatment with pegvisomant: observations from 2090 acromegaly patients in ACROSTUDY. Eur J Endocrinol 179(6):419–427

[125] Schreiber I, Buchfelder M, Droste M, et al. German Pegvisomant Investigators. Treatment of acromegaly with the GH receptor antagonist pegvisomant in clinical practice: safety and efficacy evaluation from the German Pegvisomant Observational Study. Eur J Endocrinol. 2007; 156(1): 75–82

[126] Trainer PJ, Drake WM, Katznelson L, et al. Treatment of acromegaly with the growth hormone-receptor antagonist pegvisomant. N Engl J Med. 2000; 342 (16):1171–1177

[127] Neggers SJ, de Herder WW, Janssen JA, Feelders RA, van der Lely AJ. Combined treatment for acromegaly with long-acting somatostatin analogs and pegvisomant: long-term safety for up to 4.5 years (median 2.2 years) of follow-up in 86 patients. Eur J Endocrinol. 2009; 160(4): 529–533

8 Natural History and Management Options for Cushing's Disease

Benjamin H.M. Hunn and James A.J. King

Abstract

Cushing's disease is caused by excess secretion of adrenocorticotropic hormone from a pituitary adenoma, which causes high serum cortisol. Excess serum cortisol causes a variety of metabolic and psychiatric disturbances, including hypertension, type 2 diabetes mellitus, obesity, depression, and insomnia. Rarely, Cushing's disease may first come to attention due to local mass effect of the pituitary adenoma causing visual disturbance or hyrocephalus. Historically, survival of untreated Cushing's disease is less than 5 years. Mortality in Cushing's disease is chiefly due to cardiovascular disease and systemic malignancy. Surgical resection of the causative pituitary adenoma is the primary therapy for Cushing's disease and reduces the rate of mortality. Resection of the pituitary adenoma can be performed by microscopic or endoscopic approaches, and outcomes are similar. For pituitary macroadenomas, the endoscopic approach is associated with a higher rate of remission than the microscopic approach. Radiotherapy and medications have also been used to treat Cushing's disease; however, remission rates are lower than those demonstrated by surgery. In general, recurrence of Cushing's disease following transsphenoidal surgery should prompt repeat transsphenoidal surgery. When transsphenoidal surgery fails twice, is declined, or is contraindicated, radiotherapy, bilateral adrenalectomy, or medical therapy should be considered.

Keywords: pituitary, adenoma, Cushing's disease, surgery, transsphenoidal

8.1 Introduction

Cushing's disease is caused by a pituitary adenoma that secretes excess adrenocorticotropic hormone (ACTH; sometimes known as corticotropin; see ▶ Fig. 8.1). ACTH stimulates the production of cortisol from the zona fasciculata of the adrenal gland. The manifestations of Cushing's disease arise from supraphysiological serum cortisol levels caused by excess ACTH. Cushing's disease is rare, with an estimated incidence of 1 to 2 cases per million people per year.[1,2] Females are affected at least three times more frequently.[1,2] The incidence of Cushing's disease peaks at approximately 40 years of age (▶ Table 8.1).[1,2]

Harvey Cushing first described the constellation of signs caused by elevated serum cortisol and attributed them to a basophil pituitary adenoma in his patient Minnie G.[5,6] Typically, Cushing's disease is used to refer to hypercortisolism caused by a corticotroph pituitary adenoma, whereas Cushing's syndrome refers to signs and symptoms resulting from any other cause of increased serum cortisol. Overproduction of cortisol causes multiple deleterious effects in patients, with the typical features as follows[7]:

- *Symptoms*: Depression, fatigue, menstrual abnormalities, and insomnia.
- *Signs*: Hirsutism, facial fullness and plethora, obesity, dorsocervical fat pad, abdominal striae, bruising tendency, and proximal myopathy.
- *Associated diseases*: Hypertension, type 2 diabetes mellitus, and osteoporosis.
- *In pediatric patients*: Short stature and precocious or delayed puberty.

Pituitary adenomas, including those causing Cushing's disease, are often separated based on size. Pituitary adenomas less than 10 mm in size are referred to as microadenomas and those greater than 10 mm in size are referred to as macroadenomas (▶ Fig. 8.1). Rarely, Cushing's disease presents due to a macroadenoma causing local mass effect. Symptoms of mass effect include the following[8]:

- *Compression of the optic chiasm*: Classically produces bitemporal hemianopia but can produce unilateral visual deficits or reductions in visual acuity.
- *Compression of the third ventricle*: Can cause obstructive hydrocephalus.
- *Compression of the cavernous sinus*: Can cause diplopia (cranial nerves III, IV and VI), facial pain (cranial nerves V_1, V_2), or proptosis (occlusion of the cavernous sinus).

Genetic abnormalities may underlie the development of ACTH-secreting pituitary adenomas. Cushing's disease is a rare feature of multiple endocrine neoplasia type 1 (MEN1), which is caused by mutations in *menin*.[9] Somatic mutations in the genes encoding or regulating the growth hormone receptor, the epidermal growth factor receptor, and *P53* may also be associated with the development of corticotroph pituitary adenomas.[10,11]

Diagnosis of Cushing's disease can be complex, and should involve a multidisciplinary team including a neurosurgeon, endocrinologist, neuroradiologist, and neuropathologist. In most instances, when Cushing's disease is suspected based on signs and symptoms, an assay that assesses serum cortisol is performed. This may be a 24-hour urinary cortisol study, a low-dose dexamethasone-suppression test, or late-night salivary cortisol.[7] Following the demonstration of pathologically heightened cortisol, further investigations should be performed to investigate the cause of cortisol hypersecretion. A key distinction is between ACTH-dependent and ACTH-independent causes, and this can be examined by measuring serum ACTH levels, or performing a high-dose dexamethasone-suppression test or a corticotrophin-releasing hormone test. Once ACTH-dependent hypercortisolism is established, a magnetic resonance imaging (MRI) to examine for the presence of a corticotroph pituitary adenoma is indicated. Thin-cut coronal and axial sequences are necessary to examine for microadenomas. If no adenoma is detectable on MRI, some centers use inferior petrosal sinus sampling (IPSS) to determine if there is a central to peripheral ACTH gradient, indicating a likely pituitary source of ACTH. IPSS can also be used to determine whether the right or left pituitary is producing excess ACTH and, therefore, provide a target for

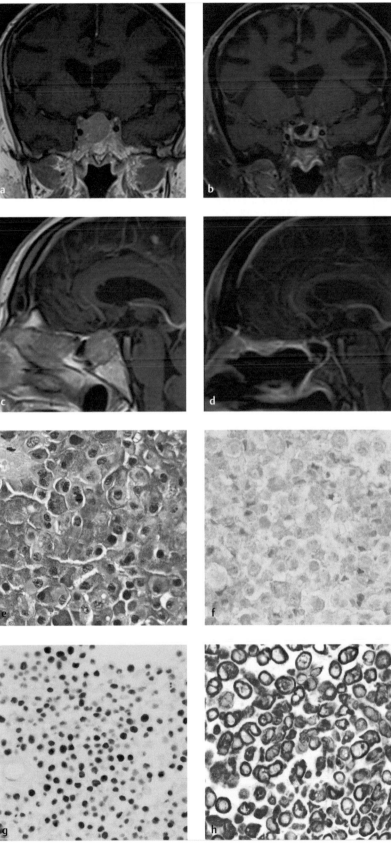

Fig. 8.1 Radiological and histological features of Cushing's disease. **(a)** Preoperative and **(b)** postoperative contrast-enhanced T1-weighted coronal magnetic resonance imaging (MRI) of a patient with a corticotroph cell pituitary macroadenoma causing Cushing's disease. **(c)** Preoperative and **(d)** postoperative contrast-enhanced T1-weighted sagittal MRI of a patient with a corticotroph cell pituitary macroadenoma causing Cushing's disease. **(e)** Hematoxylin and eosin staining demonstrating a moderately cellular pituitary adenoma with Crooke's hyaline change in several cells (×600). **(f)** ACTH immunostaining demonstrating moderate positive staining in tumor cells consistent with granulated corticotroph cell adenoma (×400). **(g)** T-pit transcription factor immunostaining demonstrating strong positive staining in tumor cell nuclei confirming corticotroph cell lineage (×400). **(h)** Section immunostained for low-molecular-weight cytokeratin CAM5.2 highlighting perinuclear Crooke's hyaline change (×400). (The photomicrographs are provided courtesy of Michael Gonzales, Associate Professor, Royal Melbourne Hospital.)

Table 8.1 Characteristics of Cushing's disease patients in published studies

Study	Period	n	Female (%)	Age, mean (y)	Initial TSS (%)	Remission (%)	Follow-up (y)	SMR if cured	SMR not cured
Swearingen et al[20]	1978–1996	161	80	38	100	93	5.7	NA	NA
Lindholm et al[1]	1985–1995	73	68	41[a]	54	62	8.1	0.3	5.1
Hammer et al[19]	1975–1998	289	83	36[b]	100	82	11.1	1.2	2.8
Dekkers et al[22]	1977–2005	74	76	39[b]	100	80	12.8	1.8	4.4
Bolland et al[4] (macroadenoma)	1960–2005	30	73	45	NA	93	6.9	2.3	5.7
Bolland et al[4] (microadenoma)	1960–2005	158	77	36	NA	91	7.5	3.1	2.4
Clayton et al[18]	1958–2010	60	85	NA	58	90	1.3	3.3	16
Hassan-Smith et al[17]	1988–2009	72	79	40	100	72	4.6	2.5	4.1
Ntali et al[15]	1967–2009	182	75	40[a]	87	62[c]	12	10	NA
Yaneva et al[16]	1965–2010	240	82	38	66	55[d]	7.1	1.7	4.6
Weighted SMR (95% CI)								2.5 (1.4–4.2)	4.6 (2.9–77.3)

Abbreviations: CI, confidence interval; SMR, standardized mortality ratio; TSS, transsphenoidal surgery.
Source: Adapted from van Haalen et al.[3] The study by Bolland et al[4] separated patients based on tumor size with no pooled data.
[a]Median.
[b]Age at operation, not diagnosis.
[c]Of 159 undergoing initial transsphenoidal surgery.
[d]Of 154 undergoing initial transsphenoidal surgery.

surgery when an adenoma is not radiologically identifiable. It should be noted, however, that IPSS correctly predicts tumor laterality in only 70% of cases.[12]

The mainstay of Cushing's disease treatment is surgical resection of the causative pituitary adenoma, as this achieves key goals of treatment: biochemical normalization of cortisol levels with acceptable morbidity, reversal of clinical signs and symptoms, and long-term remission.[13] However, several other treatment options are available or under investigation, most notably pituitary irradiation, bilateral adrenalectomy, and drug therapies.

8.2 Selected Papers on the Natural History of Cushing's Disease

- Cushing H. The basophil adenomas of the pituitary body and their clinical manifestations (pituitary basophilism). Bull Johns Hopkins Hosp 1932;50:137–195
- Lindholm J, Juul S, Jørgensen JO, et al. Incidence and late prognosis of cushing's syndrome: a population-based study. J Clin Endocrinol Metab 2001;86(1):117–123
- van Haalen FM, Broersen LHA, Jorgensen JO, Pereira AM, Dekkers OM. Management of endocrine disease: mortality remains increased in Cushing's disease despite biochemical remission—a systematic review and meta-analysis. Eur J Endocrinol 2015;172(4):R143–R149

8.3 The Natural History of Cushing's Disease

Cushing's disease is associated with significant mortality and morbidity. In Cushing's original series, the median survival of untreated Cushing's disease was 4.6 years.[5] A summary of contemporary studies that examine mortality in Cushing's disease is provided in ▶ Table 8.1.[1,14,15,16,17,18,19,20] The data from these

Table 8.2 Common comorbidities in Cushing's disease at the time of diagnosis

Disease	Percentage affected
Hypertension	58–85
Obesity	32–41
Diabetes mellitus	20–47
Depression	50–81
Osteoporosis	31–50
Dyslipidemia	38–71

Source: Data adapted from Feelders et al.[21]

studies examine patients with treated Cushing's disease, with the data pertaining to patients with relapsed Cushing's disease perhaps the best proxy for the natural history of the disease. A well-designed and conducted meta-analysis by van Haalen et al of a pooled group of 776 Cushing's disease patients showed that patients who were not cured had a standardized mortality ratio (SMR) of 4.6 (95% confidence interval [CI]: 2.9–7.3) compared to an age- and sex-matched population, indicating patients with Cushing's disease were 4.6 times more likely to die compared to patients without Cushing's disease.[3] Successful treatment lowered the SMR to 2.5 (95% CI: 1.4–4.2).

Mortality in Cushing's disease is predominantly secondary to cardiovascular disease (30–62.7%, depending on series), manifesting mainly as ischemic heart disease or stroke. Other common causes of death in Cushing's disease are systemic malignancy (7.7–25%) and infection (3.9–21.4%). Older age at diagnosis and male sex both predict mortality.[4,15,16,18,19,20]

Common comorbid diseases are those caused by cortisol excess, and are listed in ▶ Table 8.2.[21] When compared to patients with nonfunctioning pituitary adenomas, patients with Cushing's disease have poorer outcomes, suggesting that there are factors intrinsic to the disease that cause increased morbidity and mortality.[22]

8.4 Selected Papers on the Treatment Outcomes of Cushing's Disease

- Broersen LHA, Biermasz NR, van Furth WR, et al. Endoscopic vs. microscopic transsphenoidal surgery for Cushing's disease: a systematic review and meta-analysis. Pituitary 2018;21(5):524–534
- Sonino N, Zielezny M, Fava GA, Fallo F, Boscaro M. Risk factors and long-term outcome in pituitary-dependent Cushing's disease. J Clin Endocrinol Metab 1996;81(7):2647–2652
- Nelson DH, Meakin JW, Thorn GW. ACTH-producing pituitary tumors following adrenalectomy for Cushing's syndrome. Ann Intern Med 1960;52:560–569

8.5 Treatment of Cushing's Disease

8.5.1 Surgical Resection

Transsphenoidal surgical resection of the causative pituitary adenoma is the cornerstone of modern treatment in Cushing's disease. Meta-analysis of data from 6,695 patients treated using transsphenoidal surgery demonstrates an 80% remission rate.[23] In this dataset, which included 5,711 patients operated on using microscopic techniques and 984 patients undergoing endoscopic pituitary resection, there was no difference in rate of remission based on surgical technique.

In general, types of operative complications differ between the microscopic and endoscopic techniques. The rates of common complications are detailed in ▶ Table 8.3.[23] It should be noted that endoscopic techniques are newer, and earlier endoscopic cases included in meta-analyses may have higher rates of complications. Cerebrospinal fluid (CSF) leak is reported more frequently following endoscopic surgery, complicating 12.9% of cases, compared with 4.0% for the microscopic approach.[23] Use of a nasal septal flap to close dural defects reduces the rate of CSF leak, and this is recommended in the cases where CSF leak is seen at the time of surgery.[24]

There are some data to suggest that the risk of postoperative DVT is increased in Cushing's disease, with rates as high as 4% in some series.[25,26] This may be related to a postsurgical hypercoagulable state that is heightened in Cushing's disease, as well as obesity in Cushing's disease patients. Special care must therefore be taken in these patients to minimize DVT risk in the postoperative period.

The achievement of remission following transsphenoidal surgery for Cushing's disease is a primary concern. Longer exposure to elevated cortisol is associated with higher mortality; similarly, patients who relapse have worse outcomes.[19,27] Rates of relapse are reduced for microadenomas compared with macroadenomas.[23] Notably, the rate of remission for macroadenomas treated with the endoscopic technique is 76.3%, significantly greater than macroadenomas operated on microscopically (59.9%).[23] These data suggest that endoscopic techniques may be preferred for macroadenoma resection. Other authors have noted that use of the endoscope expands the visualized operative field, and this may be responsible for improved macroadenoma resection rates.[28,29,30] Expectedly, low postoperative serum cortisol is a consistent predictor of long-term remission.[31,32,33,34] If in remission, patients can be profoundly hypocortisolemic, and typically will require oral corticosteroid supplementation for 3 to 12 months. A baseline MRI of the pituitary gland performed 3 months postoperatively can be helpful to determine if adenoma recurrence occurs.

Choice of surgical case is one of the key determinants of operative success. In general, macroadenomas and microadenomas identifiable on MRI are clear operative targets. A more fraught area are MRI-negative pituitary adenomas, where there is no clear consensus based on the reported data of the appropriate approach, and outcomes are worse.[19,34,35] In these cases, it is of the utmost importance that an ectopic source of ACTH is excluded. Careful reexamination and, if necessary, repeat diagnostic pituitary imaging is also important; some authors report good experience using dynamic MRI and T2-weighted sequences.[36] If there is ongoing suspicion of Cushing's disease, or IPSS evidence of a pituitary source, then surgical pituitary exploration to attempt to identify a microadenoma is indicated.[35,36,37] In some instances, a microadenoma cannot be identified at surgical exploration. In this circumstance, some authors advocate hemihypophysectomy based on IPSS evidence of laterality of ACTH secretion. It should be noted that this approach achieves relatively low rates of remission; in a series of 57 patients in whom no adenoma was found, hemihypophysectomy based on IPSS lateralization achieved remission rates of 41.4%.[38]

8.5.2 Radiation Therapy

Aside from transsphenoidal surgery, other approaches to treat Cushing's disease have been trialed, most commonly pituitary irradiation and bilateral adrenalectomy. Both alternative approaches have limitations. When compared with transsphenoidal surgery, pituitary irradiation is more likely to cause hormonal deficits and can cause damage to the visual apparatus.[39,40,41]

Table 8.3 Outcomes following microscopic and endoscopic transsphenoidal surgery for Cushing's disease

Event rate (%) by surgical technique	Microscopic (95% CI)	Endoscopic (95% CI)
Remission rate, all adenomas	80.5 (77.6–83/3)	79.2 (74.3–83.8)
Remission rate, macroadenomas	59.9 (52.0–67.6)	76.3(64.3–86.7)
Remission rate, microadenomas	85.5 (81.2–89.3)	83.9 (76.8–90.0)
Mortality	0.0 (0.0–0.2)	0.4 (0.0–2.2)
CSF leak	4.0 (2.3–6.1)	12.9 (5.8–22.1)
Meningitis	0.6 (0.1–1.3)	0.1 (0.0–1.0)
SIADH	3.5 (1.3–6.6)	5.3 (2.9–8.0)
Diabetes insipidus (permanent)	2.4 (1.1–4.1)	4.0 (2.2–6.3)
Postoperative hemorrhage	1.9 (0.7–3.5)	3.7 (0.8–8.3)

Abbreviations: CI, confidence interval; CSF, cerebrospinal fluid; SIADH, syndrome of inappropriate antidiuretic hormone secretion.
Source: Adapted from data calculated by Broersen et al.[23]

Bilateral adrenalectomy is a radical approach to eliminate endogenous cortisol secretion, and can be complicated by Nelson's syndrome—the enlargement of the existing corticotroph macroadenoma following bilateral adrenalectomy.[42,43]

Data directly comparing transsphenoidal surgery, pituitary irradiation, and bilateral adrenalectomy have rarely been published. A retrospective series by Sonino et al demonstrated that transsphenoidal surgery had a higher 10-year remission rate than pituitary irradiation (74.1 vs. 65.1%).[44] This was compared with bilateral adrenalectomy, which resulted in 71.2% of individuals free of Nelson's syndrome at 10 years.[44] Nagesser et al have reported equivalent outcomes between transsphenoidal surgery and a combined approach comprising unilateral adrenalectomy and pituitary irradiation.[45]

Several authors have examined the use of stereotactic radiosurgery to treat corticotroph pituitary adenomas, and a few large series have now been reported. Most of these series described treatment of relapsing or invasive corticotroph pituitary adenomas following transsphenoidal surgery.[46,47,48] One series reported by Wan et al used stereotactic radiosurgery as the primary treatment modality, with 19 of 68 patients with Cushing's disease achieving normalization of hormonal status.[41] More promising results have been reported by Mehta et al from a large multicenter study, with 15 of 22 patients who had radiosurgery as the primary treatment modality in remission at 10 years.[40] Transsphenoidal surgery is not a therapeutic option in some patients, as they are unfit for surgery or do not wish to consider it. In these patients, alternative therapies such as stereotactic radiosurgery or medical therapies may be considered.

8.5.3 Medical Treatment

Medical therapies for Cushing's disease have also been examined; such therapies may direct toward the pituitary gland, the adrenal gland, or the actions of cortisol may be systemically antagonized. Drug therapies are summarized in ▶ Table 8.4. Mifepristone, a systemic glucocorticoid receptor antagonist,

was assessed in the SEISMIC (Study of the Efficacy and Safety of Mifepristone in the Treatment of Endogenous Cushing's Syndrome) study, which included 43 patients with recurrent Cushing's disease in a total of 50 patients with endogenous Cushing's syndrome.[49] Overall, 87% of patients had improvement in glycemic or blood pressure control, or both. Mifepristone inhibits the action of cortisol, without decreasing cortisol levels, and therefore standard measures of remission in Cushing's disease are irrelevant.[49] Etomidate is used for short-term control of hypercortisolemia in critically ill patients, without the intention of causing remission; it is administered as a low-dose intravenous infusion.[50]

8.5.4 Recurrent Cushing's Disease

The treatment of recurrent Cushing's disease is an area where there are less data to guide practice; however, there is broad consensus in the literature that the appropriate treatment of recurrent Cushing's disease is repeat transsphenoidal surgery.[57,58,59,60] In cases of recurrent Cushing's disease, it is important that all radiologic and laboratory tests are repeated and reexamined to ensure certainty of diagnosis. Some authors advocate that repeat surgery be performed in the same hospital admission as the initial surgery if postoperative serum cortisol levels do not fall below a certain threshold (e.g., 50 nmol/L); this recommendation is supported by observational studies demonstrating that postoperative cortisol levels accurately predict long-term outcome following transsphenoidal surgery for Cushing's disease.[31,32,33,34,57,58,61,62,63] An alternative to repeat transsphenoidal surgery is proposed by Prevedello et al, who suggest recurrence of Cushing's disease following transsphenoidal surgery should be treated by stereotactic radiosurgery; if this is not successful, then bilateral adrenalectomy should be performed.[64] Remission rates using this protocol (transsphenoidal surgery, stereotactic radiosurgery, then bilateral adrenalectomy) were 95.8%. A reasonable compromise may be to perform a second, more extensive, transsphenoidal pituitary resection when Cushing's disease recurs, and if this is unsuccessful, then

Table 8.4 Commonly used medical treatments for Cushing's disease

Drug	Site of action	Drug class	Mechanism of action	Remission (%)[51]	Major adverse effects	References
Pasireotide	Pituitary	Somatostatin analog	Inhibition of somatostatin receptor subtype 5	41.1	Hyperglycemia in 50%, GH deficiency	51,52
Cabergoline	Pituitary	Dopamine receptor (D2R) agonist	Antagonizes D2 receptors, reducing ACTH production	35.7	Headache, dizziness, cardiac valve fibrosis at high doses	51,53,54,55
Ketoconazole	Adrenal	CYPIIAI and CYPIIBI inhibitor	Inhibits multiple levels of cortisol synthesis	49.0	Hepatotoxicity	51
Metyrapone	Adrenal	CYPIIBI inhibitor	Prevents conversion of 11-deoxycortisol to cortisol by inhibiting CYPIIBI (11β-hydroxylase)	60.0	Acne, hirsutism, hypertension	51
Etomidate	Adrenal	CYPIIAI and CYPIIBI inhibitor	Inhibits multiple levels of cortisol synthesis	NA	Nephrotoxicity	50,51
Mitotane	Adrenal	Adrenolytic, CYPIIAI and CYPIIBI inhibitor	Inhibits multiple levels of cortisol synthesis	81.8	Hepatotoxicity	51,56
Mifepristone	Tissues	Glucocorticoid receptor antagonist	Inhibits the effect of cortisol at its receptor	NA	Hypokalemia, hypertension	49,51

Abbreviations: ACTH, adrenocorticotrophic hormone; GH, growth hormone; NA, not applicable (see text for explanation).

consider stereotactic radiosurgery, bilateral adrenalectomy, or medical therapy in conjunction with the patient and the multidisciplinary team.

8.6 Authors' Recommendations

- Diagnosis and treatment of Cushing's disease is complex; an experienced multidisciplinary team including a neurosurgeon, endocrinologist, and other specialists is required to produce optimal patient outcomes.
- Transsphenoidal surgery is the mainstay of Cushing's disease treatment.
- Microscopic and endoscopic transsphenoidal surgeries have approximately equivalent outcomes; endoscopic resection may be preferred for macroadenomas.
- Recurrence of Cushing's disease following transsphenoidal surgery should prompt repeat transsphenoidal surgery.
- When transsphenoidal surgery fails twice, is declined, or is contraindicated, radiotherapy, bilateral adrenalectomy, or medical therapy should be considered.

References

[1] Lindholm J, Juul S, Jørgensen JO, et al. Incidence and late prognosis of cushing's syndrome: a population-based study. J Clin Endocrinol Metab. 2001; 86(1):117–123

[2] Etxabe J, Vazquez JA. Morbidity and mortality in Cushing's disease: an epidemiological approach. Clin Endocrinol (Oxf). 1994; 40(4):479–484

[3] van Haalen FM, Broersen LHA, Jorgensen JO, Pereira AM, Dekkers OM. Management of endocrine disease: mortality remains increased in Cushing's disease despite biochemical remission—a systematic review and meta-analysis. Eur J Endocrinol. 2015; 172(4):R143–R149

[4] Bolland MJ, Holdaway IM, Berkeley JE, et al. Mortality and morbidity in Cushing's syndrome in New Zealand. Clin Endocrinol (Oxf). 2011; 75(4):436–442

[5] Cushing H. The basophil adenomas of the pituitary body and their clinical manifestations (pituitary basophilism). Bull Johns Hopkins Hosp. 1932; 50:137–195

[6] Cushing H. The Pituitary Body and Its Disorders: Clinical States Produced by Disorders of the Hypophysis Cerebri. London: J. B. Lippincott Company; 1912

[7] Nieman LK, Biller BMK, Findling JW, et al. The diagnosis of Cushing's syndrome: an Endocrine Society clinical practice guideline. J Clin Endocrinol Metab. 2008; 93(5):1526–1540

[8] Greenberg MS. Handbook of Neurosurgery. New York, NY: Thieme; 2010

[9] Matsuzaki LN, Canto-Costa MH, Hauache OM. Cushing's disease as the first clinical manifestation of multiple endocrine neoplasia type 1 (MEN1) associated with an R460X mutation of the MEN1 gene. Clin Endocrinol (Oxf). 2004; 60(1):142–143

[10] Karl M, Von Wichert G, Kempter E, et al. Nelson's syndrome associated with a somatic frame shift mutation in the glucocorticoid receptor gene. J Clin Endocrinol Metab. 1996; 81(1):124–129

[11] Bilodeau S, Vallette-Kasic S, Gauthier Y, et al. Role of Brg1 and HDAC2 in GR trans-repression of the pituitary POMC gene and misexpression in Cushing disease. Genes Dev. 2006; 20(20):2871–2886

[12] Wind JJ, Lonser RR, Nieman LK, DeVroom HL, Chang R, Oldfield EH. The lateralization accuracy of inferior petrosal sinus sampling in 501 patients with Cushing's disease. J Clin Endocrinol Metab. 2013; 98(6):2285–2293

[13] Biller BMK, Grossman AB, Stewart PM, et al. Treatment of adrenocorticotropin-dependent Cushing's syndrome: a consensus statement. J Clin Endocrinol Metab. 2008; 93(7):2454–2462

[14] Clayton RN, Jones PW, Reulen RC, et al. Mortality in patients with Cushing's disease more than 10 years after remission: a multicentre, multinational, retrospective cohort study. Lancet Diabetes Endocrinol. 2016; 4(7):569–576

[15] Ntali G, Asimakopoulou A, Siamatras T, et al. Mortality in Cushing's syndrome: systematic analysis of a large series with prolonged follow-up. Eur J Endocrinol. 2013; 169(5):715–723

[16] Yaneva M, Kalinov K, Zacharieva S. Mortality in Cushing's syndrome: data from 386 patients from a single tertiary referral center. Eur J Endocrinol. 2013; 169(5):621–627

[17] Hassan-Smith ZK, Sherlock M, Reulen RC, et al. Outcome of Cushing's disease following transsphenoidal surgery in a single center over 20 years. J Clin Endocrinol Metab. 2012; 97(4):1194–1201

[18] Clayton RN, Raskauskiene D, Reulen RC, Jones PW. Mortality and morbidity in Cushing's disease over 50 years in Stoke-on-Trent, UK: audit and meta-analysis of literature. J Clin Endocrinol Metab. 2011; 96(3):632–642

[19] Hammer GD, Tyrrell JB, Lamborn KR, et al. Transsphenoidal microsurgery for Cushing's disease: initial outcome and long-term results. J Clin Endocrinol Metab. 2004; 89(12):6348–6357

[20] Swearingen B, Biller BM, Barker FG, II, et al. Long-term mortality after transsphenoidal surgery for Cushing disease. Ann Intern Med. 1999; 130(10):821–824

[21] Feelders RA, Pulgar SJ, Kempel A, Pereira AM. The burden of Cushing's disease: clinical and health-related quality of life aspects. Eur J Endocrinol. 2012; 167(3):311–326

[22] Dekkers OM, Biermasz NR, Pereira AM, et al. Mortality in patients treated for Cushing's disease is increased, compared with patients treated for nonfunctioning pituitary macroadenoma. J Clin Endocrinol Metab. 2007; 92(3):976–981

[23] Broersen LHA, Biermasz NR, van Furth WR, et al. Endoscopic vs. microscopic transsphenoidal surgery for Cushing's disease: a systematic review and meta-analysis. Pituitary. 2018; 21(5):524–534

[24] Horiguchi K, Murai H, Hasegawa Y, Hanazawa T, Yamakami I, Saeki N. Endoscopic endonasal skull base reconstruction using a nasal septal flap: surgical results and comparison with previous reconstructions. Neurosurg Rev. 2010; 33(2):235–241, discussion 241

[25] Semple PL, Laws ER, Jr. Complications in a contemporary series of patients who underwent transsphenoidal surgery for Cushing's disease. J Neurosurg. 1999; 91(2):175–179

[26] Fahlbusch R, Buchfelder M, Müller OA. Transsphenoidal surgery for Cushing's disease. J R Soc Med. 1986; 79(5):262–269

[27] Lambert JK, Goldberg L, Fayngold S, Kostadinov J, Post KD, Geer EB. Predictors of mortality and long-term outcomes in treated Cushing's disease: a study of 346 patients. J Clin Endocrinol Metab. 2013; 98(3):1022–1030

[28] Jho HD, Carrau RL. Endoscopic endonasal transsphenoidal surgery: experience with 50 patients. J Neurosurg. 1997; 87(1):44–51

[29] Apuzzo ML, Heifetz MD, Weiss MH, Kurze T. Neurosurgical endoscopy using the side-viewing telescope. J Neurosurg. 1977; 46(3):398–400

[30] Kawamata T, Iseki H, Ishizaki R, Hori T. Minimally invasive endoscope-assisted endonasal trans-sphenoidal microsurgery for pituitary tumors: experience with 215 cases comparing with sublabial trans-sphenoidal approach. Neurol Res. 2002; 24(3):259–265

[31] Sarkar S, Rajaratnam S, Chacko G, Mani S, Hesargatta AS, Chacko AG. Pure endoscopic transsphenoidal surgery for functional pituitary adenomas: outcomes with Cushing's disease. Acta Neurochir (Wien). 2016; 158(1):77–86, discussion 86

[32] Bochicchio D, Losa M, Buchfelder M. Factors influencing the immediate and late outcome of Cushing's disease treated by transsphenoidal surgery: a retrospective study by the European Cushing's Disease Survey Group. J Clin Endocrinol Metab. 1995; 80(11):3114–3120

[33] Pereira AM, van Aken MO, van Dulken H, et al. Long-term predictive value of postsurgical cortisol concentrations for cure and risk of recurrence in Cushing's disease. J Clin Endocrinol Metab. 2003; 88(12):5858–5864

[34] Bansal P, Lila A, Goroshi M, et al. Duration of post-operative hypocortisolism predicts sustained remission after pituitary surgery for Cushing's disease. Endocr Connect. 2017; 6(8):625–636

[35] Wagenmakers MAEM, Boogaarts HD, Roerink SHPP, et al. Endoscopic transsphenoidal pituitary surgery: a good and safe primary treatment option for Cushing's disease, even in case of macroadenomas or invasive adenomas. Eur J Endocrinol. 2013; 169(3):329–337

[36] Sun Y, Sun Q, Fan C, et al. Diagnosis and therapy for Cushing's disease with negative dynamic MRI finding: a single-centre experience. Clin Endocrinol (Oxf). 2012; 76(6):868–876

[37] Chandler WF, Barkan AL, Hollon T, et al. Outcome of transsphenoidal surgery for Cushing disease: a single-center experience over 32 years. Neurosurgery. 2016; 78(2):216–223

[38] Hofmann BM, Hlavac M, Martinez R, Buchfelder M, Müller OA, Fahlbusch R. Long-term results after microsurgery for Cushing disease: experience with 426 primary operations over 35 years. J Neurosurg. 2008; 108(1):9–18

[39] Höybye C, Grenbäck E, Rähn T, Degerblad M, Thorén M, Hulting A-L. Adrenocorticotropic hormone-producing pituitary tumors: 12- to 22-year follow-up after treatment with stereotactic radiosurgery. Neurosurgery. 2001; 49(2):284–291, discussion 291–292

[40] Mehta GU, Ding D, Patibandla MR, et al. Stereotactic radiosurgery for Cushing disease: results of an international, multicenter study. J Clin Endocrinol Metab. 2017; 102(11):4284–4291

[41] Wan H, Chihiro O, Yuan S. MASEP gamma knife radiosurgery for secretory pituitary adenomas: experience in 347 consecutive cases. J Exp Clin Cancer Res. 2009; 28(1):36

[42] Nelson DH, Meakin JW, Thorn GW. ACTH-producing pituitary tumors following adrenalectomy for Cushing's syndrome. Ann Intern Med. 1960; 52:560–569

[43] Nelson DH, Meakin JW, Dealy JBJ, Jr, Matson DD, Emerson K, Jr, Thorn GW. ACTH-producing tumor of the pituitary gland. N Engl J Med. 1958; 259(4): 161–164

[44] Sonino N, Zielezny M, Fava GA, Fallo F, Boscaro M. Risk factors and long-term outcome in pituitary-dependent Cushing's disease. J Clin Endocrinol Metab. 1996; 81(7):2647–2652

[45] Nagesser SK, van Seters AP, Kievit J, et al. Treatment of pituitary-dependent Cushing's syndrome: long-term results of unilateral adrenalectomy followed by external pituitary irradiation compared to transsphenoidal pituitary surgery. Clin Endocrinol (Oxf). 2000; 52(4):427–435

[46] Trifiletti DM, Xu Z, Dutta SW, et al. Endocrine remission after pituitary stereotactic radiosurgery: differences in rates of response for matched cohorts of cushing's disease and acromegaly patients. Int J Radiat Oncol Biol Phys. 2018; 102(3):e354–e355

[47] Sheehan JP, Xu Z, Salvetti DJ, Schmitt PJ, Vance ML. Results of gamma knife surgery for Cushing's disease. J Neurosurg. 2013; 119(6):1486–1492

[48] Shepard MJ, Mehta GU, Xu Z, et al. Technique of whole-sellar stereotactic radiosurgery for Cushing disease: results from a multicenter, international cohort study. World Neurosurg. 2018; 116:e670–e679

[49] Fleseriu M, Biller BMK, Findling JW, Molitch ME, Schteingart DE, Gross C, SEISMIC Study Investigators. Mifepristone, a glucocorticoid receptor antagonist, produces clinical and metabolic benefits in patients with Cushing's syndrome. J Clin Endocrinol Metab. 2012; 97(6):2039–2049

[50] Preda VA, Sen J, Karavitaki N, Grossman AB. Etomidate in the management of hypercortisolaemia in Cushing's syndrome: a review. Eur J Endocrinol. 2012; 167(2):137–143

[51] Broersen LHA, Jha M, Biermasz NR, Pereira AM, Dekkers OM. Effectiveness of medical treatment for Cushing's syndrome: a systematic review and meta-analysis. Pituitary. 2018; 21(6):631–641

[52] Colao A, Petersenn S, Newell-Price J, et al. Pasireotide B2305 Study Group. A 12-month phase 3 study of pasireotide in Cushing's disease. N Engl J Med. 2012; 366(10):914–924

[53] Palui R, Sahoo J, Kamalanathan S, Kar SS, Selvarajan S, Durgia H. Effect of cabergoline monotherapy in Cushing's disease: an individual participant data meta-analysis. J Endocrinol Invest. 2018; 41(12):1445–1455

[54] Pivonello R, Ferone D, de Herder WW, et al. Dopamine receptor expression and function in corticotroph pituitary tumors. J Clin Endocrinol Metab. 2004; 89(5):2452–2462

[55] Vilar L, Naves LA, Azevedo MF, et al. Effectiveness of cabergoline in monotherapy and combined with ketoconazole in the management of Cushing's disease. Pituitary. 2010; 13(2):123–129

[56] Luton JP, Mahoudeau JA, Bouchard P, et al. Treatment of Cushing's disease by O,p'DDD. Survey of 62 cases. N Engl J Med. 1979; 300(9):459–464

[57] Dimopoulou C, Schopohl J, Rachinger W, et al. Long-term remission and recurrence rates after first and second transsphenoidal surgery for Cushing's disease: care reality in the Munich Metropolitan Region. Eur J Endocrinol. 2013; 170(2):283–292

[58] Hameed N, Yedinak CG, Brzana J, et al. Remission rate after transsphenoidal surgery in patients with pathologically confirmed Cushing's disease, the role of cortisol, ACTH assessment and immediate reoperation: a large single center experience. Pituitary. 2013; 16(4):452–458

[59] Liubinas SV, Porto LD, Kaye AH. Management of recurrent Cushing's disease. J Clin Neurosci. 2011; 18(1):7–12

[60] Patil CG, Veeravagu A, Prevedello DM, Katznelson L, Vance ML, Laws ER, Jr. Outcomes after repeat transsphenoidal surgery for recurrent Cushing's disease. Neurosurgery. 2008; 63(2):266–270, discussion 270–271

[61] Porterfield JR, Thompson GB, Young WF, Jr, et al. Surgery for Cushing's syndrome: an historical review and recent ten-year experience. World J Surg. 2008; 32(5):659–677

[62] Feng M, Liu Z, Liu X, et al. Diagnosis and outcomes of 341 patients with Cushing's disease following transsphenoid surgery: a single-center experience. World Neurosurg. 2018; 109:e75–e80

[63] Knappe UJ, Lüdecke DK. Persistent and recurrent hypercortisolism after transsphenoidal surgery for Cushing's disease. In: Modern Neurosurgery of Meningiomas and Pituitary Adenomas. Vienna: Springer Vienna; 1996:31–34

[64] Prevedello DM, Pouratian N, Sherman J, et al. Management of Cushing's disease: outcome in patients with microadenoma detected on pituitary magnetic resonance imaging. J Neurosurg. 2008; 109(4):751–759

9 Natural History and Management Options of Traumatic Brain Injury

Stephen Honeybul

Abstract

Traumatic brain injury (TBI) is a global health care problem that consumes significant clinical and research resources and the medical and surgical management strategies continues to evolve. From a clinical perspective, the development of sophisticated web-based prediction models has provided clinically useful information regarding prognosis, and the development of sophisticated intracranial monitoring techniques has provided a considerable amount of data regarding the developing secondary brain injury. In addition, the results of several recent prospective multicenter randomized controlled trials have provided important information to guide clinical practice.

There have been considerable advances in knowledge regarding the basic science of the complex cellular response to trauma, and this has challenged the traditional classification of primary and secondary brain injury. It is also becoming increasingly apparent that TBI is a very heterogeneous disease process with areas of ischemia coexisting with mass lesions, contusions, areas with blood-brain barrier disruption as well as areas where the brain parenchyma is relatively normal. The optimal management for each type of brain injury will not necessarily be the same, and there are significant limitations when attempting to apply blanket therapies across all types of TBI. What remain to be established are either new or improved therapeutic strategies that convert the basic science and clinical information gained into clinical benefit and this is the challenge in the years ahead.

Keywords: traumatic brain injury, hypothermia, barbiturate coma, decompressive craniectomy, outcome prediction

9.1 Introduction

Traumatic brain injury (TBI) is a global health care problem that consumes significant clinical and research resources, and the medical and surgical management strategies continue to evolve. From a clinical perspective, there have been significant improvements in data gathering and statistical analysis that have enabled researchers to develop sophisticated web-based prediction models that can be used to stratify patients according to injury severity and provide clinically useful information regarding prognosis.[1,2] In addition, the continued development of sophisticated intracranial monitoring techniques has provided a considerable amount of data regarding the developing secondary brain injury.[3,4] Finally, the results of several recent prospective multicenter randomized controlled trials have provided important information to guide clinical practice.[5,6,7,8,9,10,11]

In addition to these clinical developments, there have been considerable advances in knowledge regarding the basic science of the complex cellular response to trauma and this has challenged the traditional classification of primary brain injury, which occurs at the initial trauma, and the secondary injury,

which follows in the hours and days thereafter. It is now realized that there is considerable overlap between these two processes and a substantial amount of cell death is due to a series of deleterious neurochemical cascades that are initiated at the time of injury and are amplified by secondary insults such as hypoxia or hypotension.[12,13] It is also becoming increasingly apparent that TBI is a very heterogeneous disease process with areas of ischemia coexisting with mass lesions, contusions, areas with blood–brain barrier disruption, as well as areas where the brain parenchyma is relatively normal. The optimal management for each type of brain injury will not necessarily be the same, and there are significant limitations when attempting to apply blanket therapies across all types of TBI.

What remains to be established are either new or improved therapeutic strategies that convert the basic science and clinical information gained into clinical benefit, and this is the challenge in the years ahead.

9.2 Selected Papers on the Natural History of Traumatic Brain Injury

- Mollayeva T, Kendzerska T, Mollayeva S, Shapiro CM, Colantonio A, Cassidy JD. A systematic review of fatigue in patients with traumatic brain injury: the course, predictors and consequences. Neurosci Biobehav Rev 2014;47:684–716
- Hicks AJ, Gould KR, Hopwood M, Kenardy J, Krivonos I, Ponsford JL. Behaviours of concern following moderate to severe traumatic brain injury in individuals living in the community. Brain Inj 2017;31(10):1312–1319

9.3 Natural History of Traumatic Brain Injury

The traditional classification of TBI severity is divided into mild, moderate, and severe, based on the initial Glasgow coma scale (GCS). Mild is classified as a GCS of 13 to 15, moderate as 9 to 12, and severe as less than 8. Notwithstanding some limitations of this classification, it does serve as a useful framework in which to consider the long-term outcome. There is, however, wide variation in the incidence of posttraumatic symptoms ranging from complete recovery in most patients to high rates of chronic problems.[14,15,16] This variation has been reported across all levels of injury severity and whereas this may reflect a lack of standardization when considering timing of assessment, symptom description, and a universally accepted definition of outcome, it may equally reflect the heterogeneity of the disease process.

Headache is one of the most common persisting symptoms with reported incidence ranging from 30 to 90%.[17] The mechanism of headache remains poorly understood; however, the presence of premorbid headaches appears significant. Indeed, the presence of a premorbid symptom is an important predictor of several posttraumatic symptoms, and the posttraumatic exacerbation of that particular symptom, such as headaches, may merely be a reflection of reduced tolerance brought on by the brain injury.

Fatigue is another common long-standing problem that can have a very negative effect on social, physical, and cognitive function after TBI; however, as with other posttraumatic symptoms, there is a wide range of reported prevalence from as low as 21% to as high as 73%.[14] This wide prevalence is perhaps unsurprising given the difficulties inherent in defining "fatigue." For example, "physiological fatigue" refers to a state of general tiredness due to physical or mental exertion, which can be ameliorated by rest, whereas "pathological fatigue" refers to a weariness that is unrelated to previous exertion and is not ameliorated by rest. These difficulties in symptom definition are further compounded when considering the numerous possible causes of fatigue, which may include any combination of neuroanatomical, functional, psychological, biochemical, or endocrine dysfunction. Notwithstanding several comprehensive reviews into this topic, there remains relatively limited knowledge regarding specific clinical and pathophysiological factors that predispose to posttraumatic fatigue, its natural history, and the overall health care burden of this symptom.

The same can be said of many other reported posttraumatic symptoms such as sleep dysfunction, depression, physical and cognitive impairment, and overall medical and neurological dysfunction, all of which can have a significant impact on an individual's long-term recovery.[16,17]

Finally, one of the most challenging aspects of recovery from moderate to severe TBI is the development of behavioral changes that can continue after the acute phase of recovery, becoming chronic and thereafter persistent.[18] These so-called behaviors of concern (BoCs) cover a broad spectrum ranging from apathy and social withdrawal to more challenging behaviors such as disinhibition, sexually inappropriate, aggressive, and violent behavior patterns.

There are likely to be many factors that contribute to the BoCs, but it is becoming increasingly apparent that not only do these issues persist in many individuals but they can also worsen over time and may be exacerbated when individuals become frustrated as they attempt to reintegrate into family and community life. These individuals place a significant strain on community health care resources, and recent studies investigating this issue have highlighted the lack of resources available among community-based adults who have survived many years with these issues.[18]

Overall, the long-term natural history of TBI remains difficult to predict on an individual basis and further work is required in order to gain consensus regarding issues such as precise symptom definition, timelines for assessment, and validated measures of outcome. It would also be useful to make any early determination regarding which individuals are likely to develop long-term problems and it is in this regard that more sophisticated outcome prediction models may provide some benefit.

9.4 Predicting Outcomes Following Traumatic Brain Injury

Predicting long-term outcome following TBI is important for several reasons, not least of which is the need to counsel families regarding what to expect in terms of functional recovery and the likelihood or otherwise of return of their loved one back into family life and the working environment. In addition, prognosis must be important when considering the continuation or indeed withdrawal of intensive care and neurosurgical therapy. Finally, the wider implications of equitable and sustainable use of resources need to be considered, not only in the acute phase of intervention but also when considering allocation of scarce rehabilitation facilities. Notwithstanding some limitations, prognostically important information can be obtained from the severity of the initial brain injury and thereafter the severity of the developing secondary brain injury.

9.5 Assessment of the Primary Brain Injury

Traditionally, the GCS has been used as an indicator of the severity of the initial injury, as well as clinical variables such as age, pupillary reaction, presence of extracranial injuries, and certain radiological features on initial computed tomography scan. More recently, the availability of increasing amounts of accurate baseline data, combined with advances in statistical analysis, has enabled researchers to develop sophisticated web-based prediction models that provide a mathematical calculation of a prognostic risk.[1,2] The CRASH (Corticosteroid Randomization after Significant Head Injury) collaborators' model was developed from the data collected on the 10,000 patients in the CRASH trial that investigated whether steroids were beneficial following TBI, and included mild, moderate, and severe TBI.[19] The clinical predictive variables required for the CRASH model are age, postresuscitation GCS score, pupillary response, and presence of a major extracranial injury. The radiological predictive variables are the presence of petechial hemorrhage, subarachnoid blood, midline shift, nonevacuated hematoma, and obliteration of the basal cisterns.

The IMPACT (International Mission for Prognosis and Clinical Trial) model was developed from 8,509 patients and focused on patients with moderate and severe TBI.[2] The baseline presentation data differ slightly from that of the CRASH model. Only the motor function of the GCS is required, hypoxia and hypotension are recorded separately, and epidural mass is recorded as a separate radiological finding. The model also uses the Marshall radiological classification and incorporates the prognostic significance of presentation blood glucose and hemoglobin levels.

Both models are Web based and they provide a percentage risk of unfavorable outcome at 6 months. Unfavorable outcome is defined by the Glasgow Outcome Score (GOS) of severely disabled, vegetative, or dead.[20] Several studies have demonstrated how the prediction of an unfavorable outcome may be used as a surrogate index of injury severity with which patients can be stratified according to injury severity.[21,22,23] The authors of both models emphasize that the information provided should only be used to support and not replace clinical judgment; however, the data do provide an objective assessment of injury severity and can perhaps form the basis for ethical discussions when considering lifesaving but nonrestorative surgical intervention.[24,25]

9.6 Assessment of Secondary Brain Injury

The use of intracranial pressure (ICP) monitoring has become widespread over the recent years not only to guide therapy but also to provide important prognostic information.[26,27] There is a strong correlation between outcome and the number of hours the ICP remains above 20 mm Hg, and this has been used as a threshold at which many medical therapies are introduced in a stepwise protocol-driven manner.[28] However, notwithstanding the prognostic significance, one of the fundamental challenges in neurotrauma has been the inability to demonstrate that the reduction in ICP brought about by many of these therapies is necessarily translated into an improvement in clinical outcome.

Indeed, it is becoming increasingly apparent that whereas the ICP is a useful marker of the developing injury severity, it is essentially a marker of end organ injury, and reducing the absolute number by either medical or surgical means will not reverse the effects of the pathology that precipitated the rise in ICP. What is really needed is a more acute marker of the developing secondary brain injury and this has led to the development of several multimodal monitoring techniques such as microdialysis, brain tissue oxygenation, bedside measures of autoregulation (such as the pressure reactivity index or the mean index), and continuous electroencephalography monitoring.[3,4]

Unfortunately, despite significant developments in the availability and use of these techniques, the clinical benefit gained from many of the recorded events remains undetermined. What is becoming increasingly apparent is that information obtained from a single modality that is interpreted independent from other physiological and metabolic parameters is unlikely to provide clinical benefit. In the same way that the CRASH and IMPACT models have combined individual prognostic indicators, what may now be required are advances in real-time, user-friendly data analysis and presentation that can be used to guide appropriately targeted individualized therapeutic management strategies. In addition, whereas the increasing complexity of monitoring technology must be matched with the appropriate clinical skills required to interpret the information gained, this is unlikely to improve outcome unless accompanied by new or improved therapies.

9.7 Selected Papers on the Treatment Outcomes

- Cooper DJ, Rosenfeld JV, Murray L, et al; DECRA Trial Investigators; Australian and New Zealand Intensive Care Society Clinical Trials Group. Decompressive craniectomy in diffuse traumatic brain injury. N Engl J Med 2011;364(16):1493–1502
- Hutchinson PJ, Kolias AG, Timofeev IS, et al; RESCUEicp Trial Collaborators. Trial of decompressive craniectomy for traumatic intracranial hypertension. N Engl J Med 2016;375(12):1119–1130
- Adelson PD, Wisniewski SR, Beca J, et al; Paediatric Traumatic Brain Injury Consortium. Comparison of hypothermia and normothermia after severe traumatic brain injury in children

(Cool Kids): a phase 3, randomised controlled trial. Lancet Neurol 2013;12(6):546–553
- Andrews PJ, Sinclair HL, Rodriguez A, et al; Eurotherm3235 Trial Collaborators. Hypothermia for intracranial hypertension after traumatic brain injury. N Engl J Med 2015;373(25):2403–2412

9.8 Treatment Options

In general terms, the management of patients with mild and moderate TBI is supportive with an emphasis placed on the prevention of secondary brain injury due to hypoxia or hypotension combined with clinical surveillance to detect any neurological deterioration. The management strategies for these patients have changed little over the recent years; however, the management of severe TBI has evolved considerably.

9.9 Medical Management of Severe Traumatic Brain Injury

Management of TBI in the neurointensive care setting is targeted at optimizing cerebral perfusion and oxygenation with a view to minimizing secondary insults. Endotracheal intubation, sedation, and ventilation allow full control of cerebral perfusion and oxygenation, prevent agitation due to pain and distress, and facilitate ICP monitoring. The aim of ICP monitoring is to identify those patients who develop either surgical lesions requiring evacuation or progressive cerebral swelling, which would preclude from early weaning. This ICP-targeted approach also aims to maintain the cerebral perfusion pressure (mean arterial blood pressure minus the ICP) below a certain threshold using several interventions that are introduced in a stepwise protocol-driven manner.[28]

Once the ICP starts to rise above 20 mm Hg, initial management strategies include head elevation, further sedation and paralysis, cerebrospinal fluid (CSF) drainage, and osmotherapy with either mannitol or more recently hypertonic saline. These have been part of protocolized management for many years and continue to do so; however, many other therapies that once formed the cornerstone of neurointensive care management have had to be reevaluated in the light of recent clinical evidence.

For many years, patients who developed intracranial hypertension were routinely hyperventilated, placed in a barbiturate coma, or more recently rendered hypothermic.[29,30,31,32] The rationale was that lowering the ICP would improve cerebral perfusion, reduce secondary brain injury, and improve clinical outcome. However, despite numerous clinical studies demonstrating the use of these therapies in the management of raised ICP, none have demonstrated a conclusive improvement in outcome. Indeed, the recent randomized controlled trials investigating the role of hypothermia have shown a tendency to increased mortality in those patients randomized to the treatment arms of the trial.[6,7,8,9,10,11] The Hutchison et al pediatric trial showed a higher death rate and incidence of poor neurological outcome in the hypothermia group (23 of 108 [21%] patients in the hypothermia group died vs. 14 [12%] in the normothermia group).[8] The National Acute Brain Injury Study:

Hypothermia II (NABISH II) trial investigated early cooling within 2 hours of injury, and the outcomes were worse in the hypothermia group, although this was not statistically significant.[9] The "Cool Kids" trial was stopped on the grounds of futility because hypothermia initiated early, used globally for 48 to 72 hours, and with a slow rewarming did not improve mortality at 3 months and again there was a tendency to increased mortality in the hypothermia group (6 of 39 [15%] patients in the hypothermia group vs. 2 [5%] in the normothermia group).[10] Finally, the most recent multicenter trial by Andrews et al failed to show not only that hypothermia provided clinical benefit but also that there was a tendency to cause harm such that the trial also had to be halted early.[11] Sixty nine of the 192 patients (36.5%) in the control group achieved a favorable outcome compared with 49 patients (25.7%) in the hypothermia arm of the trial. In addition, there was, again, an increased mortality in the hypothermia group (68 [34.9%] patients died vs. 51 [26.6%] in the normothermia group).

On face value, these findings would appear counterintuitive; however, studies investigating the effect that these three therapies have on cerebral blood flow indicate a probable reason. There is little doubt that barbiturates and hypothermia have the potential to be neuroprotective due to their influence on many aspects of the cellular response to injury, including calcium-mediated toxicity, glutamate excitotoxicity, free radical peroxidation, and cellular apoptosis.[33,34,35] However, the mechanism by which these three therapies produce the often-rapid fall in ICP that occurs after their application is predominantly a result of cerebral vasoconstriction, and the subsequent reduction in cerebral blood flow has been clearly demonstrated by a number of studies.[36,37,38] This does not necessarily mean that use of these therapies should be abandoned but rather their use should be far more judicious and should be generally reserved for intractable intracranial hypertension that is unresponsive to the aforementioned medical therapies. Their use must be tempered with the realization that any reduction in ICP may come at a cost of an increase in treatment morbidity and in these circumstances, consideration is often given to the use of decompressive craniectomy.

9.10 Surgical Management of Severe Traumatic Brain Injury

In some respects, the surgical management of severe TBI has changed over the recent years. The importance of early diagnosis of a clinically significant mass lesion such as an acute extradural, subdural, or parenchymal hematoma is well recognized and the need for expedient surgical evacuation is unquestioned. However, the past three decades have seen considerable debate regarding the use of decompressive craniectomy. The procedure itself is technically straightforward and first became popular in the management of severe TBI in the early 1970s. However, its use was almost abandoned in the latter part of that decade due to a combination of poor clinical outcomes and experimental studies that seemed to suggest that decompression may worsen cerebral edema.[39,40] Despite these early setbacks, interest in the procedure returned throughout the 1980s and 1990s, and there was a progressive increase in the number of publications reporting surgical efficacy of the procedure.[41,42,43] Overall, there

appeared to be little doubt that surgical intervention could reduce mortality; however, there has always been a concern that surgical intervention would convert death into survival with severe disability and dependency.[39] In an attempt to address this issue, the last decade has seen two prospective multicenter randomized controlled trials investigating this issue.

9.11 Decompressive Craniectomy Following Severe Traumatic—not Hemicraniectomy Brain Injury

The DECompressive CRAniectomy (DECRA) study investigated the role of early bifrontal decompressive craniectomy in the context of diffuse cerebral swelling, and it demonstrated that outcomes were worse in those patients in the surgical arm of the trial.[5] The results of the study evoked considerable debate, and one of the key criticisms was that the ICP threshold at which patients were randomised (20 mm Hg for more than 15 minutes in the hour) was not representative of current clinical practice (which is to intervene at higher ICP thresholds). While in hindsight, this may be a valid observation, it fails to acknowledge the trial hypothesis, which was that early decompression would improve cerebral perfusion, reduce secondary insults, and improve clinical outcome.

Given the enrolment at a relatively low ICP threshold, it is unsurprising that the trial did not demonstrate a survival benefit for those patients randomized to the surgical arm of the trial. However, the trial did clearly show that at that ICP threshold (20 mm Hg for > 15 min/h) there was insufficient ongoing secondary brain injury and therefore any potential benefit obtained from improved cerebral perfusion was offset by the now well-recognized surgical morbidity of the initial decompressive procedure and subsequent reconstructive cranioplasty. While the patients in the trial may not have been representative of current clinical practice, if the trial had shown benefit, these patients would have come to represent the *clinical practice of the future* and this would have had significant impact on neurosurgical resources.[44]

It is in this regard that the results of the recently published Randomized Evaluation of Surgery with Craniectomy for Uncontrollable Elevation of ICP (RESCUEicp) are particularly relevant as it was felt to be more reflective of current clinical practice.[6] The trial compared last-tier secondary decompressive craniectomy with continued medical management in patients with a higher ICP threshold (25 mm Hg for 1–12 hours despite maximal medical treatment, except for barbiturates). It was conducted over a 10-year period between 2004 and 2014 and 409 patients were randomized among 2,008 eligible patients, at 52 centers in 20 countries. The trial demonstrated a clear survival benefit in those patients randomized to surgical decompression; however, this reduction in mortality came as an almost direct result of an increase in the number of survivors either in a vegetative state or with severe disability. At 12 months of follow-up, there was a small increase, albeit statistically insignificant in the number of patients with a favorable outcome from 34.6% in the medical arm of the trial to 42% ($p = 0.12$) in the surgical arm of the trial. However, this small increase was only possible by including patients with upper levels of severe disability within the favorable outcome category. Without this recategorization, the number of patients who survived with lower moderate disability or better (traditionally a favorable outcome) was very similar (32% favorable in the surgical arm of the trial and 28.5% favorable in the medical arm).

A further, ethically challenging finding was the increase in the number of survivors in a vegetative state. At 6 months, the number of vegetative survivors increased from 4 of 188 patients (2.1%) randomized to the medical arm of the trial to 17 of 201 patients (8.5%) randomized to the surgical arm. This finding is even more ethically problematic when considering outcome findings at 12 months because six of these patients subsequently died (five patients in the surgical arm and one patient in the medical arm). The psychological distress for families involved in these circumstances and the resource implications cannot be underestimated. A final issue that must be taken into consideration is high crossover of patients from the medical arm of the trial to the surgical arm. Among the 196 patients randomized to receive medical therapy, 73 went on to have a decompressive procedure. How that should affect the interpretation of the results is difficult to determine, but as the authors stated, the observed treatment effect may be somewhat diluted. Indeed, it could be argued that there is a strong ethical imperative to assess the outcome in those patients randomized to the medical arm who subsequently underwent surgical decompression. If many of these patients went on to make a good long-term recovery, there would be grounds to argue in favor of the ongoing use of decompressive craniectomy for those with failed second-tier therapy resulting in intractable intracranial hypertension. Conversely, if there was a significant number of survivors in this group of patients had either severe disability or in a vegetative state (and who were analyzed in the medical arm of the trial), the support for the ongoing use of the procedure would be seriously called into question.

Overall, the results of these studies represent overwhelming evidence for efficacy of decompressive craniectomy as a lifesaving intervention; however, these recent studies clearly demonstrate that surgical intervention will not reverse the pathophysiology of the primary neurological insult and any reduction in mortality will come as a result of an increase in the number of survivors with significant disability.[45]

This raises several important ethical issues and the question remains as to the ongoing role of decompressive craniectomy and the direction of future research into clinical efficacy of the procedure. Given the significant reduction in mortality, it would appear unlikely that further randomized controlled trials comparing surgical decompression with standard medical therapy will be possible. Currently in most institutions, surgical intervention is usually performed when patients either have failed or are in the process of failing medical management, and randomizing patients in these circumstances is problematic as was clearly demonstrated in the RESCUEicp trial. However, there does appear to be a subset of patients who require surgical decompression, who survive and go on to make a good long-term recovery. In addition, some individuals seem to adapt to a level of disability and dependency that they might previously have thought to be unacceptable. The difficulty has always been how to accurately predict long-term outcome, and it is in this regard that observation cohort studies and the use of the aforementioned prediction models may be beneficial.

Over the recent years, several observational cohort studies in Western Australia have used the percentage prediction of unfavorable outcome provided by either the CRASH or IMPACT model as a surrogate index of injury severity with which to stratify patients according to injury severity.[21,22,23,46] Comparing the prediction of unfavorable outcome with the observed long-term outcome provides an objective assessment of the most likely outcome either for those patients who require surgical intervention to evacuate a mass lesion (primary decompression) or in those patients who develop intractable intracranial hypertension (secondary decompression; ▶ Fig. 9.1 and ▶ Fig. 9.2). Notwithstanding the limitations of applying population-based data to individual clinical cases, this type of objective assessment may act as a prompt to initiate discussions regarding realistic long-term outcome expectations.

In the emotionally charged circumstances of acute neurotrauma, it would certainly be impractical and potentially inappropriate to discuss detailed statistical data; however, once the prediction of an unfavorable outcome exceeds 80%, discussions regarding outcome cannot be dichotomized into life or death because to do so would fail to recognize that the most likely outcome if the patient survives is that of severe disability and dependency. Conversely for patients who develop intractable intracranial hypertension and have a prediction of unfavorable outcome less than 60%, while acknowledging some uncertainty, it may be reassuring that surgical decompression should proceed given the survival advantage and the possibility of a favorable outcome. The obvious difficulty comes when the prediction is between 60 and 80% because the observed outcomes are distributed evenly between death and a good outcome. In these circumstances, the most likely outcome is statistically almost impossible to predict, and discussions regarding long-term outcome must be reflective of the uncertainty.

The decision to perform decompressive craniectomy will always be challenging, and there will never be a one-size-fits-all approach to these ethically challenging decisions. However, this type of methodology may provide prognostic assistance and in certain circumstances prompt appropriate discussions regarding the possibility and acceptability of this outcome and perhaps guide clinically and ethically appropriate decisions.

There is certainly a need to continue research into TBI; however, the direction of clinical research may move away from randomized controlled trials, which are expensive and difficult to design and execute. There has recently been a move to so-called comparative effectiveness research, which aims to gather large quantities of clinical, radiological, and blood biospecimens along with outcome data. By detailing the entire clinical course of patient's injury details, treatment, outcome, and health costs, it is hoped that (cost-)effective medical care will be identified and a resource for further research provided. There is little doubt that these initiatives will provide invaluable information regarding efficacy of treatment currently provided for the "silent epidemic" that is a significant global health care issue. However, what is really required are new therapies that can halt or repair the multifactorial disease process that is traumatic brain and this must also continue to be a focus of research in the future.

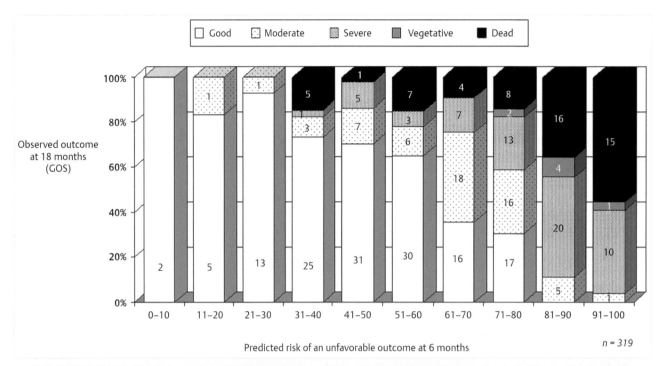

Fig. 9.1 The CRASH (Corticosteroid Randomization after Significant Head Injury) collaborators' prediction model. The prediction of an unfavorable outcome at 6 months (*x* axis) and the observed outcome at 18 months among the 319 patients for whom 18-month follow-up was available. Numbers within the bar chart represent absolute patient numbers. (Reproduced with permission of Elsevier from Honeybul S, Ho KM. Predicting long-term neurological outcomes after severe traumatic brain injury requiring decompressive craniectomy: a comparison of the CRASH and IMPACT prognostic models. Injury. 2016; 47(9):1886–1892.)

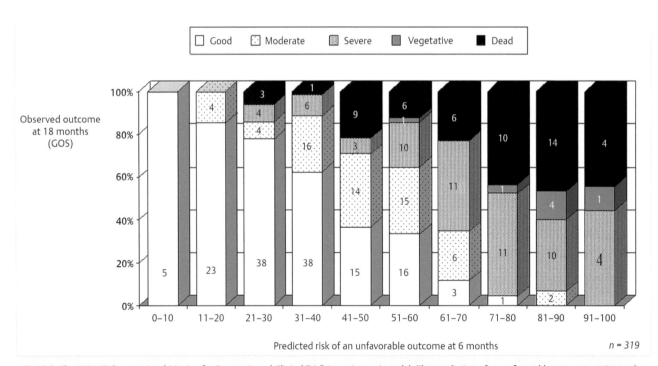

Fig. 9.2 The IMPACT (International Mission for Prognosis and Clinical Trial) investigators' model. The prediction of an unfavorable outcome at 6 months (*x* axis) and the observed outcome at 18 months among the 319 patients on whom 18-month follow-up was available. Numbers within the bar chart represent absolute patient numbers. (Reproduced with permission of Elsevier from Honeybul S, Ho KM. Predicting long-term neurological outcomes after severe traumatic brain injury requiring decompressive craniectomy: a comparison of the CRASH and IMPACT prognostic models. Injury. 2016; 47(9):1886–1892.)

9.12 Authors' Recommendations

- The development and refinement of outcome prediction models may provide clinically useful information regarding initial injury severity.
- The use of ICP monitoring should continue as it provides a useful marker of the developing secondary brain injury.
- An ICP of greater than 20 mm Hg should be the threshold to consider stepwise application medical therapies such as head elevation, osmotherapy, and further sedation and neuromuscular paralysis.
- Use of hyperventilation, barbiturates, and hypothermia may be considered for intractable intracranial hypertension.
- Decompressive craniectomy may be used in circumstances where a patient is thought otherwise unlikely to survive.
- Prediction models may provide useful information to guide ethical discussions when considering lifesaving but nonrestorative surgical decompression.

References

[1] Perel P, Arango M, Clayton T, et al. MRC CRASH Trial Collaborators. Predicting outcome after traumatic brain injury: practical prognostic models based on large cohort of international patients. BMJ. 2008; 336(7641):425–429

[2] Murray GD, Butcher I, McHugh GS, et al. Multivariable prognostic analysis in traumatic brain injury: results from the IMPACT study. J Neurotrauma. 2007; 24(2):329–337

[3] Citerio G, Oddo M, Taccone FS. Recommendations for the use of multimodal monitoring in the neurointensive care unit. Curr Opin Crit Care. 2015; 21(2):113–119

[4] Honeybul S. An update on the management of traumatic brain injury. J Neurosurg Sci. 2011; 55(4):343–355

[5] Cooper DJ, Rosenfeld JV, Murray L, et al. DECRA Trial Investigators, Australian and New Zealand Intensive Care Society Clinical Trials Group. Decompressive craniectomy in diffuse traumatic brain injury. N Engl J Med. 2011; 364(16):1493–1502

[6] Hutchinson PJ, Kolias AG, Timofeev IS, et al. RESCUEicp Trial Collaborators. Trial of decompressive craniectomy for traumatic intracranial hypertension. N Engl J Med. 2016; 375(12):1119–1130

[7] Clifton GL, Miller ER, Choi SC, et al. Lack of effect of induction of hypothermia after acute brain injury. N Engl J Med. 2001; 344(8):556–563

[8] Hutchison JS, Ward RE, Lacroix J, et al. Hypothermia Pediatric Head Injury Trial Investigators and the Canadian Critical Care Trials Group. Hypothermia therapy after traumatic brain injury in children. N Engl J Med. 2008; 358(23):2447–2456

[9] Clifton GL, Valadka A, Zygun D, et al. Very early hypothermia induction in patients with severe brain injury (the National Acute Brain Injury Study: Hypothermia II): a randomised trial. Lancet Neurol. 2011; 10(2):131–139

[10] Adelson PD, Wisniewski SR, Beca J, et al. Paediatric Traumatic Brain Injury Consortium. Comparison of hypothermia and normothermia after severe traumatic brain injury in children (Cool Kids): a phase 3, randomised controlled trial. Lancet Neurol. 2013; 12(6):546–553

[11] Andrews PJ, Sinclair HL, Rodriguez A, et al. Eurotherm3235 Trial Collaborators. Hypothermia for intracranial hypertension after traumatic brain injury. N Engl J Med. 2015; 373(25):2403–2412

[12] Sahuquillo J, Poca MA, Amoros S. Current aspects of pathophysiology and cell dysfunction after severe head injury. Curr Pharm Des. 2001; 7(15):1475–1503

[13] Johnson VE, Stewart W, Smith DH. Axonal pathology in traumatic brain injury. Exp Neurol. 2013; 246:35–43

[14] Mollayeva T, Kendzerska T, Mollayeva S, Shapiro CM, Colantonio A, Cassidy JD. A systematic review of fatigue in patients with traumatic brain injury: the course, predictors and consequences. Neurosci Biobehav Rev. 2014; 47:684–716

[15] van der Naalt J, Timmerman ME, de Koning ME, et al. Early predictors of outcome after mild traumatic brain injury (UPFRONT): an observational cohort study. Lancet Neurol. 2017; 16(7):532–540

[16] Jaeger M, Deiana G, Nash S, et al. Prognostic factors of long-term outcome in cases of severe traumatic brain injury. Ann Phys Rehabil Med. 2014; 57(6–7):436–451

[17] Lucas S, Smith BM, Temkin N, Bell KR, Dikmen S, Hoffman JM. Comorbidity of headache and depression after mild traumatic brain injury. Headache. 2016; 56(2):323–330

[18] Hicks AJ, Gould KR, Hopwood M, Kenardy J, Krivonos I, Ponsford JL. Behaviours of concern following moderate to severe traumatic brain injury in individuals living in the community. Brain Inj. 2017; 31(10):1312–1319

[19] Roberts I, Yates D, Sandercock P, et al. CRASH trial collaborators. Effect of intravenous corticosteroids on death within 14 days in 10008 adults with clinically significant head injury (MRC CRASH trial): randomised placebo-controlled trial. Lancet. 2004; 364(9442):1321–1328

[20] Jennett B, Bond M. Assessment of outcome after severe brain damage. Lancet. 1975; 1(7905):480–484

[21] Honeybul S, Ho KM, Lind CRP, Corcoran T, Gillett GR. The retrospective application of a prediction model to patients who have had a decompressive craniectomy for trauma. J Neurotrauma. 2009; 26(12):2179–2183

[22] Honeybul S, Ho KM, Lind CRP, Gillett GR. Observed versus predicted outcome for decompressive craniectomy: a population-based study. J Neurotrauma. 2010; 27(7):1225–1232

[23] Honeybul S, Ho KM. Predicting long-term neurological outcomes after severe traumatic brain injury requiring decompressive craniectomy: a comparison of the CRASH and IMPACT prognostic models. Injury. 2016; 47(9):1886–1892

[24] Gillett GR, Honeybul S, Ho KM, Lind CR. Neurotrauma and the RUB: where tragedy meets ethics and science. J Med Ethics. 2010; 36(12):727–730

[25] Honeybul S, Gillett GR, Ho K. Futility in neurosurgery: a patient-centered approach. Neurosurgery. 2013; 73(6):917–922

[26] Juul N, Morris GF, Marshall SB, Marshall LF, The Executive Committee of the International Selfotel Trial. Intracranial hypertension and cerebral perfusion pressure: influence on neurological deterioration and outcome in severe head injury. J Neurosurg. 2000; 92(1):1–6

[27] Marmarou A, Anderson R, Ward JD, et al. Impact of ICP instability and hypotension on outcome in patients with severe head trauma. J Neurosurg. 1991; 75:s59–s66

[28] Bratton SL, Chestnut RM, Ghajar J, et al. Brain Trauma Foundation, American Association of Neurological Surgeons, Congress of Neurological Surgeons, Joint Section on Neurotrauma and Critical Care, AANS/CNS. Guidelines for the management of severe traumatic brain injury. J Neurotrauma. 2007; 24 (Suppl 1):S55–S58

[29] Muizelaar JP, Marmarou A, Ward JD, et al. Adverse effects of prolonged hyperventilation in patients with severe head injury: a randomized clinical trial. J Neurosurg. 1991; 75(5):731–739

[30] Curley G, Kavanagh BP, Laffey JG. Hypocapnia and the injured brain: more harm than benefit. Crit Care Med. 2010; 38(5):1348–1359

[31] Eisenberg HM, Frankowski RF, Contant CF, Marshall LF, Walker MD. High-dose barbiturate control of elevated intracranial pressure in patients with severe head injury. J Neurosurg. 1988; 69(1):15–23

[32] Ward JD, Becker DP, Miller JD, et al. Failure of prophylactic barbiturate coma in the treatment of severe head injury. J Neurosurg. 1985; 62(3):383–388

[33] Koizumi H, Povlishock JT. Posttraumatic hypothermia in the treatment of axonal damage in an animal model of traumatic axonal injury. J Neurosurg. 1998; 89(2):303–309

[34] Sutcliffe IT, Smith HA, Stanimirovic D, Hutchison JS. Effects of moderate hypothermia on IL-1 beta-induced leukocyte rolling and adhesion in pial microcirculation of mice and on proinflammatory gene expression in human cerebral endothelial cells. J Cereb Blood Flow Metab. 2001; 21(11):1310–1319

[35] Koerner IP, Brambrink AM. Brain protection by anesthetic agents. Curr Opin Anaesthesiol. 2006; 19(5):481–486

[36] Rosomoff HL, Holaday DA. Cerebral blood flow and cerebral oxygen consumption during hypothermia. Am J Physiol. 1954; 179(1):85–88

[37] Nordström CH, Messeter K, Sundbärg G, Schalén W, Werner M, Ryding E. Cerebral blood flow, vasoreactivity, and oxygen consumption during barbiturate therapy in severe traumatic brain lesions. J Neurosurg. 1988; 68(3):424–431

[38] Yundt KD, Diringer MN. The use of hyperventilation and its impact on cerebral ischemia in the treatment of traumatic brain injury. Crit Care Clin. 1997; 13(1):163–184

[39] Cooper PR, Rovit RL, Ransohoff J. Hemicraniectomy in the treatment of acute subdural hematoma: a re-appraisal. Surg Neurol. 1976; 5(1):25–28

[40] Cooper PR, Hagler H, Clark WK, Barnett P. Enhancement of experimental cerebral edema after decompressive craniectomy: implications for the management of severe head injuries. Neurosurgery. 1979; 4(4):296–300

[41] Polin RS, Shaffrey ME, Bogaev CA, et al. Decompressive bifrontal craniectomy in the treatment of severe refractory posttraumatic cerebral edema. Neurosurgery. 1997; 41(1):84–92, discussion 92–94

[42] Guerra WK, Gaab MR, Dietz H, Mueller JU, Piek J, Fritsch MJ. Surgical decompression for traumatic brain swelling: indications and results. J Neurosurg. 1999; 90(2):187–196

[43] Aarabi B, Hesdorffer DC, Ahn ES, Aresco C, Scalea TM, Eisenberg HM. Outcome following decompressive craniectomy for malignant swelling due to severe head injury. J Neurosurg. 2006; 104(4):469–479

[44] Honeybul S, Ho KM, Lind CR. What can be learned from the DECRA study. World Neurosurg. 2013; 79(1):159–161

[45] Honeybul S, Ho KM, Gillett GR. Long-term outcome following decompressive craniectomy: an inconvenient truth? Curr Opin Crit Care. 2018; 24(2):97–104

[46] Honeybul S, Ho KM, Lind CR, Gillett GR. Validation of the CRASH model in the prediction of 18-month mortality and unfavorable outcome in severe traumatic brain injury requiring decompressive craniectomy. J Neurosurg. 2014; 120(5):1131–1137

10 Natural History and Management Options of Angionegative Subarachnoid Hemorrhage

Jorn Van Der Veken, Aye Aye Gyi, and Amal Abou-Hamden

Abstract

Angionegative subarachnoid hemorrhage (SAH) is a subset of nontraumatic SAH, in which there is no underlying cause detected on the initial vascular imaging. Compared to its aneurysmal SAH counterpart, angionegative SAH has a more favorable natural history. This impacts the overall inpatient hospital management, timing, and the degree of follow-up required.

Keywords: angionegative, subarachnoid hemorrhage, perimesencephalic bleed, diffuse subarachnoid hemorrhage, nontraumatic subarachnoid hemorrhage

10.1 Introduction

In 15 to 20% of patients presenting with a nontraumatic subarachnoid hemorrhage (SAH), a cause for the hemorrhage cannot be detected on the initial vascular imaging. This group is referred to as the angionegative SAH group. There is no consensus on the timing, number, and type of investigations needed to define an angionegative SAH. Digital subtraction angiography (DSA) has been the imaging modality of choice, but with the advent of high-quality 3D computed tomography angiography (CTA) and magnetic resonance angiography (MRA), routine use of this more conventional and invasive investigation has been challenged. Based on radiological findings, angionegative SAHs are further classified into the following:

- *Perimesencephalic SAH (PMSAH)*: It was initially described by van Gijn et al in 1985[1] and has a characteristic radiographic pattern of hemorrhage restricted to the perimesencephalic cisterns on CTB.[1,2]
- *Non-PMSAH or diffuse SAH (dSAH)*: This is characterized by a more widespread distribution of SAH with a visible extension into the anterior part of the ambient cistern or to the basal part of the Sylvian fissures, mimicking an aneurysmal SAH.[1,2]

This classification refers to the initial computed tomography of the brain (CTB) ideally performed within 24 hours after the ictus, as delayed imaging might mimic a PMSAH due to blood resorption.[1,2] Although often considered a single pathological entity, distinguishing non-PMSAH from PMSAH is particularly important as they have a different natural course and management.

In a recent systematic review and meta-analysis, demographic characteristics of patients (n = 3,853) were described in 49 of 58 included studies.[3] The mean age of included patients was 53.8 years. Forty-five studies including 3,530 patients reported diagnoses stratified by bleeding pattern and found that 1,763/3,530 (49.9%) had a PMSAH and 1,577/3,530 (44.7%) had a non-PMSAH.[3] Unlike aneurysmal SAH, there is a male predominance in angionegative SAH (54.3%). A summary of demographic data from the systematic review is presented in ► Table 10.1.[3]

Table 10.1 General demographics of the study patients adapted from Mohan et al[3]

Studies	Type of study	No. of patients	Mean age (y)	Male (%)
Rinkel et al[4]	Retro	65	53.0	61.5%
Goergen et al[5]	Retro	18	NR	NR
Van Calenbergh et al[6]	Retro	62	47.0	40.0%
Hütter et al[7]	Retro	20	49.0	NR
Canhão et al[8]	Pros and retro	71	49.9	56.0%
Tatter et al[9]	Retro	40	NR	NR
Duong et al[10]	Pros	92	49.0	54.0%
Berdoz et al[11]	Retro	52	52.8	65.0%
Linn et al[12]	Pros	23	56.0	74.0%
Madureira et al[13]	Pros	18	NR	NR
Marquardt et al[14]	Pros	21	55.0	52.0%
Franz et al[15]	Retro	34	50.1	52.0%
Ildan et al[16]	Retro	84	49.5	NR
Alén et al[17]	Pros	44	51.9	63.6%
Lang et al[18]	Pros	57	54.7	56.0%
Topcuoglu et al[19]	Retro	86	54.3	63.0%
Caeiro et al[20]	Pros	33	NR	NR
Jung et al[21]	Pros	143	52.3	42.0%
Matsuyama et al[22]	Pros	9	50.0	57.0%
Andaluz and Zuccarello[23]	Retro	92	49.4	34.0%
Kang et al[24]	Retro	52	55.4	53.8%

(Continued)

Table 10.1 (*Continued*) General demographics of the study patients adapted from Mohan et al[3]

Studies	Type of study	No. of patients	Mean age (y)	Male (%)
Whiting et al[25]	Retro	89	56.0	51.0%
Beseoglu et al[26]	Retro	21	57.2	60.0%
Caeiro et al[27]	Pros	37	NR	43.0%
Nayak et al[28]	Retro	190	57.0	61.6%
Alfieri et al[29]	Pros	38	44.3	NR
Fontanella et al[30]	Retro	102	53.0	62.7%
Kong et al[31]	Pros	31	49.7	NR
Oda et al[32]	Retro	15	NR	NR
Pyysalo et al[33]	Retro	97	52.0	36.0%
Cánovas et al[34]	Retro	108	52.4	44.9%
Delgado Almandoz et al[35]	Retro	72	53.1	36.1%
Gross et al[36]	Retro	77	59.8	48.0%
Kostić et al[37]	Pros	36	48.3	55.6%
Lin et al[38]	Pros	68	59.5	51.5%
Maslehaty et al[39]	Pros and retro	179	NR	60.0%
Yu et al[40]	Retro	28	60.3	51.1%
Zhong et al[41]	Retro	49	54.0	49.0%
Boswell et al[42]	Retro	31	56.3	55.0%
Dalyai et al[43]	Retro	254	NR	NR
Khan et al[44]	Retro	50	52.5	60.0%
Muehlschlegel et al[45]	Retro	93	54.0	59.0%
Prat et al[46]	Retro	63	52.4	54.0%
Tsermoulas et al[47]	Retro	62	51.0	51.2%
Woodfield et al[48]	Retro	240	51.0	62.0%
Ellis et al[49]	Pros	173	55.0	55.0%
Konczalla et al[50]	Pros	125	56.0	70.0%
Kumar et al[51]	Pros	39	50.5	69.0%
Mensing et al[52]	Pros	79	53.0	54.0%
Qureshi et al[53]	Retro	5	59.8	NR
Canneti et al[54]	Retro	41	55.0	51.0%
Dalbjerg et al[55]	Retro	95	53.0	48.4%
Konczalla et al[56]	Retro	152	58.0	59.0%
Konczalla et al[57]	Pros	173	56.0	NR
Sprenker et al[58]	Retro	26	NR	NR
Walcott et al[59]	Retro	138	55.6	53.6%
Konczalla et al[60]	Retro	225	57.0	NR
Moscovici et al[61]	Retro	56	53.4	54.0%

Abbreviations: NR, not reported; Pros, prospective; Retro, retrospective; WFNS, World Federation of Neurosurgical Societies.

A pooled analysis of data from 9 studies with 646 patients showed that a significantly greater number of patients in the non-PMSAH group had a poor-grade SAH (World Federation of Neurosurgical Societies [WFNS] grade >2) than PMSAH group (24.6 vs. 7.2%; ▶ Table 10.2).[3]

10.2 Selected Papers on the Natural History of Angionegative SAH

- Mohan M, Islim AI, Rasul FT, et al; British Neurosurgical Trainee Research Collaborative. Subarachnoid haemorrhage

with negative initial neurovascular imaging: a systematic review and meta-analysis. Acta Neurochir (Wien) 2019;161(10):2013–2026
- Hui FK, Tumialán LM, Tanaka T, Cawley CM, Zhang YJ. Clinical differences between angiographically negative, diffuse subarachnoid hemorrhage and perimesencephalic subarachnoid hemorrhage. Neurocrit Care 2009;11(1):64–70

10.3 Natural History

The natural history of angionegative SAH is generally more favorable compared to their angiopositive counterparts. However, complications are well recognized and these include vasospasm,

Table 10.2 Proportion of study participants with poor grade SAH (WFNS grade greater than 2)[3]

Studies	Total patients	Poor WFNS grade, PMSAH	Poor WFNS grade, non-PMSAH
Van Calenbergh et al[6]	44	3/20	9/24
Berdoz et al[11]	52	0/22	9/30
Beseoglu et al[26]	26	1/17	4/9
Kostić et al[37]	34	1/18	4/16
Khan et al[44]	40	1/17	3/23
Moscovici et al[61]	56	0/25	22/31
Konczalla et al[50]	125	7/73	12/52
Konczalla et al[57]	173	8/87	15/86
Sprenker et al[58]	96	1/25	6/71
Total	646	22/304 (7.2%)	84/342 (24.6%)

Abbreviations: PMSAH, perimesencephalic subarachnoid hemorrhage; WFNS, World Federation of Neurosurgical Societies.

Table 10.3 Pooled analysis of published data on the complications stratified by bleeding pattern

Complications	Studies	Events/no. of patients (%)	PMSAH (%)	non-PMSAH (%)
Rebleed	Hui et al[62]	NR	NR	NR
	Mohan et al[3]	56/1,675 (3.3%)	4/506 (1.1%)	16/530 (3.5%)
Hydrocephalus	Hui et al[62]	36/94 (38.3%)	3/36 (9.6%)	33/36 (50.8%)
	Mohan et al[3]	469/2,399 (19.5%)	104/915 (9.0%)	241/924 (25.5%)
Radiological vasospasm	Hui et al[62]	22/94 (23.4%)	3/22 (9.6%)	19/22 (28.6%)
	Mohan et al[3]	180/1,435 (12.5%)	49/530 (8.3%)	116/630 (14.0%)
Seizures	Hui et al[62]	NR	NR	NR
	Mohan et al[3]	12/379 (3.2%)	3/164 (2.5%)	8/179 (5.2%)

Abbreviations: NR, not reported; PMSAH, perimesencephalic subarachnoid hemorrhage.

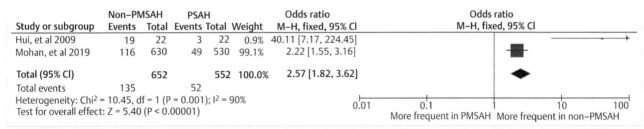

Fig. 10.1 Forest plots of complications data in perimesencephalic subarachnoid hemorrhage (PMSAH) versus non-PMSAH comparing **(a)** hydrocephalus and **(b)** radiological vasospasm.

hydrocephalus, permanent ischemic complications, chronic headaches, and rehemorrhage.[3,62] A pooled analysis of published data (▶ Table 10.3) suggests that the incidence of rebleeding in the non-PMSAH group was approximately 3.5% compared to 1.1% in PMSAH group. Development of hydrocephalus was found to be considerably worse in the non-PMSAH group (25.5 vs. 9.0%) with requirement for external ventricular drainage (41 vs. 9.6%), and eventual permanent cerebrospinal fluid diversion (20.6 vs. 0%).[3] Furthermore, non-PMSAH patients had higher rates of radiological

vasospasm (14.0 vs. 8.3%) and seizures (5.2 vs. 2.5%) when compared to those with PMSAH patients.[3] Another publication reported a higher rate of hydrocephalus and radiological vasospasm for the non-PMSAH group.[62] A forest plot meta-analysis of available complications data from both studies[3,62] showed a higher risk of overall hydrocephalus (odds ratio [OR], 2.69; 95% confidence interval [CI], 2.10–3.45) and radiological vasospasm (OR, 2.57; 95% CI, 1.82–3.62) for the non-PMSAH group (▶ Fig. 10.1).

Table 10.4 Length of stay (days) for patients with angionegative SAH stratified by SAH types

Study	Total		Subgroups					
	n	LOS	PMSAH (n)	LOS	Non-PMSAH (n)	LOS	Radiologically negative (n)	LOS
Goergen et al[5]	18	NR	9	12[a]	NR	NA	NR	NA
Andaluz and Zuccarello[23]	92	6.3[b]	45	4.3[b]	47	8.3[b]	0	NA
Beseoglu et al[26]	21	15.3[b]	12	11.2[b]	9	20.7[b]	0	NA
Nayak et al[28]	190	14	NR	NA	NR	NA	NR	NA
Delgado Almandoz et al[35]	25	2–7[a]	15	2–7[a]	8	2–7[a]	2	2–7
	34	8–14[a]	12	8–14[a]	20	8–14[a]	2	8–14[a]
	13	≥15[a]	2	≥15[a]	11	≥15[a]	0	≥15
Boswell et al[42]	31	NR	14	12.5[b]	16	13.2[b]	1	NR
Khan et al[44]	50	NR	17	8.3	23	10	10	5
Muehlschlegel et al[45]	93	11	36	NR	48	NR	9	NR
Canneti et al[54]	41	21.1[b]	17	17[b]	24	24[b]	0	

Abbreviations: LOS, length of stay; NA, not applicable; NR, not reported; PMSAH, perimesencephalic subarachnoid hemorrhage.
Source: adapted from Mohan et al.[3]
[a]Discharge within days of admission.
[b]Mean/median.

A pooled analysis of functional outcome data stratified by bleeding patterns reported in the systematic review suggested that the non-PMSAH patients were more likely to experience poor functional outcomes (modified Rankin Scale [mRS] ≥3) than those with PSAH at 3 to 6 months (12.8 vs. 6.1%) and ≥1 year (14.4 vs. 7.3%).[3] Ultimately, only 76% of the non-PMSAH patients achieved complete recovery and independent living, compared to 96.7% of the PMSAH patients.[3]

The length of hospital stay was reported in 9 studies (608 patients) with median and mean values of 10 and 8.3 days in PMSAH patients versus 8.3 and 4 days in non-PMSAH patients (▶ Table 10.4).[3]

10.4 Selected Papers on the Management Options of Angionegative SAH

- Geng B, Wu X, Brackett A, Malhotra A. Meta-analysis of recent literature on utility of follow-up imaging in isolated perimesencephalic hemorrhage. Clin Neurol Neurosurg 2019;180:111–116
- Dalyai R, Chalouhi N, Theofanis T, et al. Subarachnoid hemorrhage with negative initial catheter angiography: a review of 254 cases evaluating patient clinical outcome and efficacy of short- and long-term repeat angiography. Neurosurgery 2013;72(4):646–652, discussion 651–652

10.5 Treatment Options

A recent 2019 meta-analysis of 13 studies including 588 patients assessed the utility of follow-up imaging for aneurysm detection in PMSAH after a negative initial angiographic study.[63] The findings of the study revealed that out of the 588 patients, an intracranial aneurysm or other causes of hemorrhage were identified only in 3 patients (2 aneurysms and 1 vasculitis).[64] The findings suggested that there is limited utility to perform a DSA after an initial CTA in PMSAH cohort.[63] The summary of the findings are presented in ▶ Table 10.5.

A conservative approach with follow-up using CTA may be an alternative option in cases of some uncertainty. For the non-PMSAH cohort, the diagnostic yield is much higher, and further investigation involving a repeat six-vessel DSA and magnetic resonance imaging (MRI)/MRA of the cervical region is recommended. In a retrospective review of 254 patients with initially negative DSA examination, angiograms were performed at the time of initial hemorrhage, at 1 week, and again at 6 weeks. The overall detection rate of a responsible intracranial lesion by the repeated DSA was 12.5% in the non-PMSAH group and 0% in the PMSAH group. A repeat DSA study is therefore strongly advised for patients with the non-PMSAH pattern.[43]

Data supporting the role of nimodipine in improving outcomes in angionegative SAH patients are limited. With clinical vasospasm being rather anecdotal in PMSAH, the role of nimodipine in this group seems unnecessary. With vasospasm being more frequently encountered in the non-PMSAH groups and a clinical course like aneurysmal SAH, there is a potential role for nimodipine.[63]

No studies investigating ideal blood pressure targets were found. Extrapolating aneurysmal SAH guidelines to non-PMSAH seems appropriate for the above-mentioned reasons.[64]

There is a marked heterogeneity of data in the literature as to which imaging modalities to use for repeat imaging and the time frame for when this repeat imaging should be undertaken. The preference at our institution is that unless the initial CT scan with high-quality vascular imaging is completed within several hours after the onset of symptoms, PMSAH patients need at least one DSA to exclude a vascular abnormality. For non-PMSAH patients, it is advisable to investigate and follow up more comprehensively and as early as possible to optimize the chances of identifying a vascular abnormality as recommended in the flow chart in ▶ Fig. 10.2.

Table 10.5 Summary of the data from the meta-analysis of 13 studies regarding the utility of follow-up imaging in PMSAH[6]

Studies	Total patients (females)	Age (y)	Initial CTA performed	Initial CTA yield	Initial DSA performed	Initial DSA yield	Repeat imaging modality	Repeat imaging performed	Repeat imaging yield
Almandoz et al[65]	82 (40)	55.4 ± 9.6	12	0	12	0	CTA/DSA	12	0
Kumar et al[51]	131 (53)	53	22	0	22	0	DSA	22	0
Woodfield et al[48]	17 (8)	51.5 ± 9.4	90	0	90	0	DSA	20	0
Canneti et al[54]	90 (NR)	NR	15	0	2	0	DSA	17	0
Yap et al[66]	33 (NR)	NR	39	0	2	0	DSA	35	0
Akcakaya et al[67]	41 (NR)	NR			33	0	DSA	33	0
Coelho et al[68]	62 (NR)	NR	29	0			CTA/DSA	26	0
Heit et al[64]	24 (12)	53.0 ± 12.0	71	0	71	0	DSA	71	3
Mortimer et al[69]	72 (24)	52.7 ± 10.8	72	0			DSA	72	0
Potter et al[70]	22 (7)	52.5			131	0	DSA	131	0
Sahin et al[71]	71 (33)	NR			24	1	DSA	22	
Song et al[72]	29 (16)	52.4 ± 11.8			62	0	CTA/DSA	45	0
Xu et al[73]	12 (5)	NR	82	0	82	0	DSA	82	0

Abbreviations: CTA, computed tomography angiography; DSA, digital subtraction angiography; NR, not reported; PMSAH, perimesencephalic subarachnoid hemorrhage.

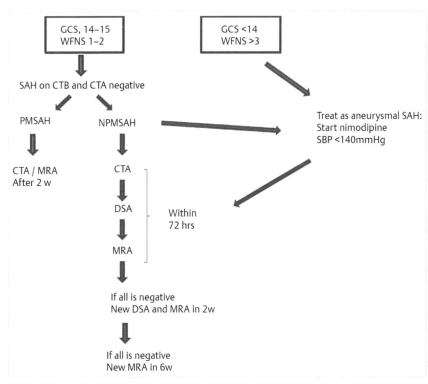

Fig. 10.2 Recommended treatment flow chart for the management of non-aneurysmal subarachnoid hemorrhages (CTA, computed tomography angiography; CTB, CT of the brain; DSA, digital subtraction angiography; GCS, Glasgow Coma Scale; MRA, magnetic resonance angiography; NPMSAH, non-PMSAH; PMSAH, perimesencephalic SAH; SAH, subarachnoid hemorrhage; SBP, systolic blood pressure; WFNS, World Federation of Neurosurgical Societies).

10.6 Authors' Recommendations

- Rather than using the term angionegative SAH, we recommend using either PMSAH or non-PMSAH as these two groups have a very different natural course and management options.
- The PMSAH group usually has a benign clinical course and a repeat DSA very seldom reveals a culprit intracranial aneurysm. Therefore, a repeat DSA may not be needed in case of PMSAH.
- In contrast, the non-PMSAH group appears to have an increased risk of complications, such as rebleeding, hydrocephalus, cerebral vasospasm, and a worse neurological outcome compared to the PMSAH group. Therefore, we recommend vascular imaging assessment including DSA in patients with a non-PMSAH pattern on initial imaging. If these imaging studies are negative, further investigation involving a new DSA and MRI/MRA of the cervical region should be performed within 2 weeks. If no diagnosis was identified on this imaging, a new MRI/A is recommended in 6 weeks.

References

[1] van Gijn J, van Dongen KJ, Vermeulen M, Hijdra A. Perimesencephalic hemorrhage: a nonaneurysmal and benign form of subarachnoid hemorrhage. Neurology. 1985; 35(4):493–497

[2] van Gijn J, Rinkel GJ. Subarachnoid haemorrhage: diagnosis, causes and management. Brain. 2001; 124(Pt 2):249–278

[3] Mohan M, Islim AI, Rasul FT, et al. British Neurosurgical Trainee Research Collaborative. Subarachnoid haemorrhage with negative initial neurovascular imaging: a systematic review and meta-analysis. Acta Neurochir (Wien). 2019; 161(10):2013–2026

[4] Rinkel GJ, Wijdicks EF, Vermeulen M, Hasan D, Brouwers PJ, van Gijn J. The clinical course of perimesencephalic nonaneurysmal subarachnoid hemorrhage. Ann Neurol. 1991; 29(5):463–468

[5] Goergen SK, Barrie D, Sacharias N, Waugh JR. Perimesencephalic subarachnoid haemorrhage: negative angiography and favourable prognosis. Australas Radiol. 1993; 37(2):156–160

[6] Van Calenbergh F, Plets C, Goffin J, Velghe L. Nonaneurysmal subarachnoid hemorrhage: prevalence of perimesencephalic hemorrhage in a consecutive series. Surg Neurol. 1993; 39(4):320–323

[7] Hütter BO, Gilsbach JM, Kreitschmann I. Is there a difference in cognitive deficits after aneurysmal subarachnoid haemorrhage and subarachnoid haemorrhage of unknown origin? Acta Neurochir (Wien). 1994; 127(3–4):129–135

[8] Canhão P, Ferro JM, Pinto AN, Melo TP, Campos JG. Perimesencephalic and nonperimesencephalic subarachnoid haemorrhages with negative angiograms. Acta Neurochir (Wien). 1995; 132(1–3):14–19

[9] Tatter SB, Crowell RM, Ogilvy CS. Aneurysmal and microaneurysmal "angiogram-negative" subarachnoid hemorrhage. Neurosurgery. 1995; 37(1):48–55

[10] Duong H, Melançon D, Tampieri D, Ethier R. The negative angiogram in subarachnoid haemorrhage. Neuroradiology. 1996; 38(1):15–19

[11] Berdoz D, Uske A, de Tribolet N. Subarachnoid haemorrhage of unknown cause: clinical, neuroradiological and evolutive aspects. J Clin Neurosci. 1998; 5(3):274–282

[12] Linn FH, Rinkel GJ, Algra A, van Gijn J. Headache characteristics in subarachnoid haemorrhage and benign thunderclap headache. J Neurol Neurosurg Psychiatry. 1998; 65(5):791–793

[13] Madureira S, Canhão P, Guerreiro M, Ferro JM. Cognitive and emotional consequences of perimesencephalic subarachnoid hemorrhage. J Neurol. 2000; 247(11):862–867

[14] Marquardt G, Niebauer T, Schick U, Lorenz R. Long term follow up after perimesencephalic subarachnoid haemorrhage. J Neurol Neurosurg Psychiatry. 2000; 69(1):127–130

[15] Franz G, Brenneis C, Kampfl A, Pfausler B, Poewe W, Schmutzhard E. Prognostic value of intraventricular blood in perimesencephalic nonaneurysmal subarachnoid hemorrhage. J Comput Assist Tomogr. 2001; 25(5):742–746

[16] Ildan F, Tuna M, Erman T, Göçer AI, Cetinalp E. Prognosis and prognostic factors in nonaneurysmal perimesencephalic hemorrhage: a follow-up study in 29 patients. Surg Neurol. 2002; 57(3):160–165, discussion 165–166

[17] Alén JF, Lagares A, Lobato RD, Gómez PA, Rivas JJ, Ramos A. Comparison between perimesencephalic nonaneurysmal subarachnoid hemorrhage and subarachnoid hemorrhage caused by posterior circulation aneurysms. J Neurosurg. 2003; 98(3):529–535

[18] Lang EW, Khodair A, Barth H, Hempelmann RG, Dorsch NWC, Mehdorn HM. Subarachnoid hemorrhage of unknown origin and the basilar artery configuration. J Clin Neurosci. 2003; 10(1):74–78

[19] Topcuoglu MA, Ogilvy CS, Carter BS, Buonanno FS, Koroshetz WJ, Singhal AB. Subarachnoid hemorrhage without evident cause on initial angiography studies: diagnostic yield of subsequent angiography and other neuroimaging tests. J Neurosurg. 2003; 98(6):1235–1240

[20] Caeiro L, Menger C, Ferro JM, Albuquerque R, Figueira ML. Delirium in acute subarachnoid haemorrhage. Cerebrovasc Dis. 2005; 19(1):31–38

[21] Jung JY, Kim YB, Lee JW, Huh SK, Lee KC. Spontaneous subarachnoid haemorrhage with negative initial angiography: a review of 143 cases. J Clin Neurosci. 2006; 13(10):1011–1017

[22] Matsuyama T, Okuchi K, Seki T, Higuchi T, Murao Y. Perimesencephalic nonaneurysmal subarachnoid hemorrhage caused by physical exertion. Neurol Med Chir (Tokyo). 2006; 46(6):277–281, discussion 281–282

[23] Andaluz N, Zuccarello M. Yield of further diagnostic work-up of cryptogenic subarachnoid hemorrhage based on bleeding patterns on computed tomographic scans. Neurosurgery. 2008; 62(5):1040–1046, discussion 1047

[24] Kang DH, Park J, Lee SH, Park SH, Kim YS, Hamm IS. Does non-perimesencephalic type non-aneurysmal subarachnoid hemorrhage have a benign prognosis? J Clin Neurosci. 2009; 16(7):904–908

[25] Whiting J, Reavey-Cantwell J, Velat G, et al. Clinical course of nontraumatic, nonaneurysmal subarachnoid hemorrhage: a single-institution experience. Neurosurg Focus. 2009; 26(5):E21

[26] Beseoglu K, Pannes S, Steiger HJ, Hänggi D. Long-term outcome and quality of life after nonaneurysmal subarachnoid hemorrhage. Acta Neurochir (Wien). 2010; 152(3):409–416

[27] Caeiro L, Santos CO, Ferro JM, Figueira ML. Neuropsychiatric disturbances in acute subarachnoid haemorrhage. Eur J Neurol. 2011; 18(6):857–864

[28] Nayak S, Kunz AB, Kieslinger K, Ladurner G, Killer M. Classification of non-aneurysmal subarachnoid haemorrhage: CT correlation to the clinical outcome. Clin Radiol. 2010; 65(8):623–628

[29] Alfieri A, Gazzeri R, Pircher M, Unterhuber V, Schwarz A. A prospective long-term study of return to work after nontraumatic nonaneurysmal subarachnoid hemorrhage. J Clin Neurosci. 2011; 18(11):1478–1480

[30] Fontanella M, Rainero I, Panciani PP, et al. Subarachnoid hemorrhage and negative angiography: clinical course and long-term follow-up. Neurosurg Rev. 2011; 34(4):477–484

[31] Kong Y, Zhang JH, Qin X. Perimesencephalic Subarachnoid Hemorrhage: Risk Factors, Clinical Presentations, and Outcome. Vienna: Springer; 2011:197–201

[32] Oda S, Shimoda M, Hoshikawa K, Osada T, Yoshiyama M, Matsumae M. Cortical subarachnoid hemorrhage caused by cerebral venous thrombosis. Neurol Med Chir (Tokyo). 2011; 51(1):30–36

[33] Pyysalo LM, Niskakangas TT, Keski-Nisula LH, Kähärä VJ, Öhman JE. Long term outcome after subarachnoid haemorrhage of unknown aetiology. J Neurol Neurosurg Psychiatry. 2011; 82(11):1264–1266

[34] Cánovas D, Gil A, Jato M, de Miquel M, Rubio F. Clinical outcome of spontaneous non-aneurysmal subarachnoid hemorrhage in 108 patients. Eur J Neurol. 2012; 19(3):457–461

[35] Delgado Almandoz JE, Jagadeesan BD, Refai D, et al. Diagnostic yield of computed tomography angiography and magnetic resonance angiography in patients with catheter angiography-negative subarachnoid hemorrhage. J Neurosurg. 2012; 117(2):309–315

[36] Gross BA, Lin N, Frerichs KU, Du R. Vasospasm after spontaneous angiographically negative subarachnoid hemorrhage. Acta Neurochir (Wien). 2012; 154(7):1127–1133

[37] Kostić A, Stojanov D, Stefanović I, et al. Complications after angiogram-negative subarachnoid haemorrhage: comparative study of pretruncal and nonpretruncal hemorrhage patients. Srp Arh Celok Lek. 2012; 140(1–2):8–13

[38] Lin N, Zenonos G, Kim AH, et al. Angiogram-negative subarachnoid hemorrhage: relationship between bleeding pattern and clinical outcome. Neurocrit Care. 2012; 16(3):389–398

[39] Maslehaty H, Petridis AK, Barth H, Mehdorn HM. Diagnostic value of magnetic resonance imaging in perimesencephalic and nonperimesencephalic subarachnoid hemorrhage of unknown origin. J Neurosurg. 2011; 114(4):1003–1007

[40] Yu D-W, Jung YJ, Choi BY, Chang CH. Subarachnoid hemorrhage with negative baseline digital subtraction angiography: is repeat digital subtraction angiography necessary? J Cerebrovasc Endovasc Neurosurg. 2012; 14(3):210–215

[41] Zhong W, Zhao P, Wang D, et al. Different clinical characteristics between perimesencephalic subarachnoid hemorrhage and diffuse subarachnoid hemorrhage with negative initial angiography. Turk Neurosurg. 2014; 24(3):327–332

[42] Boswell S, Thorell W, Gogela S, Lyden E, Surdell D. Angiogram-negative subarachnoid hemorrhage: outcomes data and review of the literature. J Stroke Cerebrovasc Dis. 2013; 22(6):750–757

[43] Dalyai R, Chalouhi N, Theofanis T, et al. Subarachnoid hemorrhage with negative initial catheter angiography: a review of 254 cases evaluating patient clinical outcome and efficacy of short- and long-term repeat angiography. Neurosurgery. 2013; 72(4):646–652, discussion 651–652

[44] Khan AA, Smith JDS, Kirkman MA, et al. Angiogram negative subarachnoid haemorrhage: outcomes and the role of repeat angiography. Clin Neurol Neurosurg. 2013; 115(8):1470–1475

[45] Muehlschlegel S, Kursun O, Topcuoglu MA, Fok J, Singhal AB. Differentiating reversible cerebral vasoconstriction syndrome with subarachnoid hemorrhage from other causes of subarachnoid hemorrhage. JAMA Neurol. 2013; 70(10):1254–1260

[46] Prat D, Goren O, Bruk B, Bakon M, Hadani M, Harnof S. Description of the vasospasm phenomena following perimesencephalic nonaneurysmal subarachnoid hemorrhage. BioMed Res Int. 2013; 2013(3):371063

[47] Tsermoulas G, Flett L, Gregson B, Mitchell P. Immediate coma and poor outcome in subarachnoid haemorrhage are independently associated with an aneurysmal origin. Clin Neurol Neurosurg. 2013; 115(8):1362–1365

[48] Woodfield J, Rane N, Cudlip S, Byrne JV. Value of delayed MRI in angiogram-negative subarachnoid haemorrhage. Clin Radiol. 2014; 69(4):350–356

[49] Ellis JA, McDowell MM, Mayer SA, Lavine SD, Meyers PM, Connolly ES, Jr. The role of antiplatelet medications in angiogram-negative subarachnoid hemorrhage. Neurosurgery. 2014; 75(5):530–535, discussion 534–535

[50] Konczalla J, Platz J, Schuss P, Vatter H, Seifert V, Güresir E. Non-aneurysmal non-traumatic subarachnoid hemorrhage: patient characteristics, clinical outcome and prognostic factors based on a single-center experience in 125 patients. BMC Neurol. 2014; 14(1):140

[51] Kumar R, Das KK, Sahu RK, et al. Angio negative spontaneous subarachnoid hemorrhage: Is repeat angiogram required in all cases? Surg Neurol Int. 2014; 5:125

[52] Mensing LA, Ruigrok YM, Greebe P, Vlak MHM, Algra A, Rinkel GJE. Risk factors in patients with perimesencephalic hemorrhage. Eur J Neurol. 2014; 21(6):816–819

[53] Qureshi AI, Jahangir N, Qureshi MH, et al. A population-based study of the incidence and case fatality of non-aneurysmal subarachnoid hemorrhage. Neurocrit Care. 2015; 22(3):409–413

[54] Canneti B, Mosqueira AJ, Nombela F, Gilo F, Vivancos J. Spontaneous subarachnoid hemorrhage with negative angiography managed in a stroke unit: clinical and prognostic characteristics. J Stroke Cerebrovasc Dis. 2015; 24(11):2484–2490

[55] Dalbjerg SM, Larsen CC, Romner B. Risk factors and short-term outcome in patients with angiographically negative subarachnoid hemorrhage. Clin Neurol Neurosurg. 2013; 115(8):1304–1307

[56] Konczalla J, Schuss P, Platz J, Vatter H, Seifert V, Güresir E. Clinical outcome and prognostic factors of patients with angiogram-negative and non-perimesencephalic subarachnoid hemorrhage: benign prognosis like perimesencephalic SAH or same risk as aneurysmal SAH? Neurosurg Rev. 2015; 38(1):121–127, discussion 127

[57] Konczalla J, Schmitz J, Kashefiolasl S, Senft C, Seifert V, Platz J. Non-aneurysmal subarachnoid hemorrhage in 173 patients: a prospective study of long-term outcome. Eur J Neurol. 2015; 22(10):1329–1336

[58] Sprenker C, Patel J, Camporesi E, et al. Medical and neurologic complications of the current management strategy of angiographically negative nontraumatic subarachnoid hemorrhage patients. J Crit Care. 2015; 30(1):216.e7–216.e11

[59] Walcott BP, Stapleton CJ, Koch MJ, Ogilvy CS. Diffuse patterns of nonaneurysmal subarachnoid hemorrhage originating from the Basal cisterns have predictable vasospasm rates similar to aneurysmal subarachnoid hemorrhage. J Stroke Cerebrovasc Dis. 2015; 24(4):795–801

[60] Konczalla J, Kashefiolasl S, Brawanski N, et al. Cerebral vasospasm and delayed cerebral infarctions in 225 patients with non-aneurysmal subarachnoid hemorrhage: the underestimated risk of Fisher 3 blood distribution. J Neurointerv Surg. 2016; 8(12):1247–1252

[61] Moscovici S, Fraifeld S, Ramirez-de-Noriega F, et al. Clinical relevance of negative initial angiogram in spontaneous subarachnoid hemorrhage. Neurol Res. 2013; 35(2):117–122

[62] Hui FK, Tumialán LM, Tanaka T, Cawley CM, Zhang YJ. Clinical differences between angiographically negative, diffuse subarachnoid hemorrhage and perimesencephalic subarachnoid hemorrhage. Neurocrit Care. 2009; 11 (1):64–70

[63] Geng B, Wu X, Brackett A, Malhotra A. Meta-analysis of recent literature on utility of follow-up imaging in isolated perimesencephalic hemorrhage. Clin Neurol Neurosurg. 2019; 180:111–116

[64] Heit JJ, Pastena GT, Nogueira RG, et al. Cerebral angiography for evaluation of patients with CT angiogram-negative subarachnoid hemorrhage: an 11-year experience. AJNR Am J Neuroradiol. 2016; 37(2): 297–304

[65] Delgado Almandoz JE, Kadkhodayan Y, Crandall BM, et al. Diagnostic yield of delayed neurovascular imaging in patients with subarachnoid hemorrhage, negative initial CT and catheter angiograms, and a negative 7 day repeat catheter angiogram. Journal of Neurointerventional Surgery 2014;6:637–64

[66] Yap, L, Dyde, RA, Hodgson, TJ, Patel, UI, and Coley, SC. Spontaneous subarachnoid hemorrhage and negative initial vascular imaging – should further investigation depend upon the pattern of hemorrhage on the presenting CT? Acta Neurochirurgica. 2015; 157(9), 1477-1484. https://doi.org/10.1007/S00701-015-2506-5

[67] Akcakaya MO, Aydoseli A, Aras Y, et al. Clinical course of non-traumatic non-aneurysmal subarachnoid hemorrhage: a single institution experience over 10 years and review of the contemporary literature. Turk Neurosurg. 2017;27(5):732–742

[68] Coelho LG, Costa JM, Silva EI. Non-aneurysmal spontaneous subarachnoid hemorrhage: perimesencephalic versus non-perimesencephalic. Hemorragia subaracnóidea espontânea não aneurismática: perimesencefálica versus não perimesencefálica. Rev Bras Ter Intensiva. 2016;28(2):141-146. doi:10.5935/0103-507X.20160028

[69] Mortimer AM, Appelman AP, Renowden SA. The negative predictive value of CT angiography in the setting of perimesencephalic subarachnoid hemorrhage. J Neurointerv Surg. 2016 Jul;8(7):728-31. doi: 10.1136/neurintsurg-2015-011814. Epub 2015 Jun 4. PMID: 26044985

[70] Potter CA, Fink KR, Ginn AL, Haynor DR. Perimesencephalic Hemorrhage: Yield of Single versus Multiple DSA Examinations-A Single-Center Study and Meta-Analysis. Radiology. 2016 Dec;281(3):858-864. doi: 10.1148/radiol.2016152402. Epub 2016 May 27. PMID: 27232640

[71] Sahin S, Delen E, Korfali E. Perimesencephalic subarachnoid hemorrhage: Etiologies, risk factors, and necessity of the second angiogram. Asian J Neurosurg. 2016;11(1):50-53. doi:10.4103/1793-5482.165793

[72] Song JP, Ni W, Gu YX, Zhu W, Chen L, Xu B, Leng B, Tian YL, Mao Y. Epidemiological Features of Nontraumatic Spontaneous Subarachnoid Hemorrhage in China: A Nationwide Hospital-based Multicenter Study. Chin Med J (Engl). 2017 Apr 5;130(7):776-781. doi: 10.4103/0366-6999.202729. PMID: 28345540; PMCID: PMC5381310

[73] Xu L, Fang Y, Shi X, et al. Management of Spontaneous Subarachnoid Hemorrhage Patients with Negative Initial Digital Subtraction Angiogram Findings: Conservative or Aggressive? Biomed Res Int. 2017;2017:2486859. doi:10.1155/2017/2486859

11 Natural History and Management Options of Low-Grade Glioma

Rebecca J. Limb, Cristian Gragnaniello, and Leon T. Lai

Abstract

This chapter aims to summarize the most up-to-date literature on the clinical management of low-grade glioma, including the impact of surgical resection and adjuvant therapies on patient survival. In recent years, emerging evidence has somewhat modified practice worldwide, and with the advent of detailed molecular characterization, predicting tumor behavior may allow better prognosis and better guidance for therapy.

Keywords: low-grade glioma, natural history, extent of resection, radiotherapy, chemotherapy

11.1 Introduction

Low-grade gliomas (LGGs) are World Health Organization (WHO) grade II glial series tumors and represent a heterogenous group of neoplasms with astrocytic, oligodendroglial, ependymal, or mixed cellular histology. Worldwide incidence in adults is estimated to be 0.26 to 0.75 per 100,000[3] and they account for approximately 15% of all brain tumors.[1] There is a slight male predominance and a biphasic age distribution with the first peak occurring during childhood (ages 6–12 years) and a second peak in adulthood (between the third and fifth decades). The median age of presentation in adults is 35 years.

With growing use of neuroimaging, incidental LGGs are increasingly being diagnosed, which poses significant management dilemmas for these asymptomatic patients. Symptomatic LGGs often present with partial or generalized seizures. It is thought that these tumors produce factors that either mimic glutamate or increase the circulating levels of glutamate, which is neuroexcitatory acting via alpha-amino-3-hydroxy-5-methyl-4-isoxazolepropionic acid (AMPA) and N-methyl-D-aspartate (NDMA) receptors. Most LGGs, and in particular diffuse astrocytoma (DA) and oligodendroglioma (OG), show a predilection for the supratentorial compartments, namely (in decreasing order of frequency) frontal, temporal, insula, parietal, and occipital lobes.

The prognosis for LGG is generally favorable compared to their high-grade counterpart, although in recent years a growing body of evidence suggests these pathologies are part of a continuous genetic and molecular spectrum, as opposed to separate disease entities (▶ Fig. 11.1). Long-term survival for LGGs ranges from 5 to 13 years depending on the histological and molecular tumor profile.[2]

11.2 Selected Papers on the Natural History of LGG

- Smits A, Jakola AS. Clinical presentation, natural history, and prognosis of diffuse low-grade gliomas. Neurosurg Clin N Am 2019;30(1):35–42[4]
- Opoku-Darko M, Eagles ME, Cadieux M, Isaacs AM, Kelly JJP. Natural history and growth patterns of incidentally discovered diffusely infiltrating low-grade gliomas: a volumetric study. World Neurosurg 2019;132:e133–e139
- Gui C, Kosteniuk SE, Lau JC, Megyesi JF. Tumor growth dynamics in serially-imaged low-grade glioma patients. J Neurooncol 2018;139(1):167–175
- Potts MB, Smith JS, Molinaro AM, Berger MS. Natural history and surgical management of incidentally discovered low-grade gliomas. J Neurosurg 2012;116(2):365–372

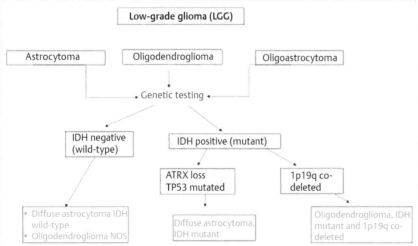

Fig. 11.1 Summary of WHO (2016) low-grade glioma classification pathway.[3] (IDH, isocitrate dehydrogenase; NOS, not otherwise specified.)

11.3 Natural History of Low-Grade Glioma

The natural history of LGG is not well characterized in the literature, in part owing to the lack of long-term observational studies and the propensity for treatment bias. Contemporary evidence suggests LGGs display an asymptomatic (silent) phase, during which time the tumor may grow slowly at an estimated rate of 2 to 4 mm/y.[5,7] This may then be followed by a symptomatic phase, characterized by seizures in 70 to 90%,[5] and finally, a progressive phase during which the tumor may grow exponentially.[6,7] At this point, increasing mass effect may be the main driver of neurological signs and symptoms, requiring surgical intervention to alleviate. The time periods between these stages are usually measured in years or months but are difficult to predict.[5] Clinically silent tumors are more likely to be of lower volume, located in less eloquent areas, and therefore have a better prognosis following treatment.[8]

Increasingly, molecular rather than histological characteristics are becoming valuable in predicting LGG behavior[3]:

- Isocitrate dehydrogenase 1 (IDH-1 and IDH-2) enzyme gene mutation absence, that is, "negative" status in LGG (the so-called wild-type variant) confers more aggressive clinical behavior and rapid tumor progression.
- In OG, the presence of chromosomal co-deletion of 1p/19q along with IDH-1 mutant (positive) status is associated with a less aggressive clinical course.
- Other molecular markers, such as ATRX mutation, TERT (upregulating) promoter mutation, TP53 mutation, and MGMT methylation status, are not required for diagnosis but are adjuncts in predicting clinical behavior. ATRX and TP53 inactivating mutations are found in the majority of LGGs, but their role in prognostication is complex and appears to be more relevant in combination with other molecular subtypes, for example, IDH mutations. Similarly, TERT promoter mutations in combination with IDH-negative (wild-type) status confer a worse prognosis in LGGs. MGMT methylation

is associated with improved tumor response to temozolomide (TMZ) chemotherapy, but its role in LGG prognostication is currently less clear than in high-grade gliomas (HGGs).[32]

Median long-term survival ranges from 10 to 15 years for grade 2 OG, and 6 to 8 years for DA (although this is heavily influenced by IDH-1 mutation status, and some estimates state median survival to be as high as 10 years in the presence of an IDH-1 mutation).

11.4 Rate of Progression to High-Grade Glioma

Rates of progression to HGG are difficult to quantify, as available observational data are confounded by the effect of treatment bias (▶ Table 11.1). However, malignant progression following treatment is heterogeneously reported and can be as high as 72% over a median follow-up of 8 years.[9] A more recent study reported a 17% transformation rate among 486 LGG patients over a median 5-year follow-up. However, treatment modalities were variable, ranging from observation only to radiotherapy alone, chemotherapy alone (TMZ), and a combination of postoperative radiotherapy and chemotherapy. Factors associated with malignant transformation (MT) were male sex, tumor size >5 cm, IDH-1 negative mutation status, IDH-1 mutation positive but 1p19q noncodeleted, and TMZ therapy.[10] Interestingly, few laboratory studies have correlated TMZ with increased rate of MT in LGG. This is thought to relate to hypermutation causing "selection pressure" on LGG cells, thereby enhancing the ability of more aggressive mutations to arise.[11] For this reason, TMZ chemotherapy in some centers is increasingly being reserved for tumors that have already undergone MT, and other chemotherapeutic agents (e.g., vincristine, nimustine, procarbazine, lomustine, or CCNU) are more favored for the treatment of "lower-risk" LGG tumors with a favorable molecular profile.[1,2] However, some centers still advocate the use of TMZ as a preferred first-line agent.[12] The role of greater extent of resection

Table 11.1 Summary of the literature on factors affecting malignant transformation in LGG [10,13,15,16,17,18,20,21,22,23,24,26]

Studies	Study type	Patients	FU (y)	MT rate (%)	Evidence level (NHMRC)
Ius et al[24]	Retro	190	4.7	32.6	IV
Jakola et al[26]	Pros	153	7.0	Biopsy + surveillance 56 Early resection 37	III
Gozé et al[23]	Retro	131	4.6	42.1	IV
Duffau[22]	Pros	16	11.0	0	IV
Leu et al[21]	Retro	210	20.0	33	IV
Murphy et al[20]	Retro	599	7.4	21	III-IV
Fukuya et al[17]	Pros	81	6.7	47	IV
Jansen et al[16]	Retro	110	10.5	65.5	IV
Kavouridis et al[13]	Retro	326	5.4	24.5	IV
Morshed et al[18]	Retro	26	5.2	34.6	III-IV
Tom et al[10]	Retro	486	5.3	17	IV
Jakola et al[15]	Retro	43	-	44	IV

Abbreviations: FU, follow-up; MT, malignant transformation; NHMRC, National Health and Medical Research Council; Pros, prospective; Retro, retrospective.

Note: Where information was missing or not studied, a blank space has been left.

(EOR) on malignant progression-free survival (MPFS) has also been extensively studied in recent years, and found overall to be associated with delayed time to malignant progression, as well as longer progression-free survival (PFS) and overall survival (OS).[13,14,16,17,19,20,21,23,25,26]

11.5 Selected Papers on the Treatment Outcomes of LGGs

- Ghaffari-Rafi A, Samandouras G. Effect of treatment modalities on progression-free survival and overall survival in molecularly subtyped WHO grade II diffuse gliomas: a systematic review. World Neurosurg 2020;133:366–380.e2
- Hervey-Jumper SL, Berger MS. Evidence for improving outcome through extent of resection. Neurosurg Clin N Am 2019;30(1):85–93
- Brown TJ, Bota DA, van Den Bent MJ, et al. Management of low-grade glioma: a systematic review and meta-analysis. Neurooncol Pract 2019;6(4):249–258
- Darlix A, Mandonnet E, Freyschlag CF, et al. Chemotherapy and diffuse low-grade gliomas: a survey within the European Low-Grade Glioma Network. Neurooncol Pract 2019;6(4):264–273
- Young JS, Gogos AJ, Morshed RA, Hervey-Jumper SL, Berger MS. Molecular characteristics of diffuse lower grade gliomas: what neurosurgeons need to know. Acta Neurochir (Wien) 2020;162(8):1929–1939
- Gogos AJ, Young JS, Pereira MP, et al. Surgical management of incidentally discovered low-grade gliomas. J Neurosurg 2020 (e-pub ahead of print). doi:10.3171/2020.6.JNS201296

11.6 Treatment Options

Management options for LGGs include radiological surveillance, biopsy, or surgical resection. Operative strategy may include partial resection (PR), subtotal resection (STR), or gross total resection (GTR), depending on tumor location and patient factors. Adjuvant therapy may follow after either biopsy or resection, in the form of fractionated or unfractionated radiotherapy, and chemotherapy separately or in combination. Predicting the natural history of an LGG based on its underlying molecular subtype is paramount in guiding clinical decision-making. The optimal management approach is not always clear and relies on a well-considered multidisciplinary neuro-oncological approach. Among these, EOR has been found to correlate with better survival rates.

11.6.1 Surveillance Alone

Close radiological surveillance, with 6-monthly magnetic resonance imaging (MRI) scans for the first few years, may be acceptable when a tumor is small, asymptomatic, and is located in an eloquent area. Such lesions are increasingly being discovered incidentally on neuroimaging. This management strategy is supported by some authors, and surgery is deferred until the patient experiences symptoms or has imaging findings suggestive of growth or high-grade transformation.[12] In the case of a low-risk lesion (e.g., suspected tectal plate glioma) that has

demonstrated radiological and clinical stability for more than a few years, an extended surveillance MRI scan interval of once every 1 to 2 years is appropriate.

11.6.2 Radical Surgical Resection

Studies published over the last several decades have demonstrated that in LGGs, significant improvements in OS, PFS, and delays in MT can be achieved with maximal safe resection (▶ Table 11.2).[1,13,14,16,17,19,20,21,23,24,25,26,36] In 2012, a landmark *JAMA* study demonstrated that maximal safe resection versus biopsy alone conferred a significant improvement in OS for LGGs.[26] A recent meta-analysis also demonstrated that GTR versus STR was associated with a significant survival benefit at 2, 5, and 10 years. However, the authors highlighted that the strength of this recommendation must be tempered by the low quality of the existing evidence (▶ Fig. 11.2).[1] A large case series published in 2020 of LGGs undergoing maximal safe resection indicated significantly greater EOR for incidental tumors, which translated into significantly improved OS.[36] In the cases where the lesion is easily surgically accessible and noneloquent, GTR should be considered. Surgical adjuncts that are becoming standard of care to maximize safe resection include electrocorticography (ECOG) to perform asleep motor mapping or awake surgery with speech and/or motor mapping. This requires specialized anesthetic and surgical teams, the availability of which is not universal worldwide. Other important adjuncts to maximize surgical resection include intraoperative imaging such as intraoperative MRI (iMRI) or ultrasound (▶ Table 11.3). One of the obvious disadvantages with iMRI is safety concerns, necessitating procedures that can add hours to a surgical case. In recent years, the technology surrounding navigated intraoperative ultrasound probes has advanced significantly, which circumvents any safety issues and allows real-time images via a hand-held device that is easy for the surgeon to use. It may be therefore that intraoperative ultrasound will replace intraoperative MRI as a tool to maximize EOR in the future.

11.6.3 Radiotherapy

In recent years, radiotherapy has become a key treatment consideration for LGG, as evidence has emerged demonstrating improved outcomes. The European Organization for Research and Treatment of Cancer (EORTC) 22845 randomized trial published in 2005 suggested that early radiotherapy following surgical resection (vs. delayed radiotherapy once progression was confirmed) was associated with improved PFS but not OS.[9] Similarly, a recent meta-analysis identified a PFS benefit at 2, 5, and 10 years with postoperative radiation (▶ Fig. 11.3).[1] Adverse effects of radiotherapy relate to radiotoxicity and the potential for neurocognitive side effects; therefore, the optimal timing of radiotherapy treatment for LGGs is not clear. Delaying radiotherapy treatment until tumor progression does not negatively impact on OS, but it may affect PFS. Recent evidence suggests that moderate dose radiation (45–55 Gy) appears to be as effective as higher-dose radiation (59–65 Gy) and decreases the risk of radiation toxicity without compromising on efficacy.[1]

Table 11.2 Summary of the literature on the relationship between EOR and survival in LGG[10,13,15,16,17,18,20,21,22,23,24,26]

Studies	EOR (%)	5-y OS (%)	5-y PFS (%)	OS and PFS (y)	Association between unfavorable molecular subtypes/histological subtypes and MT	Study conclusion(s)	Evidence level (NHMRC)
Ius et al[24]	79–91	80.0%	59.0%	–	–	OS improved by EOR	IV
Jakola et al[26]	–	60.0% (biopsy) 74.0% (resection)	–	–	–	Early surgical resection associated with better OS	III
Gozé et al[23]	STR: 37.0 GTR: 14.0 biopsy/PR: 14.0	82%	–	–	Yes	Tumor expansion rate and IDH-1 mutation are independent predictors of MT	IV
Duffau[22]	>100.0	100%	50.0%	–	–	Supratotal resection may reduce MT	IV
Leu et al[21]	–	–	–	4.8 IDH⁻ 11 IDH⁺	Yes	Molecular markers impact on MT and OS	IV
Murphy et al[20]	GTR: 35.0 NTR: 6.0 STR: 22.0 Biopsy: 34.0 Other: 3.0	75% (with MT) 87% (without MT)	30% with MT 60% without MT		Yes	Older age, male sex, chemotherapy alone and multifocality were predictive for MT	III–IV
Fukuya et al[17]	90.0		–	PFS: 3.3 OS: 12.6	Yes	IDH: LGG prone to early progression Greater EOR: more favorable patterns of recurrence	IV
Jansen et al[16]	GTR: 52.7 STR: 25.5 Biopsy: 21.8	88.0%	38.0%		Yes	Molecular profile strongest predictor of progression Greater EOR increases time to progression and MT	IV
Kavouridis et al[13]	77.8	88.3%	30.0%		Yes	EOR affects survival and MT, more so in IDH⁻ and IDH⁺ astrocytoma	IV
Morshed et al[18]	75.4	–	–	PFS: 2.0 OS: 5.2	Yes	Association between greater age and unfavorable LGG mutations, shorter PFS	III-IV
Tom et al[10]	GTR: 42.0 STR: 21.0 Biopsy: 33.0 unknown: 4.0	82.0%	86.0%		Yes	TMZ associated with higher rates of MT	IV
Jakola et al[15]	–	–	–		Yes	MT occurs locally in >90%	IV

Abbreviations: EOR, extent of resection; GTR, gross total resection; LGG, low-grade glioma; MT, malignant transformation; NHMRC, National Health and Medical Research Council; OS, overall survival; NTR, near-total resection; PFS, progression-free survival; PR, partial resection; STR, subtotal resection; TMZ, temozolomide therapy.
Note: Where information was missing or not studied, a blank space has been left.

11.6.4 Chemotherapy

The role of chemotherapy is less clear in the treatment of LGG, mainly due to the lack of standardized chemotherapeutic regimens in the literature. However, there is some evidence to suggest it may confer significant survival benefit when combined with radiotherapy as an adjuvant treatment. Any potential survival benefit, however, must be weighed against the risk of toxicity, particularly with alkylating chemotherapy regimens, that is, procarbazine, CCNU, and vincristine (PCV). A recent randomized controlled trial (RCT)[2] reported a 5.5-year median OS and PFS benefit in LGG patients undergoing postoperative radiotherapy plus PCV chemotherapy versus radiotherapy alone. This treatment benefit was observed to be greatest in OG or oligoastrocytoma patients, and those with an IDH-1 mutation.[2] Additional evidence is provided by the Radiation Therapy Oncology Group (RTOG) 9802 study, which demonstrated that in LGG patients older than 40 years or who have undergone STR, radiotherapy plus PCV chemotherapy significantly improves OS and PFS compared to radiotherapy alone. However, molecular

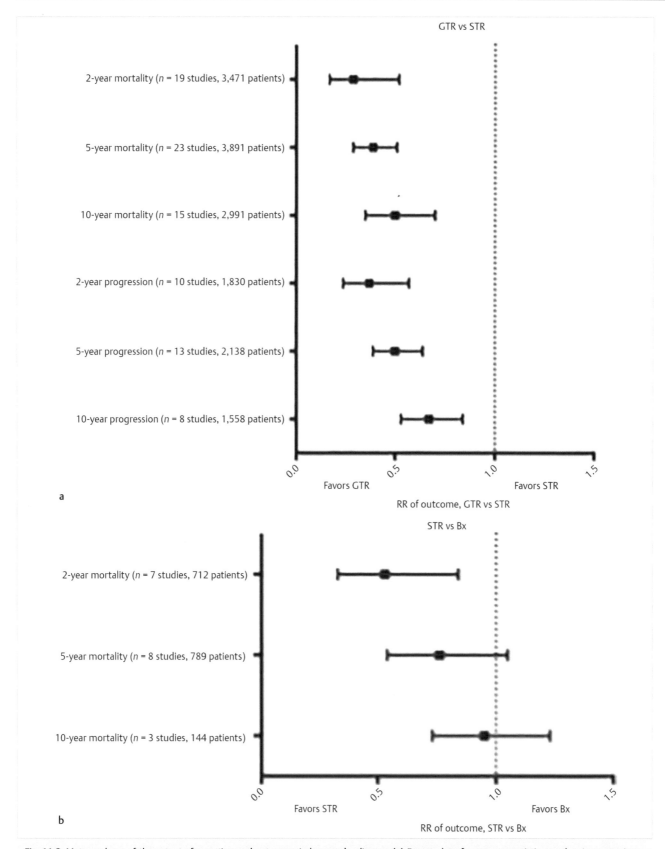

Fig. 11.2 Meta-analyses of the extent of resection and outcomes in low-grade gliomas. **(a)** Forest plot of summary statistics on the six comparisons regarding outcomes of patients who received gross total resection (GTR) compared to those who received subtotal resection (STR). Values plotted are relative risks (RR) with 95% confidence intervals. Summary statistics that do not cross X = 1 indicate a benefit favoring GTR over STR. **(b)** Forest plot of summary statistics of STR versus biopsy (Bx). (Adapted from Brown et al.[1] by permission of the Oxford University Press.)

Table 11.3 Summary of evidence-based surgical adjuncts maximizing EOR[33,34,35]

Surgical adjunct	Benefits	Disadvantages
iMRI[33]	Accurate radiological assessment (FLAIR sequence for LGG)	Increased operative time Not universally available Expensive Safety concerns
Awake surgery and/or ECOG[34]	Early recognition and avoidance of deficit Lower cost than iMRI and iUSS	Patient tolerance Anesthetic considerations Not 100% effective in preventing permanent deficit
iUSS[35]	Real-time tumor data No significant safety risk Lower cost than iMRI	Not universally available Specialist hardware and software required

Abbreviations: ECOG, electrocorticography; EOR, extent of resection; FLAIR, fluid-attenuated inversion recovery; iMRI, intraoperative MRI; iUSS, intraoperative ultrasound.

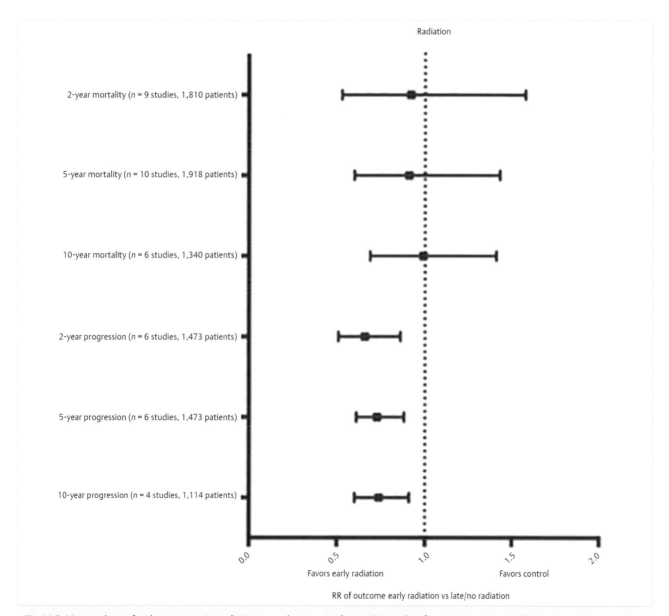

Fig. 11.3 Meta-analyses of early postoperative radiation versus late or no radiation. Forest plot of summary statistics on the six comparisons regarding outcomes of patients who received early postoperative radiation compared to those who received late or no radiation. Values plotted are relative risks (RR) with 95% confidence intervals. Summary statistics that do not cross X = 1 indicate a benefit favoring early radiation over late or no radiation. (Adapted from Brown et al.[1] by permission of the Oxford University Press.)

features such as IDH mutation or 1p19q codeletion status were not considered in this study.[27] A recent meta-analysis also demonstrated a 5- and 10-year survival benefit with the addition of adjuvant chemotherapy with radiotherapy versus radiotherapy alone (▶ Fig. 11.4).[1] It has previously been reported that presence of an IDH-1 mutation has been associated with improved response to radiotherapy combined with chemotherapy in grade 2 glioma.[28] The EORTC 22033 study highlighted the importance of molecular diagnostics in the characterization of LGGs and suggested a possible survival benefit in giving chemotherapy alone as initial therapy for IDH-1 mutated and 1p19q codeleted low-grade gliomas. However, this was nonsuperior to treatment with radiotherapy alone.[29]

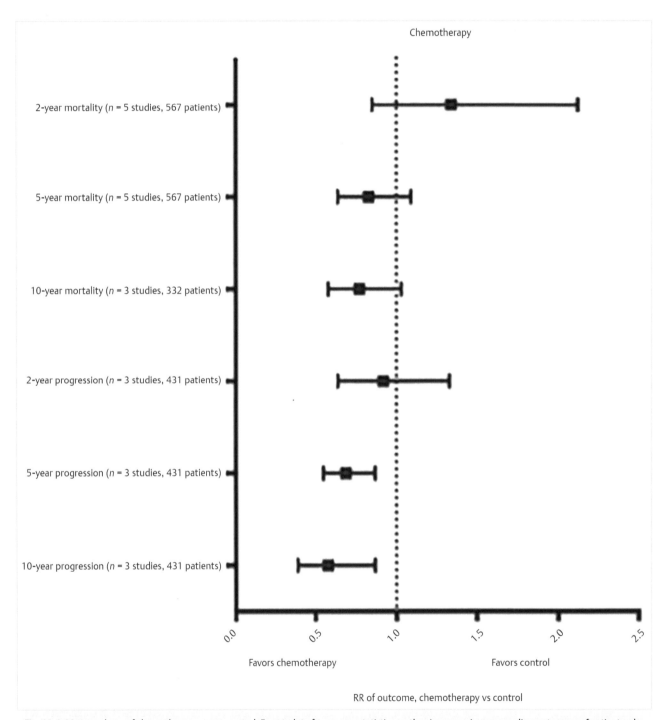

Fig. 11.4 Meta-analyses of chemotherapy versus control. Forest plot of summary statistics on the six comparisons regarding outcomes of patients who received chemotherapy. Values plotted are relative risks (RR) with 95% confidence intervals. Summary statistics that do not cross X = 1 indicate a benefit favoring chemotherapy. (Adapted from Brown et al.[1] by permission of the Oxford University Press.)

11.7 Prognostication

The EORTC and RTOG have both independently developed prognostic scores to identify risk factors and aid clinicians.[30] High-risk patients according to the EORTC (Pignatti) score are those aged ≥ 40 years, histological finding of astrocytoma, presence of neurological deficits before surgery, tumor diameter of ≥ 6 cm, and tumor crossing the midline (▶ Table 11.4). The authors categorized patients either as low risk in the presence of zero to two factors or high risk when three to five factors were present, and the OS was 7.80 versus 3.67 years for low- and high-risk patients, respectively (▶ Table 11.4).[31] The RTOG score considers only two clinical factors: age ≥ 40 years and an STR of the tumor, both of which independently denote "high-risk" LGG status.

A later meta-analysis in 2019 identified that maximum tumor diameter > 5 cm, eloquent tumor location, lack of an IDH mutation (wild-type status), lack of 1p19q codeletion, and a Karnofsky Performance Scale (KPS) ≤ 80% either before or after surgery are associated with poorer OS and may guide decision-making regarding adjuvant therapies.[1] Molecular profiles of LGGs are becoming increasingly important with regard to prognostication.[32]

Table 11.4 Pignatti (EORTC) Score for prognostication in low-grade glioma

Criterion	Points (Yes/No)	0-2 Points = Low Risk: Median Survival 7.8 yrs 3-5 Points = High Risk: Median Survival 3.7 yrs
Age ≥ 40	1/10	
Astrocytoma histology	1/10	
Maximum diameter ≥ 6 cm	1/10	
Tumor crossing midline	1/10	
Neurological deficit pre-op	1/10	

Source: Modified from Pignatti et al.[31]

11.8 Authors' Recommendations (▶ Fig. 11.5)

- LGGs display three phases of natural history (silent, symptomatic, and growth). Therefore, consideration needs to be given to which of these phases patients present with to guide clinical recommendations.
- A well-considered multidisciplinary neuro-oncological team approach is necessary to optimize treatment outcomes.
- EOR has been found to correlate with better survival rates. Therefore, intraoperative adjuncts should be used to optimize resection margins.
- Consideration of adjuvant chemoradiotherapy tailored to the molecular characteristics of the tumor, stratifying patients into "high-risk" or "low-risk" LGG group.
- Close monitoring with serial MRI scans on a 6- to 12-monthly basis, with the expectation that progression and possible MT will eventuate.

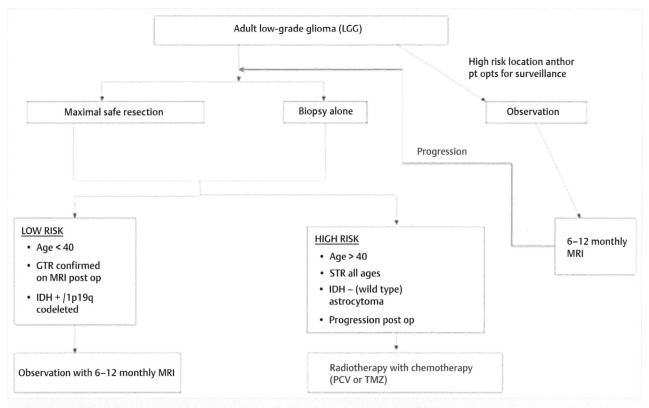

Fig. 11.5 Authors' proposed treatment algorithm for the management of low-grade glioma (LGG).

References

[1] Brown TJ, Bota DA, van Den Bent MJ, et al. Management of low-grade glioma: a systematic review and meta-analysis. Neurooncol Pract. 2019; 6(4):249–258

[2] Buckner JC, Shaw EG, Pugh SL, et al. Radiation plus procarbazine, CCNU, and vincristine in low-grade glioma. N Engl J Med. 2016; 374(14):1344–1355

[3] Louis DN, Ohgaki H, Wiestler OD, et al. WHO Classification of Tumours of the Central Nervous System. 4th ed. Lyon: IARC; 2016

[4] Xiao J, Jin Y, Nie J, Chen F, Ma X. Diagnostic and grading accuracy of 18F-FDOPA PET and PET/CT in patients with gliomas: a systematic review and meta-analysis. BMC Cancer. 2019; 19(1):767

[5] Smits A, Jakola AS. Clinical presentation, natural history, and prognosis of diffuse low-grade gliomas. Neurosurg Clin N Am. 2019; 30(1):35–42

[6] Opoku-Darko M, Eagles ME, Cadieux M, Isaacs AM, Kelly JJP. Natural history and growth patterns of incidentally discovered diffusely infiltrating low-grade gliomas: a volumetric study. World Neurosurg. 2019; 132:e133–e139

[7] Gui C, Kosteniuk SE, Lau JC, Megyesi JF. Tumor growth dynamics in serially-imaged low-grade glioma patients. J Neurooncol. 2018; 139(1):167–175

[8] Potts MB, Smith JS, Molinaro AM, Berger MS. Natural history and surgical management of incidentally discovered low-grade gliomas. J Neurosurg. 2012; 116(2):365–372

[9] van den Bent MJ, Afra D, de Witte O, et al. EORTC Radiotherapy and Brain Tumor Groups and the UK Medical Research Council. Long-term efficacy of early versus delayed radiotherapy for low-grade astrocytoma and oligodendroglioma in adults: the EORTC 22845 randomised trial. Lancet. 2005; 366(9490):985–990

[10] Tom MC, Park DYJ, Yang K, et al. Malignant transformation of molecularly classified adult low-grade glioma. Int J Radiat Oncol Biol Phys. 2019; 105(5):1106–1112

[11] Johnson BE, Mazor T, Hong C, et al. Mutational analysis reveals the origin and therapy-driven evolution of recurrent glioma. Science. 2014; 343(6167):189–193

[12] Darlix A, Mandonnet E, Freyschlag CF, et al. Chemotherapy and diffuse low-grade gliomas: a survey within the European Low-Grade Glioma Network. Neurooncol Pract. 2019; 6(4):264–273

[13] Kavouridis VK, Boaro A, Dorr J, et al. Contemporary assessment of extent of resection in molecularly defined categories of diffuse low-grade glioma: a volumetric analysis. J Neurosurg. 2020; 133(5):1291–1301

[14] Hervey-Jumper SL, Berger MS. Evidence for improving outcome through extent of resection. Neurosurg Clin N Am. 2019; 30(1):85–93

[15] Jakola AS, Bouget D, Reinertsen I, et al. Spatial distribution of malignant transformation in patients with low-grade glioma. J Neurooncol. 2020; 146(2):373–380

[16] Jansen E, Hamisch C, Ruess D, et al. Observation after surgery for low grade glioma: long-term outcome in the light of the 2016 WHO classification. J Neurooncol. 2019; 145(3):501–507

[17] Fukuya Y, Ikuta S, Maruyama T, et al. Tumor recurrence patterns after surgical resection of intracranial low-grade gliomas. J Neurooncol. 2019; 144(3):519–528

[18] Morshed RA, Han SJ, Hervey-Jumper SL, et al. Molecular features and clinical outcomes in surgically treated low-grade diffuse gliomas in patients over the age of 60. J Neurooncol. 2019; 141(2):383–391

[19] Yang K, Nath S, Koziarz A, et al. Biopsy versus subtotal versus gross total resection in patients with low-grade glioma: a systematic review and meta-analysis. World Neurosurg. 2018; 120:e762–e775

[20] Murphy ES, Leyrer CM, Parsons M, et al. Risk factors for malignant transformation of low-grade glioma. Int J Radiat Oncol Biol Phys. 2018; 100(4):965–971

[21] Leu S, von Felten S, Frank S, Boulay JL, Mariani L. IDH mutation is associated with higher risk of malignant transformation in low-grade glioma. J Neurooncol. 2016; 127(2):363–372

[22] Duffau H. Long-term outcomes after supratotal resection of diffuse low-grade gliomas: a consecutive series with 11-year follow-up. Acta Neurochir (Wien). 2016; 158(1):51–58

[23] Gozé C, Blonski M, Le Maistre G, et al. Imaging growth and isocitrate dehydrogenase 1 mutation are independent predictors for diffuse low-grade gliomas. Neuro-oncol. 2014; 16(8):1100–1109

[24] Ius T, Isola M, Budai R, et al. Low-grade glioma surgery in eloquent areas: volumetric analysis of extent of resection and its impact on overall survival. A single-institution experience in 190 patients: clinical article. J Neurosurg. 2012; 117(6):1039–1052

[25] Ghaffari-Rafi A, Samandouras G. Effect of treatment modalities on progression-free survival and overall survival in molecularly subtyped WHO grade II diffuse gliomas: a systematic review. World Neurosurg. 2020; 133:366–380.e2

[26] Jakola AS, Myrmel KS, Kloster R, et al. Comparison of a strategy favoring early surgical resection vs a strategy favoring watchful waiting in low-grade gliomas. JAMA. 2012; 308(18):1881–1888

[27] Buckner JC, Pugh SL, Shaw EG, et al. Phase III study of radiation therapy (RT) with or without procarbazine, CCNU, and vincristine (PCV) in low-grade glioma: RTOG 9802 with alliance, ECOG, and SWOG. J Clin Oncol. 2014; 32(15_suppl):2000

[28] Okita Y, Narita Y, Miyakita Y, et al. IDH1/2 mutation is a prognostic marker for survival and predicts response to chemotherapy for grade II gliomas concomitantly treated with radiation therapy. Int J Oncol. 2012; 41(4):1325–1336

[29] Baumert BG, Hegi ME, van den Bent MJ, et al. Temozolamide chemotherapy versus radiotherapy in high-risk low-grade glioma (EORTC 22033–26033): a randomised, open-label, phase 3 intergroup study. Lancet Oncol. 2016; 17(11):1521–1532

[30] Lanese A, Franceschi E, Brandes AA. The risk assessment in low-grade gliomas: an analysis of the European Organization for Research and Treatment of Cancer (EORTC) and the Radiation Therapy Oncology Group (RTOG) criteria. Oncol Ther. 2018; 6(2):105–108

[31] Pignatti F, van den Bent M, Curran D, et al. European Organization for Research and Treatment of Cancer Brain Tumor Cooperative Group, European Organization for Research and Treatment of Cancer Radiotherapy Cooperative Group. Prognostic factors for survival in adult patients with cerebral low-grade glioma. J Clin Oncol. 2002; 20(8):2076–2084

[32] Young JS, Gogos AJ, Morshed RA, Hervey-Jumper SL, Berger MS. Molecular characteristics of diffuse lower grade gliomas: what neurosurgeons need to know. Acta Neurochir (Wien). 2020; 162(8):1929–1939

[33] Yahanda AT, Patel B, Shah AS, et al. Impact of intraoperative magnetic resonance imaging and other factors on surgical outcomes for newly diagnosed grade II astrocytomas and oligodendrogliomas: a multicenter study. Neurosurgery. 2020; 88(1):63–73

[34] Szelényi A, Bello L, Duffau H, et al. Workgroup for Intraoperative Management in Low-Grade Glioma Surgery within the European Low-Grade Glioma Network. Intraoperative electrical stimulation in awake craniotomy: methodological aspects of current practice. Neurosurg Focus. 2010; 28(2):E7

[35] Bø HK, Solheim O, Kvistad KA, et al. Intraoperative 3D ultrasound-guided resection of diffuse low-grade gliomas: radiological and clinical results. J Neurosurg. 2019; 132(2):518–529

[36] Gogos AJ, Young JS, Pereira MP, et al. Surgical management of incidentally discovered low-grade gliomas. J Neurosurg. 2020 Oct 2:1-8. doi: 10.3171/2020.6.JNS201296. Epub ahead of print. PMID: 33007758

12 Natural History and Management Options of Nonfunctional Pituitary Adenoma

Vincent Dodson, Neil Majmundar, Wayne D. Hsueh, Jean Anderson Eloy, and James K. Liu

Abstract

Nonfunctional pituitary adenomas are "benign" neoplasms of the pituitary gland which may cause mass effect upon the surrounding neurovascular structures. Symptoms include headaches, visual field defects, and potentially pituitary hormonal disturbances secondary to compression of the pituitary gland and/or stalk. Routine work-up for patients with these lesions includes laboratory testing (including pituitary hormone levels), preoperative visual field testing, and advanced imaging (CT head and MRI brain). Treatment options include endoscopic endonasal transsphenoidal surgery and radiosurgery.

Keywords: pituitary tumor, pituitary adenoma, nonfuctioning pituitary adenoma, transphenoidal, endoscopic endonasal, radiosurgery

12.1 Introduction

Pituitary adenomas are benign neoplasms of the pituitary gland, which can cause mass effect upon surrounding neurovascular structures. The prevalence ranges between 14 and 54%, with equal distribution between genders and age groups.[1,2] Pituitary adenomas may be functional (actively hormone secreting) or nonfunctional (inactive). The symptoms exhibited by functional pituitary adenomas are directly associated with the hormone being secreted. Nonfunctional pituitary adenomas (NFPAs) are often asymptomatic or demonstrate symptoms secondary to mass effect (▶ Fig. 12.1), which includes headaches and visual field defects from optic chiasm compression.[3] NFPAs may also cause hypopituitarism as a result of compression of the pituitary gland and stalk, which can result in hypogonadal symptoms such as loss of libido, oligomenorrhea, and erectile dysfunction.[4]

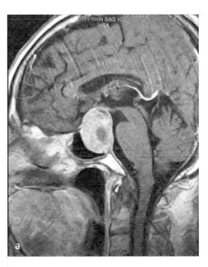
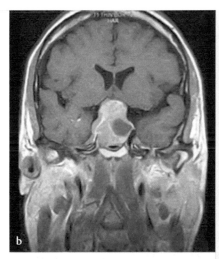
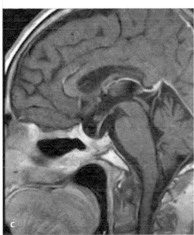
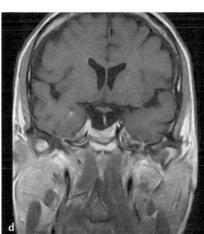

Fig. 12.1 (a) Sagittal and (b) coronal views of preoperative postgadolinium T1-weighted magnetic resonance imaging (MRI) of a nonfunctioning pituitary adenoma with suprasellar extension causing bitemporal hemianopsia due to optic chiasm compression. The patient was also presented with lower than normal baseline cortisol levels. The tumor was completely removed via an endoscopic endonasal transsphenoidal approach with preservation of the pituitary gland and stalk. (c) Sagittal and (d) coronal views of postoperative postgadolinium T1-weighted MRI showing complete removal without residual tumor. The optic chiasm is decompressed and well visualized.

12.2 Selected Papers on the Natural History of NFPAs

- Imran SA, Yip C-E, Papneja N, et al. Analysis and natural history of pituitary incidentalomas. Eur J Endocrinol 2016;175(1):1–9
- Fernández-Balsells MM, Murad MH, Barwise A, et al. Natural history of nonfunctioning pituitary adenomas and incidentalomas: a systematic review and metaanalysis. J Clin Endocrinol Metab 2011;96(4):905–912

12.3 Natural History of NFPAs

Patients with NFPAs most commonly present with headaches or symptoms related to pituitary dysfunction, typically hypogonadism.[6] Most discovered NFPAs are greater than 10 mm as these are more likely to be symptomatic.[5] NFPAs may be further classified by their size. Tumors less than 10 mm are referred to as microadenomas and tumors greater than 10 mm are referred to as macroadenomas. While studies examining the natural course of untreated NFPAs are scarce, macroadenomas are more likely to exhibit tumor growth and complications.[6]

Growth rates of NFPAs can vary widely, with most NFPAs either increasing in size or remaining the same size. While many patients who are found to have growth of their NFPAs may remain asymptomatic, they may experience symptoms secondary to mass effect upon the local neurovascular structures. These symptoms include visual field deficits secondary to compression of the optic apparatus, hypopituitarism secondary to mass effect on the gland or stalk, and pituitary apoplexy secondary to intratumoral hemorrhage and/or infarction. While hypopituitarism may be associated with tumor growth, Imran et al found that the presentation of secondary hormonal deficiency was not related to initial size of the NFPA at presentation, and most nonsurgical patients (88%) experienced no change in their secondary hormonal deficiency on follow-up.[5]

Pituitary apoplexy, although rare, is the most serious complication that can lead to ophthalmoplegia and vision loss. Fernández-Balsells et al found in their meta-analysis that the incidence of pituitary apoplexy is 0.2 per 100 person-years.[6] Treatment with hormone analogs is a risk factor for developing apoplexy as the analogs can abruptly cause an increase in metabolic activity and subsequent tumor infarction.[7] Multiple retrospective studies of patients with pituitary adenomas found that having an NFPA was a risk factor among several others for pituitary apoplexy.[8,9,10] Another exceedingly rare sequela of NFPAs is the malignant transformation to nonfunctioning pituitary carcinomas. Prognosis of this condition is generally poor, and the pathogenesis of the malignant transformation of NFPAs is not well understood.[11]

Although all risk factors for the growth of NFPAs are not well understood, a retrospective study found that NFPAs have a higher risk of enlargement compared to nonpituitary sellar masses, such as Rathke's cleft cysts, craniopharyngiomas, and meningiomas.[5] Among NFPAs, macroadenomas are also at a higher risk of growth than microadenomas.[6,12] Furthermore, age may play a role in the rate of tumor growth.[13] Watts et al found in their retrospective analysis of surgically treated patients with NFPAs that age was a significant risk factor for tumor regrowth, with younger patients more likely to experience a higher rate of regrowth. Their study found for every year older a patient was at presentation, there was an associated 3% reduction in regrowth rate. When patients were grouped by age, they found that patients who were ≤41 years old had a 4.2 times higher regrowth rate than patients who were ≥41 years old.[13] Remission after surgery is also lowest in patients with NFPAs compared to patients with functioning adenomas, perhaps because they are more likely discovered when they have become too big to make curative surgery a possibility.[14]

12.4 Selected Papers on the Management Options of NFPAs

- Lucas JW, Bodach ME, Tumialan LM, et al. Congress of neurological surgeons systematic review and evidence-based guideline on primary management of patients with nonfunctioning pituitary adenomas. Neurosurgery 2016;79(4):E533–E535
- Kuo JS, Barkhoudarian G, Farrell CJ, et al. Congress of neurological surgeons systematic review and evidence-based guideline on surgical techniques and technologies for the management of patients with nonfunctioning pituitary adenomas. Neurosurgery 2016;79(4):E536–E538

12.5 Management Options

12.5.1 Endocrine Evaluation

The first step in evaluating a pituitary adenoma is to determine whether it is a functioning or a nonfunctioning adenoma. This step is critical in determining whether the pituitary adenoma is a prolactinoma, as prolactinomas can be treated medically in most cases, whereas NFPAs are more often treated surgically.[17] Given that the development of secondary hormonal deficiency is a common complication in patients presenting with NFPAs, these patients should receive routine endocrine evaluation. NFPAs may cause hyperprolactinemia by causing compression of the pituitary stalk disrupting dopamine release. While no specific cutoff exists for serum prolactin levels to make the distinction between prolactinomas and NFPAs, patients with prolactinomas generally have higher levels of serum prolactin than those with NFPAs and concomitant hyperprolactinemia. Hong et al found that patients with NFPAs and concomitant hyperprolactinemia generally have serum prolactin levels less than 100 ng/mL.[18]

In addition to potentially causing hyperprolactinemia, NFPAs may also cause deficiencies of anterior pituitary function. Growth hormone deficiency, central hypothyroidism, central hypogonadism, and adrenal insufficiency have all been reported as possible sequelae of NFPAs. As the prevalence of these deficiencies is common in patients with NFPAs, routine endocrine axis testing is indicated for newly diagnosed patients and during follow-up.

12.5.2 Ophthalmologic Evaluation

The preoperative assessment of vision in patients with NFPAs can be helpful in tracking postoperative visual improvement. Visual testing is particularly important in older patients, as visual symptoms may go unnoticed in this age group.[19] Earlier detection of visual deficits can help preserve visual function after surgery. While visual field testing can assess the degree of impairment caused by the NFPA and track postoperative visual recovery, its use as a prognostic factor for predicting postoperative visual function is less understood. Optic atrophy detected by funduscopy was identified by Schmalisch et al as a prognostic factor. They found that among patients who exhibited chiasmal syndrome prior to surgery, those without optic atrophy on preoperative evaluation had a visual improvement rate of 81.6%, whereas those with unilateral or bilateral optic atrophy improved at a rate of 66.7 and 57.1%, respectively.[20] Although further studies need to be conducted to assess the prognostic value of preoperative visual testing, it is nonetheless important for tracking postoperative visual improvement.

12.5.3 Surgery

Surgery is the most studied intervention for NFPAs. Multiple retrospective studies have demonstrated that surgery is both safe and effective. However, the literature is less clear on which patients should receive surgery. Studies that have examined the natural history of NFPAs based the decision to operate upon clinical presentation. In the study by Imran et al, indications for surgical intervention included impaired vision, radiographic evidence of tumor growth, or contact of the tumor with the optic chiasm.[5] Even when there is no contact of the tumor with the optic apparatus, surgery may still be an option. Dekkers et al recommend that the decision to operate should be individualized, and the factors that should guide this decision include age of the patient, distance between the tumor and the optic apparatus, fertility status, and patient preference.[21]

Although the guidelines for surgical management of NFPAs are not clear, the benefits of surgery are well documented. In a series of 114 patients with NFPAs, Berkmann et al reported that 42 of 83 patients (50.6%) recovered endocrine function, 64 of 68 patients (94.1%) improved initial visual field deficits, and 55 of 59 patients (93.2%) improved initial visual acuity deficits.[22] Dehdashti et al found that of the 80 patients who had visual problems and were subsequently treated with endoscopic transsphenoidal surgery; in their study, 89% of the patients experienced either total or partial visual improvement.[23] Fleseriu et al demonstrated that the surgical removal of NFPAs resulted in the resolution or improvement of headache in 12 of 15 patients.[24] Compared to the resolution of other symptoms, the recovery of secondary hormonal deficiency is not as robust after surgery. Imran et al found that from the NFPA patients who underwent surgery, 71% experienced no change in their secondary hormonal deficiency status.[5]

The options for surgical approach for resection of NFPAs are microsurgical or endoscopic transsphenoidal surgery.[16] Both options are safe and comparable in efficacy, though minor differences in clinical outcome and complications have been observed in some studies. Dallapiazza et al found that although both approaches are comparable in extent of tumor resection, microsurgery more often requires the use of a lumbar drain postoperatively.[25] The endoscopic technique can be successfully implemented via the endonasal transsphenoidal approach. Several studies have demonstrated that the endoscopic approach can achieve gross total resection in the majority of cases.[23,26,27]

12.5.4 Radiation Therapy

Although Gamma Knife treatment plays a role in the treatment of NFPAs, it does not seem to be as effective in treating NFPAs as it is for hormone-secreting pituitary adenomas.[28] Losa et al found that the recurrence rate after adjuvant Gamma Knife surgery treatment was 9.6% in patients with NFPAs compared to 4.8% in patients with hormone-secreting adenomas. Furthermore, the 10-year progression-free survival rate was 78.7% in patients with NFPAs and 93.3% in patients with hormone-secreting adenomas.[28]

Several other studies have demonstrated that Gamma Knife surgery is a safe and effective form of initial treatment of NFPAs.[29,30,31] In general, Gamma Knife surgery is reserved for patients for whom surgery would pose significant risk. Target lesions for Gamma Knife therapy should also be smaller than 3 cm, and the distance from critical neurological structures such as the optic chiasm should exceed 2 mm.[28] Park et al utilized Gamma Knife as primary treatment for 15 patients with advanced age or significant surgical risk, and achieved tumor reduction in 9 patients.[31] Lee et al found that in similar patients for whom Gamma Knife surgery was used as initial therapy, control of tumor growth at 10 years was achieved in 85% of the patients.[30]

Gamma Knife surgery is also useful as an adjuvant therapy following initial surgical resection and has been shown to successfully control long-term tumor growth.[32,33] In a large, multicenter study of 512 patients, Gamma Knife surgery was performed in patients with recurrent or residual NFPAs. This group found that the progression-free tumor survival following Gamma Knife surgery was associated with smaller adenoma volumes and the absence of suprasellar extension.[34] Whether the Gamma Knife surgery is administered as an adjuvant therapy or as delayed therapy (i.e., administered when tumor progression is observed on follow-up) also seems to make a clinically significant difference. Pomeraniec et al found that NFPA patients who received delayed Gamma Knife therapy had a greater risk of tumor progression, though the timing of the Gamma Knife surgery seems not to impact the onset of endocrinopathy.[35]

Although Gamma Knife surgery is generally safe, it is not without its complications. Optic neuropathy has been previously reported, so it is best to perform Gamma Knife surgery when there is sufficient space between the tumor margin and the optic pathways. Sheehan et al reported that 41 of 442 (9.3%) patients who underwent Gamma Knife surgery experienced a new cranial nerve dysfunction, with dysfunction of the optic nerve being the most common.[34] New-onset hypopituitarism is also a relatively common complication of Gamma Knife surgery.[36] In the same study, 92 of 435 patients demonstrated some degree of new-onset or worsened hypopituitarism, with hypothyroidism being the most common.[34] As with any therapy involving radiation, the theoretical risk of inducing secondary tumors must always be considered, though these instances are rare.

12.5.5 Medical Therapy

Although medical therapy is not likely to play a significant role in the treatment of NFPAs, interest in medical therapy is bolstered by research suggesting that NFPAs express dopamine and somatostatin receptors. These receptors may act as potential targets for pharmacotherapy.

Dopamine agonists are commonly used to treat prolactinomas, but there is limited evidence to suggest that they may also be useful in the treatment of NFPAs.[37,38] In one of the few randomized clinical trials testing the efficacy of cabergoline, a dopamine agonist, in the treatment of NFPAs, Batista et al found that the group treated for 2 years with cabergoline after surgery had a tumor shrinkage rate of 28.8% and a tumor enlargement rate of 5.1%, whereas the control group experienced a tumor shrinkage rate of 10.5% and a tumor enlargement rate of 15.8%.[39]

Somatostatin analogs such as octreotide have also been investigated as potential treatment for NFPAs. Fusco et al used a long-term regimen of octreotide in patients with an unresectable NFPA remnant and found that 5 of 26 (19.2%) patients in the treated group experienced tumor growth, whereas 7 of 13 (53.8%) in the control group experienced tumor growth.[40] Interestingly, although there is modest evidence to support the use of somatostatin analogs to treat NFPAs, the use of growth hormone replacement therapy in NFPA patients deficient in growth hormone does not seem to increase the risk of tumor growth.[41] Although surgery remains the mainstay of treatment for NFPAs, alternative methods of treatment are important, especially in the cases where gross total surgical resection cannot be achieved or in the cases where there is recurrence. The evidence for the efficacy of medical treatment of NFPAs is largely limited to small prospective observational studies, so more robust studies such as placebo-controlled randomized clinical trials need to be performed to fully investigate the benefit of medical therapy.

12.6 Authors' Recommendations

- Imaging studies (CT, CTA, and MRI) should be carefully reviewed to assess tumor size and degree of extension. The tumor's relationship with the optic apparatus, bilateral internal carotid arteries, and the pituitary gland and stalk should be carefully studied.
- Routine preoperative laboratory testing for pituitary hormone levels should be ordered to assess the functionality of the tumor (FH, LSH, ACTH, cortisol, TSH, T3, Free T4, prolactin, GH, IGF-1, and testosterone in men).
- Preoperative visual field testing should be performed in all patients.
- Endoscopic transsphenoidal surgery remains the mainstay of treatment for NFPAs. Surgery should be pursued if there is evidence of impaired vision, radiographic evidence of tumor growth, or contact of the tumor with the optic chiasm.
- Gamma Knife surgery should be reserved for patients with advanced age or significant surgical risk or residual tumor in the cavernous sinus.
- Patients should undergo postoperative and annual MRI to track degree of tumor resection, evidence of tumor residual, or recurrence.
- Patients should also undergo neuro-ophthalmological evaluation as well as routine endocrine assessment during the postoperative period.

References

[1] Molitch ME. Nonfunctioning pituitary tumors and pituitary incidentalomas. Endocrinol Metab Clin North Am. 2008; 37(1):151–171, xi

[2] Ntali G, Wass JA. Epidemiology, clinical presentation and diagnosis of non-functioning pituitary adenomas. Pituitary. 2018; 21(2):111–118

[3] Asa SL, Ezzat S. The pathogenesis of pituitary tumors. Annu Rev Pathol. 2009; 4:97–126

[4] Ferrare E, Ferraroni M, Castrignanò T, et al. Non-functioning pituitary adenoma database: a useful resource to improve the clinical management of pituitary tumors. Eur J Endocrinol. 2006; 155(6):823–829

[5] Imran SA, Yip C-E, Papneja N, et al. Analysis and natural history of pituitary incidentalomas. Eur J Endocrinol. 2016; 175(1):1–9

[6] Fernández-Balsells MM, Murad MH, Barwise A, et al. Natural history of nonfunctioning pituitary adenomas and incidentalomas: a systematic review and metaanalysis. J Clin Endocrinol Metab. 2011; 96(4):905–912

[7] Sasagawa Y, Tachibana O, Nakagawa A, Koya D, Iizuka H. Pituitary apoplexy following gonadotropin-releasing hormone agonist administration with gonadotropin-secreting pituitary adenoma. J Clin Neurosci. 2015; 22(3):601–603

[8] Liu ZH, Tu PH, Pai PC, Chen NY, Lee ST, Chuang CC. Predisposing factors of pituitary hemorrhage. Eur J Neurol. 2012; 19(5):733–738

[9] Möller-Goede DL, Brändle M, Landau K, Bernays RL, Schmid C. Pituitary apoplexy: re-evaluation of risk factors for bleeding into pituitary adenomas and impact on outcome. Eur J Endocrinol. 2011; 164(1):37–43

[10] Zhu X, Wang Y, Zhao X, et al. Incidence of pituitary apoplexy and its risk factors in Chinese people: a database study of patients with pituitary adenoma. PLoS One. 2015; 10(9):e0139088

[11] Lenders N, McCormack A. Malignant transformation in non-functioning pituitary adenomas (pituitary carcinoma). Pituitary. 2018; 21(2):217–229

[12] Molitch ME. Management of incidentally found nonfunctional pituitary tumors. Neurosurg Clin N Am. 2012; 23(4):543–553

[13] Watts AK, Easwaran A, McNeill P, Wang YY, Inder WJ, Caputo C. Younger age is a risk factor for regrowth and recurrence of nonfunctioning pituitary macroadenomas: results from a single Australian centre. Clin Endocrinol (Oxf). 2017; 87(3):264–271

[14] Roelfsema F, Biermasz NR, Pereira AM. Clinical factors involved in the recurrence of pituitary adenomas after surgical remission: a structured review and meta-analysis. Pituitary. 2012; 15(1):71–83

[15] Lucas JW, Bodach ME, Tumialan LM, et al. Congress of neurological surgeons systematic review and evidence-based guideline on primary management of patients with nonfunctioning pituitary adenomas. Neurosurgery. 2016; 79(4):E533–E535

[16] Kuo JS, Barkhoudarian G, Farrell CJ, et al. Congress of neurological surgeons systematic review and evidence-based guideline on surgical techniques and technologies for the management of patients with nonfunctioning pituitary adenomas. Neurosurgery. 2016; 79(4):E536–E538

[17] Fleseriu M, Bodach ME, Tumialan LM, et al. Congress of neurological surgeons systematic review and evidence-based guideline for pretreatment endocrine evaluation of patients with nonfunctioning pituitary adenomas. Neurosurgery. 2016; 79(4):E527–E529

[18] Hong JW, Lee MK, Kim SH, Lee EJ. Discrimination of prolactinoma from hyperprolactinemic non-functioning adenoma. Endocrine. 2010; 37(1):140–147

[19] Jahangiri A, Lamborn KR, Blevins L, Kunwar S, Aghi MK. Factors associated with delay to pituitary adenoma diagnosis in patients with visual loss. J Neurosurg. 2012; 116(2):283–289

[20] Schmalisch K, Milian M, Schimitzek T, Lagrèze WA, Honegger J. Predictors for visual dysfunction in nonfunctioning pituitary adenomas - implications for neurosurgical management. Clin Endocrinol (Oxf). 2012; 77(5):728–734

[21] Dekkers OM, Pereira AM, Romijn JA. Treatment and follow-up of clinically nonfunctioning pituitary macroadenomas. J Clin Endocrinol Metab. 2008; 93(10):3717–3726

[22] Berkmann S, Fandino J, Müller B, Kothbauer KF, Henzen C, Landolt H. Pituitary surgery: experience from a large network in Central Switzerland. Swiss Med Wkly. 2012; 142:w13680

[23] Dehdashti AR, Ganna A, Karabatsou K, Gentili F. Pure endoscopic endonasal approach for pituitary adenomas: early surgical results in 200 patients and comparison with previous microsurgical series. Neurosurgery. 2008; 62(5):1006–1015, discussion 1015–1017

[24] Fleseriu M, Yedinak C, Campbell C, Delashaw JB. Significant headache improvement after transsphenoidal surgery in patients with small sellar lesions. J Neurosurg. 2009; 110(2):354–358

[25] Dallapiazza R, Bond AE, Grober Y, et al. Retrospective analysis of a concurrent series of microscopic versus endoscopic transsphenoidal surgeries for Knosp Grades 0–2 nonfunctioning pituitary macroadenomas at a single institution. J Neurosurg. 2014; 121(3):511–517

[26] Gondim JA, Schops M, de Almeida JP, et al. Endoscopic endonasal transsphenoidal surgery: surgical results of 228 pituitary adenomas treated in a pituitary center. Pituitary. 2010; 13(1):68–77

[27] Messerer M, De Battista JC, Raverot G, et al. Evidence of improved surgical outcome following endoscopy for nonfunctioning pituitary adenoma removal. Neurosurg Focus. 2011; 30(4):E11

[28] Losa M, Spatola G, Albano L, et al. Frequency, pattern, and outcome of recurrences after Gamma Knife radiosurgery for pituitary adenomas. Endocrine. 2017; 56(3):595–602

[29] Hasegawa T, Shintai K, Kato T, Iizuka H. Stereotactic radiosurgery as the initial treatment for patients with nonfunctioning pituitary adenomas. World Neurosurg. 2015; 83(6):1173–1179

[30] Lee CC, Kano H, Yang HC, et al. Initial Gamma Knife radiosurgery for nonfunctioning pituitary adenomas. J Neurosurg. 2014; 120(3):647–654

[31] Park KJ, Kano H, Parry PV, et al. Long-term outcomes after Gamma Knife stereotactic radiosurgery for nonfunctional pituitary adenomas. Neurosurgery. 2011; 69(6):1188–1199

[32] El-Shehaby AM, Reda WA, Tawadros SR, Abdel Karim KM. Low-dose Gamma Knife surgery for nonfunctioning pituitary adenomas. J Neurosurg. 2012; 117 Suppl:84–88

[33] Gopalan R, Schlesinger D, Vance ML, Laws E, Sheehan J. Long-term outcomes after Gamma Knife radiosurgery for patients with a nonfunctioning pituitary adenoma. Neurosurgery. 2011; 69(2):284–293

[34] Sheehan JP, Starke RM, Mathieu D, et al. Gamma Knife radiosurgery for the management of nonfunctioning pituitary adenomas: a multicenter study. J Neurosurg. 2013; 119(2):446–456

[35] Pomeraniec IJ, Kano H, Xu Z, et al. Early versus late Gamma Knife radiosurgery following transsphenoidal surgery for nonfunctioning pituitary macroadenomas: a multicenter matched-cohort study. J Neurosurg. 2018; 129(3):648–657

[36] Zibar Tomšić K, Dušek T, Kraljević I, et al. Hypopituitarism after Gamma Knife radiosurgery for pituitary adenoma. Endocr Res. 2017; 42(4):318–324

[37] Even-Zohar N, Greenman Y. Management of NFAs: medical treatment. Pituitary. 2018; 21(2):168–175

[38] Greenman Y, Cooper O, Yaish I, et al. Treatment of clinically nonfunctioning pituitary adenomas with dopamine agonists. Eur J Endocrinol. 2016; 175(1):63–72

[39] Batista RL, Musolino NRC, Cescato VAS, et al. Cabergoline in the management of residual nonfunctioning pituitary adenoma: a single-center, open-label, 2-year randomized clinical trial. Am J Clin Oncol. 2019; 42(2):221–227

[40] Fusco A, Giampietro A, Bianchi A, et al. Treatment with octreotide LAR in clinically non-functioning pituitary adenoma: results from a case-control study. Pituitary. 2012; 15(4):571–578

[41] van Varsseveld NC, van Bunderen CC, Franken AA, Koppeschaar HP, van der Lely AJ, Drent ML. Tumor recurrence or regrowth in adults with nonfunctioning pituitary adenomas using GH replacement therapy. J Clin Endocrinol Metab. 2015; 100(8):3132–3139

13 Natural History and Management Options of Craniopharyngioma

Harshad R. Purandare and Basant K. Misra

Abstract

Craniopharyngioma is benign, slow-growing, cystic epithelial tumor that arises from the remnants of the Rathke's pouch. Most tumors grow out of the sella with variable midline suprasellar extension, compressing the optic chiasma and tracts, and may reach the floor of the third ventricle. There remains ongoing controversy relating to the type of treatment, surgical approaches, and the need for postsurgical adjuvant therapy. Specific treatment strategy should be tailored according to the institution and surgical expertise, with increasing emphasis on the quality of life in contemporary practice.

Keywords: craniopharyngioma, adamantinomatous, papillary, cystic tumor

13.1 Introduction

Craniopharyngioma is among the most challenging intracranial lesions to manage surgically and medically, with significant morbidity and recurrence, despite advances in surgical techniques, adjuvant therapy, and endocrinological care.[1] The tumor is thought to arise from the squamous cell rests of the embryonic hypophyseal–pharyngeal duct (craniopharyngeal duct; ▸ Fig. 13.1). Another hypothesis suggests origin of the tumor due to squamous metaplasia of the existing cells of the adenohypophysis. This is supported by predominant development of papillary tumors in adults.[2]

Craniopharyngioma accounts for 2 to 5% of all primary intracranial tumors and up to 10 to 15% of intracranial tumors in children.[3] It is a World Health Organization (WHO) grade I tumor. There is no genetic susceptibility or predisposition. The disease has a slight male preponderance and has a bimodal peak with increased incidence between 5 and 14 years and 65 and 74 years of age.[4]

There are two distinct histological and genomic types: adamantinomatous craniopharyngioma (ACP) and papillary craniopharyngioma (PCP). ACP is a more common subtype (86.2% cases), predominantly occurring in children and exhibits characteristic microcystic spaces, palisading columnar epithelium

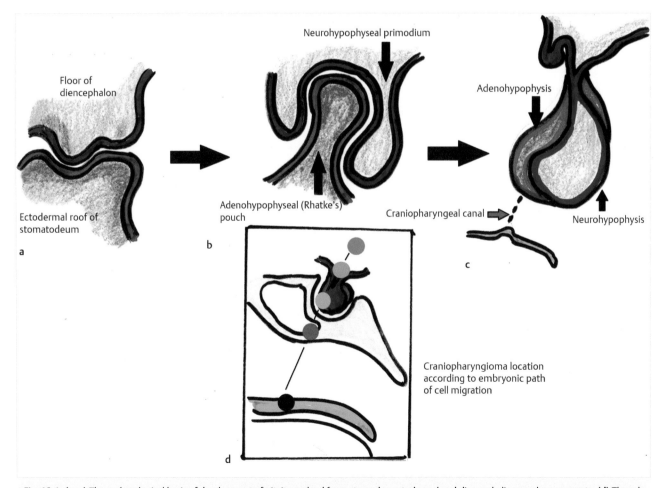

Fig. 13.1 (a–c) The embryological basis of development of pituitary gland from stomodea ectodermal and diencephalic neural components. **(d)** Though the sellar and suprasellar locations are the commonest, an uncommon location such as the pure intraventricular or sphenoid sinus is occasionally seen.

with basal nuclei, stellate reticulin, and wet keratin. PCP shows monomorphic papillary growth pattern with nonkeratinizing squamous epithelium over fibrovascular cores and scattered capillary network. Mixed or transitional forms (2.5% cases) have occasionally been reported. Tumors in the pediatric population are almost exclusively ACPs, whereas papillary tumors constitute 15 to 40% of all adult craniopharyngiomas.[5,6]

Most lesions are heterogenous with predominantly solid (18–39%), predominantly cystic (46–64%), or mixed solid and cystic (8–36%) morphology.[7,8] The cyst contains fluid described in appearance variably from "machinery oil" to "shimmering yellow cholesterol-laden" fluid. It consists of desquamated epithelium, membrane lipids, and cytoskeletal keratin. Calcification (seen in 40% of adults and 95% of pediatric cases) can be diffuse and speckled to firm, large, and chunky.[2,9] The latter is difficult to resect and amounts to significant morbidity if the same is attempted.[10]

Craniopharyngiomas form micropapillary extensions into surrounding neuroparenchymas, which elicit a gliotic reaction causing adhesion and subsequent surgical difficulty and morbidity with attempted gross total resection (GTR).[11] The difference in rate of recurrence in the adult and pediatric groups may be explained by the predominant pathological variants occurring among these tumors. PCPs and tumors in adults tend to be more indolent. ACPs are more aggressive and exhibit more brain invasion with extensive and firmer adhesions to adjacent structures.[5,6,10]

Ninety-four percent of ACPs exhibit dysregulation of the nucleocytoplasmic Wnt/β-catenin pathway in the form of CTNNB1 mutation, whereas BRAF-V600E mutations are characteristic of 96% PCPs.[1,12] Although histologically benign, rare cases of malignant transformation have been reported. While the mechanism of anaplastic transformation is unclear, animal studies suggest delayed p53 mutation developing after radiation as a possible cause.[13]

The location of the tumor in close proximity to the visual pathways, hypothalamic pituitary axis, and the limbic systems results in a wide spectrum of visual, endocrine, vegetative, and cognitive dysfunction either at presentation or as a consequence of treatment.[2,9,14]

The most common clinical presentation is visual deterioration (67%), followed by raised intracranial pressure (hydrocephalus with headache, vomiting) in 29 to 45% cases, endocrinopathies in 30 to 65% cases (panhypopituitarism with gonadal insufficiency being the commonest), hypothalamic dysfunction, and neurocognitive impairment.[9,10,15] Headache is also a common symptom, seen in 50% cases. Neurological deficits in the form of seizures, ataxia, cranial nerve palsies, and altered sensorium are seen in 17% of cases.[16] The various endocrinopathies at presentation include growth hormone (GH) deficiency (35–95%), follicle-stimulating hormone (FSH)/luteinizing hormone (LH) deficiency (38–82%), adrenocorticotropic hormone (ACTH)/cortisol (21–62%), thyroid-stimulating hormone (TSH; 21–42%), and antidiuretic hormone (ADH) diabetes insipidus (6–38%). In numerous studies, the predominant endocrine presentation in 93% of children was growth dysfunction (delayed puberty, obesity, short stature, precocious puberty), whereas the most prevalent disorders in adults were related to menstruation and sexual function.[17] Hydrocephalus is seen in 29 to 45% cases. Definitive long-term treatment for hydrocephalus was needed in 40% cases.[4,7,14]

Diagnosis and referral are often delayed for months or years (mean duration: 10 months; range: 1–108 months) due to slow growth of the lesion and insidious onset of symptoms.[17,18] Patients with hydrocephalus and neurological deficits presented earlier. Patients presenting only with endocrine deficits had a longer duration of symptoms before diagnosis. Visual impairment, hydrocephalus, and neurological deficits at initial presentation were usually associated with poorer long-term survival and outcomes. Among the pediatric population, infants and young children more frequently presented with features of raised intracranial pressure and neurological deficits, whereas elder children presented with growth failure, weight gain, or endocrine dysfunction.[19]

Computed tomography (CT) scan in ACP shows cysts of near cerebrospinal fluid (CSF) density, soft-tissue density solid component with enhancement seen in 90% cases, and stippled calcification, which is often peripherally located. Occasionally, large and chunky basally located calcification is seen. Cysts in PCP are small and often insignificant; the solid component is the dominant element and shows a more vivid and homogenous enhancement and calcification is uncommon. Magnetic resonance imaging (MRI) is the definitive diagnostic imaging to characterize the lesion and study its location and relation to the adjacent structures. Solid tumor is iso- to hypointense on T1 and mixed hypo- to hyperintensity on T2 images with patchy and reticular enhancement. Cysts have an enhancing wall, and the content shows variable T1 and T2 intensities based on their protein and cholesterol content. Giant craniopharyngiomas are tumors greater than 5 cm in diameter and have a multicompartmental extension.[18,20]

Numerous classification and grading systems have been proposed by Hoffman, Samii, Yasargil, Pudget, Kassam, etc. Although none have gained widespread acceptance, all the systems are primarily based on location and anatomical relations guiding the surgical approach.[2]

13.2 Selected Papers on the Natural History of Craniopharyngioma

- Karavitaki N, Brufani C, Warner JT, et al. Craniopharyngiomas in children and adults: systematic analysis of 121 cases with long-term follow-up. Clin Endocrinol (Oxf) 2005;62(4):397–409
- Wijnen M, van den Heuvel-Eibrink MM, Janssen JAMJL, et al. Very long-term sequelae of craniopharyngioma. Eur J Endocrinol 2017;176(6):755–767
- Zacharia BE, Bruce SS, Goldstein H, Malone HR, Neugut AI, Bruce JN. Incidence, treatment and survival of patients with craniopharyngioma in the surveillance, epidemiology and end results program. Neuro-oncol 2012;14(8):1070–1078

13.3 Natural History of Craniopharyngioma

Literature data on the natural history of craniopharyngioma are sparse as almost all tumors undergo inevitable treatment following diagnosis.[2] The age-adjusted incidence rate of craniopharyngioma ranges between 1.3 and 1.7 cases per 1,000,000 person-years.[21]

Most tumors grow out of the sella with variable midline suprasellar extension (94% cases), compressing the optic chiasma and tracts, and may reach the floor of the third ventricle. Purely intrasellar tumors occur in 4% cases only, whereas 75% cases are purely suprasellar. Posterior growth results in extension to the interpeduncular cistern with splaying of the peduncles. Supratentorial hydrocephalus results from occlusion of the foramen of Monroe or the aqueduct of Sylvius. Lateral extensions would result in subfrontal or mesial temporal mass effect and even occasional extension to the lateral ventricle. Rare locations include purely third ventricular, purely mesial temporal, pineal, and cerebellopontine angle.[22]

The huge heterogeneity regarding the location, shape, speed of growth, formation of cysts, and compliance of brain tissue to progressive displacements makes us reconsider the classic division into pediatric and adult subgroups of lesions in favor of the concept of "individual" lesion, based on clinical and pathological objective data. It highlights the requirement for multidisciplinary follow-up involving neuropsychological and psychosocial assessment and support, exercise, and lifestyle counseling commencing early in the postoperative period and regular medical review by the treating neurosurgeon, radiation oncologist, endocrinologists, and ophthalmologists.[23]

The growth rate of craniopharyngiomas is variable, and hence, no reliable clinical, histological, or radiological predictors of recurrence or behavior exist. A good evaluation of risk of recurrence requires a long follow-up as it is a slow-growing tumor. A minimum follow-up of 5 years is required, with a 10-year follow-up being preferred.[8] Most recurrences occur within the first 3 to 5 years.[4,24,25] Risk of recurrence is noted to be higher with incomplete primary resection, cystic tumors (due to capsular adhesion), supradiaphragmatic lesions, hypothalamic involvement (leading to incomplete resection), and in tumors with higher MIB index.[4,15,19,26]

Recurrent tumors are associated with decreased rates of GTR and overall survival (OS) with increased rate of mortality and morbidity, including higher risk of visual deterioration, due to severe adhesions to the surrounding critical structures.[8,17,19,26,27]

Because of the benign nature of the disease and excellent short-term survival, data on OS are scant in the literature. Because these lesions often exhibit aggressive local recurrence, progression-free survival is typically used as the benchmark when evaluating various treatment paradigms. Yet craniopharyngiomas have a substantially reduced OS, with mortality risk being three to six times that of the general population.[28]

The OS rates, which reflect the effect of multiple treatments described in exclusively pediatric series, ranged from 83 to 96% at 5 years, 65 to 100% at 10 years, and averaging 62% at 20 years. In adults or a broad age range population (adults and children) series, the OS rates ranged from 54 to 96% at 5 years, 40 to 93% at 10 years, and 66 to 85% at 20 years.[16] Younger age, small tumors, subtotal resection, and radiation therapy were found to be associated with improved OS in a multivariate analysis. Men and women had similar survival rates. Black patients had poorer OS.[23]

Despite the survival data, the long-term morbidity is quite severe. A prospective study of craniopharyngioma survivors demonstrated that whereas cognitive function per se was not severely impacted, behavioral problems and affect disturbances were prominent, resulting in significant impairment of global functioning in most patients.[22] Numerous studies have confirmed a high incidence of reduced quality of life and social functioning.[29,30] A cohort of 128 patients having a median follow-up of 13 years exhibited pituitary deficiencies in 98% cases, visual disturbances in 75% cases, and obesity in 56% cases.[31] Morbid obesity was seen in 16% cases.[32]

Hypothalamic obesity in craniopharyngioma is significant not only because it has been shown to severely impact quality of life but also due to the associated high risk of metabolic syndrome, cardiovascular disease, and multisystem morbidity. Weight gain results from damage to the ventromedial hypothalamus, which leads, variably, to a low resting metabolic rate, autonomic imbalance, endocrine deficits, reduced physical activity and impaired functional capacity, and insomnia.[16] Patients with higher body mass index (BMI) prior to surgery are at particular risk. Pharmacotherapy is ineffective in controlling obesity and hence surgical preservation of hypothalamic integrity is mandatory to minimize this devastating sequelae.[26,27]

Disease-related mortality can occur even many years after treatment. Causes of late mortality include progressive disease with multiple recurrences, chronic hypothalamic insufficiency, hormonal deficiencies, cerebrovascular disease, and seizures; decreased mineral bone density with fractures; and nonalcoholic steatohepatitis, leading to liver cirrhosis in some cases.[4,7,14,33]

13.4 Selected Papers on the Management of Craniopharyngioma

- Fahlbusch R, Honegger J, Paulus W, Huk W, Buchfelder M. Surgical treatment of craniopharyngiomas: experience with 168 patients. J Neurosurg 1999;90(2):237–250
- Van Effenterre R, Boch AL. Craniopharyngioma in adults and children: a study of 122 surgical cases. J Neurosurg 2002;97(1):3–11
- Morisako H, Goto T, Goto H, Bohoun CA, Tamrakar S, Ohata K. Aggressive surgery based on an anatomical subclassification of craniopharyngiomas. Neurosurg Focus 2016;41(6):E10
- Yaşargil MG, Curcic M, Kis M, Siegenthaler G, Teddy PJ, Roth P. Total removal of craniopharyngiomas. Approaches and long-term results in 144 patients. J Neurosurg 1990;73(1):3–11
- Cavallo LM, Frank G, Cappabianca P, et al. The endoscopic endonasal approach for the management of craniopharyngiomas: a series of 103 patients. J Neurosurg 2014;121(1):100–113

13.5 Treatment Options

Optimal therapeutic approach for craniopharyngiomas is not well defined. Some authors recommend GTR as a primary goal if it can be attained with minimal or limited morbidity, thus aiming to limit long-term recurrence. On the contrary, other authors routinely advocate a subtotal resection followed by adjuvant therapy to minimize complications and preserve maximum functionality.[6,7,20,34,35] The risk of recurrence and regrowth is as high as 80%; hence, adjuvant therapy is often essential.

GTR is associated with increased risk of developing neurological deficits and endocrinopathies (three to five times).[6,14,36] Patients undergoing surgery for tumor more than 3 cm in size and those with hypothalamic invasion experienced more endocrine and neurological morbidity such as panhypopituitarism (32–48% cases), diabetes insipidus (40–55% cases), morbid obesity (25–30% cases), disorders of hunger and thirst, poikilothermia, somnolence, and a range of neurocognitive deficits.[10,14,19,37] Patients with postoperative deficits report an overall deterioration of quality of life.[38,39] Many studies have shown that less aggressive resection does not have a significant impact on overall recurrence rates and has an overall superior functional outcome. Hence, decision-making has to be individualized with the contemporary strategy of maximal but safe resection, followed by RT being favored by a majority.[4,6,10,31,40,41,42,43]

13.5.1 Surgery

Patients presenting with obtundation and obstructive hydrocephalus will need to undergo an external drainage to save life before definitive tumor treatment can be undertaken. An upfront shunt procedure before tumor excision is usually avoided. Preoperatively, stabilization of the endocrine axis with administration of steroids and thyroxine supplementation and correction of electrolyte abnormalities related to diabetes insipidus are essential and may take around 3 to 7 days to do so. Detailed neuro-ophthalmological evaluation including assessment of visual acuity and perimetry is mandatory for prognostication and as a baseline for follow-up evaluation after treatment.[2]

Transcranial microsurgical resection forms the first line of treatment for most craniopharyngiomas. A select subset can be resected through an endonasal approach. The transcranial approaches include anterior approach (unilateral subfrontal, bifrontal basal interhemispheric, bifrontal transbasal), anterolateral approaches (pterional, frontotemporal, and orbitozygomatic), and superior approach (interhemispheric transcallosal transventricular and transcortical transventricular; ▶ Fig. 13.2). To achieve maximal safe resection, the choice of surgical approach is critical and this is determined by a detailed preoperative evaluation of the imaging studies for tumor size, location, extent, calcification, cystic components, invasion, presence or absence of hydrocephalus, and relation to adjacent structures, specifically the optic apparatus, the circle of Willis, and the hypothalamus.[2,3,4,7,30,44,45,46] The surgeon's preference, comfort, and experience are also other relevant factors.

▶ Table 13.1 compares surgical outcomes and complications in some of the large series of surgical management of craniopharyngiomas published in literature.

Transcranial Microsurgical Approaches

The unilateral subfrontal approach is the least traumatic due to limited cortical handling and can be used for small to moderate-sized midline lesions in prechiasmatic location with extension to anterior fossa and suprasellar region (▶ Fig. 13.3).[2,4,7,47,48,49,50,51,52,53] It maintains midline orientation. Tumor in the third ventricle can be approached through the lamina terminalis. Ipsilateral olfactory nerve is at risk of damage in the approach. Conventionally, the pterional approach has been favored for most small to moderate-sized

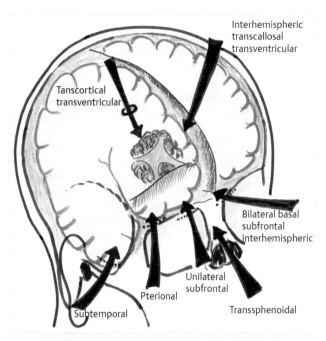

Fig. 13.2 Diagrammatic representation of the various surgical approaches for craniopharyngioma excision.

craniopharyngiomas having superior or lateral extensions. With multiple trajectories through the interoptic, opticocarotid, and lateral carotid corridors combined with translamina terminalis corridor, tumor going up to the anterior aspect of the third ventricle, the interpeduncular fossa, and the lateral regions can be resected (▶ Fig. 13.4). The approach is limited by "blind areas" under the ipsilateral optic nerve limiting retrochiasmatic resection, ipsilateral posterior and superior third ventricular regions, and ipsilateral extreme lateral mesial temporal regions. The visualization of the contralateral carotid is compromised, and operating between perforator vessels may prove hazardous. A modified approach combining the pterional and lateral subfrontal approach is often sufficient for more radical extensions, whereas a combination approach with transcallosal or transcortical transventricular surgery may be employed for large suprasellar and intraventricular extensions. The orbitozygomatic approach, an extension of the pterional approach, provides a more anteroinferior to posterosuperior trajectory to approach suprasellar lesions with reduced brain retraction.

The anterior basal bifrontal interhemispheric approach is appropriate for moderate to large retrochiasmatic and suprasellar tumors with retrosellar extension (▶ Fig. 13.5). Though needing more extensive dissection, retraction, and hence being more technically challenging, the approach avoids the blind spots related to unilateral approach. Performing a bifrontal craniotomy right up to the anterior cranial fossa floor, even at the cost of opening the frontal sinus, just above the nasion reduces brain retraction. Additional removal of the supraorbital bony ridge provides a more inferior to superior trajectory. Bifrontal lobe retraction provides a panoramic view of all the tumor compartments. Morbidity is related to bifrontal retraction, venous congestion and infarction, and potential anterior cerebral artery injuries. The authors do not favor this approach.

Table 13.1 Surgical outcomes and complications in major case series

Studies	Patients (% adults)	Mean f/u (y)	GTR/NTR (%)	Surgical Cx (%)	% CSF leak (% meningitis)	Surgical mortality (%)	Long-term mortality (%)	Long-term poor outcomes/poor QOL (%)	Permanent endocrine dysfunction (%)	Vision nonimprovement/ deterioration (%)	Recurrence (%)
Baskin et al[54]	74	4.0	8.0	12.0	5.4	4.1	6.7	22.2	45.0	8.0	9.0
Yasargil et al[41]	144 (51.4)	0–22	90.1	16.7		2.1	16.7	15.9	79.2	34.0	11.0
Fahlbusch et al[4]	168 (80)	5.4	49.0	11.7	1.8 (1.8)	1.2	9.5	7.4		20.8	13.1
Duff et al[17]	121 (74)	10.0	57.0	19.0		1.7	12.4	39.7		24.3	24.0
Van Effenterre et al[8]	122 (76)	7.0	79.0	19.0		2.5	17	15.0	46.0	15.0	24.0
Zhao et al[27]	214	5.2	70.3	26.0		5.1	12.6	20.5	78.5	21.3	21.8
Mortini et al[36]	112 (70)	5.5	71.6	26.6		2.7	9.7	14.3	90.0	39.0	24.5
Hoffman et al[55]	73		83.1	13.8	6.2 (1.5)	0				9.6	12.3
Cavallo et al[65]	103	4.0	68.9	9.6	14.6	1.9	3.8	12.4	46.2	20.2	22.3
Bao et al[24]	52	2.6	84.6			3.85	18.0	51.9	53.3	14.0	17.3
Du et al[56]	177 (68)	3.9	94.3			1.9	12.9	7.4	81.2	23.0	
Morisako et al[26]	72 (75)	4.7	98.6	5.2	1.7	0	4.2		88.9	6.9	20.8
Park et al[57]	116 (99)	3.2	85.0	23.0	11.2 (6.0)	1.6	NA	21.6	46.6	6.9	14.7
Guo et al[58]	335 (75)	2.7	79.1	20.4	2.1 (1.5)	2.69	9.7	9.7		28.0	17.2

Abbreviations: CSF, cerebrospinal fluid; Cx, complications; f/u, follow-up; GTR, gross total resection; NTR, near total resection; QOL, quality of life.

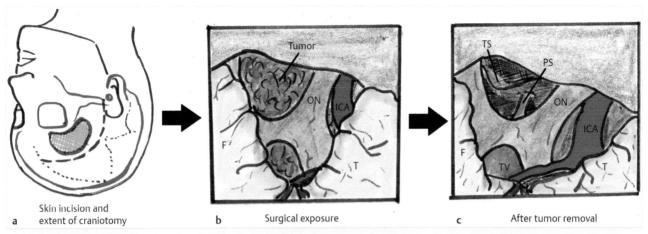

a   Skin incision and extent of craniotomy   b   Surgical exposure   c   After tumor removal

Fig. 13.3 The unilateral subfrontal approach. **(a)** The location of the skin flap and the extent of craniotomy. **(b)** The exposure obtained. **(c)** The view after resection of the tumor (F, frontal lobe; ICA, right supraclinoid internal carotid artery; ON, right optic nerve; PS, pituitary stalk; T, temporal lobe; TS, tuberculum sella; TV, third ventricle after opening lamina terminalis).

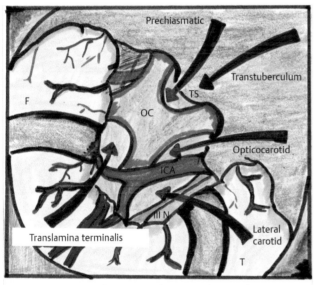

Surgical corridors in the pterional approach

Fig. 13.4 The various surgical corridors obtained through the right pterional approach (F, frontal lobe; ICA, right supraclinoid internal carotid artery; OC, optic chiasma; T, temporal lobe; TS, tuberculum sella; III-N, right third nerve).

Occasional craniopharyngiomas predominantly in the third ventricle (3–10% cases) and reaching high up to the foramen of Monroe and causing obstructive hydrocephalus can be satisfactorily resected through the interhemispheric transcallosal transventricular approach or the frontal transcortical transventricular approach. The approach has limitations in resecting the infrachiasmatic, sellar, and posterior third ventricular extension of the tumor, which would require a combination with a basal approach. The neurocognitive deterioration risks related to corpus callosum and fornix handling, manipulation of intraventricular veins, and medial frontal retraction are specific to this approach.

Transsphenoidal Approach

Transcranial approaches have a common risk of brain retraction and of manipulation of the optic nerve as it is placed between the surgeon and the tumor (▶ Fig. 13.6). The ability to see the most superior pole of the tumor is often lacking and over manipulating. The endonasal approach avoids these drawbacks. The refinement of the transsphenoidal approach with advancement in endoscopic instrumentation has provided additional armamentarium to the surgeon in the form of endoscopic endonasal and extended endoscopic endonasal approach (via transtuberculum, transplanum, and transclival corridors after bone drilling).[59,60,61,62,63] This approach is suitable for cases with widened sella having purely sellar lesions or sellar–suprasellar or retrosellar median infradiaphragmatic lesions with retrochiasmatic extension into the third ventricle. The approach exposes the tumor along its longitudinal axis up to its apex and eliminates brain retraction. Its inferior to superior tumor direction of debulking relaxes the optic apparatus before handling of the nerves. Large tumors, multicompartment tumors, and tumors with lateral extension beyond the carotid bifurcation are poor candidates for this approach and are best managed transcranially. There is a significantly higher risk of CSF rhinorrhea (18–26% against 0–2% in transcranial approaches) due to direct opening of the third ventricle though the nasal route and may need a repeat surgery to repair the same. The use of vascularized nasoseptal flaps in sellar floor reconstruction has enabled significant reduction in leak rate. Need of expertise, technical support, specialized instrumentation, prolonged operative time, and slow learning curve have restricted the routine use of this technique only to specialized centers.[3,4,8,51,64,65]

Endonasal surgery scores over transcranial surgery in postoperative visual outcomes. Intraoperative early handling of stretched optic nerves and inadvertent damage to superior hypophyseal trunk or branches during tumor resection in transcranial approach leads to visual deterioration in 11 to 18% cases as compared to their preoperative status. Moreover, improvement of the preoperative visual deficit is seen in 25 to 42% cases.[3,50,61,66,67,68] On the contrary, endoscopic endonasal series

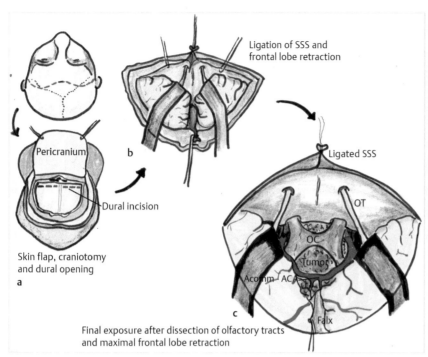

Fig. 13.5 The various steps in the anterior basal bifrontal interhemispheric approach. **(a)** The bicoronal skin flap with elevation of the pericranial flap for floor repair at the end of surgery. Note the craniotomy taken well down to the level of the frontal sinus and basal opening of the dura. **(b)** The ligation and division of the anterosuperior sagittal sinus and gradual elevation of the frontal lobes to show the olfactory tracts, which are carefully separated by sharp arachnoid dissection. **(c)** The panoramic exposure of the tumor after maximal retraction of the frontal lobes (Acomm ACA, anterior communicating artery anterior cerebral artery complex; OC, optic chiasma; OT, olfactory tract; SSS, superior sagittal sinus).

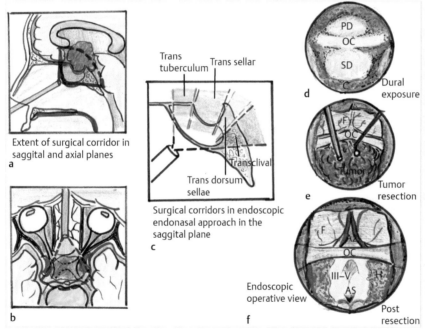

Fig. 13.6 Endonasal endoscopic approach to craniopharyngioma. Extent and limits of the exposure obtained as seen in the **(a)** sagittal and **(b)** axial planes. **(c)** The various corridors of the approach in the sagittal plane. The sequential surgical steps shown include **(d)** sellar and presellar dural exposure and the endoscopic view **(e)** during removal of a retrochiasmatic tumor and **(f)** after complete removal of the tumor with visualization of the third ventricular cavity (A2, bilateral A2 segments of anterior cerebral artery; AS, aqueduct of Sylvius; F, frontal lobes; H, hypothalamus; III–V, third ventricular cavity; OC, optic chiasma; PD, presellar dura; SD, sellar dura).

report overall improvement in 56 to 92% cases and deterioration in less than 2% cases.[4,6,7,10,18,30,40]

Although a meta-analysis suggested that surgical approach did not have any statistically significant effect on rate of recurrence, analysis of literature in adult craniopharyngiomas puts the average rate of long-term recurrence with GTR, subtotal resection (STR) + RT, and STR alone at 17, 27, and 45%, respectively. The comparative analysis did not reach statistical significance. On the other hand, reviews by Yang as well as Clarke et al analyzing mixed series of adult and pediatric or predominantly pediatric population yield similar 5-year progression-free survival of 67 to 77% and 69 to 73% in GTR and SRT + XRT groups, respectively. The surgical mortality ranges from 0 to 5.4%.[2,4,6,8,14,20,31,32] Wang et al performed a meta-analysis of survival outcomes of GTR versus STR with RT for craniopharyngioma. A systematic search was performed for articles published until October 2017 in the PubMed, Embase, and Cochrane Central databases. A total of 744 patients (seven cohort studies) were enrolled for analyses. There were no significant differences between the GTR and STR with RT groups when the authors compared the pooled hazard ratios (HRs) at the end of the follow-up period. OS (pooled HR = 0.76; 95%

Table 13.2 Extent of resection and recurrence rates in major case series

Studies	No. of cases	Mean f/u (y)	Recurrence (%)		
			GTR	NTR/STR	NTR/STR + RT/SRS
Fahlbusch et al[4]	168	5.4	11	51	NA
Van Effenterre et al[8]	122	4	13	33–69	RT not given
Duff et al[17]	121	10	18	50	9
Karavitaki et al[7]	121	8.6	0	61	24
Mortini et al[36]	106	6.9	14	54	NA
Zhao et al[27]	214	5.2	10.1	92.3	31.3
Lee et al[92]	90	5.8	33	73	53
Morisako et al[26]	72	4.7	9.3	27.3	66.7
Park et al[57]	116	3.3	9.3	22.7	16.7

Abbreviations: f/u, follow-up; GTR, gross total resection; NTR, near total resection; RT, radiation therapy; SRS, stereotactic radiosurgery; STR, subtotal resection.

Table 13.3 Rate of GTR, surgical mortality and morbidity reported in resection of new and recurrent craniopharyngiomas

Series	Total no. of cases	New				Recurrent			
		No. of cases	GTR/NTR (%)	Sx/long-term mortality	Sx morbidity	No. of cases	GTR/NTR (%)	Sx/long-term mortality	Sx morbidity
Fahlbusch et al[4]	163	129	56.6		11.6	34	35.3		14.7
Elliot et al[68]	86	57	100	7	26.2	29	62	32	45.4
Zhao et al[93]	219	189	74.6	6.6		30	43.3	26.7	

Abbreviations: GTR, gross total resection; NTR, near total resection; Sx, surgery.

confidence interval [CI]: 0.46–1.25; p = 0.28) and progression-free survival (pooled HR = 1.52; 95% CI: 0.42–5.44; p = 0.52) were similar between the two groups.[69]

▶ Table 13.2 presents the relationship of recurrence rates to extent of resection and adjuvant therapy in some major case series.

Recurrent tumors are difficult to manage due to extensive scarring and adhesions. Redo surgery has a lesser likelihood of radical decompression and is associated with higher morbidity and mortality, especially in the adult population.[4,6,7,70,71,72] Recurring cysts with mass effect may be considered for stereotactic aspiration or Ommaya chamber placement.

▶ Table 13.3 presents the rates of GTR, surgical mortality, and morbidity reported in resection of new and recurrent craniopharyngiomas in some major series.

Radiotherapy

Technological improvements in radiation planning and conformal dose delivery have reduced the risks of radiation injury to adjacent normal tissues. Small residual tumors away from the visual pathway are best treated with Gamma Knife radiosurgery (GKRS). However, for residual tumors with close proximity to the optic apparatus, the preferred modality is photon-based intensity-modulated RT (IMRT). The superior dose profile obtained using proton beam therapy (PBT) has resulted in its increased use. RT is delivered in doses of 50 to 54 Gy at 1.8 Gy per fraction.[35,43,73,74,75,76,77] All techniques have equivalent tumor control rates and OS ranging from 83 to 91% in most series. Bishop et al compared PBT with IMRT for pediatric

craniopharyngioma in terms of OS, disease control, cyst dynamics, and toxicity. At 59.6 months' median follow-up (PBT: 33 months vs. IMRT: 106 months), the 3-year outcomes were 96% for OS and neither OS, disease control nor toxicity differed between treatment groups.[73] Harrabi et al analyzed effects of fractionated stereotactic RT (FSRT) in 55 patients for postoperative residual or progressive disease. A median dose of 52.2 (50–57.6) Gy was applied with typical dose per fraction of 1.8 Gy five times per week. During median follow-up of 128 months, local control rate was 95.3% after 5 years, 92.1% after 10 years, and 88.1% after 20 years. OS after 10 years was 83.3%, and after 20 years was 67.8%.[78] Hasegawa et al reported 100 patients with 109 craniopharyngiomas treated with GKRS with marginal doses varying from 10 to 18 (median: 11.4) Gy and maximum dose to any part of the optic apparatus varied from 2 to 18 (median: 10) Gy. The actuarial 5- and 10-year OS rates of tumor progression after GKRS were 93 and 88%, respectively, whereas the actuarial 5- and 10-year progression-free survival rates were 62 and 52%, respectively. Radiation-induced optic neuropathy was noted in 5% cases.[79] Jeon et al published their experience of RT in 50 patients with craniopharyngioma. RT consisted of FRT (37 patients) and GKRS (13 patients). The total dose delivered for FRT was 50.2 (range: 50–60) Gy, with a daily dose of 2 Gy. The GKRS dose varied from 10 to 12 Gy at 50% isodose (median dose: 11 Gy). The actuarial 5- and 10-year survival was 91.1 and 86.1%, respectively. Progression-free survival rates at 5 and 10 years were 56.7 and 45.3%, respectively. Univariate analysis revealed that treatment modality (FRT or GKRS) was not associated with tumor recurrence.[80]

After RT, although solid or nodular tumor growth is a definite evidence of tumor progression, cystic growth is often confounding, and cystic changes may be preexisting, may occur during RT, or after RT. This may alter dose planning and may impact the overall dose delivered. Early cystic changes, which are asymptomatic, are often transient and will subside with no intervention. Delayed or late cyst development with persistence or progression beyond 3 years of treatment is often regarded as disease progression. In a cohort of pediatric gliomas treated with RT, the 3-year nodular progression-free survival was 95%, whereas the 3-year cystic progression-free survival rate was only about 76%. Post-RT, new endocrinopathies occurred in over 80% cases with panhypopituitarism in 30% cases and morbid obesity in 25 to 28% cases. A delay in use of RT, however, as an adjuvant therapy till the time of disease progression is seen to have more morbidity. Patients undergoing STR +XRT had poorer visual outcomes as compared to patients undergoing STR only. This is most likely due to successive injury to optic apparatus during surgical handling as well as by radiation. This can be partially mitigated by a planned STR targeted toward achieving maximum separation of the residual tumor from the optic pathways so that the optic apparatus exposure is well within the safe limits.[14,81]

Other Therapeutic Options

Considering the morbid outcomes with surgical decompression as well as radiation, minimally invasive therapeutic options are being explored. The role of intracavitary RT (brachytherapy) in cystic craniopharyngiomas has thus been deemed promising by using beta radiation emitting radioisotopes isotopes, mainly utilizing yttrium-90 or phosphorus-32.[82,83] With a therapeutic range of only a few millimeters, they have a potential to be precise with minimal long-term toxicity due to limited exposure of surrounding healthy brain to ionizing radiation. Brachytherapy aims to reduce the cyst size with decompression of the ventricles and relief of mass effect on hypothalamus and optic structures. The agents are instilled via stereotactic guidance or endoscopically.[84] Some authors prefer placement of Ommaya reservoir and subsequent injection as it reduces the risk of radioisotope leakage. The dose administered locally is in the range of 90 to 300 Gy and has been shown to achieve cyst control in 67 to 88% cases.[74,85] Extra cavitary leakage of radioactive material despite all precautions is a major drawback. Radiation-induced visual deterioration including blindness, panhypopituitarism, and recurrence due to continued growth of the associated solid component are major associated complications.[86]

Other minimally invasive therapeutic options for cystic lesions include stereotactic aspiration followed by intralesional bleomycin or interferon alpha.[87]

Craniopharyngioma Genetics and Targeted Intervention: A Novel Approach

Identification of specific genetic mutations in craniopharyngiomas has opened a new window of therapeutic modality.[1,88,89,90,91] Most of the mutations are single clonal driver mutations, and this genetic simplicity of craniopharyngiomas holds promise for being of therapeutic potential. Trials of targeted therapy in PCP using BRAF inhibition using kinase inhibitors like dabrafenib and vemurafenib along with simultaneous downstream inhibition of the MAP kinase (MEK) pathway using trametinib to overcome the problem of resistance have given promising results in small case studies primarily involving recurrent tumors, achieving symptomatic relief, and reduced tumor volume. On the other hand, the ubiquity of the Wnt/β-catenin pathway and its activation of multiple downstream cascades make targeted therapy in ACPs a challenge and agents are still under development and need further studies.

13.6 Our Experience

The senior author has operated on 141 craniopharyngioma patients till 2018. A retrospective analysis of cases operated between 1995 and 2012 at P.D. Hinduja National Hospital & Medical Research Centre (PDHNH) had yielded 86 patients and the following text is our early and long-term results based on 75 patients in whom detailed follow-up data were available. There were 52 males and 23 females, and the age ranged from 1 to 66 years with a mean age of 25.6 years. The follow-up ranged from 3 to 144 months (mean: 40 months). One hundred and sixteen operations were done in 75 cases and the philosophy was safe radical excision. The majority (109) were operated on through a transcranial approach and only 7 cases were operated on through a transsphenoidal route. Though a higher percentage of patients today are operated on through endonasal route in our practice, transcranial approach is still done in the majority of the cases. The lateral subfrontal or a combined pterional-lateral subfrontal (PLSF) approach was the commonest approach (99 procedures). A PLSF gives a wide corridor to midline, parasellar, and retrochiasmal extensions. Using the various corridors, prechiasmal, opticocarotid, carotid-oculomotor most anterior, and parasellar components could be removed. Retrochiasmal tumors are adequately and preferably removed through a translamina terminalis approach. Endoscopic assistance helps in a more complete clearance. One must employ extreme caution while operating through the opticocarotid space to avoid vascular injury. The various other transcranial approaches were supraorbital keyhole (5), interhemispheric transcallosal (2), bifrontal (2), and midline suboccipital (1). The authors do not advocate any bifrontal approach. Currently, the authors rarely perform the supraorbital keyhole approach. The endonasal transsphenoidal approach is performed in (1) purely sellar lesion, (2) predominantly cystic lesion, (3) predominantly retrochiasmal tumor in the midline, and (4) multicompartmental lesions when the goal is only decompression or as the first stage to be followed by a transcranial lesion.

A radical total or near-total excision was achieved in 86% of patients. Significant improvement of vision was achieved in 75% of patients. Eighty-two percent of patients required hormone replacement in the immediate postoperative period. In the long term, hormone replacement was required for glucocorticoid (63%), thyroid (57%), desmopressin (DDAVP; 30%), testosterone (15%), and GH (10%). There was one postoperative mortality because of hypothalamic disturbances. Eleven patients received post-op radiation, 7 RT, and 4 Gamma Knife radiosurgery. Recurrence of tumor was seen in 25% of patients.

13.7 Authors' Recommendations

- Craniopharyngioma is a benign tumor that has generated much controversy. Debates over subtotal/radical excision, transcranial/transsphenoidal approach, and adjuvant upfront/on recurrence radiation continue.
- There is no class 1 or strong evidence in favor of a particular strategy. Today quality of life (QOL) has gained significant attention. Hence, each team must develop its own strategy depending on the availability of expertise and resources.
- A patient in a resource-limited facility is probably best managed by safe subtotal excision and adjunct radiation to reduce postoperative intensive care unit (ICU) and frequent follow-up surveillance. This strategy would also be appropriate for a young neurosurgeon early in his or her practice.
- A more experienced surgeon with all the facility and expertise can afford to be more radical in an attempt to have a long recurrence-free survival. Either way, it is a long-term commitment if one wants to manage a patient with craniopharyngioma.

References

[1] Gupta S, Bi WL, Giantini Larsen A, Al-Abdulmohsen S, Abedalthagafi M, Dunn IF. Craniopharyngioma: a roadmap for scientific translation. Neurosurg Focus. 2018; 44(6):E12

[2] King James AJ, Mehta V, Black PM. Craniopharyngioma. In: Youmans JR, Winn HR, eds. Youmans Neurological Surgery. 6th ed. Philadelphia, PA: Saunders/Elsevier; 2011

[3] Komotar RJ, Starke RM, Raper DM, Anand VK, Schwartz TH. Endoscopic endonasal compared with microscopic transsphenoidal and open transcranial resection of craniopharyngiomas. World Neurosurg. 2012; 77(2):329–341

[4] Fahlbusch R, Honegger J, Paulus W, Huk W, Buchfelder M. Surgical treatment of craniopharyngiomas: experience with 168 patients. J Neurosurg. 1999; 90(2):237–250

[5] Pekmezci M, Louie J, Gupta N, Bloomer MM, Tihan T. Clinicopathological characteristics of adamantinomatous and papillary craniopharyngiomas: University of California, San Francisco experience 1985–2005. Neurosurgery. 2010; 67(5):1341–1349, discussion 1349

[6] Dandurand C, Sepehry AA, Asadi Lari MH, Akagami R, Gooderham P. Adult Craniopharyngioma: case series, systematic review, and meta-analysis. Neurosurgery. 2018; 83(4):631–641

[7] Karavitaki N, Brufani C, Warner JT, et al. Craniopharyngiomas in children and adults: systematic analysis of 121 cases with long-term follow-up. Clin Endocrinol (Oxf). 2005; 62(4):397–409

[8] Van Effenterre R, Boch AL. Craniopharyngioma in adults and children: a study of 122 surgical cases. J Neurosurg. 2002; 97(1):3–11

[9] Karavitaki N, Cudlip S, Adams CB, Wass JA. Craniopharyngiomas. Endocr Rev. 2006; 27(4):371–397

[10] Weiner HL, Wisoff JH, Rosenberg ME, et al. Craniopharyngiomas: a clinicopathological analysis of factors predictive of recurrence and functional outcome. Neurosurgery. 1994; 35(6):1001–1010, discussion 1010–1011

[11] Kawamata T, Kubo O, Hori T. Histological findings at the boundary of craniopharyngiomas. Brain Tumor Pathol. 2005; 22(2):75–78

[12] Martinez-Gutierrez JC, D'Andrea MR, Cahill DP, Santagata S, Barker FG, II, Brastianos PK. Diagnosis and management of craniopharyngiomas in the era of genomics and targeted therapy. Neurosurg Focus. 2016; 41(6):E2

[13] Narla S, Govindraj J, Chandrasekar K, Sushama P. Craniopharyngioma with malignant transformation: Review of literature. Neurol India. 2017; 65(2):418–420

[14] Sughrue ME, Yang I, Kane AJ, et al. Endocrinologic, neurologic, and visual morbidity after treatment for craniopharyngioma. J Neurooncol. 2011; 101(3):463–476

[15] Karavitaki N. Management of craniopharyngiomas. J Endocrinol Invest. 2014; 37(3):219–228

[16] Larijani B, Bastanhagh MH, Pajouhi M, Kargar Shadab F, Vasigh A, Aghakhani S. Presentation and outcome of 93 cases of craniopharyngioma. Eur J Cancer Care (Engl). 2004; 13(1):11–15

[17] Duff J, Meyer FB, Ilstrup DM, Laws ER, Jr, Schleck CD, Scheithauer BW. Long-term outcomes for surgically resected craniopharyngiomas. Neurosurgery. 2000; 46(2):291–302, discussion 302–305

[18] Prieto R, Pascual JM, Rosdolsky M, et al. Craniopharyngioma adherence: a comprehensive topographical categorization and outcome-related risk stratification model based on the methodical examination of 500 tumors. Neurosurg Focus. 2016; 41(6):E13

[19] Hoffmann A, Boekhoff S, Gebhardt U, et al. History before diagnosis in childhood craniopharyngioma: associations with initial presentation and long-term prognosis. Eur J Endocrinol. 2015; 173(6):853–862

[20] Salzman KL, Rees JH. Craniopharyngioma. In: Osborn AG, Salzman KL, Jhaveri MD, eds. Diagnostic Imaging: Brain. 3rd ed. Philadelphia PA: Elsevier; 2016

[21] Daubenbüchel AM, Hoffmann A, Gebhardt U, Warmuth-Metz M, Sterkenburg AS, Muller HL. Hydrocephalus and hypothalamic involvement in pediatric patients with craniopharyngioma or cysts of Rathke's pouch: impact on long-term prognosis. Eur J Endocrinol. 2015; 172(5):561–569

[22] Larkin SJ, Ansorge O. Pathology and pathogenesis of craniopharyngiomas. Pituitary. 2013; 16(1):9–17

[23] Rath SR, Lee S, Kotecha RS, Taylor M, Junckerstorff RC, Choong CS. Childhood craniopharyngioma: 20-year institutional experience in Western Australia. J Paediatr Child Health. 2013; 49(5):403–408

[24] Bao Y, Pan J, Qi ST, Lu YT, Peng JX. Origin of craniopharyngiomas: implications for growth pattern, clinical characteristics, and outcomes of tumor recurrence. J Neurosurg. 2016; 125(1):24–32

[25] Tomita T, McLone DG. Radical resections of childhood craniopharyngiomas. Pediatr Neurosurg. 1993; 19(1):6–14

[26] Morisako H, Goto T, Goto H, Bohoun CA, Tamrakar S, Ohata K. Aggressive surgery based on an anatomical subclassification of craniopharyngiomas. Neurosurg Focus. 2016; 41(6):E10

[27] Zhao X, Yi X, Wang H, Zhao H. An analysis of related factors of surgical results for patients with craniopharyngiomas. Clin Neurol Neurosurg. 2012; 114(2):149–155

[28] Zacharia BE, Bruce SS, Goldstein H, Malone HR, Neugut AI, Bruce JN. Incidence, treatment and survival of patients with craniopharyngioma in the surveillance, epidemiology and end results program. Neuro-oncol. 2012; 14(8):1070–1078

[29] Pierre-Kahn A, Recassens C, Pinto G, et al. Social and psycho-intellectual outcome following radical removal of craniopharyngiomas in childhood. A prospective series. Childs Nerv Syst. 2005; 21(8–9):817–824

[30] Müller HL, Bruhnken G, Emser A, et al. Longitudinal study on quality of life in 102 survivors of childhood craniopharyngioma. Childs Nerv Syst. 2005; 21(11):975–980

[31] Wijnen M, van den Heuvel-Eibrink MM, Janssen JAMJL, et al. Very long-term sequelae of craniopharyngioma. Eur J Endocrinol. 2017; 176(6):755–767

[32] Müller HL, Gebhardt U, Etavard-Gorris N, et al. Prognosis and sequela in patients with childhood craniopharyngioma: results of HIT-ENDO and update on KRANIOPHARYNGEOM 2000. Klin Padiatr. 2004; 216(6):343–348

[33] Visser J, Hukin J, Sargent M, Steinbok P, Goddard K, Fryer C. Late mortality in pediatric patients with craniopharyngioma. J Neurooncol. 2010; 100(1):105–111

[34] Kawamata T, Amano K, Aihara Y, Kubo O, Hori T. Optimal treatment strategy for craniopharyngiomas based on long-term functional outcomes of recent and past treatment modalities. Neurosurg Rev. 2010; 33(1):71–81

[35] Schoenfeld A, Pekmezci M, Barnes MJ, et al. The superiority of conservative resection and adjuvant radiation for craniopharyngiomas. J Neurooncol. 2012; 108(1):133–139

[36] Mortini P, Losa M, Pozzobon G, et al. Neurosurgical treatment of craniopharyngioma in adults and children: early and long-term results in a large case series. J Neurosurg. 2011; 114(5):1350–1359

[37] Müller HL. Consequences of craniopharyngioma surgery in children. J Clin Endocrinol Metab. 2011; 96(7):1981–1991

[38] Okada T, Fujitsu K, Ichikawa T, et al. Radical resection of craniopharyngioma: discussions based on long-term clinical course and histopathology of the dissection plane. Asian J Neurosurg. 2018; 13(3):640–646

[39] Tan TSE, Patel L, Gopal-Kothandapani JS, et al. The neuroendocrine sequelae of paediatric craniopharyngioma: a 40-year meta-data analysis of 185 cases from three UK centres. Eur J Endocrinol. 2017; 176(3):359–369

[40] Crowley RK, Hamnvik OP, O'Sullivan EP, et al. Morbidity and mortality in patients with craniopharyngioma after surgery. Clin Endocrinol (Oxf). 2010; 73(4):516–521

[41] Fjalldal S, Holmer H, Rylander L, et al. Hypothalamic involvement predicts cognitive performance and psychosocial health in long-term survivors of childhood craniopharyngioma. J Clin Endocrinol Metab. 2013; 98(8):3253–3262

[42] Elowe-Gruau E, Beltrand J, Brauner R, et al. Childhood craniopharyngioma: hypothalamus-sparing surgery decreases the risk of obesity. J Clin Endocrinol Metab. 2013; 98(6):2376–2382

[43] Clark AJ, Cage TA, Aranda D, et al. A systematic review of the results of surgery and radiotherapy on tumor control for pediatric craniopharyngioma. Childs Nerv Syst. 2013; 29(2):231–238

[44] Komotar RJ, Roguski M, Bruce JN. Surgical management of craniopharyngiomas. J Neurooncol. 2009; 92(3):283–296

[45] Yaşargil MG, Curcic M, Kis M, Siegenthaler G, Teddy PJ, Roth P. Total removal of craniopharyngiomas. Approaches and long-term results in 144 patients. J Neurosurg. 1990; 73(1):3–11

[46] Zhang YQ, Ma ZY, Wu ZB, Luo SQ, Wang ZC. Radical resection of 202 pediatric craniopharyngiomas with special reference to the surgical approaches and hypothalamic protection. Pediatr Neurosurg. 2008; 44(6):435–443

[47] Nanda A, Narayan V, Mohammed N, Savardekar AR, Patra DP. Microsurgical resection of suprasellar craniopharyngioma: technical purview. J Neurol Surg B Skull Base. 2018; 79 Suppl 3:S247–S248

[48] Liu JK, Sevak IA, Carmel PW, Eloy JA. Microscopic versus endoscopic approaches for craniopharyngiomas: choosing the optimal surgical corridor for maximizing extent of resection and complication avoidance using a personalized, tailored approach. Neurosurg Focus. 2016; 41(6):E5

[49] Pascual JM, González-Llanos F, Barrios L, Roda JM. Intraventricular craniopharyngiomas: topographical classification and surgical approach selection based on an extensive overview. Acta Neurochir (Wien). 2004; 146 (8):785–802

[50] Dehdashti AR, de Tribolet N. Frontobasal interhemispheric trans-lamina terminalis approach for suprasellar lesions. Neurosurgery. 2008; 62(6) Suppl 3:1233–1239

[51] Hori T, Kawamata T, Amano K, Aihara Y, Ono M, Miki N. Anterior interhemispheric approach for 100 tumors in and around the anterior third ventricle. Neurosurgery. 2010; 66(3) Suppl Operative:65–74

[52] Golshani KJ, Lalwani K, Delashaw JB, Selden NR. Modified orbitozygomatic craniotomy for craniopharyngioma resection in children. J Neurosurg Pediatr. 2009; 4(4):345–352

[53] Behari S, Banerji D, Mishra A, et al. Intrinsic third ventricular craniopharyngiomas: report on six cases and a review of the literature. Surg Neurol. 2003; 60(3):245–252, discussion 252–253

[54] Baskin DS, Wilson CB. Surgical management of craniopharyngiomas. A review of 74 cases. J Neurosurg. 1986 Jul;65(1):22–7. doi: 10.3171/jns.1986.65.1.0022. PMID: 3712025

[55] Hofmann BM, Höllig A, Strauss C, Buslei R, Buchfelder M, Fahlbusch R. Results after treatment of craniopharyngiomas: further experiences with 73 patients since 1997. J Neurosurg. 2012 Feb;116(2):373–84. doi: 10.3171/2011.6.JNS081451. Epub 2011 Sep 23. PMID: 21942724

[56] Du C, Feng CY, Yuan XR, Liu Q, Peng ZF, Jiang XJ, Li XJ, Xiao GL, Li YF, Xiong T. Microsurgical management of craniopharyngiomas via a unilateral subfrontal approach: a retrospective study of 177 continuous cases. World Neurosurg. 2016 Jun;90:454–468. doi: 10.1016/j.wneu.2016.03.002. Epub 2016 Mar 10. Erratum in: World Neurosurg. 2018 Aug;116:541. PMID: 26970477

[57] Park HR, Kshettry VR, Farrell CJ, Lee JM, Kim YH, Won TB, Han DH, Do H, Nyguist G, Rosen M, Kim DG, Evans JJ, Paek SH. Clinical outcome after extended endoscopic endonasal resection of craniopharyngiomas: two-institution experience. World Neurosurg. 2017 Jul;103:465–474. doi: 10.1016/j.wneu.2017.04.047. Epub 2017 Apr 19. PMID: 28433845

[58] Guo F, Wang G, Suresh V, Xu D, Zhang X, Feng M, Wang F, Liu X, Song L. Clinical study on microsurgical treatment for craniopharyngioma in a single consecutive institutional series of 335 patients. Clin Neurol Neurosurg. 2018 Apr;167:162–172. doi: 10.1016/j.clineuro.2018.02.034. Epub 2018 Mar 16. PMID: 29501046

[59] Gardner PA, Kassam AB, Snyderman CH, et al. Outcomes following endoscopic, expanded endonasal resection of suprasellar craniopharyngiomas: a case series. J Neurosurg. 2008; 109(1):6–16

[60] Alli S, Isik S, Rutka JT. Microsurgical removal of craniopharyngioma: endoscopic and transcranial techniques for complication avoidance. J Neurooncol. 2016; 130(2):299–307

[61] Schwartz TH, Anand VK. The endoscopic endonasal transsphenoidal approach to the suprasellar cistern. Clin Neurosurg. 2007; 54:226–235

[62] Sankhla SK, Jayashankar N, Khan GM. Endoscopic endonasal transplanum transtuberculum approach for retrochiasmatic craniopharyngiomas: operative nuances. Neurol India. 2015; 63(3):405–413

[63] Wannemuehler TJ, Rubel KE, Hendricks BK, et al. Outcomes in transcranial microsurgery versus extended endoscopic endonasal approach for primary resection of adult craniopharyngiomas. Neurosurg Focus. 2016; 41(6):E6

[64] Jeswani S, Nuño M, Wu A, et al. Comparative analysis of outcomes following craniotomy and expanded endoscopic endonasal transsphenoidal resection of craniopharyngioma and related tumors: a single-institution study. J Neurosurg. 2016; 124(3):627–638

[65] Cavallo LM, Frank G, Cappabianca P, et al. The endoscopic endonasal approach for the management of craniopharyngiomas: a series of 103 patients. J Neurosurg. 2014; 121(1):100–113

[66] Leng LZ, Greenfield JP, Souweidane MM, Anand VK, Schwartz TH. Endoscopic, endonasal resection of craniopharyngiomas: analysis of outcome including extent of resection, cerebrospinal fluid leak, return to preoperative productivity, and body mass index. Neurosurgery. 2012; 70(1):110–123, discussion 123–124

[67] Koutourousiou M, Gardner PA, Fernandez-Miranda JC, Tyler-Kabara EC, Wang EW, Snyderman CH. Endoscopic endonasal surgery for craniopharyngiomas: surgical outcome in 64 patients. J Neurosurg. 2013; 119(5):1194–1207

[68] Elliott RE, Jane JA, Jr, Wisoff JH. Surgical management of craniopharyngiomas in children: meta-analysis and comparison of transcranial and transsphenoidal approaches. Neurosurgery. 2011; 69(3):630–643, discussion 643

[69] Wang G, Zhang X, Feng M, Guo F. Comparing survival outcomes of gross total resection and subtotal resection with radiotherapy for craniopharyngioma: a meta-analysis. J Surg Res. 2018; 226:131–139

[70] Minamida Y, Mikami T, Hashi K, Houkin K. Surgical management of the recurrence and regrowth of craniopharyngiomas. J Neurosurg. 2005; 103(2):224–232

[71] Turel MK, Tsermoulas G, Gonen L, et al. Management and outcome of recurrent adult craniopharyngiomas: an analysis of 42 cases with long-term follow-up. Neurosurg Focus. 2016; 41(6):E11

[72] Wisoff JH. Surgical management of recurrent craniopharyngiomas. Pediatr Neurosurg. 1994; 21 Suppl 1:108–113

[73] Bishop AJ, Greenfield B, Mahajan A, et al. Proton beam therapy versus conformal photon radiation therapy for childhood craniopharyngioma: multi-institutional analysis of outcomes, cyst dynamics, and toxicity. Int J Radiat Oncol Biol Phys. 2014; 90(2):354–361

[74] Zhang C, Verma V, Lyden ER, et al. The role of definitive radiotherapy in craniopharyngioma: a SEER analysis. Am J Clin Oncol. 2018; 41(8):807–812

[75] Boehling NS, Grosshans DR, Bluett JB, et al. Dosimetric comparison of three-dimensional conformal proton radiotherapy, intensity-modulated proton therapy, and intensity-modulated radiotherapy for treatment of pediatric craniopharyngiomas. Int J Radiat Oncol Biol Phys. 2012; 82(2):643–652

[76] Clark AJ, Cage TA, Aranda D, Parsa AT, Auguste KI, Gupta N. Treatment-related morbidity and the management of pediatric craniopharyngioma: a systematic review. J Neurosurg Pediatr. 2012; 10(4):293–301

[77] Minniti G, Esposito V, Amichetti M, Enrici RM. The role of fractionated radiotherapy and radiosurgery in the management of patients with craniopharyngioma. Neurosurg Rev. 2009; 32(2):125–132, discussion 132

[78] Harrabi SB, Adeberg S, Welzel T, et al. Long term results after fractionated stereotactic radiotherapy (FSRT) in patients with craniopharyngioma: maximal tumor control with minimal side effects. Radiat Oncol. 2014; 9:203

[79] Hasegawa T, Kobayashi T, Kida Y. Tolerance of the optic apparatus in single-fraction irradiation using stereotactic radiosurgery: evaluation in 100 patients with craniopharyngioma. Neurosurgery. 2010; 66(4):688–694, discussion 694–695

[80] Jeon C, Kim S, Shin HJ, et al. The therapeutic efficacy of fractionated radiotherapy and gamma-knife radiosurgery for craniopharyngiomas. J Clin Neurosci. 2011; 18(12):1621–1625

[81] Kim YH, Kim CY, Kim JW, et al. Longitudinal analysis of visual outcomes after surgical treatment of adult craniopharyngiomas. Neurosurgery. 2012; 71(3):715–721

[82] Bartels U, Laperriere N, Bouffet E, Drake J. Intracystic therapies for cystic craniopharyngioma in childhood. Front Endocrinol (Lausanne). 2012; 3:39

[83] Mrowczynski OD, Langan ST, Rizk EB. Craniopharyngiomas: A systematic review and evaluation of the current intratumoral treatment landscape. Clin Neurol Neurosurg. 2018; 166:124–130

[84] Kickingereder P, Maarouf M, El Majdoub F, et al. Intracavitary brachytherapy using stereotactically applied phosphorus-32 colloid for treatment of cystic craniopharyngiomas in 53 patients. J Neurooncol. 2012; 109(2):365–374

[85] Pollock BE, Lunsford LD, Kondziolka D, Levine G, Flickinger JC. Phosphorus-32 intracavitary irradiation of cystic craniopharyngiomas: current technique and long-term results. Int J Radiat Oncol Biol Phys. 1995; 33(2): 437–446

[86] Voges J, Sturm V, Lehrke R, Treuer H, Gauss C, Berthold F. Cystic craniopharyngioma: long-term results after intracavitary irradiation with stereotactically applied colloidal beta-emitting radioactive sources. Neurosurgery. 1997; 40(2):263–269, discussion 269–270

[87] Hukin J, Steinbok P, Lafay-Cousin L, et al. Intracystic bleomycin therapy for craniopharyngioma in children: the Canadian experience. Cancer. 2007; 109 (10):2124–2131

[88] Martinez-Gutierrez JC, D'Andrea MR, Cahill DP, Santagata S, Barker FG, II, Brastianos PK. Diagnosis and management of craniopharyngiomas in the era of genomics and targeted therapy. Neurosurg Focus. 2016; 41(6):E2

[89] Aylwin SJ, Bodi I, Beaney R. Pronounced response of papillary craniopharyngioma to treatment with vemurafenib, a BRAF inhibitor. Pituitary. 2016; 19(5):544–546

[90] Robinson LC, Santagata S, Hankinson TC. Potential evolution of neurosurgical treatment paradigms for craniopharyngioma based on genomic and transcriptomic characteristics. Neurosurg Focus. 2016; 41(6):E3

[91] Omay SB, Chen YN, Almeida JP, et al. Do craniopharyngioma molecular signatures correlate with clinical characteristics? J Neurosurg. 2018; 128(5): 1473–1478

[92] Lee MH, Kim SH, Seoul HJ, Nam DH, Lee JI, Park K, Kim JH, Kong DS. Impact of maximal safe resection on the clinical outcome of adults with craniopharyngiomas. J Clin Neurosci. 2012 Jul;19(7):1005-8. doi: 10.1016/j.jocn.2011.09.033. Epub 2012 May 16. PMID: 22595354

[93] Zhao X, Yi X, Wang H, Zhao H. An analysis of related factors of surgical results for patients with craniopharyngiomas. Clin Neurol Neurosurg. 2012 Feb;114(2):149-55. doi: 10.1016/j.clineuro.2011.10.004. Epub 2011 Nov 5. PMID: 22056762

14 Natural History and Management Options of Idiopathic Intracranial Hypertension

Kevin Liu and Helen V. Danesh-Meyer

Abstract

Idiopathic intracranial hypertension is a disease of raised intracranial pressure causing headache and visual changes.

Epidemiology: Incidence rate of 0.5-2 per 100,000 person years in the general population with higher rates seen in obese women of childbearing age.

Natural History: Vision loss can manifest both early or late in the disease course and often does so without the patient realising. Visual field defects can be observed in up to 87% of patients, though 67% of patients can be asymptomatic with mild/minimal defects. Visual prognosis is good with treatment in up to 60% of patients and only 10% experience worsening visual function. Rate of blindness or severe visual impairment range between 1 and 10%. Recurrence rates vary between 8.3 and 52% and more commonly associated with treatment nonadherence, pregnancy, or weight gain. Three percent patients have a fulminant variant with rapid vision loss from symptom onset, have poor visual prognosis, and often require surgical intervention.

Management: Weight loss is a successful treatment associated with improvement in vision and reduction in headaches. This can also be achieved through bariatric surgery especially in cases where regaining of weight is associated with relapse of disease.

Medical treatment includes acetazolamide with the strongest evidence followed by topiramate and furosemide as alternatives. Corticosteroids are not recommended as long term or routine therapy as withdrawal is associated with rebound in intracranial pressure as well as weight gain. Serial lumbar punctures are not routinely recommended but have a role for those awaiting surgery or avoiding medical treatment in pregnant patients.

Surgical treatment includes optic nerve sheath fenestration, ventriculoperitoneal shunts or lumboperitoneal shunts, and venous sinus stenting. They are generally more indicated in patients in whom vision loss is rapid, have severe symptoms, or the disease is uncontrolled by medical management. There is no evidence to suggest clear superiority of one over another, though choice often depends on individual patient presentation and expertise of the center.

Keywords: idiopathic intracranial hypertension, pseudotumor cerebri, papilloedema, bariatric surgery, optic nerve sheath fenestration, venitriculoperitoneal shunt, lumboperitoneal shunt, venous sinus stenting

14.1 Introduction

Idiopathic intracranial hypertension (IIH), also known as pseudotumor cerebri, is a condition characterized by (1) clinical features of raised intracranial pressure (ICP), (2) normal cerebrospinal fluid (CSF) composition, and (3) absence of abnormal findings on neuroimaging.[1]

IIH typically affects young obese women, often with menstrual irregularities.[2,3] The overall incidence is between 0.5 and 2.0 per 100,000 person-years. The rate is higher among obese women of childbearing age (incidence between 12 and 20 per 100,000 person-years).[2] This incidence is predicted to worsen in parallel with increasing future rates of obesity globally as they have both already demonstrated to have done so for 25 years since 1990.[3,4]

Patients usually present with a variety of symptoms indicative of elevated ICP, the more common ones being headache, transient visual obscurations, and pulsatile tinnitus.[5,6,7] Patients with IIH may develop diplopia secondary to unilateral or bilateral sixth nerve palsy (a false localizing sign). Other common nonvisual symptoms include nausea, vomiting, dizziness, and neck and back pain. Less common visual symptoms are retrobulbar pain and sustained visual loss.

Clinical examination reveals papilledema with an otherwise normal neurological examination. The importance of papilledema is that it raises the possibility of damage to optic nerve function if the disc swelling is sustained. It is important to remember that visual acuity is preserved in early papilledema. Visual field testing may reveal an enlarged blind spot, which reflects the papilledema rather than decreased optic nerve function. However, prolonged or extremely elevated ICP may result in optic nerve compromise. This manifests as visual field defects in the early stages. With progression of optic nerve damage, there is decreased visual acuity and loss of color vision.[5] The most important long-term sequela of IIH is visual loss; therefore, it is critical to perform regular assessment of optic nerve function, which includes visual acuity, visual field (formal automated testing), color vision, and fundus examination.

The diagnosis of IIH requires normal neuroimaging, which includes either a computed tomography (CT) venogram or magnetic resonance (MR) venogram so that venous sinus stenosis/thrombosis can be excluded. In addition, it is important to exclude space-occupying lesion or abnormal meningeal enhancement. Neuroimaging findings that are consistent with elevated ICP include flattening of the globes, fluid in the subarachnoid space around the optic nerves, an empty sellae, and small ventricles (▶ Fig. 14.1). Venous sinus narrowing may also be a sign of raised ICP, although in some cases it may be the underlying cause.

If papilledema is present in the presence of normal neuroimaging, then a lumbar puncture is required to both measure the opening pressure and to evaluate the CSF composition. The diagnosis of IIH requires normal CSF composition and elevated opening pressure (1) greater than 250 mm H_2O in adults; (2) greater than 280 mm H_2O in children and adolescents; or (3) 250 mm H_2O for nonobese, nonsedated children.[8]

There have been multiple secondary causes for pseudotumor cerebri noted in the literature. There is a long list of medications that have been reported to be associated with or causative of

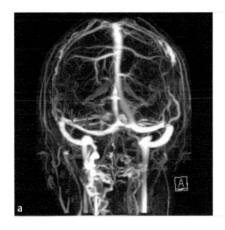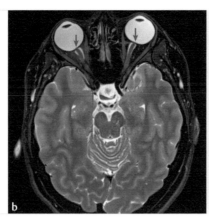

Fig. 14.1 Neuroimaging features of idiopathic intracranial hypertension (IIH). **(a)** Magnetic resonance imaging (MRI) venography showing narrowing of the left transverse sinus (*arrows*). **(b)** T2-weighted MRI, axial, and flattening of the globes (*vertical arrows*) and distension of optic nerve sheaths (*horizontal arrows*).

IIH. Of these, the most common and relevant include tetracycline antibiotics and vitamin A and its metabolites. Tetracycline has been suggested as a precipitant to IIH with between 7 and 9% of patients found to be taking tetracycline concurrently. Withdrawal of the medication may result in resolution of the IIH in some cases; however, persistent IIH has also been reported.[9,10,11] Excess vitamin A and its metabolites (retinoids) have been suggested in multiple reports to also act as another secondary cause; however, the recent IIH Treatment Trial (IIHTT) with the Neuro-Ophthalmology Research Disease Investigator Consortium (NORDIC) Idiopathic Intracranial Hypertension Study Group produced conflicting evidence where toxicity from vitamin A and retinoids is unlikely to be contributory based on their measurements of vitamin A metabolites in the serum and CSF of their study patients.[12] Other medications have also included thyroxine, growth hormone, tamoxifen, corticosteroids, lithium, and ciclosporin.[2] Nitrofurantoin, sulfonamides, and nalidixic acid have been reported as a secondary cause for children.[2,13,14]

For medical disorders associated with pseudotumor cerebri, chronic anemia has been shown to have an incidence association of 10.3% with resolution of this illness upon correction of anemia.[15] Other disorders include Addison's disease, obstructive sleep apnea, and systemic lupus erythematous.[2,16,17]

14.2 Selected Papers on Natural History

- Corbett JJ, Savino PJ, Thompson HS, et al. Visual loss in pseudotumor cerebri. Follow-up of 57 patients from five to 41 years and a profile of 14 patients with permanent severe visual loss. Arch Neurol 1982;39(8):461–474
- Wall M, George D. Idiopathic intracranial hypertension. A prospective study of 50 patients. Brain 1991;114(Pt 1A): 155–180
- Shah VA, Kardon RH, Lee AG, Corbett JJ, Wall M. Long-term follow-up of idiopathic intracranial hypertension: the Iowa experience. Neurology 2008;70(8):634–640
- Wall M, Kupersmith MJ, Thurtell MJ, Moss HE, Moss EA, Auinger P; NORDIC Idiopathic Intracranial Hypertension Study Group. The longitudinal idiopathic intracranial hypertension trial: outcomes from months 6–12. Am J Ophthalmol 2017;176:102–107

14.3 Natural History of Idiopathic Intracranial Hypertension

There are no prospective series of large study size evaluating the natural history of IIH. There are only relatively small retrospective reviews with selected populations, for example, males with IIH. There is a recent multicenter trial of IIH, the Idiopathic Intracranial Hypertension Trial (IIHT), which is a randomized prospective multicenter trial recruiting 165 participants with mild IIH. Natural history data are beginning to emerge from this study although they remain limited at this stage. The data summarized below are based on the available evidence as depicted in ▶ Fig. 14.2.

Vision loss can manifest both early and late in the disease course and often does so without the patient realizing it.[18,19] Such vision loss commonly occurs over a long course of months to years and can range from mild defects with enlarged blind spots, nasal defects, and generalized depressions to permanent blindness, which is the main morbidity associated with IIH.[6] Visual field defects were observed in monitored patients (75-87% on Goldmann perimetry and 56-80% on automated perimetry). Sixty-seven percent of these defects were mild/minimal and patients were reportedly asymptomatic with these defects.[19] In general, visual prognosis appears to be good with treatment, with 51 to 60% of patients found to have stable or improved visual fields and only 10% experiencing worsening visual function.[6,18] However, the risk of blindness is variable depending on the population and the treatment. Corbett[18] found that 24.6% developed blindness in one or both eyes, with 78% of those with persistent vision loss at initial assessment found to be blind on follow-up. Other more recent studies report lower rates of blindness/severe visual impairment or treatment failure, occurring in 1 to 13.8% of observed patients.[6,20,21,22,23] The NORDIC IIHTT showed a treatment failure rate of 1% in patients on acetazolamide and a weight loss diet compared to 10% on weight loss diet only.[21,24]

Recurrence of IIH has been found to occur in patients after resolution of symptoms and recovery from the first episode or after stability of months and years at a reported rate of between 8.3 and 52%.[25,26,27,28] Recurrence mainly occurred in the context of cessation of acetazolamide treatment due to noncompliance or intolerance of the medication.[25] In some studies, weight gain has also been shown to have an association with recurrence.[27,28]

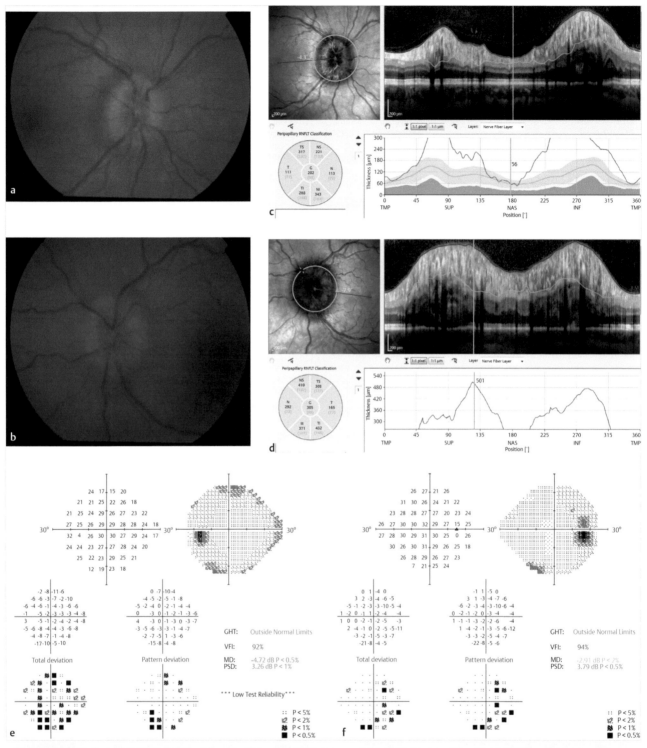

Fig. 14.2 Fundus photographs and optical coherence tomography (OCT) can contribute to diagnosis and monitoring of idiopathic intracranial hypertension (IIH) and papilledema. **(a)** Fundal photograph of the right eye and **(b)** fundal photograph of the left eye with corresponding OCT scans of the **(c)** right and **(d)** left eyes. Humphrey visual fields of the same **(e)** left and **(f)** right eyes. **(a)** and **(b)** show optic disc swelling with elevated discs and peripapillary haloes. **(c)** and **(d)** show increases in retinal nerve fiber layer thickness (RNFL). Both **(e)** and **(f)** show enlarged blind spots and **(d)** shows early stages of generalized constriction of the visual field.

Approximately 3% of patients with IIH experience a fulminant variant of the disease with rapid vision loss within 4 weeks of symptom onset, requiring surgical intervention, but unfortunately this group of patients have been shown to have very poor visual outcomes with 50% blindness in a study's patients, particularly in those with greater surgical delay, and 100% of patients left with severe visual field defects.[29]

14.3.1 Factors Predicting Blindness or Poor Visual Outcome

Patients at initial assessment who were found to have persistent vision loss with poor visual acuity and those with high-grade papilledema were found to be at greater risk of vision loss.[21,24] Papilledema and treatment effect were best found to be monitored by photographic disc area from fundus photos and volume on optical coherence tomography (OCT) rather than the Frisén score (a clinical score for papilledema).[30] Papilledema can also be monitored with the assistance of OCT, which is a noninvasive technique that measures the peripapillary retinal nerve fiber layer thickness.[31,32] This allows a quantitative measure of optic nerve head swelling. One caveat is that the nerve swelling may resolve for two reasons[1]: resolution of the papilledema or[2] death of ganglion cells, which results in loss of retinal nerve fiber layer; therefore, there is less nerve fiber tissue to become swollen.

Men who make up less than 10% of IIH patients have greater risk of treatment failure and severe visual impairment in one or both eyes with the risk found to be up to 26 times that of women.[21,33] Obesity is well known to be associated with a greater risk of IIH; in addition, a higher percentage of weight gain in the year prior to symptom onset in both obese and nonobese patients was reported to have a greater risk.[34] Szewka et al, in a study of 414 patients, found that those who were morbidly obese were likely to have severe papilledema on initial assessment, which is associated with greater risk of severe vision loss and every increase in 10 kg/m^2 of body mass index (BMI) increased the risk of severe vision loss by 1.4 times.[35] Patients of black race were also found to have increased risk of blindness and worse visual outcomes despite equal access to health care and treatment than nonblacks with relative risk of 3.5 for blindness in one eye and 4.8 in both eyes.[22] Systemic hypertension has been observed as another risk factor for poor visual outcomes, with between 62 and 80% of patients who developed blindness having systemic hypertension.[18,22] Onset of IIH during puberty was associated with greater moderate to poor visual outcomes compared to prepubescent, teenage/young adult, and adult age groups.[36] The results of the IIHTT) showed that the presence nerve fiber layer hemorrhages in at least one eye correlated with the severity of papilledema and with failed treatment outcomes/poorer visual outcomes.[37] Another finding from the IIHTT trial also showed that patients with more than 30 transient visual obscurations per month were 10.59 times more likely to have treatment failure compared to those with less than 30 per month.[21]

14.4 Selected Papers on Management Options for Idiopathic Intracranial Hypertension

- Lai LT, Danesh-Meyer HV, Kaye AH. Visual outcomes and headache following interventions for idiopathic intracranial hypertension. J Clin Neurosci 2014;21(10):1670–1678
- Menger RP, Connor DE Jr, Thakur JD, et al. A comparison of lumboperitoneal and ventriculoperitoneal shunting for idiopathic intracranial hypertension: an analysis of economic impact and complications using the nationwide inpatient sample. Neurosurg Focus 2014;37(5):E4
- Piper RJ, Kalyvas AV, Young AMH, Hughes MA, Jamjoom AAB, Fouyas IP. Interventions for idiopathic intracranial hypertension. Cochrane Database Syst Rev 2015;(8):CD003434
- Manfield JH, Yu KK, Efthimiou E, Darzi A, Athanasiou T, Ashrafian H. Bariatric surgery or non-surgical weight loss for idiopathic intracranial hypertension? A systematic review and comparison of meta-analyses. Obes Surg 2017;27(2):513–521
- Nicholson P, Brinjikji W, Radovanovic I, et al. Venous sinus stenting for idiopathic intracranial hypertension: a systematic review and meta-analysis. J Neurointerv Surg 2019;11(4):380–385

14.5 Management Options for Idiopathic Intracranial Hypertension

With the current evidence and literature, universally accepted recommendations for the management of IIH are limited due to the paucity of randomized controlled trials (RCTs), prospective trials, and strong evidence.[38] The treatment of IIH has two major goals: preservation of vision and the alleviation of symptoms, most commonly headache. If causative medication or agents are identified, they should be ceased. Patients with IIH require regular follow-up to monitor response to treatment as well as to prevent visual loss. Intervals for follow-up visits are individualized depending on the severity of disease.

Some patients with normal vision and minimal symptoms require no treatment other than monitoring. We can categorize management options into three groups: (1) weight loss (including bariatric surgery), (2) pharmaceutical treatments, and (3) surgical treatments.

14.5.1 Weight Loss Including Bariatric Surgery

Weight loss has been shown to be a successful treatment.[27,28,34,35] A 2017 systematic review and meta-analysis was performed containing 8 studies and 277 patients for nonsurgical weight loss interventions (medical, behavioral, and lifestyle).[39] The results show a decrease in 4.2 kg/m^2 BMI, 66.7% improvement in papilledema, 75.4% improvement in visual fields, and 23.2% improvement in headaches though they acknowledge the lack of prospective and randomized trials in the current literature.[39]

Bariatric surgery is an alternative option to achieving weight loss with evidence of great effectiveness in achieving and maintaining weight loss in the long term.[40] One of the concerns with conservative weight loss methods is the significant risk of regaining weight and subsequently evoking a relapse/recurrence of IIH.[28] Two systematic reviews for bariatric surgery as an intervention for IIH reviewed 6 studies and 12 case reports, totaling 67 patients, which showed a decrease in 17 kg/m^2 in BMI in 25 patients and a decrease of 18.9-cm H_2O in 12 patients. Papilledema resolved completely in 27 patients, and 92% improvement in headache symptoms (36/39) and 93% improvement in visual fields (14/15) were observed.[39,41] The mortality rate of bariatric surgery ranges between 0.05 and 0.14% and major complication rate between 2 and 6%.[42] However, it is the most costly compared to other surgical interventions for IIH and is dependent on the availability of the procedure being offered at the surgical service of the patient's location as well as the patient's appropriateness and their eligibility to qualify for the surgery there.[43] Like conservative weight loss methods, there is insufficient reliable evidence to establish its long-term and comparative effectiveness.

Currently, there is the Idiopathic Intracranial Hypertension Weight Trial (IIH:WT), a multicenter open-label RCT of 64 IIH participants with BMI over 35 kg/m^2, which will compare bariatric surgery to dietary weight loss program with 5-year follow-up and is currently in the preresults stage.[42] This trial hopefully will provide insight into the long-term disease-modifying role of weight loss in managing IIH as well as cost-effectiveness and promote the generation of treatment guidelines.

14.5.2 Pharmaceutical Treatments

Treatment of IIH with medications typically begins with acetazolamide, a carbonic anhydrase inhibitor, given the evidence generated from the IIHTT randomized control trial in 2014.[24] IIHTT was a double-masked RCT of 165 participants in 38 centers in North America and recruited IIH patients aged between 18 and 60 years with mild visual field loss (–2 and –7 dB perimetric mean deviation [PMD]). The study compared acetazolamide with placebo, with all participants taking a low-sodium and weight-reduction diet. IIHTT showed improvement in both groups in visual field measures over 6 months with an increase in PMD of 1.43 versus 0.71 dB for acetazolamide versus placebo. The study also demonstrated greater reduction in papilledema weight (–7.5 vs. –3.45 kg) and improvements in vision-related quality of life compared to placebo. There was reported greater decrease in lumbar CSF opening pressure in the acetazolamide group versus placebo at 6 months measured in 48 to 55% of patients in each group that agreed to have a lumbar puncture at 6 months (–11.23 vs. –5.24 cm H$_2$O). There were no differences in headache disability score between the two groups though both had improved from baseline. The six of the seven patients in total who were considered treatment failure were from the placebo group.

The adverse effects that occurred in more than 5% of participants in the acetazolamide group were paresthesia, dysgeusia, fatigue, hypocapnia, nausea, vomiting, diarrhea, and tinnitus. Nine participants of 86 (10.5%) had adverse events that were classified as serious and average adherence was 89% in the acetazolamide group versus 93% in placebo. Dosing of acetazolamide was 2.5 g/d on average with more than 40% receiving 4 g/d.

The continuation of this trial, the Longitudinal Idiopathic Intracranial Hypertension Trial (LIIHT), picked up after the 6-month visit and all placebo patients changed to acetazolamide and all participants were evaluated again at 12 months.[44] Both groups continued to improve with respect to visual fields, papilledema, vision related quality though there were greater improvements in the placebo group that had changed to acetazolamide. Headache disability score also appeared to improve

more in the initial placebo group that switched over to acetazolamide, suggesting a possible benefit of acetazolamide for managing headache. Overall from this study, it demonstrated evidence that acetazolamide in addition to a low-sodium and weight loss diet was effective in treating IIH patients with mild visual loss and was relatively well tolerated. Acetazolamide has long-term complications, most notably, increasing the risk of kidney stones. In addition, patients need to have their potassium monitored as acetazolamide can cause potassium depletion.

Furosemide, a loop diuretic, has been used as an adjunct to acetazolamide in patients with IIH with a potential additive effect in animal studies and small case series.[45,46] Topiramate is an antiseizure and migraine prophylactic medication has been shown in an open label study in Turkey of topiramate versus acetazolamide in 40 randomized IIH patients to have similar improvements in visual fields to acetazolamide with also greater weight loss seen in the topiramate group.[47] It is thought to act as a carbonic anhydrase inhibitor in reducing ICP, which has also been demonstrated in rat studies.[48,49] Its role as a prophylactic migraine medication contributes to headache management and its side effect profile also contains appetite suppression, which can contribute to weight loss; however, it is worth noting up to 10% of patients report cognition problems as an adverse event.[50] Fatigue and distal paresthesia are reported side effects like acetazolamide.[47]

Corticosteroids were first described as a treatment since 1961; however, it not recommended as long-term or routine therapy for IIH given that withdrawal of steroids has shown severe rebound in ICPs and vision loss in addition to the weight gain associated with corticosteroids.[51,52,53,54]

Serial lumbar punctures are another treatment option although it has a limited role as CSF reforms within 6 hours unless there is a leak. In addition, lumbar puncture tends to be uncomfortable with risk of complications such as low-pressure headache, CSF leak, and infection. However, it is sometimes useful in anticipation of surgery or in pregnancy who wish to avoid medical therapy.[55]

14.5.3 Surgical Treatments

Surgical treatment of IIH has been shown to be undertaken in less than 9% of patients with IIH from the data of 23,182 IIH patients in the United Kingdom between the years 2002 and 2016.[4] The general indication for surgical intervention has been for cases with rapid onset and severe vision loss (fulminant IIH), progressive vision loss despite full medical therapy, or patients who do not tolerate medical therapy and are debilitated by symptoms.[4] Current surgical options include optic nerve sheath fenestration (OSNF), CSF diversion or shunting procedures (ventriculoperitoneal shunts [VPS] or lumboperitoneal shunts [LPS]), and venous sinus stenting (VSS). Systematic reviews have shown there is a lack of robust evidence to suggest clear superiority of one surgical treatment modality over another as there are no studies with great designs directly comparing these treatments to one another in the same population.[43,56] Choice of procedure is often dependent on the expertise of the center. The strength of the evidence gathered from combining data from mostly case series and case reports is limited due to statistical heterogeneity, publication bias, and selection bias related to the retrospective nature of some studies. Combining data of studies where there are different indications for surgery in the study patients and different outcomes measured also contributes to the limitations of our available evidence.

OSNF involves an incision of the optic nerve sheath to produce an opening releasing CSF and consequently reducing ICP. The procedure has shown significant improvements in vision with medically refractive IIH patients with those with severe vision loss, papilledema, and minimal headache being the most appropriate to undergo ONSF.[57] The data from two recent large meta-analyses for OSNF[43,57] show 75 to 89% of patients receiving OSNF as the first surgical procedure for medical refractory IIH. There was improvement in vision in 59 to 67% of eyes, and 84 to 95% of eyes had stable or improved visual acuity after the procedure. Overall, 64 to 68% of eyes (470/688) demonstrated improvement in visual fields, 41 to 44% of patients displayed improvement in headaches, and papilledema improved in 80 to 95% of patients. The complication rate was found to be 18 to 26% (1.5% major complications and 16.4% minor complications in the Satti et al[57] meta-analysis) with the most common complications being diplopia (26–43%), pupillary complications (9.7–25%; tonic pupil), late failure (10%), cranial nerve III or VI palsy (7.2%), orbital hematoma (7.2%), and corneal dellen (2.2–6%). Most complications were found to be transient in nature and nondisabling. Repeat OSNFs were found to be undertaken in a variable range between 9.21 and 69.8% of patients though these figures are greatly affected by the length of follow-up in the included studies. Fifty-three percent of patients had OSNF in only one eye as there is evidence that doing the intervention in one eye produces benefits for both eyes.[58] OSNF has also been suggested as the least expensive among the surgical interventions for IIH.[43] Endoscopic optic nerve decompression has shown some preliminary benefits in a small sample of patients with fewer risks.[59]

CSF diversion procedures include two types of procedures: VPS or LPS. Benefits from either shunt procedure has been shown to result in improvement in vision in 54%, headaches in up to 95%, and papilledema in 70%.[57,60] Two further meta-analyses comparing LPS versus VPS postoperatively showed similar improvements in visual acuity (56.6–67 vs. 49.3–55%), visual field (71 vs. 69%), headache (75.2–96 vs. 62.5–94%), and papilledema (91 vs. 90%).[43,56] However, a 10-year retrospective review showed that headaches persisted in 77 and 79% of patients at 1 and 2 years postoperatively.[61] Overall, 32 to 43% of patients receiving CSF shunts were reported to require at least one additional surgery after their initial surgery with similar rates for LPS and VPS.[43,56,57] Some studies suggest that LPS has a slightly higher failure rate than VPS.[62] On average, patients who experienced shunt failure needed 2.78 additional procedures.[57] The rate for major and minor complications were 7.6 and 32.9%, respectively, with the main complications being shunt infection, tonsillar herniation, subdural hematoma, CSF fistula, abdominal and back pain, low-pressure headache/CSF leak, and shunt dysfunction.[57] Overall compared to OSNF, CSF diversion has a worse complication profile and greater cost but addresses headache, which OSNF does not.[43]

VSS is a relatively newer approach in invasively managing IIH as there has been some focus on the stenosis of intracranial transverse venous sinuses and pressure gradient found across the stenotic segments in relation to IIH.[63] The largest and most recent meta-analysis of 474 patients in 18 centers found 78% of the patients undergoing VSS as primary treatment with an average pressure gradient of 21 mm Hg.[63] Results showed 93.7% improvement in papilledema, 79.6% improvement in headache, 90.3% improvement in tinnitus, 12.4% required a repeat procedure with 9% requiring repeat VSS and 3% requiring CSF shunt surgery, and finally 9.8% was the overall rate of recurrence. For complications, overall mortality was 0% and major complication rate was 1.9% (subdural hematoma, subarachnoid hemorrhage during or immediately after VSS) and all those patients made a long-term recovery without long-term morbidity. However, these rates are from centers with experience in this procedure and who undertake VSS at regular frequency. In these centers, VSS shows an excellent complication profile, low relapse rate, lower need for repeat procedure/revision, and comparatively satisfactory results in improvements in vision, papilledema, and headache with better outcomes compared with OSNF and CSF diversion.[43,56,57,63] The initial cost of the first VSS procedure is similar to that of the initial CSF diversion procedures; however, given the lower rate of repeat procedures, it can be seen as more cost effective.[43] However, VSS is indicated for patients with a confirmed pressure gradient between stenotic segments of the venous sinuses and these results may not apply to all patients with IIH. Furthermore, given a lack of randomized controlled studies for the surgical interventions for IIH, we are unable to provide robust evidence in recommending VSS as a more mainstream/first-line treatment for IIH, and we would require future studies to explore this.

14.6 Authors' Recommendations

- Although studies on the natural history of IIH are limited, there is some evidence that risk factors for severe and permanent vision loss include being male, morbidly obese, or African American. In addition, other risk factors that may be relevant include systemic hypertension, higher grade of papilledema, presence of nerve fiber layer hemorrhage, over 30 transient visual obscurations a month, and disease onset during puberty.
- Recurrence of IIH can occur with weight gain, during pregnancy, or cessation of acetazolamide treatment.
- There is definitive evidence to show weight loss with dieting and/or treatment with acetazolamide are effective treatments for IIH.
- Bariatric surgery is potentially an effective method of achieving and maintaining weight loss; however, it comes with its greater surgical risks and costs.
- Furosemide and topiramate have been used as adjuncts and/or alternatives to acetazolamide with some effect demonstrated in the literature.
- We do not recommend steroids in the routine or long-term treatment of IIH.
- Serial lumbar punctures have a more limited niche role when used while awaiting surgery or for pregnant patients wishing to avoid medical therapy. Generally, it is not recommended for routine treatment.
- Surgical interventions have shown improvements in visual outcomes and headache though they are more indicated in the cases where vision loss is rapid and severe or progressing despite full medical treatment or in patients not tolerating medical therapy.

- Current available surgical interventions that have been studied are ONSF (and endoscopic optic nerve decompression), VPS, LPS, and VSS. Systematic reviews so far have yielded no robust evidence to suggest clear superiority of one intervention over another. The decision often depends on the experience of the center.
- OSNF is suggested to be preferable for patients with mainly visual symptoms and minimal headache. Endoscopic approach to decompression shows promise but will require more studies and evidence.
- CSF diversion procedures are superior to OSNF with managing headache; however, they come with a greater complication profile and revision rate.
- VSS is a potential treatment for patients with stenosis of the venous sinuses and has the lowest complication profile and comparable improvement results with OSNF and CSF shunting. However, stronger evidence in the form of RCTs will be necessary before recommending it as the mainstream/first-line treatment.
- CSF drainage is needed in the minority of patients with IIH who undergo unsuccessful conservative management.

References

[1] Friedman DI, Jacobson DM. Diagnostic criteria for idiopathic intracranial hypertension. Neurology. 2002; 59(10):1492–1495

[2] Markey KA, Mollan SP, Jensen RH, Sinclair AJ. Understanding idiopathic intracranial hypertension: mechanisms, management, and future directions. Lancet Neurol. 2016; 15(1):78–91

[3] Kilgore KP, Lee MS, Leavitt JA, et al. Re-evaluating the incidence of idiopathic intracranial hypertension in an era of increasing obesity. Ophthalmology. 2017; 124(5):697–700

[4] Mollan SP, Aguiar M, Evison F, Frew E, Sinclair AJ. The expanding burden of idiopathic intracranial hypertension. Eye (Lond). 2019; 33(3):478–485

[5] Wall M, Kupersmith MJ, Kieburtz KD, et al. NORDIC Idiopathic Intracranial Hypertension Study Group. The idiopathic intracranial hypertension treatment trial: clinical profile at baseline. JAMA Neurol. 2014; 71(6):693–701

[6] Wall M, George D. Idiopathic intracranial hypertension. A prospective study of 50 patients. Brain. 1991; 114 Pt 1A:155–180

[7] Giuseffi V, Wall M, Siegel PZ, Rojas PB. Symptoms and disease associations in idiopathic intracranial hypertension (pseudotumor cerebri): a case-control study. Neurology. 1991; 41(2 (Pt 1)):239–244

[8] Friedman DI, Liu GT, Digre KB. Revised diagnostic criteria for the pseudotumor cerebri syndrome in adults and children. Neurology. 2013; 81 (13):1159–1165

[9] Friedman DI, Gordon LK, Egan RA, et al. Doxycycline and intracranial hypertension. Neurology. 2004; 62(12):2297–2299

[10] Kesler A, Goldhammer Y, Hadayer A, Pianka P. The outcome of pseudotumor cerebri induced by tetracycline therapy. Acta Neurol Scand. 2004; 110(6): 408–411

[11] Sundholm A, Burkill S, Sveinsson O, Piehl F, Bahmanyar S, Nilsson Remahl AIM. Population-based incidence and clinical characteristics of idiopathic intracranial hypertension. Acta Neurol Scand. 2017; 136(5):427–433

[12] Libien J, Kupersmith MJ, Blaner W, et al. NORDIC Idiopathic Intracranial Hypertension Study Group. Role of vitamin A metabolism in IIH: results from the idiopathic intracranial hypertension treatment trial. J Neurol Sci. 2017; 372:78–84

[13] Riyaz A, Aboobacker CM, Sreelatha PR. Nalidixic acid induced pseudotumour cerebri in children. J Indian Med Assoc. 1998; 96(10):308–314

[14] Cohen DN. Intracranial hypertension and papilledema associated with nalidixic acid therapy. Am J Ophthalmol. 1973; 76(5):680–682

[15] Mollan SP, Ball AK, Sinclair AJ, et al. Idiopathic intracranial hypertension associated with iron deficiency anaemia: a lesson for management. Eur Neurol. 2009; 62(2):105–108

[16] Man BL, Mok CC, Fu YP. Neuro-ophthalmologic manifestations of systemic lupus erythematosus: a systematic review. Int J Rheum Dis. 2014; 17(5): 494–501

[17] Condulis N, Germain G, Charest N, Levy S, Carpenter TO. Pseudotumor cerebri: a presenting manifestation of Addison's disease. Clin Pediatr (Phila). 1997; 36(12):711–713

[18] Corbett JJ, Savino PJ, Thompson HS, et al. Visual loss in pseudotumor cerebri. Follow-up of 57 patients from five to 41 years and a profile of 14 patients with permanent severe visual loss. Arch Neurol. 1982; 39(8):461–474

[19] Rowe FJ, Sarkies NJ. Assessment of visual function in idiopathic intracranial hypertension: a prospective study. Eye (Lond). 1998; 12(Pt 1):111–118

[20] Bulens C, De Vries WA, Van Crevel H. Benign intracranial hypertension. A retrospective and follow-up study. J Neurol Sci. 1979; 40(2–3):147–157

[21] Wall M, Falardeau J, Fletcher WA, et al. NORDIC Idiopathic Intracranial Hypertension Study Group. Risk factors for poor visual outcome in patients with idiopathic intracranial hypertension. Neurology. 2015; 85(9):799–805

[22] Bruce BB, Preechawat P, Newman NJ, Lynn MJ, Biousse V. Racial differences in idiopathic intracranial hypertension. Neurology. 2008; 70(11):861–867

[23] Best J, Silvestri G, Burton B, Foot B, Acheson J. the incidence of blindness due to idiopathic intracranial hypertension in the UK. Open Ophthalmol J. 2013; 7:26–29

[24] Wall M, McDermott MP, Kieburtz KD, et al. NORDIC Idiopathic Intracranial Hypertension Study Group Writing Committee. Effect of acetazolamide on visual function in patients with idiopathic intracranial hypertension and mild visual loss: the idiopathic intracranial hypertension treatment trial. JAMA. 2014; 311(16):1641–1651

[25] Taktakishvili O, Shah VA, Shahbaz R, Lee AG. Recurrent idiopathic intracranial hypertension. Ophthalmology. 2008; 115(1):221

[26] Shah VA, Kardon RH, Lee AG, Corbett JJ, Wall M. Long-term follow-up of idiopathic intracranial hypertension: the Iowa experience. Neurology. 2008; 70(8):634–640

[27] Kesler A, Hadayer A, Goldhammer Y, Almog Y, Korczyn AD. Idiopathic intracranial hypertension: risk of recurrences. Neurology. 2004; 63(9): 1737–1739

[28] Ko MW, Chang SC, Ridha MA, et al. Weight gain and recurrence in idiopathic intracranial hypertension: a case-control study. Neurology. 2011; 76(18): 1564–1567

[29] Thambisetty M, Lavin PJ, Newman NJ, Biousse V. Fulminant idiopathic intracranial hypertension. Neurology. 2007; 68(3):229–232

[30] Sheils CR, Fischer WS, Hollar RA, Blanchard LM, Feldon SE, NORDIC Idiopathic Intracranial Hypertension Study Group. The relationship between optic disc volume, area, and frisén score in patients with idiopathic intracranial hypertension. Am J Ophthalmol. 2018; 195:101–109

[31] Huang-Link Y, Eleftheriou A, Yang G, et al. Optical coherence tomography represents a sensitive and reliable tool for routine monitoring idiopathic intracranial hypertension with and without papilledema. Eur J Neurol. 2019; 26(5):808–e57

[32] Eren Y, Kabatas N, Guven H, Comoglu S, Gurdal C. Evaluation of optic nerve head changes with optic coherence tomography in patients with idiopathic intracranial hypertension. Acta Neurol Belg. 2019; 119(3):351–357

[33] Bruce BB, Kedar S, Van Stavern GP, et al. Idiopathic intracranial hypertension in men. Neurology. 2009; 72(4):304–309

[34] Daniels AB, Liu GT, Volpe NJ, et al. Profiles of obesity, weight gain, and quality of life in idiopathic intracranial hypertension (pseudotumor cerebri). Am J Ophthalmol. 2007; 143(4):635–641

[35] Szewka AJ, Bruce BB, Newman NJ, Biousse V. Idiopathic intracranial hypertension: relation between obesity and visual outcomes. J Neuroophthalmol. 2013; 33(1):4–8

[36] Stiebel-Kalish H, Kalish Y, Lusky M, Gaton DD, Ehrlich R, Shuper A. Puberty as a risk factor for less favorable visual outcome in idiopathic intracranial hypertension. Am J Ophthalmol. 2006; 142(2):279–283

[37] Wall M, Thurtell MJ, NORDIC Idiopathic Intracranial Hypertension Study Group. Optic disc haemorrhages at baseline as a risk factor for poor outcome in the idiopathic intracranial hypertension treatment trial. Br J Ophthalmol. 2017; 101(9):1256–1260

[38] Piper RJ, Kalyvas AV, Young AMH, Hughes MA, Jamjoom AAB, Fouyas IP. Interventions for idiopathic intracranial hypertension. Cochrane Database Syst Rev. 2015(8):CD003434

[39] Manfield JH, Yu KK, Efthimiou E, Darzi A, Athanasiou T, Ashrafian H. Bariatric surgery or non-surgical weight loss for idiopathic intracranial hypertension? A systematic review and comparison of meta-analyses. Obes Surg. 2017; 27 (2):513–521

[40] Garb J, Welch G, Zagarins S, Kuhn J, Romanelli J. Bariatric surgery for the treatment of morbid obesity: a meta-analysis of weight loss outcomes for laparoscopic adjustable gastric banding and laparoscopic gastric bypass. Obes Surg. 2009; 19(10):1447–1455

[41] Handley JD, Baruah BP, Williams DM, Horner M, Barry J, Stephens JW. Bariatric surgery as a treatment for idiopathic intracranial hypertension: a systematic review. Surg Obes Relat Dis. 2015; 11(6):1396–1403

[42] Ottridge R, Mollan SP, Botfield H, et al. Randomised controlled trial of bariatric surgery versus a community weight loss programme for the sustained treatment of idiopathic intracranial hypertension: the Idiopathic Intracranial Hypertension Weight Trial (IIH:WT) protocol. BMJ Open. 2017; 7 (9):e017426

[43] Kalyvas AV, Hughes M, Koutsarnakis C, et al. Efficacy, complications and cost of surgical interventions for idiopathic intracranial hypertension: a systematic review of the literature. Acta Neurochir (Wien). 2017; 159(1):33–49

[44] Wall M, Kupersmith MJ, Thurtell MJ, Moss HE, Moss EA, Auinger P, NORDIC Idiopathic Intracranial Hypertension Study Group. The longitudinal idiopathic intracranial hypertension trial: outcomes from months 6–12. Am J Ophthalmol. 2017; 176:102–107

[45] McCarthy KD, Reed DJ. The effect of acetazolamide and furosemide on cerebrospinal fluid production and choroid plexus carbonic anhydrase activity. J Pharmacol Exp Ther. 1974; 189(1):194–201

[46] Schoeman JF. Childhood pseudotumor cerebri: clinical and intracranial pressure response to acetazolamide and furosemide treatment in a case series. J Child Neurol. 1994; 9(2):130–134

[47] Celebisoy N, Gökçay F, Sirin H, Akyürekli O. Treatment of idiopathic intracranial hypertension: topiramate vs acetazolamide, an open-label study. Acta Neurol Scand. 2007; 116(5):322–327

[48] Leniger T, Thöne J, Wiemann M. Topiramate modulates pH of hippocampal CA3 neurons by combined effects on carbonic anhydrase and Cl-/HCO3-exchange. Br J Pharmacol. 2004; 142(5):831–842

[49] Scotton WJ, Botfield HF, Westgate CS, et al. Topiramate is more effective than acetazolamide at lowering intracranial pressure. Cephalalgia. 2019; 39(2):209–218

[50] Mula M. Topiramate and cognitive impairment: evidence and clinical implications. Ther Adv Drug Saf. 2012; 3(6):279–289

[51] Liu GT, Glaser JS, Schatz NJ. High-dose methylprednisolone and acetazolamide for visual loss in pseudotumor cerebri. Am J Ophthalmol. 1994; 118(1):88–96

[52] Neville BG, Wilson J. Benign intracranial hypertension following corticosteroid withdrawal in childhood. BMJ. 1970; 3(5722):554–556

[53] Liu GT, Kay MD, Bienfang DC, Schatz NJ. Pseudotumor cerebri associated with corticosteroid withdrawal in inflammatory bowel disease. Am J Ophthalmol. 1994; 117(3):352–357

[54] Paterson R, Depasquale N, Mann S. Pseudotumor cerebri. Medicine (Baltimore). 1961; 40:85–99

[55] Yiangou A, Mitchell J, Markey KA, et al. Therapeutic lumbar puncture for headache in idiopathic intracranial hypertension: minimal gain, is it worth the pain? Cephalalgia. 2019; 39(2):245–253

[56] Lai LT, Danesh-Meyer HV, Kaye AH. Visual outcomes and headache following interventions for idiopathic intracranial hypertension. J Clin Neurosci. 2014; 21(10):1670–1678

[57] Satti SR, Leishangthem L, Chaudry MI. Meta-analysis of CSF diversion procedures and dural venous sinus stenting in the setting of medically refractory idiopathic intracranial hypertension. AJNR Am J Neuroradiol. 2015; 36(10):1899–1904

[58] Alsuhaibani AH, Carter KD, Nerad JA, Lee AG. Effect of optic nerve sheath fenestration on papilledema of the operated and the contralateral nonoperated eyes in idiopathic intracranial hypertension. Ophthalmology. 2011; 118(2):412–414

[59] Tarrats L, Hernández G, Busquets JM, et al. Outcomes of endoscopic optic nerve decompression in patients with idiopathic intracranial hypertension. Int Forum Allergy Rhinol. 2017; 7(6):615–623

[60] McGirt MJ, Woodworth G, Thomas G, Miller N, Williams M, Rigamonti D. Cerebrospinal fluid shunt placement for pseudotumor cerebri-associated intractable headache: predictors of treatment response and an analysis of long-term outcomes. J Neurosurg. 2004; 101(4):627–632

[61] Sinclair AJ, Kuruvath S, Sen D, Nightingale PG, Burdon MA, Flint G. Is cerebrospinal fluid shunting in idiopathic intracranial hypertension worthwhile? A 10-year review. Cephalalgia. 2011; 31(16):1627–1633

[62] Menger RP, Connor DE, Jr, Thakur JD, et al. A comparison of lumboperitoneal and ventriculoperitoneal shunting for idiopathic intracranial hypertension: an analysis of economic impact and complications using the nationwide inpatient sample. Neurosurg Focus. 2014; 37(5):E4

[63] Nicholson P, Brinjikji W, Radovanovic I, et al. Venous sinus stenting for idiopathic intracranial hypertension: a systematic review and meta-analysis. J Neurointerv Surg. 2019; 11(4):380–385

15 Natural History and Management Options of Chronic Subdural Hematoma

Dana C. Holl, Angelos G. Kolias, Ruben Dammers, and Ivan Timofeev

Abstract

Chronic subdural hematoma (CSDH) is a frequent pathological entity in daily clinical practice. The incidence is expected to double over the next 30 years, but evidence-based CSDH guidelines are lacking. Currently, surgery is the mainstay in CSDH treatment. Middle meningeal artery embolization and nonsurgical treatments have also been suggested in the management of CSDH. High-quality randomized controlled trials are currently ongoing in order to provide class I evidence on the clinical and cost-effectiveness of (non)surgical treatments.

Keywords: chronic subdural hematoma, pathophysiology, surgical, nonsurgical, middle meningeal artery embolization

15.1 Introduction

Chronic subdural hematoma (CSDH) is an abnormal collection of blood, blood breakdown products, and cerebrospinal fluid in the subdural space. It is an increasingly common neurological condition among the elderly, with a preponderance among men (male-to-female ratio across all age groups of 2:1).[1,2,3,4,5,6,7] Its incidence has increased over time from 1.7 to 31.2 per 100,000 persons per year (before 2000)[7,8,9] to 20.6 to 79.6 per 100,000 persons per year (from 2000 onward).[7,10,11,12] With the growing aging population, availability of neuroimaging, and the mounting use of antiplatelet medication and anticoagulant, the incidence of CSDH is expected to increase.[13,14]

Clinical manifestations of CSDH are variable and mainly caused by immediate intracranial compression through expansion of the hematoma. CSDH has an indolent course of disease progression with an average latent period of weeks or even months[3,15,16] until patients present with slowly progressive symptoms, such as headache, behavioral disturbance (cognitive decline, acute confusion), gait disturbance and falls, limb weakness, drowsiness, or coma. Aphasia, collapse, seizure, incontinence, visual disturbance, and vomiting have also been reported.[3,5,17,18]

The increasing incidence of CSDH underscores the importance of understanding the pathophysiology, natural history, and the available treatment options. Whereas treatment goals for CSDH are well established, several important aspects of its clinical management remain controversial. This chapter examines available literature on the natural history and treatment options for CSDH.

15.2 Selected Papers on the Natural History of Chronic Subdural Hematoma

- Edlmann E, Giorgi-Coll S, Whitfield PC, Carpenter KLH, Hutchinson PJ. Pathophysiology of chronic subdural haematoma: inflammation, angiogenesis and implications for pharmacotherapy. J Neuroinflammation 2017;14(1):108

- Holl DC, Volovici V, Dirven CMF, et al; Dutch Chronic Subdural Hematoma Research Group (DSHR). Pathophysiology and nonsurgical treatment of chronic subdural hematoma: from past to present to future. World Neurosurg 2018;116:402–411.e2

15.3 Natural History

Studies looking at the natural history of CSDH are sparse and are predominantly of low level of evidence. The natural history of CSDH remains unclear and is only described in case reports or small case series.

A recent phase 2 placebo-controlled trial of atorvastatin as primary therapy enrolled patients with a CSDH and mild symptoms (90% had a Glasgow Coma Scale [GCS] of 15 and no neurological deficits) found that the rate of progression to surgery due to increased CSDH volume and/or neurological worsening was 23.5% in the control group (74% within the first month and 26% during months 2–4).[21] It has to be noted that the baseline CSDH volume was 62 mL in this study, which is substantially less than the baseline CSDH volume in most surgical series. Without any treatment, few CSDHs have been reported to regress spontaneously, whereas 40% of all patients may eventually recover on medical management without surgical intervention. At least 20% of patients undergoing conservative management will experience clinical deterioration and require surgical intervention. However, it seems that there are no clear clinical or radiological signs indicating whether the CSDH will resolve spontaneously or not.

CSDH is often preceded by a minor head trauma, which can cause cleavage of the dural border cell layer (▶ Fig. 15.1).[18,19,20] This cell layer is a sublayer of the dura mater consisting of flattened fibroblasts with minimal extracellular collagen.[22,23,24] Damage of the dural border cell layer leads to the formation of the subdural space with an external and an internal membrane, which develop within 1 and 3 weeks, respectively.[25,26] In contrast to the internal membrane, the external membrane is abundant with highly permeable capillaries, which leads to extravasation of vascular contents into the newly formed subdural space. In addition, the external membrane is thicker, with layers of active fibroblasts and collagen fibrils, a source of angiogenic and inflammatory mediators.[18,19,20,24] Once the dural border cell layer is damaged, CSF and/or small quantities of blood are interposed within this cell layer. This leads to a vicious cycle resulting in enlargement of the subdural space and the formation of a CSDH.[19,20]

Three pathophysiological processes can be distinguished within the vicious CSDH cycle: inflammation, angiogenesis, and hyperfibrinolysis (▶ Fig. 15.2).[19,20]

15.3.1 Inflammation

Damaged dural cells, fibroblasts, and endothelial cells release chemokines and cytokines, which activate a range of inflammatory cells, among which are neutrophils, eosinophils,

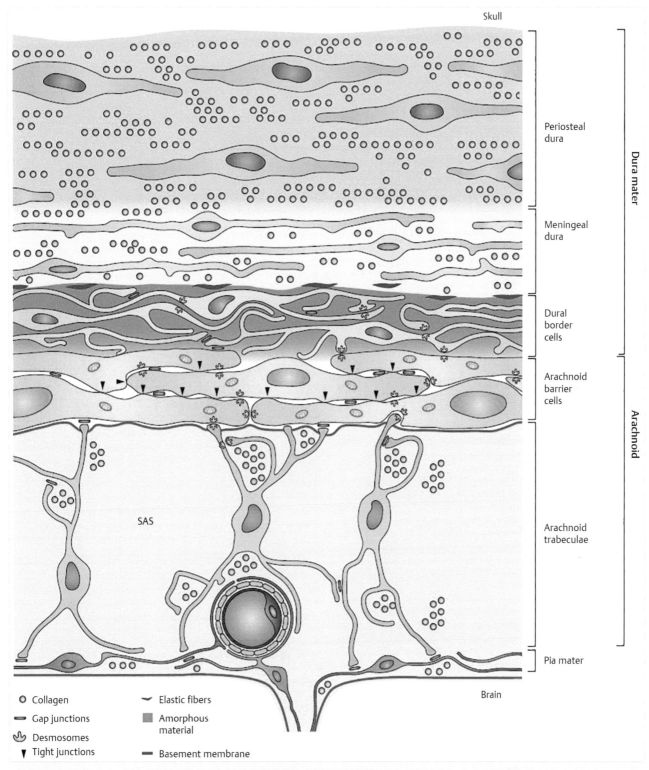

Fig. 15.1 Dural border cell layer (SAS, subarachnoid space). (Adapted from Haines.[23])

lymphocytes, and macrophages.[19,20,27,28,29,30,31,32,33] Cytokines, such as interleukin-6 (IL-6), IL-8, and the anti-inflammatory IL-10, are present in the CSDH at higher concentrations than in serum.[34,35,36,37,38] CSDH is, therefore, a local inflammatory process, and does not inflict a systemic responses such as elevation of erythrocyte sedimentation rate (ESR) and C-reactive protein (CRP). Inflammatory IL-6 is secreted within the subdural space by fibroblasts, monocytes, and endothelial cells[39] in response to cell injury and hemorrhage.[40,41] It provides an acute response to inflammation with B and T cell differentiation, enhancement of leucocyte recruitment, and acute phase protein induction.[39,40] In addition, it increases platelet production and

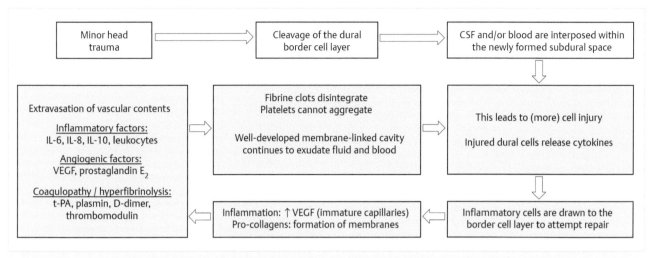

Fig. 15.2 The pathophysiology of the chronic subdural hematoma (CSDH), characterized by inflammation, angiogenesis, and hyperfibrinolysis. This cycle perpetuates (CSF, cerebrospinal fluid; IL, interleukin; t-PA, tissue plasminogen activator; VEGF, vascular endothelial growth factor).

enlarges endothelial gap junctions with subsequent increased vascular permeability.[42] Proinflammatory IL-8 attracts inflammatory cells, among which are neutrophils, to the inflammation site.[43] IL-8 also acts as an angiogenic factor.[38,44] Anti-inflammatory IL-10 deactivates T cells, monocytes, and macrophages, and reduces proinflammatory cytokine production.[45,46]

15.3.2 Angiogenesis

Vascular endothelial growth factor (VEGF) is one of the proangiogenic factors, which is found at significantly higher concentrations in the external membrane and in CSDH fluid compared to serum and cerebrospinal fluid.[28,29,30,47,48,49,50] It has been suggested that the probability of CSDH recurrence is higher in patients with a strong VEGF expression in the external membrane.[34] VEGF is produced by macrophages and vascular endothelial cells within the external membrane. This production is stimulated by prostaglandin E2 and by hypoxia-inducible factor 1, present in the external membrane. It activates several pathways[51,52,53] that induce angiogenesis and increase vascular permeability. VEGF, in combination with angiopoietin 2, leads to the formation of immature capillaries.

15.3.3 Hyperfibrinolysis

Inflammation causes the release of tissue plasminogen activator (t-PA) from endothelial cells. The level of t-PA is significantly higher in CSDH fluid than in plasma.[54] When relatively high concentrations of t-PA are found in the CSDH, the risk of recurrence is higher.[55,56] t-PA activates plasminogen, which is converted into plasmin. This causes degradation of coagulation factors V, VIII, and XI. Plasmin also breaks down fibrin clots into fibrinogen degradation products, among which is D-dimer, a platelet aggregation inhibitor.[57,58] The external membrane is also considered a source of thrombomodulin, which is found in high levels in CSDH fluid and enhances fibrinolysis.[59] This thrombin receptor inhibits blood clotting by binding with thrombin and the activated protein C.[37] Fibrin clots disintegrate and platelets cannot aggregate. This produces more cell injury and results in a higher inflammatory response and increased VEGF production.

The pathophysiological processes, in some patients, create a vicious cycle with the subdural collection gradually enlarging. High levels of inflammatory, angiogenic, and fibrinolytic factors are present in this newly formed subdural space. This can lead to gradual but progressive neurological deterioration in some patients. In order to break this pathological cycle, treatment is usually required. Surgical treatment is aimed at drainage and irrigation of the subdural space to decrease the mass effect and to reduce the levels of the inflammatory, angiogenic, and fibrinolytic factors. Nonsurgical treatments aim to control these processes pharmacologically. Conservative management with simple observation can also be used in some patients, especially those with very mild or no symptoms. However, to date it is unknown which factors contribute to the spontaneous resolution of CSDHs or may affect the balance between progression and spontaneous resolution. An increase or decrease in hematoma volume depends on the rebleed absorption rate and on the maturation and stabilization of the neomembrane.[60]

15.4 Selected Papers on the Management of Chronic Subdural Hematoma

- Kolias AG, Chari A, Santarius T, Hutchinson PJ. Chronic subdural haematoma: modern management and emerging therapies. Nat Rev Neurol 2014;10(10):570–578
- Almenawer SA, Farrokhyar F, Hong C, et al. Chronic subdural hematoma management: a systematic review and meta-analysis of 34,829 patients. Ann Surg 2014;259(3):449–457
- Brennan PM, Kolias AG, Joannides AJ, et al; British Neurosurgical Trainee Research Collaborative. The management and outcome for patients with chronic subdural hematoma: a prospective, multicenter, observational cohort study in the United Kingdom. J Neurosurg 2017;127(4):732–739

15.5 Treatment Options

Both surgical and nonsurgical approaches have been employed in the management of CSDH. Nevertheless, surgery remains the mainstay of management of patients with significant symptoms or enlarging collections. Further research on the pathophysiology and complexity of the CSDH is necessary to assess which treatment is most beneficial for individual patients. Several prospective trials have already been set up to provide class I evidence on the management of CSDH.[63]

In general, patients with significant symptoms or neurological deficits (e.g., hemiplegia) that can be attributed to a sizable CSDH will be offered surgical evacuation, if their premorbid status is reasonable. Patients with a poor premorbid status (e.g., dependent on others for activities of daily living and with several comorbidities) require careful consideration of the available options, including the option not to intervene. Patients with minimal symptoms or subtle deficits (e.g., slight pronator drift) can be managed expectantly or with pharmacotherapy (e.g., steroids).

15.5.1 Surgical

In general, three surgical techniques may be used to treat CSDH, namely, bur hole craniostomy (BHC), twist-drill craniostomy (TDC), and craniotomy.[64] There are ongoing debates as to which of these techniques best influence on operative morbidity, mortality, recurrence rates, and overall outcome. The comparative effectiveness of these three surgical procedures remains poorly characterized and class I evidence is sparse. Retrospective studies are at high risk of bias, since treatment decisions are often based on the patients' preoperative performance and on the individual preference of the treating physician.

Worldwide, BHC is the most employed procedure. Differences in effects on outcomes of BHC, TDC, and craniotomy are summarized in ▶ Table 15.1. In craniotomy, reported morbidity and mortality are higher compared to BHC and TDC; however, recurrence rates are substantially lower compared to TDC and BHC.[61,65,66,67] Craniotomy is mostly reserved for CSDH with large acute components and in CSDH with multiple membranes, or as a secondary treatment in recurrent CSDH and in subdural empyema after BHC or TDC. This might lead to higher morbidity and mortality numbers in this treatment group. Mini-craniotomy as primary surgical technique might, however, be an effective surgical technique for all types of CSDH and is the first-line option for some surgeons.[68]

Surgery-related complications include surgical site infection, subdural empyema, pneumocephalus, acute subdural hematoma, and cortical/parenchymal damage due to drains or vigorous washout. Other complications, not directly related to surgery, include respiratory and urinary infections, venous thromboembolisms, cardiac impairment, seizures, and stroke.[66,69]

The only intervention supported by class I evidence to date in the treatment of CSDH is the intraoperative placement of a soft subdural drain that remains in situ for up to 48 hours after bur hole evacuation.[5] This is associated with reduced recurrence and reduced mortality at 6 months[5,70,71,72] and with statistically significant improvements in both short- and long-term functional outcomes.[70] The role of the position (subdural, subgaleal) of the drain, the type of drain, and the

duration of drainage requires further evaluation, as a number of recent studies have contradictory findings.[4,64,73,74,75,76,77]

Recently, there has been some controversy regarding the use of subgaleal/subperiosteal versus subdural drains. A randomized trial published in 2019 found fewer recurrences in the former group (8.3%) versus the subdural drain group (12%), but due to the prespecified noninferiority hypothesis and the limited sample size, the study concluded that "the insertion of a subperiosteal drain causes at most 5.3% more recurrences compared to the insertion of a subdural drain."[78] Misplacement of the subdural drain occurred in 17% of patients, which is substantially higher than the misplacement rate in our practice (unpublished data). This is probably due to the fact that the authors inserted the subdural drain from the parietal bur hole until it reached the frontal bur hole.

In general, we advocate for the use of a subdural drain inserted via the frontal bur hole directed anteriorly, unless the brain has re-expanded fully. In such cases, a subgaleal drain can

Table 15.1 Surgical outcomes of CSDH

	Bur hole craniostomy (%)	Twist drill craniostomy (%)	Craniotomy (%)
Mortality			
Almenawer et al[61]	3.5	3.6	6.8
Weigel et al[67]	2.7	2.9	4.6
Ducruet et al[65]	3.8	5.1	12.2
Lega et al[66]	2.5	3.1	4.7
Lowest–highest	2.5–3.8	2.9–5.1	4.6–12.2
Morbidity			
Almenawer et al[61]	7.2	5.5	10.2
Weigel et al[67]	3.8	3.0	12.3
Ducruet et al[65]	3.8	3.0	12.0
Lega et al[66]	n.a.	n.a.	n.a.
Lowest–highest	3.8–7.2	3.0–5.5	10.2–12.3
Recurrence			
Almenawer et al[61]	10.5	14.5	6.2
Weigel et al[67]	12.1	18.0	10.8
Ducruet et al[65]	11.7	28.1	19.4
Lega et al[66]	10.5	31.3	11.9
Lowest–highest	10.5–12.1	14.5–31.3	6.2–19.4
Good outcome			
Almenawer et al[61]	86.0	90.2	80.3
Weigel et al[67]	79.1	88.2	67.8
Ducruet et al[65]	86.4	93.5	74.4
Lega et al[66]	80.8	61.2	78.1
Lowest–highest	79.1–86.4	61.2–93.5	67.8–80.3
Complications			
Almenawer et al[61]	n.a.	n.a.	n.a.
Weigel et al[67]	n.a.	n.a.	n.a.
Ducruet et al[65]	9.3	2.5	3.9
Lega et al[66]	6.2	4.4	5.3
Lowest–highest	6.2–9.3	2.5–4.4	3.9–5.3

Abbreviation: CSDH, chronic subdural hematoma.

be used. Insertion of a subdural drain via the parietal bur hole with the aim of reaching the frontal bur hole should be avoided as it risks injury of the cortex/cortical vessels during insertion and/or removal.

Outcomes

Surgical outcomes are in general favorable. The Cambridge CSDH drain trial found that 84% of patients in the intervention arm had a favorable modified Rankin Scale (mRS) score (0–3) on discharge and at 6 months. These findings were broadly corroborated by a United Kingdom–wide prospective multicenter study that demonstrated that 78% of patients had a favorable mRS at discharge. Factors associated with a favorable outcome include the use of a drain, better admission mRS, younger age, and avoidance of postoperative bed rest.[5,62]

Literature suggests that intraoperative irrigation of the subdural space may lead to a better outcome.[79,80,81,82] However, further evaluation on the type of irrigation fluids is needed. Also, there is no class I evidence on other possible modifiable factors such as the number of bur holes to be used in BHC, early mobilization after surgery, and the timing of resumption of anticoagulants.

15.5.2 Middle Meningeal Artery Embolization for Chronic Subdural Hematoma

An emerging but promising treatment modality for CSDH is endovascular embolization of the middle meningeal artery (MMA). The MMA gives rise to capillary feeders of hematomas. Therefore, embolization of this artery is thought to prevent blood flow into the pathologic structures, control bleeding from the CSDH membrane, and facilitate resolution of the hematoma. MMA embolization has been introduced as a minimally invasive alternative or adjunct to the conventional surgical treatments. A recent meta-analysis,[83] which examined three double-arm studies comparing embolization and conventional surgery groups, and three single-arm case series, reported an overall lower hematoma recurrence rate in the embolization group compared to surgery (2.1 vs. 27.7%; odds ratio [OR] = 0.087; 95% confidence interval [CI]: 0.025–0.292, $p < 0.001$). Surgical complication rates were similar between groups (2.1 vs. 4.4%; OR = 0.563; 95% CI: 0.107–2.96; $p = 0.497$). The results underscored the therapeutic potential of MMA embolization in cSDH and a number of randomized clinical trials are currently underway.

15.5.3 Nonsurgical

Pharmacological treatment, as monotherapy or as an adjunct to surgery, has been suggested in the management of CSDH. Nonsurgical treatment might be more cost-effective and of higher value in some situations, although this needs to be backed up by evidence of a comparable clinical effectiveness to surgical evacuation. Pharmacological agents that have been used, mostly in the context of research, are corticosteroids, statins, angiotensin-converting enzyme inhibitors (ACEIs), and tranexamic acid.

Retrospective data suggested that corticosteroids (e.g., dexamethasone and methylprednisolone) may inhibit the inflammatory and angiogenic mechanisms of the pathophysiological vicious cycle.[1,19,20,69,84,85,86,87,88,89,90,91,92] However, in 2020, results were published of the first multicenter, placebo-controlled, randomized trial of a 2-week tapering course of dexamethasone, which enrolled 748 patients with a symptomatic CSDH.[92] This trial confirmed that the risk of reoperation for recurrence was lower in patients receiving additional dexamethasone (1.7 vs. 7.1% in the placebo group). However, a favorable outcome, measured with the modified Rankin Scale at 6 months, was lower in the group receiving dexamethasone; 286 of 341 patients (83.9%) versus 306 of 339 patients (90.3%) in the placebo group. Based on these results, we recommend not to use corticosteroids in the standard management of CSDH. It should be noted that 94% of patients in this study underwent surgery according to standard practice. Therefore, no definite conclusions could be drawn regarding the effect of dexamethasone as a method of conservative management to avoid surgery. The ongoing DECSA trial will provide further insight on this matter.[93]

Statins (e.g., atorvastatin) is studied in animals and small patient cohorts.[19,20,21,89,93,94,95,96,97,98,99,100,101] In a low dose, atorvastatin had an antiangiogenic and anti-inflammatory effect and might be a safe and (cost-) effective alternative in the conservative management of CSDH. Higher doses of atorvastatin might lead to higher VEGF levels and increased inflammatory factors.

ACEIs are suggested to have an antiangiogenic effect on the CSDH,[19,20,89,102] although this has not yet been demonstrated in recent studies.[103,104,105]

Tranexamic acid has an inhibitory effect on the fibrinolytic and inflammatory mechanisms of the pathophysiological vicious cycle.[19,20,89,106] Small studies indicate a possible positive effect of tranexamic acid.[107,108]

There is insufficient class I evidence available on the pharmacological treatment. However, adequately sized multicenter randomized controlled trials are needed in order to unravel which treatment is best in each individual patient.

15.6 Authors' Recommendations

- The importance of CSDH should not be underestimated. The complication and recurrence rates are relatively high and can significantly affect the quality of life and outcome of elderly patients. Similarly, costs associated with the increasing incidence are high.
- Treatment is warranted when there are significant and progressive clinical symptoms and corresponding radiological finding of substantial subdural collection exerting mass effect on the underlying brain.
- Surgery is the mainstay of treatment for CSDH. Both BHC and TDC are considered effective treatment options and in some cases, craniotomy may be required. However, there is no level I evidence comparing these three techniques.
- There is level I evidence that placement of a subdural drain during BHC is associated with reduced recurrence and mortality.
- Good outcomes and a return to previous functional baseline can be achieved in many patients but not all.

- Complication rates are also relatively high and need to be anticipated, diagnosed, and treated in a timely manner.
- MMA embolization for CSDH is emerging as a minimally invasive alternative or adjunct to the conventional surgical treatments.
- Since the incidence of CSDH is expected to double over the next 30 years, class I evidence on the clinical and cost-effectiveness of surgical and nonsurgical treatments is highly important. High-quality randomized controlled trials are needed to provide reliable data to refine clinical decision-making.

References

[1] Berghauser Pont LM, Dammers R, Schouten JW, Lingsma HF, Dirven CM. Clinical factors associated with outcome in chronic subdural hematoma: a retrospective cohort study of patients on preoperative corticosteroid therapy. Neurosurgery. 2012; 70(4):873–880, discussion 880

[2] Forster MT, Mathé AK, Senft C, Scharrer I, Seifert V, Gerlach R. The influence of preoperative anticoagulation on outcome and quality of life after surgical treatment of chronic subdural hematoma. J Clin Neurosci. 2010; 17(8):975–979

[3] Gelabert-González M, Iglesias-Pais M, García-Allut A, Martínez-Rumbo R. Chronic subdural haematoma: surgical treatment and outcome in 1000 cases. Clin Neurol Neurosurg. 2005; 107(3):223–229

[4] Glancz LJ, Poon MTC, Coulter IC, et al. Does drain position and duration influence outcomes in patients undergoing burr-hole evacuation of chronic subdural hematoma? Lessons from a UK multicenter prospective cohort study. Neurosurgery. 2019; 85(4):486–493

[5] Santarius T, Kirkpatrick PJ, Ganesan D, et al. Use of drains versus no drains after burr-hole evacuation of chronic subdural haematoma: a randomised controlled trial. Lancet. 2009; 374(9695):1067–1073

[6] Wada M, Yamakami I, Higuchi Y, et al. Influence of antiplatelet therapy on postoperative recurrence of chronic subdural hematoma: a multicenter retrospective study in 719 patients. Clin Neurol Neurosurg. 2014; 120:49–54

[7] Rauhala M, Luoto TM, Huhtala H, et al. The incidence of chronic subdural hematomas from 1990 to 2015 in a defined Finnish population. J Neurosurg. 2019; 132(4):1147–1157

[8] Foelholm R, Waltimo O. Epidemiology of chronic subdural haematoma. Acta Neurochir (Wien). 1975; 32(3–4):247–250

[9] Kudo H, Kuwamura K, Izawa I, Sawa H, Tamaki N. Chronic subdural hematoma in elderly people: present status on Awaji Island and epidemiological prospect. Neurol Med Chir (Tokyo). 1992; 32(4):207–209

[10] Adhiyaman V, Chattopadhyay I, Irshad F, Curran D, Abraham S. Increasing incidence of chronic subdural haematoma in the elderly. QJM. 2017; 110(6):375–378

[11] Balser D, Farooq S, Mehmood T, Reyes M, Samadani U. Actual and projected incidence rates for chronic subdural hematomas in United States Veterans Administration and civilian populations. J Neurosurg. 2015; 123(5):1209–1215

[12] Karibe H, Kameyama M, Kawase M, Hirano T, Kawaguchi T, Tominaga T. Epidemiology of chronic subdural hematomas. No Shinkei Geka. 2011; 39 (12):1149–1153

[13] United Nations Department of Economic and Social Affairs, Population Division. World Population Ageing 2015 (ST/ESA/SER.A/390). New York, NY: United Nations, Department of Economic and Social Affairs, Population Division; 2015

[14] Vacca VM, Jr, Argento I. Chronic subdural hematoma: a common complexity. Nursing. 2018; 48(5):24–31

[15] Adhiyaman V, Asghar M, Ganeshram KN, Bhowmick BK. Chronic subdural haematoma in the elderly. Postgrad Med J. 2002; 78(916):71–75

[16] Stroobandt G, Fransen P, Thauvoy C, Menard E. Pathogenetic factors in chronic subdural haematoma and causes of recurrence after drainage. Acta Neurochir (Wien). 1995; 137(1–2):6–14

[17] Iliescu IA, Constantinescu AI. Clinical evolutional aspects of chronic subdural haematomas—literature review. J Med Life. 2015; 8(Spec Issue):26–33

[18] Kolias AG, Chari A, Santarius T, Hutchinson PJ. Chronic subdural haematoma: modern management and emerging therapies. Nat Rev Neurol. 2014; 10(10):570–578

[19] Edlmann E, Giorgi-Coll S, Whitfield PC, Carpenter KLH, Hutchinson PJ. Pathophysiology of chronic subdural haematoma: inflammation, angiogenesis and implications for pharmacotherapy. J Neuroinflammation. 2017; 14(1):108

[20] Holl DC, Volovici V, Dirven CMF, et al. Dutch Chronic Subdural Hematoma Research Group (DSHR). Pathophysiology and nonsurgical treatment of chronic subdural hematoma: from past to present to future. World Neurosurg. 2018; 116:402–411.e2

[21] Jiang R, Zhao S, Wang R, et al. Safety and efficacy of atorvastatin for chronic subdural hematoma in Chinese patients: a randomized ClinicalTrial. JAMA Neurol. 2018; 75(11):1338–1346

[22] Haines DE, Harkey HL, al-Mefty O. The "subdural" space: a new look at an outdated concept. Neurosurgery. 1993; 32(1):111–120

[23] Haines DE. On the question of a subdural space. Anat Rec. 1991; 230(1):3–21

[24] Mehta V, Harward SC, Sankey EW, Nayar G, Codd PJ. Evidence based diagnosis and management of chronic subdural hematoma: a review of the literature. J Clin Neurosci. 2018; 50:7–15

[25] Munro D. Surgical pathology of the subdural hematoma. Based on a study of one hundred and five cases. Archives of Neurology and Psychology.. 1936; 35:64–78

[26] Yamashima T. The inner membrane of chronic subdural hematomas: pathology and pathophysiology. Neurosurg Clin N Am. 2000; 11(3):413–424

[27] Moskala M, Goscinski I, Kaluza J, et al. Morphological aspects of the traumatic chronic subdural hematoma capsule: SEM studies. Microsc Microanal. 2007; 13(3):211–219

[28] Hara M, Tamaki M, Aoyagi M, Ohno K. Possible role of cyclooxygenase-2 in developing chronic subdural hematoma. J Med Dent Sci. 2009; 56(3):101–106

[29] Shono T, Inamura T, Morioka T, et al. Vascular endothelial growth factor in chronic subdural haematomas. J Clin Neurosci. 2001; 8(5):411–415

[30] Nanko N, Tanikawa M, Mase M, et al. Involvement of hypoxia-inducible factor-1alpha and vascular endothelial growth factor in the mechanism of development of chronic subdural hematoma. Neurol Med Chir (Tokyo). 2009; 49(9):379–385

[31] Sarkar C, Lakhtakia R, Gill SS, Sharma MC, Mahapatra AK, Mehta VS. Chronic subdural haematoma and the enigmatic eosinophil. Acta Neurochir (Wien). 2002; 144(10):983–988, discussion 988

[32] Müller W, Firsching R. Significance of eosinophilic granulocytes in chronic subdural hematomas. Neurosurg Rev. 1990; 13(4):305–308

[33] Shinde AV, Frangogiannis NG. Fibroblasts in myocardial infarction: a role in inflammation and repair. J Mol Cell Cardiol. 2014; 70:74–82

[34] Hong HJ, Kim YJ, Yi HJ, Ko Y, Oh SJ, Kim JM. Role of angiogenic growth factors and inflammatory cytokine on recurrence of chronic subdural hematoma. Surg Neurol. 2009; 71(2):161–165, discussion 165–166

[35] Stanisic M, Lyngstadaas SP, Pripp AH, et al. Chemokines as markers of local inflammation and angiogenesis in patients with chronic subdural hematoma: a prospective study. Acta Neurochir (Wien). 2012; 154(1):113–120, discussion 120

[36] Frati A, Salvati M, Mainiero F, et al. Inflammation markers and risk factors for recurrence in 35 patients with a posttraumatic chronic subdural hematoma: a prospective study. J Neurosurg. 2004; 100(1):24–32

[37] Kitazono M, Yokota H, Satoh H, et al. Measurement of inflammatory cytokines and thrombomodulin in chronic subdural hematoma. Neurol Med Chir (Tokyo). 2012; 52(11):810–815

[38] Suzuki M, Endo S, Inada K, et al. Inflammatory cytokines locally elevated in chronic subdural haematoma. Acta Neurochir (Wien). 1998; 140(1):51–55

[39] Benveniste EN. Cytokine actions in the central nervous system. Cytokine Growth Factor Rev. 1998; 9(3–4):259–275

[40] Kishimoto T, Akira S, Taga T. Interleukin-6 and its receptor: a paradigm for cytokines. Science. 1992; 258(5082):593–597

[41] Ayala A, Wang P, Ba ZF, Perrin MM, Ertel W, Chaudry IH. Differential alterations in plasma IL-6 and TNF levels after trauma and hemorrhage. Am J Physiol. 1991; 260(1, Pt 2):R167–R171

[42] Maruo N, Morita I, Shirao M, Murota S. IL-6 increases endothelial permeability in vitro. Endocrinology. 1992; 131(2):710–714

[43] Oppenheim JJ, Zachariae CO, Mukaida N, Matsushima K. Properties of the novel proinflammatory supergene "intercrine" cytokine family. Annu Rev Immunol. 1991; 9:617–648

[44] Li A, Varney ML, Valasek J, Godfrey M, Dave BJ, Singh RK. Autocrine role of interleukin-8 in induction of endothelial cell proliferation, survival, migration and MMP-2 production and angiogenesis. Angiogenesis. 2005; 8 (1):63–71

[45] Seymour RM, Henderson B. Pro-inflammatory–anti-inflammatory cytokine dynamics mediated by cytokine-receptor dynamics in monocytes. IMA J Math Appl Med Biol. 2001; 18(2):159–192

[46] Moore KW, O'Garra A, de Waal Malefyt R, Vieira P, Mosmann TR. Interleukin-10. Annu Rev Immunol. 1993; 11:165–190

[47] Hohenstein A, Erber R, Schilling L, Weigel R. Increased mRNA expression of VEGF within the hematoma and imbalance of angiopoietin-1 and -2 mRNA within the neomembranes of chronic subdural hematoma. J Neurotrauma. 2005; 22(5):518–528

[48] Weigel R, Schilling L, Schmiedek P. Specific pattern of growth factor distribution in chronic subdural hematoma (CSH): evidence for an angiogenic disease. Acta Neurochir (Wien). 2001; 143(8):811–818, discussion 819

[49] Kalamatianos T, Stavrinou LC, Koutsarnakis C, Psachoulia C, Sakas DE, Stranjalis G. PlGF and sVEGFR-1 in chronic subdural hematoma: implications for hematoma development. J Neurosurg. 2013; 118(2):353–357

[50] Hua C, Zhao G, Feng Y, Yuan H, Song H, Bie L. Role of matrix metalloproteinase-2, matrix metalloproteinase-9, and vascular endothelial growth factor in the development of chronic subdural hematoma. J Neurotrauma. 2016; 33(1):65–70

[51] Funai M, Osuka K, Usuda N, et al. Activation of PI3 kinase/Akt signaling in chronic subdural hematoma outer membranes. J Neurotrauma. 2011; 28(6):1127–1131

[52] Osuka K, Watanabe Y, Usuda N, et al. Activation of Ras/MEK/ERK signaling in chronic subdural hematoma outer membranes. Brain Res. 2012; 1489:98–103

[53] Aoyama M, Osuka K, Usuda N, et al. Expression of mitogen-activated protein kinases in chronic subdural hematoma outer membranes. J Neurotrauma. 2015; 32(14):1064–1070

[54] Ito H, Saito K, Yamamoto S, Hasegawa T. Tissue-type plasminogen activator in the chronic subdural hematoma. Surg Neurol. 1988; 30(3):175–179

[55] Weir B, Gordon P. Factors affecting coagulation: fibrinolysis in chronic subdural fluid collections. J Neurosurg. 1983; 58(2):242–245

[56] Katano H, Kamiya K, Mase M, Tanikawa M, Yamada K. Tissue plasminogen activator in chronic subdural hematomas as a predictor of recurrence. J Neurosurg. 2006; 104(1):79–84

[57] Kwaan HC. Disorders of fibrinolysis. Med Clin North Am. 1972; 56(1):163–176

[58] Fujisawa H, Ito H, Saito K, Ikeda K, Nitta H, Yamashita J. Immunohistochemical localization of tissue-type plasminogen activator in the lining wall of chronic subdural hematoma. Surg Neurol. 1991; 35(6):441–445

[59] Murakami H, Hirose Y, Sagoh M, et al. Why do chronic subdural hematomas continue to grow slowly and not coagulate? Role of thrombomodulin in the mechanism. J Neurosurg. 2002; 96(5):877–884

[60] Lee KS. Natural history of chronic subdural haematoma. Brain Inj. 2004; 18(4):351–358

[61] Almenawer SA, Farrokhyar F, Hong C, et al. Chronic subdural hematoma management: a systematic review and meta-analysis of 34,829 patients. Ann Surg. 2014; 259(3):449–457

[62] Brennan PM, Kolias AG, Joannides AJ, et al. British Neurosurgical Trainee Research Collaborative. The management and outcome for patients with chronic subdural hematoma: a prospective, multicenter, observational cohort study in the United Kingdom. J Neurosurg. 2017; 127(4):732–739

[63] Edlmann E, Holl DC, Lingsma HF, et al. Systematic review of current randomised control trials in chronic subdural haematoma and proposal for an international collaborative approach. Acta Neurochir (Wien). 2020; 162(4):763–776

[64] Baschera D, Tosic L, Westermann L, Oberle J, Alfieri A. Treatment standards for chronic subdural hematoma: results from a survey in Austrian, German, and Swiss neurosurgical units. World Neurosurg. 2018; 116:e983–e995

[65] Ducruet AF, Grobelny BT, Zacharia BE, et al. The surgical management of chronic subdural hematoma. Neurosurg Rev. 2012; 35(2):155–169, discussion 169

[66] Lega BC, Danish SF, Malhotra NR, Sonnad SS, Stein SC. Choosing the best operation for chronic subdural hematoma: a decision analysis. J Neurosurg. 2010; 113(3):615–621

[67] Weigel R, Schmiedek P, Krauss JK. Outcome of contemporary surgery for chronic subdural haematoma: evidence based review. J Neurol Neurosurg Psychiatry. 2003; 74(7):937–943

[68] Van Der Veken J, Duerinck J, Buyl R, Van Rompaey K, Herregodts P, D'Haens J. Mini-craniotomy as the primary surgical intervention for the treatment of chronic subdural hematoma: a retrospective analysis. Acta Neurochir (Wien). 2014; 156(5):981–987

[69] Holl DC, Volovici V, Dirven CMF, et al. Corticosteroid treatment compared with surgery in chronic subdural hematoma: a systematic review and meta-analysis. Acta Neurochir (Wien). 2019; 161(6):1231–1242

[70] Alcalá-Cerra G, Young AM, Moscote-Salazar LR, Paternina-Caicedo A. Efficacy and safety of subdural drains after burr-hole evacuation of chronic subdural hematomas: systematic review and meta-analysis of randomized controlled trials. World Neurosurg. 2014; 82(6):1148–1157

[71] Guilfoyle MR, Hutchinson PJ, Santarius T. Improved long-term survival with subdural drains following evacuation of chronic subdural haematoma. Acta Neurochir (Wien). 2017; 159(5):903–905

[72] Singh AK, Suryanarayanan B, Choudhary A, Prasad A, Singh S, Gupta LN. A prospective randomized study of use of drain versus no drain after burr-hole evacuation of chronic subdural hematoma. Neurol India. 2014; 62(2):169–174

[73] Bellut D, Woernle CM, Burkhardt JK, Kockro RA, Bertalanffy H, Krayenbühl N. Subdural drainage versus subperiosteal drainage in burr-hole trepanation for symptomatic chronic subdural hematomas. World Neurosurg. 2012; 77(1):111–118

[74] Chung Chan DY, Ming Woo PY, Poon WS. Chronic subdural hematoma: to drain or not to drain, this is the question. World Neurosurg. 2014; 82(6):1007–1009

[75] Soleman J, Kamenova M, Lutz K, Guzman R, Fandino J, Mariani L. Drain insertion in chronic subdural hematoma: an international survey of practice. World Neurosurg. 2017; 104:528–536

[76] Soleman J, Lutz K, Schaedelin S, Mariani L, Fandino J. Use of subperiosteal drain versus subdural drain in chronic subdural hematomas treated with burr-hole trepanation: study protocol for a randomized controlled trial. JMIR Res Protoc. 2016; 5(2):e38

[77] Bartley A, Jakola AS, Bartek J, Jr, et al. The Swedish study of Irrigation-fluid temperature in the evacuation of Chronic subdural hematoma (SIC!): study protocol for a multicenter randomized controlled trial. Trials. 2017; 18(1):471

[78] Soleman J, Lutz K, Schaedelin S, et al. Subperiosteal vs subdural drain after burr-hole drainage of chronic subdural hematoma: a randomized clinical trial (cSDH-drain-trial). Neurosurgery. 2019; 85(5):E825–E834

[79] Ishibashi A, Yokokura Y, Adachi H. A comparative study of treatments for chronic subdural hematoma: burr hole drainage versus burr hole drainage with irrigation. Kurume Med J. 2011; 58(1):35–39

[80] Kuroki T, Katsume M, Harada N, Yamazaki T, Aoki K, Takasu N. Strict closed-system drainage for treating chronic subdural haematoma. Acta Neurochir (Wien). 2001; 143(10):1041–1044

[81] Liu W, Bakker NA, Groen RJ. Chronic subdural hematoma: a systematic review and meta-analysis of surgical procedures. J Neurosurg. 2014; 121(3):665–673

[82] Tahsim-Oglou Y, Beseoglu K, Hänggi D, Stummer W, Steiger HJ. Factors predicting recurrence of chronic subdural haematoma: the influence of intraoperative irrigation and low-molecular-weight heparin thromboprophylaxis. Acta Neurochir (Wien). 2012; 154(6):1063–1067, discussion 1068

[83] Srivatsan A, Mohanty A, Nascimento FA, et al. Middle meningeal artery embolization for chronic subdural hematoma: meta-analysis and systematic review. World Neurosurg. 2019; 122:613–619

[84] Chan DYC, Sun TFD, Poon WS. Steroid for chronic subdural hematoma? A prospective phase IIB pilot randomized controlled trial on the use of dexamethasone with surgical drainage for the reduction of recurrence with reoperation. Chinese Neurosurgical Journal.. 2015; 1(1):2

[85] Delgado-López PD, Martín-Velasco V, Castilla-Díez JM, Rodríguez-Salazar A, Galacho-Harriero AM, Fernández-Arconada O. Dexamethasone treatment in chronic subdural haematoma. Neurocirugia (Astur). 2009; 20(4):346–359

[86] Emich S, Richling B, McCoy MR, et al. The efficacy of dexamethasone on reduction in the reoperation rate of chronic subdural hematoma: the DRESH study: straightforward study protocol for a randomized controlled trial. Trials. 2014; 15:6

[87] Henaux PL, Le Reste PJ, Laviolle B, Morandi X. Steroids in chronic subdural hematomas (SUCRE trial): study protocol for a randomized controlled trial. Trials. 2017; 18(1):252

[88] Prud'homme M, Mathieu F, Marcotte N, Cottin S. A pilot placebo controlled randomized trial of dexamethasone for chronic subdural hematoma. Can J Neurol Sci. 2016; 43(2):284–290

[89] Soleman J, Nocera F, Mariani L. The conservative and pharmacological management of chronic subdural haematoma. Swiss Med Wkly. 2017; 147:w14398

[90] Sun TF, Boet R, Poon WS. Non-surgical primary treatment of chronic subdural haematoma: preliminary results of using dexamethasone. Br J Neurosurg. 2005; 19(4):327–333

[91] Yao Z, Hu X, Ma L, You C. Dexamethasone for chronic subdural haematoma: a systematic review and meta-analysis. Acta Neurochir (Wien). 2017; 159 (11):2037–2044

[92] Zhang Y, Chen S, Xiao Y, Tang W. Effects of dexamethasone in the treatment of recurrent chronic subdural hematoma. World Neurosurg. 2017; 105:115–121

[93] Araújo FA, Rocha MA, Mendes JB, Andrade SP. Atorvastatin inhibits inflammatory angiogenesis in mice through down regulation of VEGF, TNF-alpha and TGF-beta1. Biomed Pharmacother. 2010; 64(1):29–34

[94] Chan DY, Chan DT, Sun TF, Ng SC, Wong GK, Poon WS. The use of atorvastatin for chronic subdural haematoma: a retrospective cohort comparison study. Br J Neurosurg. 2017; 31(1):72–77

[95] Jiang R, Wang D, Poon WS, et al. Effect of ATorvastatin On Chronic subdural Hematoma (ATOCH): a study protocol for a randomized controlled trial. Trials. 2015; 16:528

[96] Li T, Wang D, Tian Y, et al. Effects of atorvastatin on the inflammation regulation and elimination of subdural hematoma in rats. J Neurol Sci. 2014; 341(1–2):88–96

[97] Qiu S, Zhuo W, Sun C, Su Z, Yan A, Shen L. Effects of atorvastatin on chronic subdural hematoma: a systematic review. Medicine (Baltimore). 2017; 96 (26):e7290

[98] Tang R, Shi J, Li X, et al. Effects of atorvastatin on surgical treatments of chronic subdural hematoma. World Neurosurg. 2018; 117:e425–e429

[99] Wang D, Li T, Tian Y, et al. Effects of atorvastatin on chronic subdural hematoma: a preliminary report from three medical centers. J Neurol Sci. 2014; 336(1–2):237–242

[100] Wang D, Li T, Wei H, et al. Atorvastatin enhances angiogenesis to reduce subdural hematoma in a rat model. J Neurol Sci. 2016; 362:91–99

[101] Xu M, Chen P, Zhu X, Wang C, Shi X, Yu B. Effects of atorvastatin on conservative and surgical treatments of chronic subdural hematoma in patients. World Neurosurg. 2016; 91:23–28

[102] Weigel R, Hohenstein A, Schlickum L, Weiss C, Schilling L. Angiotensin converting enzyme inhibition for arterial hypertension reduces the risk of recurrence in patients with chronic subdural hematoma possibly by an antiangiogenic mechanism. Neurosurgery. 2007; 61(4):788–792, discussion 792–793

[103] Neidert MC, Schmidt T, Mitova T, et al. Preoperative angiotensin converting enzyme inhibitor usage in patients with chronic subdural hematoma: associations with initial presentation and clinical outcome. J Clin Neurosci. 2016; 28:82–86

[104] Poulsen FR, Munthe S, Søe M, Halle B. Perindopril and residual chronic subdural hematoma volumes six weeks after burr hole surgery: a randomized trial. Clin Neurol Neurosurg. 2014; 123:4–8

[105] Bartek J, Jr, Sjåvik K, Schaible S, et al. The role of angiotensin-converting enzyme inhibitors in patients with chronic subdural hematoma: a Scandinavian population-based multicenter study. World Neurosurg. 2018; 113:e555–e560

[106] Iorio-Morin C, Blanchard J, Richer M, Mathieu D. Tranexamic Acid in Chronic Subdural Hematomas (TRACS): study protocol for a randomized controlled trial. Trials. 2016; 17(1):235

[107] Kageyama H, Toyooka T, Tsuzuki N, Oka K. Nonsurgical treatment of chronic subdural hematoma with tranexamic acid. J Neurosurg. 2013; 119(2):332–337

[108] Tanweer O, Frisoli FA, Bravate C, et al. Tranexamic acid for treatment of residual subdural hematoma after bedside twist-drill evacuation. World Neurosurg. 2016; 91:29–33

16 Natural History and Management Options of Unruptured Intracranial Aneurysms

Hugo Andrade-Barazarte, Behnam Rezai Jahromi, Felix Goehre, Ajmal Zemmar, Weixing Bai, Zhiyuan Sheng, Guangmin Duan, Zhongcan Cheng, Tianxiao Li, and Juha Hernesniemi

Abstract

Intracranial aneurysms (IAs) are acquired lesions with a prevalence of 1–3% in the general population. During the last decades, diagnosis of unruptured intracranial aneurysms (UIAs) has increased due to the use of noninvasive imaging for techniques. UIAs may remain clinically asymptomatic for a long period or rupture, causing an aneurysmal subarachnoid hemorrhage (SAH). Management of UIAs is challenging and it depends on risks factors for possible aneurysm rupture. Currently, the PHASES study represents the largest and most comprehensive data set on risk of aneurysm rupture and includes independent predictors for aneurysm rupture such as: population, arterial hypertension, patient age, aneurysm size, previous SAH from another aneurysm and aneurysm site. Besides these factors, current smoking, alcohol consumption, familial history of SAH, female sex, and presence of multiple IAs are also considered risk factors for SAH.

The decision on whether to treat (through endovascular or surgical procedures) or not an UIA should be adopted in a multidisciplinary team conformed by neurosurgeons and interventional neuroradiologists, and it should take into account all relevant patient and aneurysm-related factors for possible rupture.

Keywords: intracranial aneurysms, unruptured aneurysm, microsurgery repair, endovascular treatment, management

16.1 Introduction

Intracranial aneurysms (IAs) are acquired lesions with a prevalence of 1 to 3% in the general population.[1] A current theory for aneurysm formation acknowledges the presence of underlying endothelial dysfunction that leads to pathological remodeling with degenerative changes of vascular walls.[2] Additionally, general genome-wide linkage studies have identified several loci on chromosomes 1p34.3–p36.13, 7q11, 19q13.3, and Xp22 that may predispose to IA formation.[1,3,4] During the last decades, diagnosis of unruptured intracranial aneurysms (UIAs) has increased due to the widespread use of magnetic resonance angiography (MRA) and computed tomography angiography (CTA) as screening tools (▶ Fig. 16.1).[5] UIAs may remain clinically asymptomatic for a long period or rupture, causing an aneurysmal subarachnoid hemorrhage (SAH),[6] leading to severe neurological deficit and death in up to 40%.[7,8,9,10,11,12,13]

When an aneurysm presents with rupture, the decision is clear and the goal is to secure the aneurysm by either endovascular or surgical methods to prevent rebleeding.[14,15] However, UIAs may be managed either conservatively with serial imaging or by preventive repair (endovascular treatment or microsurgery). Therefore, these therapeutic options should be tailored and individualized to each patient according to risk factors, natural history, and possible treatment-related complications.

Data regarding natural history and management of UIAs have different levels of evidence and in several circumstances are restricted to specific geographic populations, which limits its complete applicability to estimate further risks/benefits. Thus, a multidisciplinary consensus is required to estimate the short- or long-term risks of rupture of an individual aneurysm and provide further management options.

This chapter discusses available clinical data on the natural history and management options for UIAs.

16.2 Selected Papers on Natural History of UIAs

- Korja M, Lehto H, Juvela S. Lifelong rupture risk of intracranial aneurysms depends on risk factors: a prospective Finnish cohort study. Stroke 2014;45(7):1958–1963
- Morita A, Kirino T, Hashi K, et al; UCAS Japan Investigators. The natural course of unruptured cerebral aneurysms in a Japanese cohort. N Engl J Med 2012; 366(26):2474–2482
- Greving JP, Wermer MJ, Brown RD Jr, et al. Development of the PHASES score for prediction of risk of rupture of intracranial aneurysms: a pooled analysis of six prospective cohort studies. Lancet Neurol 2014;13(1):59–66
- Hackenberg KAM, Hänggi D, Etminan N. Unruptured intracranial aneurysms. Stroke 2018;49(9):2268–2275
- Juvela S, Poussa K, Lehto H, Porras M. Natural history of unruptured intracranial aneurysms: a long-term follow-up study. Stroke 2013;44(9):2414–2421

16.3 Natural History of UIAs

Despite available evidence, the true natural history of UIAs is poorly understood and whether treatment should be offered to prevent a future rupture remains controversial.[16] The temptation to treat UIAs is based on the fear of SAH and the need to prevent a conceivable rupture.[17] However, treatment decisions should be based on comparisons between the risks associated with preventive treatments and natural history of the disease, instead of preventive treatments compare to outcomes after SAH.

Currently, the PHASES study represents the largest and most comprehensive data set on risk of aneurysm rupture.[18] This study is based on six prospective UIA cohort studies comprising of 8,382 patients and 10,272 UIAs from Europe (including Finland), North America, and Japan. In this meta-analysis, the mean observed 1-year risk of rupture was 1.4% (95% confidence interval [CI]: 1.1–1.6), and the 5-year risk of rupture was 3.4% (95% CI: 2.9–4.0).[18] Furthermore, this study identified six independent

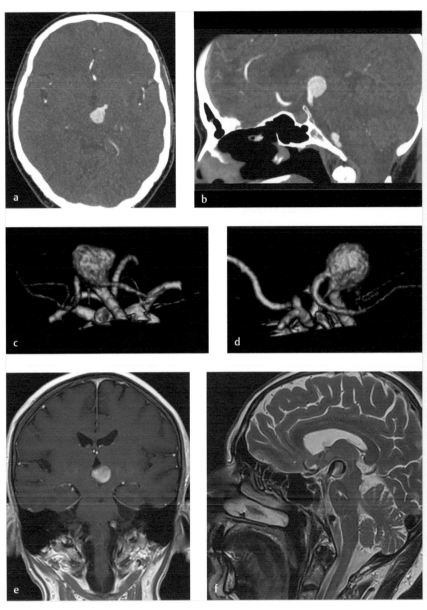

Fig. 16.1 **(a,b)** Computed tomography angiography axial and sagittal views of a large unruptured basilar artery aneurysm projecting posterior and with a wide base. **(c,d)** Three-dimensional reconstruction of computed tomography angiography. **(e,f)** Magnetic resonance imaging coronal T1-weighted with contrast and sagittal T2-weighted views demonstrating a large unruptured basilar artery aneurysm.

predictors for aneurysm rupture including (1) population, (2) arterial hypertension, (3) patient age, (4) aneurysm size, (5) previous SAH from another aneurysm, and (6) aneurysm site.

The PHASES score failed to preclude other additional known risk factors for aneurysm rupture due to lack of data or heterogeneous definitions of the data in the underlying studies.[6] ▶ Table 16.1 shows PHASES score parameters and characteristics.

16.4 Lifelong Rupture Risk of Intracranial Aneurysms Depends on Risk Factors

Data derived from population-based or case control studies identified risk factors that could be used to further estimate the relative rupture risk of patients with UIAs.[6,19,20,21,22,23,24] These

risk factors can be divided into patient-related factors (modifiable and nonmodifiable) and aneurysm-related factors.

In addition to the patient-related modifiable factors (hypertension) identified by the PHASES study, current smoking and alcohol consumption are also considered risk factors for SAH.[6,19,21,25] In a Finnish lifelong study, current smokers had an odds ratio (OR) of 3.05 (CI: 1.19–7.83) for a lifetime risk of SAH in comparison with never/ex-smokers. In addition to the current smoking activity, a large case control study with 4,701 patients reported the smoking intensity and duration associated with SAH.[26] Showing the direct correlation between smoking and SAH, several nation-wide population studies reported the decreasing incidence of SAH associated with decreasing smoking habits.[23,24] Alcohol consumption and drug abuse are also considered modifiable risk factors for SAH; however, a specific threshold regarding their detrimental effect has not been yet identified.

The PHASES study recognized some patient-related nonmodifiable risk factors for SAH such as earlier SAH from another aneurysm, age, and geographical location.[18] In addition to these

Table 16.1 PHASES score parameters and rupture risk

PHASES aneurysm risk score	Points	Change in rupture risk 95% confidence interval
(P) Population		
North American, European (other than Finnish)	0	
Japanese	3	HR: 2.8 (1.8–4.2)
Finnish	5	HR: 3.6 (2.0–6.3)
(H) Hypertension		
No	0	HR: 1.4 (1.1–1.8)
Yes	1	
(A) Age (y)		
< 70	0	HR: 1.44 (1.05–1.97)
≥ 70	1	
(S) Size of aneurysm (mm)		
< 7.0	0	HR: 1.1 (0.7–1.7)
7.0–9.9	3	HR: 2.4 (1.6–3.6)
10.0–19.9	6	HR: 5.7 (3.9–8.3)
≥ 20 mm	10	HR: 21.3 (13.5–33.8)
(E) Earlier SAH from another aneurysm		
No	0	HR: 1.4 (0.9–2.2)
Yes	1	
(S) Site of aneurysm		
ICA	0	HR: 0.5 (0.3–0.9)
MCA	2	Reference
ACA/Pcom/posterior	4	HR: 1.7 (0.7–2.6)/HR: 1.9 (1.2–2.9)/HR: 2.1 (1.4–3.0)

Abbreviations: ACA, anterior cerebral artery; HR, hazard ratio; ICA, internal carotid artery; MCA, middle cerebral artery; Pcom, posterior communicating artery; SAH, subarachnoid hemorrhage.

Currently, several studies reported that Finland have a similar incidence of SAH as compared to other Nordic countries.

16.4.1 Aneurysm-Related Risk Factors

According to the largest and most comprehensive follow-up studies of UIAs, the most important risk factors for aneurysm rupture are UIA size (> 7 mm) and location (anterior communicating, posterior communicating, or vertebrobasilar artery).[8,34,35] Additionally, an increasing number of studies including two large meta-analyses highlighted the relevance of aneurysm irregularity as an independent risk factor for rupture.[32,36] Moreover, retrospective studies have identified several morphological parameters as potential predictors of rupture including volume of the aneurysm,[37] aspect ratio,[38] bottleneck factor,[39] height-to-width ratio,[39] and volume-to-ostium area ratio (VOR).[40] A long-term follow-up prospective study by Juvela and Korja confirmed aneurysm volume, VOR, and the bottleneck factor separately as continuous variables predicted aneurysm rupture.[22] Additionally, aneurysm growth during the follow-up is associated with smoking but not with aneurysm indexes or parameters.[22]

Furthermore, UIA growth occurs in approximately 12 to 18% of patients with UIA during 2.2- to 2.7-year follow-up or approximately 45% of UIAs within 19 years and it is considered a well-established surrogate for UIA rupture.[6]

A pooled analysis comprising 10 prospective cohort studies with a total of 1,507 patients and 1,909 UIAs followed during 5,782 patient-years (median: 2.5 years; range: 0.5–14.3 years) identified earlier SAH, aneurysm location, age greater than 60 years, population, aneurysm size, and shape (ELAPSS) as independent predictors for UIA growth.[41] The ELAPSS score is helpful to identify possible aneurysm growth, thus being beneficial while considering UIA follow-up imaging.[41]

16.5 Serial Imaging Surveillance

The ELAPSS score is useful to identify patients harboring UIAs that are at risk of growth. This score allows us to estimate the 3- and 5-year risk of aneurysm growth, thus being beneficial while scheduling follow-up intervals (▶ Table 16.2 shows the ELAPSS score).[41] In a cohort of 382 patients diagnosed with UIAs followed by serial imaging (CTA and MRA), Chien et al identified that initial size and multiplicity were significant factors related to aneurysm growth. Additionally, they reported a 1.09-fold increase in risk of growth for every 1-mm increase in initial size (95% CI: 1.04–1.15; $p = 0.001$). Moreover, aneurysms in patients with multiple aneurysms were 2.43-fold more likely to grow than those in patients with single aneurysms (95% CI: 1.36–4.35; $p = 0.003$). The growth rate (speed) for UIAs ≥ 7 mm (0.085 mm/mo) was significantly higher than that for UIAs less than 3 mm (0.030 mm/mo).[42] In addition, UIAs have different tendency to grow when they are associated with different risk factors. Chien et al identified that growth (defined by size increase > 0.5–1.0 mm) in small aneurysms was difficult to detect with a 1-year follow-up imaging study.[42] Therefore, this subgroup of lesions would benefit from longer follow-up. Whereas, there are high-risk situations where patients with risk factors (smokers and suffering of hypothyroidism) in which the UIA might become greater than 7 mm within 1 year, meaning

factors, several studies have identified familial history of SAH or UIAs (defined as two or more first-degree relatives with SAH or UIA), female sex, and presence of multiple IAs as important risk factors for SAH.[6,20,25] The familial intracranial aneurysm (FIA) study demonstrated that patients with FIA carrying UIAs less than 6 mm in diameter have a 17-fold higher risk as compared to sporadic UIA carriers.[27] Additionally, several long-term prospective population-based studies have identified women to have a higher risk of SAH.[6,24,25,28,29] A long-term prospective population-based study published by Korja et al identified that multiple aneurysms are more common in women.[30] It is important to mention that aneurysm multiplicity is assumed but is not an established risk factor for rupture; therefore, more data derived from non-Japanese populations are needed to further estimate their effect.[31,32]

Two large prospective population-based studies (Finland and Japan) reported an inverse age regression for rupture, especially an increased long-term risk of rupture in patients younger than 50 years.[6,32] These findings are in contrast with the findings of the PHASES score, which recognized an increased risk of rupture in patients older than 70 years.[18]

Moreover, Finland and Japan are considered to have a higher incidence of SAH, but it remains unclear whether the increased risk is truly derived from ethnicity or rather exposure to environmental risk factors because of geographical location.[23,33]

Table 16.2 Demonstrating the ELAPSS score variables and points

Aneurysm growth risk score	Points
Earlier subarachnoid hemorrhage	
Yes	0
No	1
Location of the aneurysm	
ICA/ACA/ACOM	0
MCA	3
PCOM/posterior	5
Age (y)	
<60	0
>60 (per 5 y)	1
Population	
North America, China, and Europe	0
Japan	1
Finland	7
Size of the aneurysm (mm)	
1.0–2.9	0
3.0–4.9	4
5.0–6.9	10
7.0–9.9	13
>10	22
Aneurysm shape	
Regular	0
Irregular	4

Abbreviations: ACA, anterior cerebral artery; Acom, anterior communicating artery; ICA, internal carotid artery; MCA, middle cerebral artery; Pcom, posterior communicating artery.

that a 6-month follow-up study is critical to identify fast-growing lesions in high-risk patients.[42]

It is important to mention that the most consistent predictor of aneurysm growth is the duration of follow-up. As previously demonstrated by Juvela et al, the longer UIAs are followed, the more likely they are to enlarge.[8]

16.6 Selected Papers on Management Options for UIAs

- Backes D, Rinkel GJE, Greving JP, et al. ELAPSS score for prediction of risk of growth of unruptured intracranial aneurysms. Neurology 2017;88(17):1600–1606
- Etminan N, Brown RD Jr, Beseoglu K, et al. The unruptured intracranial aneurysm treatment score: a multidisciplinary consensus. Neurology 2015;85(10):881–889
- Bijlenga P, Gondar R, Schilling S, et al. PHASES score for the management of intracranial aneurysm: a cross-sectional population-based retrospective study. Stroke 2017;48(8):2105–2112
- Kotowski M, Naggara O, Darsaut TE, et al. Safety and occlusion rates of surgical treatment of unruptured intracranial aneurysms: a systematic review and meta-analysis of the literature from 1990 to 2011. J Neurol Neurosurg Psychiatry 2013;84(1):42–48

- Naggara ON, White PM, Guilbert F, Roy D, Weill A, Raymond J. Endovascular treatment of intracranial unruptured aneurysms: systematic review and meta-analysis of the literature on safety and efficacy. Radiology 2010;256(3):887–897

16.7 Management Options for UIAs

Treatment decision for UIAs (either by endovascular or by surgical modality) should be adopted in a multidisciplinary team conformed by neurosurgeons and interventional neuroradiologists and should take into consideration all relevant patient- and aneurysm-related factors for rupture risk.[43] Additionally, it should be based on risks and benefits to the patient when considering any management option.[43]

Due to the large variety and different levels of evidence in the management of UIAs, these decisions can often be challenging. Therefore, treatment options and follow-ups should be individualized based on previous characteristics of patients and aneurysms.

The PHASES score allows risk estimation for the possible 5-year rupture risk based on six independent parameters.[18] Therefore, treatment options and conservative management should be balanced according to rupture risk in the presence of certain risks factors (age, smoking, hypertension, hypothyroidism) and therapeutic risks of preventive repairs (endovascular and surgical complications). A recent prospective population-based study from Bijlenga et al, which included 841 patients with UIAs and ruptured IAs, identified that patients with PHASES scores less than 3 were mostly followed up with serial imaging, whereas patients with PHASES scores greater than 4 were more likely to be treated. Additionally, this group was able to identify a threshold of an absolute PHASES score of 3 to 4 to distinguish between low and high rupture risk UIA in their patients' cohort.[44]

The UIA treatment score (UIATS) is a consensus among a large multidisciplinary group of UIA specialists as an attempt to provide the best management options to UIAs.[43] This score takes in consideration patient-, aneurysm-, and treatment-related risk factors in the decision-making for or against preventive repair. The UIATS comprised two columns that contain all relevant factors for or against UIA repair. These two columns provide absolute numerical values that at the end can be used to assess the treatment recommendation or if treatment is recommended.[43]

If preventive repair is chosen, the most effective, simple, and least complicated treatment modality should be discussed within a multidisciplinary team. Additionally, it should consider patient age, comorbidities, aneurysm rupture risk, and rate of complications. Also, aneurysm-related factors for complications such as size, shape, location, and presence of calcification along the neck and parent artery.[45,46,47]

Among treatment modalities, simple coiling seems to be the preferred technique for endovascular repair and clipping the preferred technique for surgical repair.

It is generally accepted that older patients with higher comorbidity index would benefit from treatment by endovascular

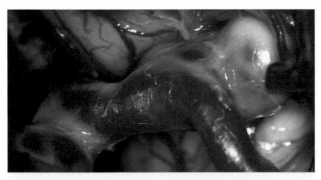

Fig. 16.2 Intraoperative view of a right-sided unruptured middle cerebral artery aneurysm.

coiling as the first-line option. On the contrary, young patients with superficial aneurysms (e.g., middle cerebral artery aneurysms) and wide-neck aneurysms should undergo surgical clipping due to the higher obliteration rate and treatment durability (▶ Fig. 16.2).[48]

16.8 Endovascular and Surgical Repair: Outcomes and Obliteration Rates

To date, there is no randomized trial regarding the best treatment option (endovascular vs. surgical repair) for UIAs. Additionally, data provided from randomized studies such as the International Subarachnoid Aneurysm Trial (ISAT) or Barrow Ruptured Intracranial Aneurysm Trial (BRAT) regarding surgical treatment or endovascular repair of ruptured aneurysms cannot be applied to UIAs.[49,50] This is probably due to the fact that patients with SAH have less favorable neurological outcomes as patients harboring UIAs, and from the surgical point of view, ruptured IAs are more challenging to handle due to the presence of blood obstructing the surgical field, artery and sac fragilities, and general brain swelling.

A large meta-analysis of surgical studies (including clipping, trapping, wrapping, and bypass), which included data from 60 studies (9 high-quality studies) comprising 9,845 patients and 10,845 UIA, reported an overall mortality of 1.7% (99% CI: 0.9–3.0) and unfavorable outcome, including death of 6.7% (99% CI: 4.9–9.0). Data on obliteration rates were available for 32% of the studies in which complete UIA occlusion was reported for 91.8% (99% CI: 90.0–93.2) of the cases.[51]

For endovascular treatment, a meta-analysis of 71 studies (including 4 with high-quality data) comprising 5,044 patients and 5,771 UIAs reported an unfavorable outcome, including death of 4.8% (99% CI: 3.9–6.0) and a mortality of 2.0% (99% CI: 1.5–2.6). In 38 of these studies, complete obliteration was achieved in 86.1% initially with recanalization rates ranging between 24.4 and 34.6% with a retreatment rate of 9.1% (99% CI: 6.2–13.1).[52] Additionally, in a subgroup analysis, unfavorable outcomes were higher in patients treated with flow-diverting stents (11.5%; 99% CI: 4.9–24.6) as compared

with patients treated with simple coiling or balloon- or stent-assisted coiling.

The safest and most effective treatment modality for UIAs remains uncertain. Therefore, treatment decisions and management options should be tailored to patient characteristics (age, risk factors), aneurysm characteristics, and local surgical and endovascular expertise for each individual aneurysm.

16.9 Authors' Recommendations

- The natural history of UIAs remains unclear.
- The lifelong rupture risk of UIAs depends on individualized patient risk profile, which can be divided into patient-related (modifiable and nonmodifiable) and aneurysm-related risk factors.
- Patient-related nonmodifiable risk factors for aneurysm rupture are age, female gender, familial history of IAs, previous presence of SAH, and geographical location.
- Patient-related modifiable risk factors are hypertension, smoking, and excessive alcohol consumption as well as use of illicit drugs.
- The most important aneurysm-related risk factors for rupture are UIA size (> 7 mm) and location (anterior communicating, posterior communicating, or vertebrobasilar artery).
- The PHASES score and the ELAPSS score are established scores to determine the 5-year risk of aneurysm rupture and the 3-/5-year risk of aneurysm growth, respectively.
- Treatment decision for UIA should be adopted in a multidisciplinary team conformed by neurosurgeons and interventional neuroradiologists and should take into consideration all relevant patient- and aneurysm-related risk factors for possible rupture.
- The UIATS is a consensus among a large multidisciplinary group of UIA specialists as an attempt to provide the best management options to UIAs. This score takes into account patient-, aneurysm-, and treatment-related risk factors in the decision-making for or against preventive repair.
- The safest and most effective treatment modality for UIAs remains uncertain. Therefore, treatment decisions and management options should be tailored to patient characteristics (age, risk factors), aneurysm characteristics, and local surgeon and endovascular expertise.

References

[1] Caranci F, Briganti F, Cirillo L, Leonardi M, Muto M. Epidemiology and genetics of intracranial aneurysms. Eur J Radiol. 2013; 82(10):1598–1605

[2] Kataoka H. Molecular mechanisms of the formation and progression of intracranial aneurysms. Neurol Med Chir (Tokyo). 2015; 55(3):214–229

[3] Foroud T, Lai D, Koller D, et al. Familial Intracranial Aneurysm Study Investigators. Genome-wide association study of intracranial aneurysm identifies a new association on chromosome 7. Stroke. 2014; 45(11):3194–3199

[4] Gaál EI, Salo P, Kristiansson K, et al. International Consortium for Blood Pressure Genome-Wide Association Studies. Intracranial aneurysm risk locus 5q23.2 is associated with elevated systolic blood pressure. PLoS Genet. 2012; 8(3):e1002563

[5] Gabriel RA, Kim H, Sidney S, et al. Ten-year detection rate of brain arteriovenous malformations in a large, multiethnic, defined population. Stroke. 2010; 41(1):21–26

[6] Korja M, Lehto H, Juvela S. Lifelong rupture risk of intracranial aneurysms depends on risk factors: a prospective Finnish cohort study. Stroke. 2014; 45 (7):1958–1963

[7] Brown RD, Jr, Broderick JP. Unruptured intracranial aneurysms: epidemiology, natural history, management options, and familial screening. Lancet Neurol. 2014; 13(4):393–404

[8] Juvela S, Poussa K, Lehto H, Porras M. Natural history of unruptured intracranial aneurysms: a long-term follow-up study. Stroke. 2013; 44(9):2414–2421

[9] Lanzino G, Brown RD, Jr. Natural history of unruptured intracranial aneurysms. J Neurosurg. 2012; 117(1):50–51, discussion 51–52

[10] Loewenstein JE, Gayle SC, Duffis EJ, Prestigiacomo CJ, Gandhi CD. The natural history and treatment options for unruptured intracranial aneurysms. Int J Vasc Med. 2012; 2012:898052

[11] Golan E, Vasquez DN, Ferguson ND, Adhikari NK, Scales DC. Prophylactic magnesium for improving neurologic outcome after aneurysmal subarachnoid hemorrhage: systematic review and meta-analysis. J Crit Care. 2013; 28(2):173–181

[12] Gray EA. Cerebral vasospasm: troubleshooting complications of treatment. Axone. 1990; 11(3):59–63

[13] Grunwald IQ, Kühn AL, Schmitt AJ, Balami JS. Aneurysmal SAH: current management and complications associated with treatment and disease. J Invasive Cardiol. 2014; 26(1):30–37

[14] Kassell NF, Torner JC, Jane JA, Haley EC, Jr, Adams HP. The International Cooperative Study on the Timing of Aneurysm Surgery. Part 2: surgical results. J Neurosurg. 1990; 73(1):37–47

[15] Korja M. ISAT: end of the debate on coiling versus clipping? Lancet. 2015; 385 (9984):2250–2251

[16] Rasmussen PA, Mayberg MR. Defining the natural history of unruptured aneurysms. Stroke. 2004; 35(1):232–233

[17] Ferguson GG, Peerless SJ, Drake CG. Natural history of intracranial aneurysms. N Engl J Med. 1981; 305(2):99

[18] Greving JP, Wermer MJ, Brown RD, Jr, et al. Development of the PHASES score for prediction of risk of rupture of intracranial aneurysms: a pooled analysis of six prospective cohort studies. Lancet Neurol. 2014; 13(1):59–66

[19] Feigin V, Parag V, Lawes CM, et al. Asia Pacific Cohort Studies Collaboration. Smoking and elevated blood pressure are the most important risk factors for subarachnoid hemorrhage in the Asia-Pacific region: an overview of 26 cohorts involving 306,620 participants. Stroke. 2005; 36(7):1360–1365

[20] Hackenberg KAM, Hänggi D, Etminan N. Unruptured intracranial aneurysms. Stroke. 2018; 49(9):2268–2275

[21] Juvela S, Hillbom M, Numminen H, Koskinen P. Cigarette smoking and alcohol consumption as risk factors for aneurysmal subarachnoid hemorrhage. Stroke. 1993; 24(5):639–646

[22] Juvela S, Korja M. Intracranial aneurysm parameters for predicting a future subarachnoid hemorrhage: a long-term follow-up study. Neurosurgery. 2017; 81(3):432–440

[23] Korja M, Lehto H, Juvela S, Kaprio J. Incidence of subarachnoid hemorrhage is decreasing together with decreasing smoking rates. Neurology. 2016; 87(11): 1118–1123

[24] Nicholson P, O'Hare A, Power S, et al. Decreasing incidence of subarachnoid hemorrhage. J Neurointerv Surg. 2019; 11(3):320–322

[25] Korja M, Silventoinen K, Laatikainen T, et al. Risk factors and their combined effects on the incidence rate of subarachnoid hemorrhage: a population-based cohort study. PLoS One. 2013; 8(9):e73760

[26] Can A, Castro VM, Ozdemir YH, et al. Association of intracranial aneurysm rupture with smoking duration, intensity, and cessation. Neurology. 2017; 89 (13):1408–1415

[27] Broderick JP, Brown RD, Jr, Sauerbeck L, et al. FIA Study Investigators. Greater rupture risk for familial as compared to sporadic unruptured intracranial aneurysms. Stroke. 2009; 40(6):1952–1957

[28] Knekt P, Reunanen A, Aho K, et al. Risk factors for subarachnoid hemorrhage in a longitudinal population study. J Clin Epidemiol. 1991; 44(9):933–939

[29] Sandvei MS, Romundstad PR, Müller TB, Vatten L, Vik A. Risk factors for aneurysmal subarachnoid hemorrhage in a prospective population study: the HUNT study in Norway. Stroke. 2009; 40(6):1958–1962

[30] Korja M, Kivisaari R, Rezai Jahromi B, Lehto H. Size and location of ruptured intracranial aneurysms: consecutive series of 1993 hospital-admitted patients. J Neurosurg. 2017; 127(4):748–753

[31] Sonobe M, Yamazaki T, Yonekura M, Kikuchi H. Small unruptured intracranial aneurysm verification study: SUAVe study, Japan. Stroke. 2010; 41(9):1969–1977

[32] Tominari S, Morita A, Ishibashi T, et al. Unruptured Cerebral Aneurysm Study Japan Investigators. Prediction model for 3-year rupture risk of unruptured cerebral aneurysms in Japanese patients. Ann Neurol. 2015; 77(6):1050–1059

[33] Korja M, Silventoinen K, McCarron P, et al. GenomEUtwin Project. Genetic epidemiology of spontaneous subarachnoid hemorrhage: Nordic Twin Study. Stroke. 2010; 41(11):2458–2462

[34] Morita A, Kirino T, Hashi K, et al. UCAS Japan Investigators. The natural course of unruptured cerebral aneurysms in a Japanese cohort. N Engl J Med. 2012; 366(26):2474–2482

[35] Wiebers DO, Whisnant JP, Huston J, III, et al. International Study of Unruptured Intracranial Aneurysms Investigators. Unruptured intracranial aneurysms: natural history, clinical outcome, and risks of surgical and endovascular treatment. Lancet. 2003; 362(9378):103–110

[36] Kleinloog R, de Mul N, Verweij BH, Post JA, Rinkel GJE, Ruigrok YM. Risk factors for intracranial aneurysm rupture: a systematic review. Neurosurgery. 2018; 82(4):431–440

[37] Juvela S, Porras M, Heiskanen O. Natural history of unruptured intracranial aneurysms: a long-term follow-up study. J Neurosurg. 1993; 79(2): 174–182

[38] Ujiie H, Tamano Y, Sasaki K, Hori T. Is the aspect ratio a reliable index for predicting the rupture of a saccular aneurysm? Neurosurgery. 2001; 48(3): 495–502, discussion 502–503

[39] Hoh BL, Sistrom CL, Firment CS, et al. Bottleneck factor and height-width ratio: association with ruptured aneurysms in patients with multiple cerebral aneurysms. Neurosurgery. 2007; 61(4):716–722, discussion 722–723

[40] Yasuda R, Strother CM, Taki W, et al. Aneurysm volume-to-ostium area ratio: a parameter useful for discriminating the rupture status of intracranial aneurysms. Neurosurgery. 2011; 68(2):310–317, discussion 317–318

[41] Backes D, Rinkel GJE, Greving JP, et al. ELAPSS score for prediction of risk of growth of unruptured intracranial aneurysms. Neurology. 2017; 88(17): 1600–1606

[42] Chien A, Callender RA, Yokota H, et al. Unruptured intracranial aneurysm growth trajectory: occurrence and rate of enlargement in 520 longitudinally followed cases. J Neurosurg. 2019; 132(4):1077–1087

[43] Etminan N, Brown RD, Jr, Beseoglu K, et al. The unruptured intracranial aneurysm treatment score: a multidisciplinary consensus. Neurology. 2015; 85(10):881–889

[44] Bijlenga P, Gondar R, Schilling S, et al. PHASES score for the management of intracranial aneurysm: a cross-sectional population-based retrospective study. Stroke. 2017; 48(8):2105–2112

[45] Andrade-Barazarte H, Kivelev J, Goehre F, et al. Contralateral approach to internal carotid artery ophthalmic segment aneurysms: angiographic analysis and surgical results for 30 patients. Neurosurgery. 2015; 77(1):104–112, discussion 112

[46] Andrade-Barazarte H, Kivelev J, Goehre F, et al. Contralateral approach to bilateral middle cerebral artery aneurysms: comparative study, angiographic analysis, and surgical results. Neurosurgery. 2015; 77(6):916–926, discussion 926

[47] Goehre F, Jahromi BR, Lehecka M, et al. Posterior cerebral artery aneurysms: treatment and outcome analysis in 121 patients. World Neurosurg. 2016; 92: 521–532

[48] Rodríguez-Hernández A, Sughrue ME, Akhavan S, Habdank-Kolaczkowski J, Lawton MT. Current management of middle cerebral artery aneurysms: surgical results with a "clip first" policy. Neurosurgery. 2013; 72(3):415–427

[49] Molyneux A, Kerr R, Stratton I, et al. International Subarachnoid Aneurysm Trial (ISAT) Collaborative Group. International Subarachnoid Aneurysm Trial (ISAT) of neurosurgical clipping versus endovascular coiling in 2143 patients with ruptured intracranial aneurysms: a randomised trial. Lancet. 2002; 360 (9342):1267–1274

[50] Spetzler RF, McDougall CG, Zabramski JM, et al. The Barrow Ruptured Aneurysm Trial: 6-year results. J Neurosurg. 2015; 123(3):609–617

[51] Kotowski M, Naggara O, Darsaut TE, et al. Safety and occlusion rates of surgical treatment of unruptured intracranial aneurysms: a systematic review and meta-analysis of the literature from 1990 to 2011. J Neurol Neurosurg Psychiatry. 2013; 84(1):42–48

[52] Naggara ON, White PM, Guilbert F, Roy D, Weill A, Raymond J. Endovascular treatment of intracranial unruptured aneurysms: systematic review and meta-analysis of the literature on safety and efficacy. Radiology. 2010; 256 (3):887–897

17 Natural History and Management Options of Aneurysmal Subarachnoid Hemorrhage

Michael A. Silva and Nirav J. Patel

Abstract

Aneurysm subarachnoid hemorrhage (aSAH) continues to impose devastating consequences on patients despite increased efforts in recent years to identify and manage aneurysms prior to rupture. The natural history of aSAH is poor with high mortality and rebleed rate. Optimal patient care should be site specific based on the proficiencies of each unique institution.

Keywords: subarachnoid hemorrhage, cerebral aneurysm, natural history, endovascular coiling, microsurgery

17.1 Introduction

Aneurysmal subarachnoid hemorrhage (aSAH) is an uncommon but potentially catastrophic neurologic disease. The prevalence of aSAH has been estimated at 2 to 3% of the population, and SAH represents 5% of all stroke.[1,2,3] The overall incidence is 9 per 100,000, although there is a high regional variability. The average age of patients presenting with SAH is the mid-50 s, with half of the patients younger than 55 years.[2,4,5] The risk of developing aSAH increases with age,[1,4] although it has been suggested that there is no significant increase in risk until the age of 80 years.[3] Smoking and hypertension are well-established modifiable risk factors for aneurysm formation and rupture. Other risk factors include female sex, family history of aneurysm, diabetes mellitus, excess alcohol consumption, atherosclerosis, and autosomal dominant polycystic kidney disease (ADPCKD).[1,3,6,7,8,9]

Most SAHs (85%) are due to aneurysmal rupture and are associated with a high mortality rate of up to 50%.[2] However, not all SAHs are due to aneurysmal rupture, and other causes of SAH such as trauma, nonaneurysmal perimesencephalic SAH, vasculopathy, or other malformations are possible.

Aneurysmal rupture often presents with a sudden-onset headache, classically described by the patient as the "worst headache of their life." It is imperative to precisely characterize the quality of the headache, which is exquisitely painful and immediate in onset, reaching its maximum intensity of less than 1 minute. One must differentiate this "thunderclap" headache from other forms of severe headache, which may gradually worsen over the course of a day or represent a particularly excruciating iteration of a patient's chronic headaches. Patients presenting with a sudden-onset severe headache, different in quality compared to prior headaches, should be taken seriously and vascular imaging should be considered. Other symptoms of aSAH include nausea, vomiting, depressed consciousness, focal neurologic deficit, and sometimes a preceding milder "sentinel" headache.[10]

A thorough history should be collected, preferably from the patient if their neurologic examination allows. Many patients with a poor Glasgow Coma Scale (GCS) score on presentation will not be able to provide a history, and imaging should be performed immediately. If possible, the patient or their family should be asked about past medical history, with special attention paid to prior known aneurysms, a history of coagulopathy or liver disease, ADPCKD, prior neurosurgical interventions, and adverse reactions to contrast. The patient's medication list should be reviewed, especially for anticoagulants or antiplatelet agents. Smoking history and family history of intracranial aneurysms should also be probed. A full neurologic examination should be performed. The Hunt-Hess score is a clinical classification that was specifically designed to stratify patients with aneurysmal rupture by mortality based on an initial series of 275 patients.[11] Along with the GCS and World Federation of Neurological Societies (WFNS) Score,[12] the Hunt–Hess score is used universally to standardize examinations across patients regardless of institution or examiner (▶ Table 17.1). Patients with a high Hunt–Hess score, especially if grade III or higher, should be considered strong candidates for prompt external ventricular drain (EVD) placement. All reversible factors contributing to a poor neurologic examination must be excluded before assigning a Hunt–Hess score. Correction of hydrocephalus, hypercarbia/hypoxemia, or metabolic factors that may be affecting the patient's examination is crucial for accurate clinical classification. This is especially true for patient's presenting with a Hunt–Hess grade V examination in whom a misleading examination due to non-SAH factors risks discouraging intervention in a

Table 17.1 Clinical grading scales for aneurysmal SAH

Hunt and Hess scale	Criteria	Mortality (%) *(per grade at admission)*	Mortality (%) *(per grade at surgery)*
Grade I	Asymptomatic, or minimal headache and slight nuchal rigidity	11	1.4
Grade II	Moderate to severe headache, nuchal rigidity, cranial nerve palsy	26	22
Grade III	Drowsiness, confusion, mild focal neurologic deficit	37	40
Grade IV	Stupor, moderate to severe hemiparesis, early decerebrate posturing	71	43
Grade V	Deep coma, decerebrate rigidity, moribund appearance	100	n/a

WFNS scale	Glasgow Coma Scale	Motor deficit
Grade I	15	Absent
Grade II	13–14	Absent
Grade III	13–14	Present
Grade IV	7–12	Present or absent
Grade V	3–6	Present or absent

Abbreviations: SAH, subarachnoid hemorrhage; WFNS, World Federation of Neurological Societies.

patient who might benefit from treatment. Correction of reversible causes, such as hydrocephalus and hematoma, can improve the neurologic examination, improve prognosis, and increase the likelihood of successful intervention.

Symptoms and history suspicious for aneurysmal rupture should prompt immediate imaging. It is imperative that new-onset, sudden, severe headaches be fully evaluated, and not sent home. Initial imaging should include a noncontrast head computed tomography (CT), which has high sensitivity for detecting hemorrhage and can accurately evaluate the extent, location, and age of subarachnoid blood, if present. The Fisher grade is a radiographic classification of the amount of subarachnoid blood seen on CT and is predominantly used as a predictor of vasospasm.[13] A modified Fisher scale is sometimes used, which dispenses of intraventricular hemorrhage as its own category and uses thin versus thick subarachnoid blood as the major differentiator between grades I to II and III to IV[14,15] (▶ Table 17.2).

If the CT is positive for subarachnoid blood, CT angiography (CTA) is unequivocally indicated to assess for an underlying vascular source (▶ Fig. 17.1). CTA is highly sensitive for detecting aneurysms; however, the gold standard is conventional angiography. Digital subtraction angiography (DSA) is exquisitely sensitive for aneurysm detection and can characterize the lesion sufficiently to guide treatment. A DSA is also useful in SAH in the setting of a negative CTA (▶ Fig. 17.2 and ▶ Fig. 17.3). The angiogram is both diagnostic and potentially therapeutic if the aneurysm is determined to be amenable to endovascular treatment. An alternative to CTA or conventional angiography in patients with contraindications to these imaging modalities is magnetic resonance angiography (MRA), which is typically performed without contrast and characterizes vascular lesions based on the effect of blood flow on magnetic resonance. However, in the acute setting, the acuity of aneurysmal rupture trumps most relative contraindications to CTA or angiography in the majority of patients.

On initial suspicion of aneurysmal rupture, certain laboratory studies and tests should be sent immediately. Coagulation studies, platelet count, platelet function assay, complete blood count (CBC), liver function tests (LFTs) to assess for liver function, and a basic metabolic panel should be part of initial laboratory studies. An electrocardiogram (EKG) is helpful to set a baseline, particularly since some patients present in mild cardiac failure, termed Takotsubo cardiomyopathy. Vital signs should be actively monitored, with particular attention paid to blood pressure. A combination of hypertension and bradycardia (Cushing's reflex) may be observed in the setting of increased intracranial pressure (ICP) and could be a sign of the need for prompt cerebrospinal fluid (CSF) diversion. Most importantly, the systolic blood pressure (SBP) should be controlled. We advocate aggressive measures to keep SBP less than 140 mm Hg to help prevent rebleeding, which carries a 80% mortality.[16]

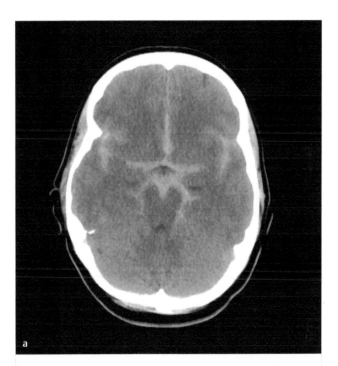

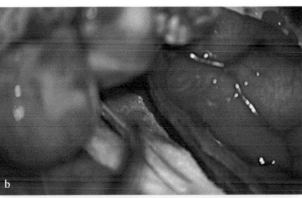

Fig. 17.1 (a) Extensive Fisher grade 4 "star-pattern" subarachnoid hemorrhage on axial noncontrast head computed tomography (CT) from a ruptured 3-mm anterior communicating artery aneurysm. Subarachnoid blood fills the interpeduncular, ambient, and crural cisterns as well as the interhemispheric and Sylvian fissures. **(b)** Intraoperative image of engorged, irritated brain parenchyma in a patient with subarachnoid hemorrhage.

Table 17.2 Radiological grading of aneurysmal SAH

Fisher scale	Subarachnoid blood			
Fisher I	None			
Fisher II	Diffuse			
Fisher III	Clot or thick layer			
Fisher IV	Intraventricular blood (diffuse or no SAH)			

Modified Fisher scale	SAH	IVH	Rate of DCI	Rate of infarction
Grade 0	None	None	0	0
Grade 1	Minimal/thin	None	12	6
Grade 2	Minimal/thin	Both lateral ventricles	21	14
Grade 3	Thick[a]	None	19	12
Grade 4	Thick	Both lateral ventricles	40	28

Abbreviations: DCI, delayed cerebral ischemia; IVH, intraventricular hemorrhage; SAH, subarachnoid hemorrhage.
[a]Completely filling ≥ 1 cistern or fissure.

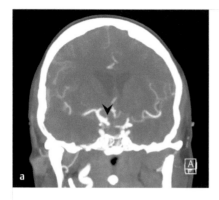
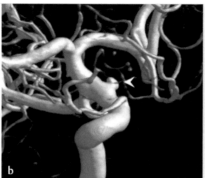
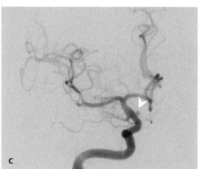
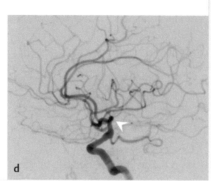

Fig. 17.2 Blister aneurysms of the internal carotid artery may be missed on imaging. They represent an important cause of aneurysmal subarachnoid hemorrhage (SAH) that must be considered in patients with negative initial imaging. Seen here is a 3-mm right internal carotid artery dorsal wall blister aneurysm on **(a)** coronal computed tomography angiography (CTA), **(b)** 3D reconstruction, **(c)** anteroposterior (AP) digital subtraction angiography (DSA), and **(d)** lateral DSA. This aneurysm was determined to be the cause of the patient's Fisher grade 3 SAH.

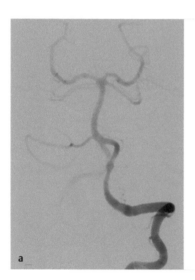
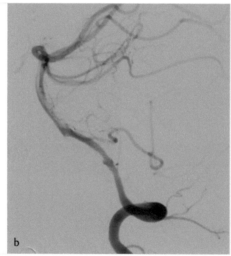

Fig. 17.3 Intracranial vertebral artery dissection, seen here on **(a)** anteroposterior (AP) and **(b)** lateral digital subtraction angiography (DSA) with injection of the left vertebral artery, is an important cause of subarachnoid hemorrhage (SAH) that should be considered in patients found to not have an aneurysm.

17.2 Selected Papers on the Natural History of Aneurysmal Subarachnoid Hemorrhage

- Nieuwkamp DJ, Setz LE, Algra A, Linn FHH, de Rooji NK, Rinkel GJ. Changes in case fatality of aneurysmal subarachnoid haemorrhage over time, according to age, sex and region: a meta-analysis. Lancet Neurol 2009;8(7): 635–642[17]
- Korja M, Kivisaari R, Rezai Jahromi B, Lehto H. Natural history of ruptured but untreated intracranial aneurysms. Stroke 2017;48(4):1081–1084

17.3 Natural History of Aneurysmal Subarachnoid Hemorrhage

Mortality after aneurysmal rupture is 50%.[2] Untreated aSAH carries a 20-day median survival and a 65% 1-year mortality.[18] For patients who survive the initial rupture event, the risk of rerupture is highest in the immediate posthemorrhage period at 8 to 23% within the first 72 hours,[19] with some studies reporting a rate of over 40% within the first 24 hours.[20] After a rebleeding event, 80% of patients die or are permanently disabled.[16] The risk of rerupture decreases progressively with each day after the initial hemorrhage down to less than 1% risk on day 21.[20] After 6 months, there is a 3.5% annual risk of rebleed, and mortality from a late repeat hemorrhage is 67%.[21]

Higher Hunt–Hess score on presentation, elevated SBP, large aneurysm size, presence of multiple aneurysms, and angiography within 6 hours are associated with increased risk of rerupture.[19,22] There is a hypothetical and controversial increased risk of rerupture after EVD placement and CSF drainage due to decreased external tamponade of the aneurysm sac resulting in increased transmural pressure[23]; however, no studies have definitively demonstrated this association.[19,22,24,25,26]

17.3.1 Vasospasm

After the immediate posthemorrhage period, patients must be monitored closely for vasospasm. Even after promptly and successfully treating a patient's aneurysm and observing an improvement in their neurologic examination, subsequent vasospasm can erase the patient's progress and leave them with lifelong debilitation. Vasospasm is one of the most feared, yet most common complications of aSAH. As many as 40% of patients experience delayed cerebral ischemia due to vasospasm after SAH, and it is associated with significant morbidity and mortality.[2,27,28,29] Predictors of vasospasm include amount (but not location) of subarachnoid blood, hypotension, hypovolemia, and loss of consciousness at the time of hemorrhage.[29,30,31,32] It is unclear whether clipping or coiling has any effect on the rate of vasospasm or infarction.[33,34,35] Magnesium is used by some groups to prevent vasospasm, but studies have shown no clear evidence of improved outcomes.[36] Nimodipine is the only vasospasm prophylaxis supported by the literature, having been shown to improve neurologic outcomes due to vasospasm when given to patients before onset of symptoms.[37,38]

The peak incidence of vasospasm occurs 4 to 14 days after aneurysm rupture.[2] Patients should be monitored for vasospasm in the hospital through this high-risk period before being discharged. The most crucial aspect of vasospasm management is precise and dependable serial neurological examination. Serial transcranial Doppler measurements (TCDs) provide a noninvasive means of screening for and monitoring vasospasm.[39] Although questions have been raised regarding the lack of sensitivity of TCDs,[40] they remain the workhorse of vasospasm monitoring. CTA or conventional angiography, as part of post-treatment follow-up imaging, may detect arterial irregularity or stenosis suggestive of vasospasm. Importantly, clinical vasospasm differs from radiographic vasospasm, and treatment of vasospasm should be reserved for patients with clinically significant vasospasm. Detailed neurologic examination of the posthemorrhage patient will identify patients with clinical vasospasm requiring treatment. If TCDs are persistently elevated, a more thorough evaluation of the extent of vasospasm can be attained with targeted CTA or conventional angiography. Hyponatremia is often a harbinger of vasospasm, as well as increased blood pressure. Finally, it is most imperative that any change in examination be taken seriously, presuming first vasospasm, and working to resolve the deficit.

The primary goal of vasospasm treatment is to prevent infarction as a result of prolonged ischemia. Intra-arterial calcium antagonists, nimodipine being the most well studied, have been shown to reduce the risk of secondary ischemia and poor clinical outcome.[41] Permissive or induced hypertension is used at some institutions to maximize cerebral perfusion in the setting of vasospasm; however, no studies have successfully demonstrated a clinical benefit for this practice.[42,43] Normovolemia should be maintained; in fact, positive fluid balance is associated with poorer outcomes.[44,45] The use of statins in patients with vasospasm is controversial.[46,47]

17.3.2 Chronic Hydrocephalus

Patients who fail EVD clamping trials and cannot be weaned off of the EVD should undergo shunt placement. Rates of chronic hydrocephalus and shunting vary wildly across institutions, ranging from 4 to 64% in the literature.[48,49] In one series of 2,842 patients, 16.3% of patients who underwent EVD placement on presentation ultimately required a shunt.[48] Predictors of shunt-dependent hydrocephalus after SAH include intraventricular hemorrhage, higher Hunt–Hess score and Fisher grade, prolonged CSF drainage, bicaudate index > 0.2, and hyperglycemia on admission.[48,50,51,52] Endoscopic third ventriculostomy (ETV) and fenestration of the lamina terminalis (FLT) during aneurysm treatment are debated as tools for reducing shunt-dependent hydrocephalus. Some studies have demonstrated a benefit, whereas others have shown no reduction in shunt dependency.[53,54]

17.3.3 Seizure

As many as 10 to 20% of patients with SAH suffer posthemorrhage seizures.[55] In a series of 7,002 patients with aSAH, 2.3% of patients experienced a seizure in the early posthemorrhage period, and an additional 5.5% of patients had late seizures.[56] Increased age, history of prior seizure, anterior circulation SAH locations, and hydrocephalus are associated with increased risk of seizure after SAH.[57] At many institutions, prophylactic antiepileptics are given; however, as previously discussed, there is insufficient evidence to support universal use of AEDs in patients with SAH. If a seizure is detected, prompt treatment and subsequent secondary prevention with AEDs should be initiated. Long-term electroencephalographic (EEG) monitoring should be considered in patients with an otherwise unexplained change in level of consciousness and neurologic examination.

17.4 Selected Papers on the Management Options for Aneurysmal Subarachnoid Hemorrhage

- Molyneux A, Kerr R, Stratton I, et al; International Subarachnoid Aneurysm Trial (ISAT) Collaborative Group. International Subarachnoid Aneurysm Trial (ISAT) of neurosurgical clipping versus endovascular coiling in 2143 patients with ruptured intracranial aneurysms: a randomised trial. Lancet 2002;360(9342):1267–1274
- McDougall CG, Spetzler RF, Zabramski JM, et al. The Barrow Ruptured Aneurysm Trial. J Neurosurg 2012;116(1):135–144

17.5 Management Options for Aneurysmal Subarachnoid Hemorrhage

Initial evaluation of the patient, assessment of Hunt–Hess or WFNS and Fisher grade, and review of key laboratory values allow for prioritization of immediate management steps. Regardless of clinical or radiographic grade, all patients should have their blood pressure closely monitored with an arterial line and systolic pressure maintained below 140 mm Hg before treatment. Central venous access should be considered in patients with a poor examination on presentation who are likely to require hypertonic agents. If a patient is on anticoagulation, reversal (if possible and safe, depending on the initial indication for anticoagulation) can be considered. Antifibrinolytic therapy might mitigate the risk of rerupture before definitive aneurysm treatment[19]; however, there is insufficient evidence in the literature to support universal use of antifibrinolytics.[58] Similarly, if the patient is on antiplatelet therapy or if laboratory studies showed low platelet count or function, platelet transfusion or desmopressin (DDAVP) can be considered. This decision should be weighed against the risk of reversing antiplatelet therapy in patients requiring it for preexisting stents or other reasons.

17.5.1 Intracranial Pressure Management

Control of ICP is critical to the management of SAH. Approximately 20% of patients with SAH develop acute hydrocephalus within 72 hours of hemorrhage.[23,59] Proposed mechanisms of hydrocephalus in the SAH patient include stimulation of choroid plexus CSF production and obstruction of CSF resorption due to interference of arachnoid granulations, but numerous other mechanisms have been proposed.[60] The typical presentation of acute hydrocephalus is depressed consciousness after an initially alert state.[61] Although 50% of patients recover spontaneously within 24 hours,[59] acute hydrocephalus after SAH is associated with a higher rate of mortality and cerebral infarction.[61]

Initial measures to control ICP should include elevating the head of the bed, relieving venous outflow compression (e.g., cervical collars), and maintaining normotension and normocapnia. Although different institutions and surgeons have diverse algorithms for timing or EVD placement, certain principles are nearly universal. Radiographic evidence of acute hydrocephalus, high Hunt–Hess score on presentation (III or higher) or WFNS score of III or higher, and decline in neurologic examination (especially development of somnolence, worsening headache, nausea, vomiting, or up-gaze palsy) should prompt repeat CT and strong consideration of EVD placement. Placement of an EVD serves several benefits beyond ICP monitoring and CSF drainage to relieve elevated ICP. The EVD can drain blood from the ventricle in Fisher grade IV patients with intraventricular extension of their SAH. The decreased ICP also relieves external pressure on the vasculature, which may be contributing to ischemia from vasospasm. The EVD should be set to drain at 20 cm H_2O to prevent malignant ICP but without excessively dropping transmural pressure and running the theoretical risk of promoting rerupture.[23,59]

Sedation (and subsequent intubation) may be required for refractory ICPs. Sedation should be used judiciously to avoid respiratory depression that would depress breathing and increase pCO_2, thus increasing ICPs. Sedation may also confound neurological examinations. Intubation and direct control of pCO_2 can combat this dilemma. If the patient becomes somnolent or is unable to maintain their airway for other reasons, intubation should be pursued. Administration of mannitol or hypertonic saline should be initiated if ICPs remain elevated. Close monitoring of laboratory values is essential. SAH is associated with hyper- and hyponatremia, which are each independently associated with poor outcomes.[62]

17.5.2 Seizure Prophylaxis

Seizure prophylaxis in the acute setting is controversial. A majority of institutions use antiepileptic drugs (AEDs) for seizure prophylaxis, but many do not.[63] In a retrospective propensity score-matched study of 353 patients, prophylactic AEDs did not significantly decrease the risk of seizure in SAH patients.[64] In a separate study of 7,002 patients, perioperative AEDs did not decrease seizure risk.[56] Similarly, a Cochrane review showed insufficient evidence and a lack of randomized trials to support or refute the use of AEDs as primary or secondary seizure prophylaxis in SAH patients.[65] When used, there is evidence to suggest that a brief course (3 days) of AEDs may be superior to extended seizure prophylaxis in these patients.[55]

17.5.3 Timing of Treatment

Optimal timing of treatment is not known, and no randomized controlled trials exist to study whether early or delayed treatment is best. Hunt and Hess postulated that delaying treatment in the higher-grade SAH would be beneficial, which inspired their namesake Hunt and Hess scale.[11] Although some studies have shown no difference in outcomes between early and delayed treatment,[66,67] it is generally thought that prompt treatment is beneficial.[68,69] A large observational study by Nieuwkamp et al found no significant difference between early and late observation.[67] However, Laidlaw and Siu studied outcomes after surgery within 24 hours of rupture and argue that ultra-early surgery may reduce the risk of rebleeding since the rate of rebleeding is highest in the early postrupture period.[68] This risk must be weighed against the increased surgical risk of operating in the immediate postbleed period.[11] Studies that compare outcomes between early and delayed treatment will be unavoidably confounded by the clinical improvement that patients treated early would have regardless of intervention, an effect not captured in the delayed treatment group. Ultimately, a randomized controlled trial is needed to credibly compare early versus delayed treatment, yet such a study is ethically challenging and unlikely to occur in the era of endovascular treatment, which avoids the risks of surgical intervention in the early postbleed period.

17.5.4 Overview of Treatment Modalities

The workhorses of aneurysm treatment are clipping, revascularization, endovascular coiling, and endovascular flow diversion (▶ Table 17.3). Microsurgical clipping, the oldest of these modalities, is a safe and reliable treatment option in many patients.[20,70,71,72,73,74] However, clipping carries the inherent risks of open surgery, requires manipulation of intact brain tissue when exposing the aneurysm, and can be challenging for aneurysms that are difficult to access surgically, but does lend itself to immediate and robust treatment (▶ Fig. 17.4). Endovascular coiling, the oldest and most widely used endovascular treatment modality, is a reliable and safe technique for treating most aneurysms.[75,76,77,78,79] In general, a key benefit of endovascular treatment is that it is a safe alternative for patients who are otherwise not healthy enough for open surgery or general anesthesia (▶ Fig. 17.5). Some aneurysms are not amenable to coiling due to a wide neck (which can lead to coil reflux and incomplete occlusion) or distal location (which limits catheter control). The use of endovascular treatment has expanded dramatically over the past few decades and even more so in the past several years as a result of new devices, improved outcomes data, and increased interventionist comfort with endovascular techniques. Flow diversion, such as with the Pipeline Embolization Device (PED), is a recent advancement in endovascular aneurysm treatment. Deployment of the PED stent within the parent vessel across the aneurysm neck diverts blood flow away from the aneurysm sac without directly manipulating the aneurysm sac like with clipping or coiling. Branching vessels off of the parent vessel covered by the stent remain perfused due to the pressure gradient driving flow through the stent wall into the branching vessel. Flow diversion has proven particularly useful in the treatment of wide-necked aneurysms that are not amenable to coiling. However, PED placement requires initiation of antiplatelet therapy, which is controversial in patients with aSAH.

17.5.5 Comparing Treatment Modalities

A summary of key studies on aneurysm treatment modalities is provided in ▶ Table 17.3. The International Subarachnoid Aneurysm Trial (ISAT), published in 2002, randomized 2,143 patients to clipping or coiling. This audit showed a survival benefit at 1 and 7 years posttreatment, with a higher rate of disability-free survival at 10 years for coiling, but a higher rate of rebleeding in the coiling cohort.[80,81,82] Another prospective randomized controlled trial comparing clipping to coiling in 109 patients with SAH showed comparable clinical outcomes at 1 year.[83] Similarly, the Barrow Ruptured Aneurysm Trial (BRAT) randomized 471 patients to clipping or coiling and found similar outcomes for anterior circulation aneurysms, but improved outcomes for coiling over clipping for aneurysms of the posterior circulation.[84,85] Coiling demonstrated a lower rate of occlusion and higher rate of retreatment, but there were zero cases of rerupture at 6 years of follow-up.[85] Another randomized controlled trial demonstrated no difference in clinical outcome between coiling and clipping despite a lower rate of complete occlusion, a lower rate of symptomatic vasospasm, and a lower rate of cerebral infarction in the coiling cohort[86] (▶ Table 17.3).

Flow diversion, one of the newest endovascular treatment options, has been used sparingly in the treatment of ruptured aneurysms due to concerns for the need for antiplatelet therapy after treatment in patients with a recent bleed. Some studies

Table 17.3 Summary of the treatment modalities and outcome of SBC reported in NCDB and the SEER database

Variable	Subcategory	NCDB (n = 936), %	SEER (n = 405), %
Age (y)	0–20	10.3	8.4
	21–59	62.9	63.2
	60 +	26.8	28.4
Gender	Male	56.2	54.8
	Female	43.8	45.2
Ethnicity	Caucasian	80.9	83.2
	African American	8.9	5.7
Tumor size (cm)	0–2	70.9	73.8
	2–5	1.4	0.7
	5 +	0.1	0.3
Surgery	Yes	83.4	87.2
	No	11.4	13.6
Radiation	Yes	46.8	45.4
	No	51.4	54.6
Radiation type	Proton	15.1	N/A
	Photon	11.1	
	IMRT	10.6	
	SRS	9.3	
Chemotherapy	Yes	1.6	97.5
	No	93.9	2.5
Combination treatment	RT + CT + Sx	0.3	1.7

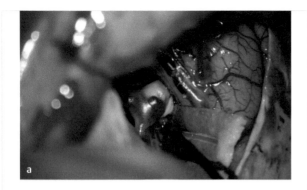

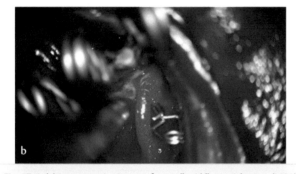

Fig. 17.4 **(a)** Intraoperative image of a small middle cranial artery (MCA) aneurysm with notable atherosclerosis. This lesion was treated with microsurgical clipping. **(b)** Intraoperative image of a different patient with multiple aneurysms, demonstrating extensive subarachnoid blood. A clip has been applied to the neck of the ruptured aneurysm.

have shown a high rate of periprocedural complications for ruptured aneurysms treated with PED.[87] However, flow diversion has demonstrated opportunity when compared to clipping and coiling for both ruptured and unruptured aneurysms.[88,89,90]

Ultimately, the choice of treatment cannot always be dictated by an external study. Each patient decision depends on patient-specific context, institutional expertise, provider proficiency, and many other factors. At our institution, we favor prompt treat for aSAH. The safest manner of achieving long-term treatment is best, but this is dependent on the patient, the case, and the team. We work to achieve excellence in endovascular, open surgical and hybrid techniques such that each is ready when the need arises. Treatment choice should be largely guided by retrospective and prospective review of outcomes by each provider at each institution, through keeping a database.

17.5.6 Procedural and Periprocedural Complications

Surgical and endovascular aneurysm treatment each carry their own risks. Intraoperative rerupture is seen with both treatment modalities[91,92]; it is associated with more favorable outcomes compared to spontaneous rupture.[91] Periprocedural complications are higher for ruptured aneurysms than unruptured aneurysms.[93] Coiling is associated with a 5.9% rate of procedural complications resulting in disability or death. Patients undergoing clipping have a higher rate of in-hospital complications, which may be related to increased length of stay[94] (▶ Table 17.3).

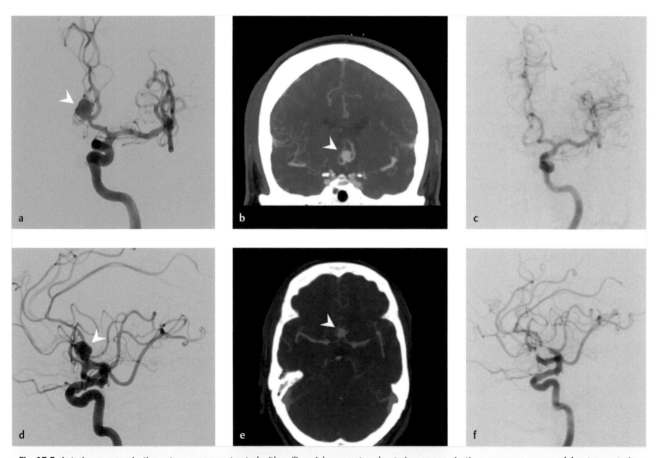

Fig. 17.5 Anterior communicating artery aneurysm treated with coiling. A large ruptured anterior communicating aneurysm seen on **(a)** anteroposterior (AP) and **(d)** lateral digital subtraction angiography (DSA) and **(b)** coronal and **(e)** axial computed tomography angiography (CTA). **(c,f)** This lesion was treated with endovascular coiling resulting in complete occlusion of the aneurysm.

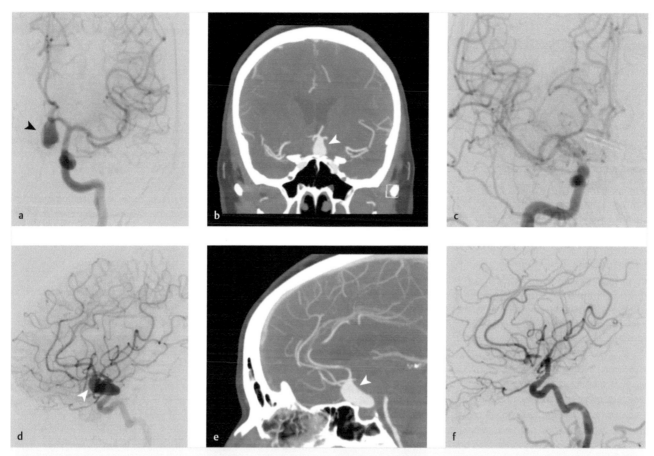

Fig. 17.6 Anterior communicating artery aneurysm treated with clipping. This patient was found to have a large, irregularly shaped anterior communicating artery aneurysm, shown here on **(a)** anteroposterior (AP) and **(d)** lateral digital subtraction angiography (DSA) and **(b)** coronal and **(e)** sagittal computed tomography angiography (CTA). **(c,f)** The lesion was treated with clipping and complete obliteration of the aneurysm was achieved.

17.5.7 Rerupture after Treatment

Assuming complete aneurysm obliteration, the rate of rerupture is low after either clipping or endovascular treatment.[95,96] Angiographically stable aneurysms have a 0.4% risk of rerupture, compared to 7.9% for recurrent aneurysms.[97] Late rebleeding (>1 month) after successfully coiled aneurysms is rare at around 1%; thus, angiographic follow-up of angiographically stable aneurysms beyond 6 months may be of limited use (▶ Fig. 17.6).[98,99]

17.6 Authors' Recommendations

Many basic principles of managing aSAH are evidence based, relatively uncontroversial, and nearly universal. However, differences in regional expertise and resources lead to distinct practice patterns across institutions. Optimal patient care should be site specific based on the proficiencies of each unique institution. Treatment algorithms should be specific to each institution and each provider such that the unique capabilities of each institution are maximally employed.

A possible paradigm of aneurysm care would be for neurovascular neurosurgeons to be well trained in both open and endovascular techniques such that they can personally offer all treatment options to patients and their families and counsel them in all options.[100,101,102] A single surgeon providing both endovascular and open vascular options does not remove bias, but can better navigate indications for applying the different technology. A potentially equivalent alternative is to have a team well versed in all options, who can work well together in an outcome-driven manner. Increased specialization within vascular neurosurgery runs the risk of limiting the scope of unbiased counseling that patients and their families can receive from a single surgeon. The obligation to offer comprehensive perspective on the scope of treatment options is particularly burdensome in the care of a ruptured aneurysms when the responsibility of management often lies with one or a handful of neurosurgeons at one institution, and the patient usually lacks the opportunity to shop around for different opinions. With these circumstantial constraints in mind, each institution should develop and embrace their own unique treatment algorithm based on transparent, prospective outcomes. This benchmarking provides direction for future decisions.

This chapter provides an overview of the basic principles of aSAH management and ruptured aneurysm treatment. By no means is this intended to be a universal guideline; rather, it represents the treatment algorithm used at one specific institution. Each provider and institution should adopt a treatment algorithm that best utilizes their unique expertise and resources.

References

[1] Rinkel GJ, Djibuti M, Algra A, van Gijn J. Prevalence and risk of rupture of intracranial aneurysms: a systematic review. Stroke. 1998; 29(1):251–256

[2] van Gijn J, Kerr RS, Rinkel GJ. Subarachnoid haemorrhage. Lancet. 2007; 369 (9558):306–318

[3] Vlak MH, Algra A, Brandenburg R, Rinkel GJ. Prevalence of unruptured intracranial aneurysms, with emphasis on sex, age, comorbidity, country, and time period: a systematic review and meta-analysis. Lancet Neurol. 2011; 10(7):626–636

[4] Epidemiology of aneurysmal subarachnoid hemorrhage in Australia and New Zealand: incidence and case fatality from the Australasian Cooperative Research on Subarachnoid Hemorrhage Study (ACROSS). Stroke. 2000; 31 (8):1843–1850

[5] Hop JW, Rinkel GJ, Algra A, van Gijn J. Case-fatality rates and functional outcome after subarachnoid hemorrhage: a systematic review. Stroke. 1997; 28(3):660–664

[6] Andreasen TH, Bartek J, Jr, Andresen M, Springborg JB, Romner B. Modifiable risk factors for aneurysmal subarachnoid hemorrhage. Stroke. 2013; 44(12): 3607–3612

[7] De Marchis GM, Lantigua H, Schmidt JM, et al. Impact of premorbid hypertension on haemorrhage severity and aneurysm rebleeding risk after subarachnoid haemorrhage. J Neurol Neurosurg Psychiatry. 2014; 85(1):56–59

[8] Juvela S. Prehemorrhage risk factors for fatal intracranial aneurysm rupture. Stroke. 2003; 34(8):1852–1857

[9] Vlak MH, Rinkel GJ, Greebe P, Algra A. Risk of rupture of an intracranial aneurysm based on patient characteristics: a case-control study. Stroke. 2013; 44(5):1256–1259

[10] Macdonald RL, Schweizer TA. Spontaneous subarachnoid haemorrhage. Lancet. 2017; 389(10069):655–666

[11] Hunt WE, Hess RM. Surgical risk as related to time of intervention in the repair of intracranial aneurysms. J Neurosurg. 1968; 28(1):14–20

[12] Report of World Federation of Neurological Surgeons Committee on a Universal Subarachnoid Hemorrhage Grading Scale. J Neurosurg. 1988; 68 (6):985–986

[13] Fisher CM, Kistler JP, Davis JM. Relation of cerebral vasospasm to subarachnoid hemorrhage visualized by computerized tomographic scanning. Neurosurgery. 1980; 6(1):1–9

[14] Claassen J, Bernardini GL, Kreiter K, et al. Effect of cisternal and ventricular blood on risk of delayed cerebral ischemia after subarachnoid hemorrhage: the Fisher scale revisited. Stroke. 2001; 32(9):2012–2020

[15] Frontera JA, Claassen J, Schmidt JM, et al. Prediction of symptomatic vasospasm after subarachnoid hemorrhage: the modified fisher scale. Neurosurgery. 2006; 59(1):21–27, discussion 21–27

[16] Roos YB, de Haan RJ, Beenen LF, Groen RJ, Albrecht KW, Vermeulen M. Complications and outcome in patients with aneurysmal subarachnoid haemorrhage: a prospective hospital based cohort study in the Netherlands. J Neurol Neurosurg Psychiatry. 2000; 68(3):337–341

[17] Nieuwkamp DJ, Setz LE, Algra A, Linn FHH, de Rooij NK, Rinkel GJ. Changes in case fatality of aneurysmal subarachnoid haemorrhage over time, according to age, sex, and region: a meta-analysis. Lancet Neurol. 2009; 8(7):635–642

[18] Korja M, Kivisaari R, Rezai Jahromi B, Lehto H. Natural history of ruptured but untreated intracranial aneurysms. Stroke. 2017; 48(4):1081–1084

[19] Larsen CC, Astrup J. Rebleeding after aneurysmal subarachnoid hemorrhage: a literature review. World Neurosurg. 2013; 79(2):307–312

[20] Brilstra EH, Algra A, Rinkel GJ, Tulleken CA, van Gijn J. Effectiveness of neurosurgical clip application in patients with aneurysmal subarachnoid hemorrhage. J Neurosurg. 2002; 97(5):1036–1041

[21] Winn HR, Richardson AE, Jane JA. The long-term prognosis in untreated cerebral aneurysms: I. The incidence of late hemorrhage in cerebral aneurysm: a 10-year evaluation of 364 patients. Ann Neurol. 1977; 1(4):358–370

[22] Beck J, Raabe A, Szelenyi A, et al. Sentinel headache and the risk of rebleeding after aneurysmal subarachnoid hemorrhage. Stroke. 2006; 37(11):2733–2737

[23] Hasan D, Vermeulen M, Wijdicks EF, Hijdra A, van Gijn J. Management problems in acute hydrocephalus after subarachnoid hemorrhage. Stroke. 1989; 20(6):747–753

[24] Hellingman CA, van den Bergh WM, Beijer IS, et al. Risk of rebleeding after treatment of acute hydrocephalus in patients with aneurysmal subarachnoid hemorrhage. Stroke. 2007; 38(1):96–99

[25] McIver JI, Friedman JA, Wijdicks EF, et al. Preoperative ventriculostomy and rebleeding after subarachnoid hemorrhage. J Neurosurg. 2002; 97(5):1042–1044

[26] Ruijs AC, Dirven CM, Algra A, Beijer I, Vandertop WP, Rinkel G. The risk of rebleeding after external lumbar drainage in patients with untreated ruptured cerebral aneurysms. Acta Neurochir (Wien). 2005; 147(11):1157–1161, discussion 1161–1162

[27] Corsten L, Raja A, Guppy K, et al. Contemporary management of subarachnoid hemorrhage and vasospasm: the UIC experience. Surg Neurol. 2001; 56(3):140–148, discussion 148–150

[28] Otite F, Mink S, Tan CO, et al. Impaired cerebral autoregulation is associated with vasospasm and delayed cerebral ischemia in subarachnoid hemorrhage. Stroke. 2014; 45(3):677–682

[29] Rabinstein AA, Friedman JA, Weigand SD, et al. Predictors of cerebral infarction in aneurysmal subarachnoid hemorrhage. Stroke. 2004; 35(8): 1862–1866

[30] Brouwers PJ, Wijdicks EF, Van Gijn J. Infarction after aneurysm rupture does not depend on distribution or clearance rate of blood. Stroke. 1992; 23(3): 374–379

[31] Hop JW, Rinkel GJ, Algra A, van Gijn J. Initial loss of consciousness and risk of delayed cerebral ischemia after aneurysmal subarachnoid hemorrhage. Stroke. 1999; 30(11):2268–2271

[32] Ohman J, Servo A, Heiskanen O. Risks factors for cerebral infarction in good-grade patients after aneurysmal subarachnoid hemorrhage and surgery: a prospective study. J Neurosurg. 1991; 74(1):14–20

[33] Dumont AS, Crowley RW, Monteith SJ, et al. Endovascular treatment or neurosurgical clipping of ruptured intracranial aneurysms: effect on angiographic vasospasm, delayed ischemic neurological deficit, cerebral infarction, and clinical outcome. Stroke. 2010; 41(11):2519–2524

[34] Gruber A, Ungersböck K, Reinprecht A, et al. Evaluation of cerebral vasospasm after early surgical and endovascular treatment of ruptured intracranial aneurysms. Neurosurgery. 1998; 42(2):258–267, discussion 267–268

[35] Kawabata Y, Horikawa F, Ueno Y, Sawada M, Isaka F, Miyake H. Clinical predictors of delayed cerebral ischemia after subarachnoid hemorrhage: first experience with coil embolization in the management of ruptured cerebral aneurysms. J Neurointerv Surg. 2011; 3(4):344–347

[36] Dorhout Mees SM, Algra A, Wong GK, et al. writing groups of MASH-I, IMASH, MASH-II, MASH and FAST-MAG. Early Magnesium Treatment After Aneurysmal Subarachnoid Hemorrhage: Individual Patient Data Meta-Analysis. Stroke. 2015; 46(11):3190–3193

[37] Allen GS, Ahn HS, Preziosi TJ, et al. Cerebral arterial spasm—a controlled trial of nimodipine in patients with subarachnoid hemorrhage. N Engl J Med. 1983; 308(11):619–624

[38] Young AM, Karri SK, Helmy A, et al. Pharmacologic management of subarachnoid hemorrhage. World Neurosurg. 2015; 84(1):28–35

[39] Kumar G, Shahripour RB, Harrigan MR. Vasospasm on transcranial Doppler is predictive of delayed cerebral ischemia in aneurysmal subarachnoid hemorrhage: a systematic review and meta-analysis. J Neurosurg. 2016; 124 (5):1257–1264

[40] Carrera E, Schmidt JM, Oddo M, et al. Transcranial Doppler for predicting delayed cerebral ischemia after subarachnoid hemorrhage. Neurosurgery. 2009; 65(2):316–323, discussion 323–324

[41] Rinkel GJ, Feigin VL, Algra A, van den Bergh WM, Vermeulen M, van Gijn J. Calcium antagonists for aneurysmal subarachnoid haemorrhage. Cochrane Database Syst Rev. 2005(1):CD000277

[42] Gathier CS, Dankbaar JW, van der Jagt M, et al. HIMALAIA Study Group. Effects of induced hypertension on cerebral perfusion in delayed cerebral ischemia after aneurysmal subarachnoid hemorrhage: a randomized clinical trial. Stroke. 2015; 46(11):3277–3281

[43] Gathier CS, van den Bergh WM, Slooter AJ, HIMALAIA-Study Group. HIMALAIA (Hypertension Induction in the Management of AneurysmaL subArachnoid haemorrhage with secondary IschaemiA): a randomized single-blind controlled trial of induced hypertension vs. no induced hypertension in the treatment of delayed cerebral ischemia after subarachnoid hemorrhage. Int J Stroke. 2014; 9(3):375–380

[44] Kissoon NR, Mandrekar JN, Fugate JE, Lanzino G, Wijdicks EF, Rabinstein AA. Positive fluid balance is associated with poor outcomes in subarachnoid hemorrhage. J Stroke Cerebrovasc Dis. 2015; 24(10):2245–2251

[45] Martini RP, Deem S, Brown M, et al. The association between fluid balance and outcomes after subarachnoid hemorrhage. Neurocrit Care. 2012; 17(2): 191–198

[46] Kramer AH, Gurka MJ, Nathan B, Dumont AS, Kassell NF, Bleck TP. Statin use was not associated with less vasospasm or improved outcome after subarachnoid hemorrhage. Neurosurgery. 2008; 62(2):422–427, discussion 427–430

[47] Lynch JR, Wang H, McGirt MJ, et al. Simvastatin reduces vasospasm after aneurysmal subarachnoid hemorrhage: results of a pilot randomized clinical trial. Stroke. 2005; 36(9):2024–2026

[48] Lai L, Morgan MK. Predictors of in-hospital shunt-dependent hydrocephalus following rupture of cerebral aneurysms. J Clin Neurosci. 2013; 20(8):1134–1138

[49] Tso MK, Ibrahim GM, Macdonald RL. Predictors of shunt-dependent hydrocephalus following aneurysmal subarachnoid hemorrhage. World Neurosurg. 2016; 86:226–232

[50] de Oliveira JG, Beck J, Setzer M, et al. Risk of shunt-dependent hydrocephalus after occlusion of ruptured intracranial aneurysms by surgical clipping or endovascular coiling: a single-institution series and meta-analysis. Neurosurgery. 2007; 61(5):924–933, discussion 933–934

[51] Gruber A, Reinprecht A, Bavinzski G, Czech T, Richling B. Chronic shunt-dependent hydrocephalus after early surgical and early endovascular treatment of ruptured intracranial aneurysms. Neurosurgery. 1999; 44(3):503–509, discussion 509–512

[52] Rincon F, Gordon E, Starke RM, et al. Predictors of long-term shunt-dependent hydrocephalus after aneurysmal subarachnoid hemorrhage. Clinical article. J Neurosurg. 2010; 113(4):774–780

[53] Andaluz N, Zuccarello M. Fenestration of the lamina terminalis as a valuable adjunct in aneurysm surgery. Neurosurgery. 2004; 55(5):1050–1059

[54] Komotar RJ, Hahn DK, Kim GH, et al. The impact of microsurgical fenestration of the lamina terminalis on shunt-dependent hydrocephalus and vasospasm after aneurysmal subarachnoid hemorrhage. Neurosurgery. 2008; 62(1):123–132, discussion 132–134

[55] Human T, Diringer MN, Allen M, et al. A randomized trial of brief versus extended seizure prophylaxis after aneurysmal subarachnoid hemorrhage. Neurocrit Care. 2018; 28(2):169–174

[56] Raper DM, Starke RM, Komotar RJ, Allan R, Connolly ES, Jr. Seizures after aneurysmal subarachnoid hemorrhage: a systematic review of outcomes. World Neurosurg. 2013; 79(5–6):682–690

[57] Jaja BNR, Schweizer TA, Claassen J, Le Roux P, Mayer SA, Macdonald RL, SAHIT Collaborators. The SAFARI score to assess the risk of convulsive seizure during admission for aneurysmal subarachnoid hemorrhage. Neurosurgery. 2018; 82(6):887–893

[58] Baharoglu MI, Germans MR, Rinkel GJ, et al. Antifibrinolytic therapy for aneurysmal subarachnoid haemorrhage. Cochrane Database Syst Rev. 2013(8): CD001245

[59] Suarez-Rivera O. Acute hydrocephalus after subarachnoid hemorrhage. Surg Neurol. 1998; 49(5):563–565

[60] Kosteljanetz M. CSF dynamics in patients with subarachnoid and/or intraventricular hemorrhage. J Neurosurg. 1984; 60(5):940–946

[61] van Gijn J, Hijdra A, Wijdicks EF, Vermeulen M, van Crevel H. Acute hydrocephalus after aneurysmal subarachnoid hemorrhage. J Neurosurg. 1985; 63(3):355–362

[62] Qureshi AI, Suri MF, Sung GY, et al. Prognostic significance of hypernatremia and hyponatremia among patients with aneurysmal subarachnoid hemorrhage. Neurosurgery. 2002; 50(4):749–755, discussion 755–756

[63] Dewan MC, Mocco J. Current practice regarding seizure prophylaxis in aneurysmal subarachnoid hemorrhage across academic centers. J Neurointerv Surg. 2015; 7(2):146–149

[64] Panczykowski D, Pease M, Zhao Y, et al. Prophylactic antiepileptics and seizure incidence following subarachnoid hemorrhage: a propensity score-matched analysis. Stroke. 2016; 47(7):1754–1760

[65] Marigold R, Günther A, Tiwari D, Kwan J. Antiepileptic drugs for the primary and secondary prevention of seizures after subarachnoid haemorrhage. Cochrane Database Syst Rev. 2013(6):CD008710

[66] Baltsavias GS, Byrne JV, Halsey J, Coley SC, Sohn MJ, Molyneux AJ. Effects of timing of coil embolization after aneurysmal subarachnoid hemorrhage on procedural morbidity and outcomes. Neurosurgery. 2000; 47(6):1320–1329, discussion 1329–1331

[67] Nieuwkamp DJ, de Gans K, Algra A, et al. Timing of aneurysm surgery in subarachnoid haemorrhage: an observational study in The Netherlands. Acta Neurochir (Wien). 2005; 147(8):815–821

[68] Laidlaw JD, Siu KH. Ultra-early surgery for aneurysmal subarachnoid hemorrhage: outcomes for a consecutive series of 391 patients not selected by grade or age. J Neurosurg. 2002; 97(2):250–258, discussion 247–249

[69] Phillips TJ, Dowling RJ, Yan B, Laidlaw JD, Mitchell PJ. Does treatment of ruptured intracranial aneurysms within 24 hours improve clinical outcome? Stroke. 2011; 42(7):1936–1945

[70] Hammer A, Steiner A, Kerry G, et al. Efficacy and safety of treatment of ruptured intracranial aneurysms. World Neurosurg. 2017; 98:780–789

[71] Hoh BL, Topcuoglu MA, Singhal AB, et al. Effect of clipping, craniotomy, or intravascular coiling on cerebral vasospasm and patient outcome after aneurysmal subarachnoid hemorrhage. Neurosurgery. 2004; 55(4):779–786, discussion 786–789

[72] Rodríguez-Hernández A, Sughrue ME, Akhavan S, Habdank-Kolaczkowski J, Lawton MT. Current management of middle cerebral artery aneurysms: surgical results with a "clip first" policy. Neurosurgery. 2013; 72(3):415–427

[73] Samson D, Batjer HH, Kopitnik TA, Jr. Current results of the surgical management of aneurysms of the basilar apex. Neurosurgery. 1999; 44(4):697–702, discussion 702–704

[74] Sundt TM, Jr, Whisnant JP. Subarachnoid hemorrhage from intracranial aneurysms. Surgical management and natural history of disease. N Engl J Med. 1978; 299(3):116–122

[75] Ayling OG, Ibrahim GM, Drake B, Torner JC, Macdonald RL. Operative complications and differences in outcome after clipping and coiling of ruptured intracranial aneurysms. J Neurosurg. 2015; 123(3):621 628

[76] Gallas S, Pasco A, Cottier JP, et al. A multicenter study of 705 ruptured intracranial aneurysms treated with Guglielmi detachable coils. AJNR Am J Neuroradiol. 2005; 26(7):1723–1731

[77] Henkes H, Fischer S, Weber W, et al. Endovascular coil occlusion of 1811 intracranial aneurysms: early angiographic and clinical results. Neurosurgery. 2004; 54(2):268–280, discussion 280–285

[78] Lempert TE, Malek AM, Halbach VV, et al. Endovascular treatment of ruptured posterior circulation cerebral aneurysms. Clinical and angiographic outcomes. Stroke. 2000; 31(1):100–110

[79] Willinsky RA, Peltz J, da Costa L, Agid R, Farb RI, terBrugge KG. Clinical and angiographic follow-up of ruptured intracranial aneurysms treated with endovascular embolization. AJNR Am J Neuroradiol. 2009; 30(5):1035–1040

[80] Molyneux A, Kerr R, Stratton I, et al. International Subarachnoid Aneurysm Trial (ISAT) Collaborative Group. International Subarachnoid Aneurysm Trial (ISAT) of neurosurgical clipping versus endovascular coiling in 2143 patients with ruptured intracranial aneurysms: a randomised trial. Lancet. 2002; 360(9342):1267–1274

[81] Molyneux AJ, Birks J, Clarke A, Sneade M, Kerr RS. The durability of endovascular coiling versus neurosurgical clipping of ruptured cerebral aneurysms: 18 year follow-up of the UK cohort of the International Subarachnoid Aneurysm Trial (ISAT). Lancet. 2015; 385 (9969):691–697

[82] Molyneux AJ, Kerr RS, Yu LM, et al. International Subarachnoid Aneurysm Trial (ISAT) Collaborative Group. International subarachnoid aneurysm trial (ISAT) of neurosurgical clipping versus endovascular coiling in 2143 patients with ruptured intracranial aneurysms: a randomised comparison of effects on survival, dependency, seizures, rebleeding, subgroups, and aneurysm occlusion. Lancet. 2005; 366 (9488):809–817

[83] Koivisto T, Vanninen R, Hurskainen H, Saari T, Hernesniemi J, Vapalahti M. Outcomes of early endovascular versus surgical treatment of ruptured cerebral aneurysms. A prospective randomized study. Stroke. 2000; 31(10):2369–2377

[84] McDougall CG, Spetzler RF, Zabramski JM, et al. The Barrow Ruptured Aneurysm Trial. J Neurosurg. 2012; 116(1):135–144

[85] Spetzler RF, McDougall CG, Zabramski JM, et al. The Barrow Ruptured Aneurysm Trial: 6-year results. J Neurosurg. 2015; 123(3):609–617

[86] Li ZQ, Wang QH, Chen G, Quan Z. Outcomes of endovascular coiling versus surgical clipping in the treatment of ruptured intracranial aneurysms. J Int Med Res. 2012; 40(6):2145–2151

[87] Lin N, Brouillard AM, Keigher KM, et al. Utilization of Pipeline embolization device for treatment of ruptured intracranial aneurysms: US multicenter experience. J Neurointerv Surg. 2015; 7(11):808–815

[88] Becske T, Kallmes DF, Saatci I, et al. Pipeline for uncoilable or failed aneurysms: results from a multicenter clinical trial. Radiology. 2013; 267 (3):858–868

[89] Chalouhi N, Zanaty M, Whiting A, et al. Treatment of ruptured intracranial aneurysms with the pipeline embolization device. Neurosurgery. 2015; 76 (2):165–172, discussion 172

[90] Silva MA, See AP, Khandelwal P, et al. Comparison of flow diversion with clipping and coiling for the treatment of paraclinoid aneurysms in 115 patients. J Neurosurg. 2019; 130(5):1505–1512

[91] Choi HH, Ha EJ, Lee JJ, et al. Comparison of clinical outcomes of intracranial aneurysms: procedural rupture versus spontaneous rupture. AJNR Am J Neuroradiol. 2017; 38(11):2126–2130

[92] Doerfler A, Wanke I, Egelhof T, et al. Aneurysmal rupture during embolization with Guglielmi detachable coils: causes, management, and outcome. AJNR Am J Neuroradiol. 2001; 22(10):1825–1832

[93] Zheng Y, Liu Y, Leng B, Xu F, Tian Y. Periprocedural complications associated with endovascular treatment of intracranial aneurysms in 1764 cases. J Neurointerv Surg. 2016; 8(2):152–157

[94] Vergouwen MD, Fang J, Casaubon LK, et al. Investigators of the Registry of the Canadian Stroke Network. Higher incidence of in-hospital complications in patients with clipped versus coiled ruptured intracranial aneurysms. Stroke. 2011; 42(11):3093–3098

[95] Investigators C, CARAT Investigators. Rates of delayed rebleeding from intracranial aneurysms are low after surgical and endovascular treatment. Stroke. 2006; 37(6):1437–1442

[96] Schaafsma JD, Sprengers ME, van Rooij WJ, et al. Long-term recurrent subarachnoid hemorrhage after adequate coiling versus clipping of ruptured intracranial aneurysms. Stroke. 2009; 40(5):1758–1763

[97] Byrne JV, Sohn MJ, Molyneux AJ, Chir B. Five-year experience in using coil embolization for ruptured intracranial aneurysms: outcomes and incidence of late rebleeding. J Neurosurg. 1999; 90(4):656–663

[98] Sluzewski M, van Rooij WJ, Beute GN, Nijssen PC. Late rebleeding of ruptured intracranial aneurysms treated with detachable coils. AJNR Am J Neuroradiol. 2005; 26(10):2542–2549

[99] Sluzewski M, van Rooij WJ, Rinkel GJ, Wijnalda D. Endovascular treatment of ruptured intracranial aneurysms with detachable coils: long-term clinical and serial angiographic results. Radiology. 2003; 227 (3):720–724

[100] de Vries J, Boogaarts HD. Treatment of patients with ruptured aneurysm by neurosurgeons that perform both open surgical and endovascular techniques is safe and effective: results of a single centre in Europe. Acta Neurochir (Wien). 2014; 156(7):1259–1266, discussion 1266

[101] Lanzino G, Fraser K, Kanaan Y, Wagenbach A. Treatment of ruptured intracranial aneurysms since the International Subarachnoid Aneurysm Trial: practice utilizing clip ligation and coil embolization as individual or complementary therapies. J Neurosurg. 2006; 104(3):344–349

[102] Zanaty M, Chalouhi N, Starke RM, et al. Short-term outcome of clipping versus coiling of ruptured intracranial aneurysms treated by dual-trained cerebrovascular surgeon: single-institution experience. World Neurosurg. 2016; 95:262–269

18 Natural History and Management Options of Cerebral Cavernous Malformation

Juri Kivelev, Jaakko Rinne, Mika Niemela, and Juha Hernesniemi

Abstract

Natural history of cavernous malformations may be affected by genetic mutational status, ultrastructural features, location along the neural axis, and, probably, perifocal hemodynamic environment. Patients with familial forms frequently harbor multiple cavernomas, whereas those with sporadic forms mostly present with a single lesion. Low blood flow inside the cavernous malformations predisposes to stasis and thrombosis, making profuse extralesional bleeding unlikely. In current clinical practice, cavernous malformations are anticipated mostly as asymptomatic incidental findings. In general, disease is characterized by three main clinical patterns: hemorrhage, seizures, and focal neurological deficits. An acute clinical manifestation is prevalently related to hemorrhage. The risk of this event, in average 1% per patient-year, depends on the location of the cavernoma and increases in deeper lesions of the brain and in brainstem. Seizure activity occurs in up to 80% of symptomatic patients with supratentorial cavernomas most probably due to hemosiderotic impregnation of perifocal brain. Focal neurological deficits are common for lesions located in eloquent areas. In summary, modern data suggest cavernomas to be fairly benign lesions which, however, may carry risks of neurological deterioration.

Keywords: cavernoma, cavernous malformation, cavernous hemangioma, venous malformation

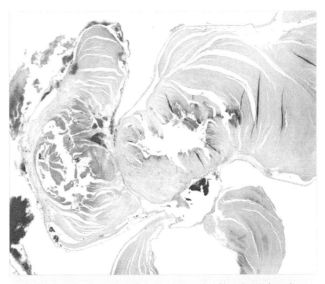

Fig. 18.1 Microscopic view of a cavernoma. The dilated vessels without intervening neural parenchyma are lined by thin endothelium and surrounded by collagenous fibrotic tissue with blue deposits of iron (hemosiderin) after hemorrhages.

18.1 Introduction

Cavernous malformations, or cavernomas, are not common but are increasingly detected as incidental findings due to widespread availability of neuroimaging. Their incidence in the general population is estimated to range between 0.16 and 0.8%.[1,2,3,4,5,6,7] Population-based annual detection rate of cavernomas has been estimated at 0.56 per 100,000 person-years for adults older than 16 years.[8] Most are diagnosed between the second and fifth decades of life and can be either sporadic or familial.[4,9,10] They occur in both genders with equal frequency.[11] Most patients present with a sporadic single lesion. However, 10 to 40% of cases are familial (or hereditary).[7,12] Familial cavernomas affect Hispanic-Americans more frequently and are typically characterized by multiple lesions. In hereditary cases, cavernomas are characterized by an autosomal dominant pattern of inheritance with incomplete penetrance. Three genes, namely, *CCM1*, *CCM2*, and *CCM3*, responsible for development of the cavernomas have been identified to date.[1]

Natural history of the disease is predetermined by cavernoma genetics, ultrastructural features, location along the neural axis, and hemodynamic alterations in the lesion and surrounding brain. ▶ Fig. 18.1 demonstrates the histological view of a cavernoma. Blood flow inside the lesions is low, predisposing to intraluminal stasis and thrombosis. Due to its fragility, a cavernoma causes repetitive microhemorrhages into the surrounding neural tissue with formation of perifocal hemosiderosis and reactive gliosis. Such local homeostatic instability produced by either genetic or reactive environmental factors (inflammation, breakdown of the blood–brain barrier, gliosis) may provoke intensive neoangiogenesis and proliferation of the sinusoids constituting cavernoma. Subsequently, lesions enlarge and grow, which may coexist with clinical progression.

Up to 40% of patients are asymptomatic.[13,14] The most frequent clinical manifestations are seizures, focal neurological deficits (FNDs), and hemorrhage. Seizure activity occurs in up to 80% of patients with supratentorial cavernomas most probably being evoked by perilesional intraparenchymal changes. FNDs are typical for cavernomas located close to eloquent regions of the brain and for spinal lesions. Headaches are a common complaint in many cavernoma patients, and usually lead to further clinical and radiological workup. However, due to their unspecific nature, it is generally accepted that headaches are not linked to the cavernoma.

18.2 Selected Papers on the Natural History of Cavernous Malformations

- Del Curling O Jr, Kelly DL Jr, Elster AD, Craven TE. An analysis of the natural history of cavernous angiomas. J Neurosurg 1991;75(5):702–708
- Kondziolka D, Lunsford LD, Kestle JR. The natural history of cerebral cavernous malformations. J Neurosurg 1995;83(5):820–824

- Horne MA, Flemming KD, Su IC, et al; Cerebral Cavernous Malformations Individual Patient Data Meta-analysis Collaborators. Clinical course of untreated cerebral cavernous malformations: a meta-analysis of individual patient data. Lancet Neurol 2016;15(2):166–173

18.3 Natural History of Cavernous Malformation

18.3.1 Risk of Hemorrhage

For supratentorial cavernomas, the estimated annual risk of hemorrhage is 1% per patient-year (range: 0.25–2.5%; ▶ Table 18.1).[3,8,15,16,17,18,19,20,21] In familial cases, bleeding rates may vary depending on the cavernoma genotype. *CCM3* carriers are more prone than *CCM2* and *CCM1* patients to develop cerebral hemorrhages, especially at a younger age.[22] Furthermore, the authors showed that in patients with multiple cavernomas *CCM1* was associated with a higher number of lesions than *CCM2* and *CCM3*. Thus, the overall risk of hemorrhage in these patients is increased due to cumulative risks from each lesion.

Infratentorial cavernomas have a higher bleeding rate with estimated annual risk ranging from 2.5 to 13.6% per patient-year.[29] This seems to be unrelated to eloquence of the region and thus easier detecting of symptomatic decline after ictus. Interestingly, larger lesion size (> 1 cm), early age at presentation (< 35 years), and coexistence of developmental venous malformation (DVA) were found to be associated with higher hemorrhage rates.[25] Nevertheless, the mechanisms of higher bleeding risk of cavernomas in the infratentorial compartment remain unclear.

Vascular permeability and iron leakage seem to play a central role in the pathogenesis of cavernomas when considering the natural history of the disease.[30] According to Girard et al, significant lesional permeability increases at follow-up correlated with interval hemorrhage or growth.[30] This corresponds with the hypothesis that enhanced vascular permeability is associated with and may drive hemorrhagic proliferation of cavernomas. Using a high magnetic resonance imaging (MRI) sensitivity technique, the authors showed higher regional brain permeability than contralateral homologous regions in anatomical locations initially lacking cavernomas, which later developed de novo lesions.

18.3.2 Risk of Rebleeding

After initial decline, caused by extralesional bleeding, many patients recover well, but some can experience rebleeding. Lesions of the brainstem seem to be more prone to rebleed. The risk of having recurrent extralesional hemorrhage in this selected group varies from 5.1 to 60% per patient-year.[29] Aiba et al found that younger women exhibited a higher incidence of rebleeding, possibly caused by hormonal factors.[26] Of note, Kalani et al in 2013 showed no increased hemorrhage risk during pregnancy, thus concluding that a history of cavernoma is not a contraindication to pregnancy or vaginal delivery.[31]

In contrast to previous studies, Barker et al proposed the concept of temporal clustering of the hemorrhages after the initial event.[32] Using sophisticated statistical analysis in 141 patients, the authors discovered quantitative evidence of a spontaneous decline in the hazard of cavernoma rehemorrhage approximately 2 years after the first hemorrhage.

Xie et al summarized published data on hemorrhage risk factors subdividing them into three groups[33]:
- *Hemorrhage risk factors*: History of previous ictus and location in brainstem.
- *Possible risk factors*: Female sex, younger age, perilesional edema on MRI, large lesion size, coexistence of DVA, hemodynamic change, or high blood pressure.
- *No risk factors*: Pregnancy, multiplicity, and antiplatelet or antithrombotic use.

This simple classification reflects modern understanding of factors that may affect cavernoma natural history. According to hese data, only a history of previous hemorrhage and brainstem location constitutes "true" increased risk of rehemorrhage, whereas other variables are not strong enough to change the natural history of the disease. Obviously further larger international multicenter prospective studies are needed to have unbiased data on disease course.

18.3.3 Risk of Seizures

Seizures are the most frequent clinical presentation of supratentorial cavernomas, occurring in 41 to 80% of patients.[1,34] For unknown reasons, cavernoma-associated seizures are more likely intractable than those related to other vascular malformations.[35,36] Temporal lobe lesions tend to cause seizures more frequently and have an obvious propensity to intractable epilepsy.[34] Less favorable seizure outcomes were noted in younger persons and women.[37] Long-lasting epileptic disorders with high frequency of seizures in certain cases can lead to development of secondary epileptogenic foci located in remote brain regions.[34] Notably, the risk of recurrent seizures appears to be as high as 5.5% per patient-year.[38]

Table 18.1 Reported symptomatic hemorrhage rates of cerebral cavernomas

Study	Annual hemorrhage rate (%)	Study design
Del Curling et al[24]	0.1	Retrospective
Robinson et al[76]	0.7	Prospective
Zabramski et al[95]	1.2	Prospective
Kondziolka et al[51]	1.3	Retrospective
	2.6	Prospective
	0.6	For incidental lesion
Aiba et al[3]	0–0.4	Prospective
Porter et al[73]	5	Retrospective
		Brainstem lesion
Labauge et al[53]	2.5	Retrospective, familial forms
Kupersmith et al[52]	2.46	Brainstem lesions
Labauge et al., 2001	4.3	Prospective, familial forms
Cantu et al[18]	1.7	Retrospective, Hispanic population
Al-Shahi Salman et al[7]	0.5	Prospective
Jeon et al[44]	4.5	Prospective

To date, there has been only one study examining seizures as an endpoint in cavernoma natural history.[1] Namely, in 2011 Josephson et al published a prospective population-based study on 139 adults diagnosed with cavernomas and found a 5-year risk of first-ever seizure to be 6% in patients presenting with cavernoma-related intracerebral hemorrhage (ICH) or FND and 4% in incidentally diagnosed cavernomas.[39] Among the adults who never experienced ICH/FND and presented with or developed epilepsy, the proportion achieving a 2-year seizure-free state over 5 years was 47%. Consequently, adults with cavernomas may have a high risk of epilepsy after the first-ever seizure and roughly half achieve 2-year seizure freedom over 5 years after epilepsy diagnosis.

18.3.4 Associated Vascular Abnormalities

Natural history of cavernomas may be affected by associated vascular abnormalities. The most frequent entity associated with cavernomas appears to be DVA.[40,41,42] It may be found in up to 25% of cavernoma patients.[43,44] Previous studies have shown conjunction of cavernoma development with venous architecture or pathophysiology related to DVA.[44,45,46,47] Brinjikji et al in their study hypothesized that the prevalence of DVA-associated cavernomas increases with age.[48] This trial included 1,689 individuals, with 116 being affected by DVA-associated cavernomas. They could identify a strong statistically significant association between age and the prevalence of DVA-associated cavernomas. Indeed, in the group of 0 to 10-year-old patients, the prevalence of DVA-associated cavernomas was 0.8%, but in the group of patients older than 70 years the rate jumped to 11.6%.[48] Based on these findings, they concluded that (1) DVA-associated cavernomas are not congenital lesions, (2) de novo cavernomas' formation associated with DVA is likely the rule rather than exception, and (3) various age-related changes in the cerebral venous system could trigger the formation of cavernomas associated with DVA.[48] These conclusions are consonant with previous reports where the trigger for microhemorrhages is generally thought to be local venous hypertension resulting from local thrombosis, stenosis, or changes in DVA architecture.[40] Moreover, severe medullary venous tortuosity, medullary venous stenosis, or sharp angles between radicular vein and the dominant medullary venous drainage are associated with a higher prevalence of cavernomas associated with DVA.[33,49]

18.4 Limitations of Studies on the Natural History of Cavernomas

Large series of untreated asymptomatic cavernoma patients with long-term follow-up are missing. A significant drawback of the current research on cavernoma natural history lies in self-limitation of retrospective studies when significant biases are established at the primary stage of collecting data. Indeed, even considered incidental, such cavernoma cases represent only a limited subset of the disease-carrier population. Accumulating literature data show enormous heterogeneity of genetic, ultrastructural, clinical, and radiological features of cavernomas. This may be related not only to intrinsic complexity of the disease but also to biased data collection and

over-/underestimating of the risks or safety of the pathology. Moreover, data collection may be altered by socioeconomic factors and local health care system organization issues such as unequal access to MRI in the general population. This may obviously disfigure understanding of disease incidence and can cause misinterpretation of factors affecting the natural history.

18.5 Selected Papers on the Treatment Outcomes for Cavernous Malformations

- Kivelev J, Laakso A, Niemelä M, Hernesniemi J. A proposed grading system of brain and spinal cavernomas. Neurosurgery 2011;69(4):807–813, discussion 813–814
- Kivelev J, Niemelä M, Hernesniemi J. Treatment strategies in cavernomas of the brain and spine. J Clin Neurosci 2012;19(4):491–497

18.6 Treatment Options for Cavernous Malformations

18.6.1 Recommendations for Treatment

Management of cavernoma patients is based on four major situational patterns[50]:

- *Conservative treatment of incidental cavernomas*: In many patients, conservative treatment of cavernomas remains the best management option due to the fairly benign clinical course of the disease. Generally speaking, in adults, asymptomatic and tiny cavernomas (nidus < 5 mm) that are radiologically stable may be observed safely, although there are some risks of developing neurological deterioration. Of note, children's cavernomas carry significant bleeding risks; conservative treatment is therefore warranted only in asymptomatic patients if on MRI the cavernoma is small and inactive.
- *Conservative treatment of symptomatic cavernomas*: Conservative treatment of cavernomas manifesting with neurological symptoms may be justified in the cases where symptoms are mild or transitional. In cases of FNDs occurring due to mass effect in eloquent regions, observation is recommended if the lesion is very small, radiologically inactive, not hemorrhagic, and not provoking further clinical deterioration. Surgical risks in these areas are increased and prophylactic lesionectomy in inexperienced hands may be more dangerous than the natural course of the lesion. In patients suffering from seizures, a conservative approach comprising administration of anticonvulsants may be sufficient treatment at least at the initial stages of the disease.[13]
- *Surgical treatment of symptomatic cavernomas*: The most common indications for surgery are seizures and overt hemorrhage. Regarding timing, we prefer to remove a cavernoma at an early stage after the first seizure, especially when a lesion exhibits signs of recent hemorrhage. In the literature, lesionectomy has been shown to be effective in

Table 18.2 Scoring in grading system of brain and spinal cavernomas

Variable	Score
Location	
Basal ganglia, infratentorial, spinal cord	2
Supratentorial	1
Focal neurological deficit	
Yes	1
No	0

Table 18.3 A proposed grading system applied to our series of 303 operated cavernoma patients

Classification	Condition at long-term follow-up		Total (%)
	Favorable outcome (%)	Unfavorable outcome (%)	
Grade 1	165 (87)	24 (13)	189 (62)
Grade 2	45 (79)	12 (21)	57 (19)
Grade 3	26 (46)	31 (54)	57 (19)

controlling seizures, particularly when accompanied by resection of the perifocal hemosiderotic parenchyma.[51,52] In these series, patients with secondary generalized seizures preoperatively were significantly less likely to achieve a seizure-free state than those with simple partial and complex partial seizures (26 vs. 65 and 52%, respectively). Cavernoma hemorrhage is frequently accompanied by FNDs, especially when located in deep brain. Gross et al published their meta-analysis of 78 studies including a total of 745 brainstem cavernoma patients; 683 patients (92%) had the lesion completely removed.[53] At the postoperative follow-up, 85% of the patients were reported to be improved or the same neurologically. The surgical mortality rate was 1.9%.

In general, the goal of operative treatment of a cavernoma is gross total resection. Partial removal can significantly increase the risk of bleeding, with consequent complications. Apart from other neurovascular pathologies, such as cerebral aneurysms and arteriovenous malformations, no rational classifications assessing surgical outcome are available in the literature. In 2011, we proposed our cavernoma grading system, which was based on a large number of consecutive patients ($n = 303$) treated at the Helsinki University Hospital in 1980 to 2009, to assist the surgeon in decision-making.[31] The follow-up assessment of these patients was performed on average 5.7 years (range: 0.2–36 years) postoperatively. A grading system is based on the results of multivariate analysis of factors predicting long-term outcome. It includes two items, location and preexisting FND, both of which were shown to be independent risk factors for unfavorable outcome. Both of these had an approximately threefold relative risk of causing some degree of disability postoperatively. Patients with 1 point were assigned to grade 1, those with 2 points to grade 2, and those with 3 points to grade 3 (▶ Table 18.2). When applied to our series, this grading system strongly correlated with outcome ($p < 0.001$, Pearson's χ^2 test; ▶ Table 18.3).

- *Surgical treatment of incidental cavernomas*: This clinical situation seems to be the most controversial in the management of cavernomas. A decision to surgically remove an incidental cavernoma should be justified by a systematic analysis of all factors potentially affecting outcome. In these cases, the role of subjective aspects regarding optimal treatment strategy is more emphasized. Indeed, if the patient prefers to avoid the risks related to natural history of the disease and the cavernoma can be safely removed, the decision to operate is rational. Furthermore, in pediatric patients, preventive surgery might be reasonable, taking into account the preponderance of cavernomas in children to bleed.

Some reports have shown the efficacy of stereotactic radiotherapy,[27] but its long-term results are still controversial and the side effects may outweigh the natural history risks, significantly limiting its use in cavernoma management.[23,54] In addition, the long-term effect of radiotherapy cannot be objectively confirmed by any reliable radiological investigation.

18.7 Authors' Recommendations

- For supratentorial cavernomas, the estimated annual risk of hemorrhage is 1% per patient-year (range: 0.25–2.5%).
- Infratentorial cavernomas have higher bleeding rates with estimated annual risk ranging from 2.5 to 13.6% per patient-year.
- The risk of rebleeding is correlated to a prior history of hemorrhage and brainstem location.
- Evidence-based management guidelines of cerebral cavernous malformations have not been established. Treatment recommendation should be based on assessment of several factors, related to the size and location of the lesion, whether the disease is familial or sporadic, patient lifestyle and preference, and surgeon experience.
- The use of radiotherapy to treat cavernomas is controversial as long-term results are lacking and treatment side effects may outweigh the natural history.

References

[1] Akers A, Al-Shahi Salman R, A Awad I, et al. Synopsis of guidelines for the clinical management of cerebral cavernous malformations: consensus recommendations based on systematic literature review by the angioma alliance scientific advisory board clinical experts panel. Neurosurgery. 2017; 80(5):665–680

[2] Al-Holou WN, O'Lynnger TM, Pandey AS, et al. Natural history and imaging prevalence of cavernous malformations in children and young adults. J Neurosurg Pediatr. 2012; 9(2):198–205

[3] Del Curling O, Jr, Kelly DL, Jr, Elster AD, Craven TE. An analysis of the natural history of cavernous angiomas. J Neurosurg. 1991; 75(5):702–708

[4] Giombini S, Morello G. Cavernous angiomas of the brain. Account of fourteen personal cases and review of the literature. Acta Neurochir (Wien). 1978; 40 (1–2):61–82

[5] Lunsford LD, Khan AA, Niranjan A, Kano H, Flickinger JC, Kondziolka D. Stereotactic radiosurgery for symptomatic solitary cerebral cavernous malformations considered high risk for resection. J Neurosurg. 2010; 113(1):23–29

[6] Moriarity JL, Wetzel M, Clatterbuck RE, et al. The natural history of cavernous malformations: a prospective study of 68 patients. Neurosurgery. 1999; 44 (6):1166–1171, discussion 1172–1173

[7] Porter RW, Detwiler PW, Spetzler RF, et al. Cavernous malformations of the brainstem: experience with 100 patients. J Neurosurg. 1999; 90(1):50–58

[8] Al-Shahi Salman R, Hall JM, Horne MA, et al. Scottish Audit of Intracranial Vascular Malformations (SAIVMs) collaborators. Untreated clinical course of

cerebral cavernous malformations: a prospective, population-based cohort study. Lancet Neurol. 2012; 11(3):217–224

[9] Takenaka N, Imanishi T, Sasaki H, et al. Delayed radiation necrosis with extensive brain edema after gamma knife radiosurgery for multiple cerebral cavernous malformations: case report. Neurol Med Chir (Tokyo). 2003; 43(8): 391–395

[10] Töpper R, Jürgens E, Reul J, Thron A. Clinical significance of intracranial developmental venous anomalies. J Neurol Neurosurg Psychiatry. 1999; 67 (2):234–238

[11] Horne MA, Flemming KD, Su IC, et al. Cerebral Cavernous Malformations Individual Patient Data Meta-analysis Collaborators. Clinical course of untreated cerebral cavernous malformations: a meta-analysis of individual patient data. Lancet Neurol. 2016; 15(2):166–173

[12] Pozzati E, Acciarri N, Tognetti F, Marliani F, Giangaspero F. Growth, subsequent bleeding, and de novo appearance of cerebral cavernous angiomas. Neurosurgery. 1996; 38(4):662–669, discussion 669–670

[13] Batra S, Lin D, Recinos PF, Zhang J, Rigamonti D. Cavernous malformations: natural history, diagnosis and treatment. Nat Rev Neurol. 2009; 5(12): 659–670

[14] Voigt K, Yaşargil MG. Cerebral cavernous haemangiomas or cavernomas. Incidence, pathology, localization, diagnosis, clinical features and treatment. Review of the literature and report of an unusual case. Neurochirurgia (Stuttg). 1976; 19(2):59–68

[15] Cantu C, Murillo-Bonilla L, Arauz A, Higuera J, Padilla J, Barinagarrementeria F. Predictive factors for intracerebral hemorrhage in patients with cavernous angiomas. Neurol Res. 2005; 27(3):314–318

[16] Hsu PW, Chang CN, Tseng CK, et al. Treatment of epileptogenic cavernomas: surgery versus radiosurgery. Cerebrovasc Dis. 2007; 24(1):116–120, discussion 121

[17] Kivelev J, Niemelä M, Hernesniemi J. Treatment strategies in cavernomas of the brain and spine. J Clin Neurosci. 2012; 19(4):491–497

[18] Kupersmith MJ, Kalish H, Epstein F, et al. Natural history of brainstem cavernous malformations. Neurosurgery. 2001; 48(1):47–53, discussion 53–54

[19] Perrini P, Lanzino G. The association of venous developmental anomalies and cavernous malformations: pathophysiological, diagnostic, and surgical considerations. Neurosurg Focus. 2006; 21(1):e5

[20] Rigamonti D, Hadley MN, Drayer BP, et al. Cerebral cavernous malformations. Incidence and familial occurrence. N Engl J Med. 1988; 319(6):343–347

[21] Yu T, Liu X, Lin X, et al. The relation between angioarchitectural factors of developmental venous anomaly and concomitant sporadic cavernous malformation. BMC Neurol. 2016; 16(1):183

[22] Denier C, Labauge P, Bergametti F, et al. Société Française de Neurochirurgie. Genotype-phenotype correlations in cerebral cavernous malformations patients. Ann Neurol. 2006; 60(5):550–556

[23] Robinson JR, Awad IA, Little JR. Natural history of the cavernous angioma. J Neurosurg. 1991; 75(5):709–714

[24] Zabramski JM, Wascher TM, Spetzler RF, et al. The natural history of familial cavernous malformations: results of an ongoing study. J Neurosurg. 1994; 80 (3):422–432

[25] Kondziolka D, Lunsford LD, Kestle JR. The natural history of cerebral cavernous malformations. J Neurosurg. 1995; 83(5):820–824

[26] Aiba T, Tanaka R, Koike T, Kameyama S, Takeda N, Komata T. Natural history of intracranial cavernous malformations. J Neurosurg. 1995; 83(1):56–59

[27] Labauge P, Brunereau L, Lévy C, Laberge S, Houtteville JP. The natural history of familial cerebral cavernomas: a retrospective MRI study of 40 patients. Neuroradiology. 2000; 42(5):327–332

[28] Jeon JS, Kim JE, Chung YS, et al. A risk factor analysis of prospective symptomatic haemorrhage in adult patients with cerebral cavernous malformation. J Neurol Neurosurg Psychiatry. 2014; 85(12):1366–1370

[29] Wurm G, Schnizer M, Fellner FA. Cerebral cavernous malformations associated with venous anomalies: surgical considerations. Neurosurgery. 2005; 57(1) Suppl:42–58, discussion 42–58

[30] Girard R, Fam MD, Zeineddine HA, et al. Vascular permeability and iron deposition biomarkers in longitudinal follow-up of cerebral cavernous malformations. J Neurosurg. 2017; 127(1):102–110

[31] Kalani MY, Zabramski JM. Risk for symptomatic hemorrhage of cerebral cavernous malformations during pregnancy. J Neurosurg. 2013; 118(1): 50–55

[32] Barker FG, II, Amin-Hanjani S, Butler WE, et al. Temporal clustering of hemorrhages from untreated cavernous malformations of the central nervous system. Neurosurgery. 2001; 49(1):15–24, discussion 24–25

[33] Xie MG, Li D, Guo FZ, et al. Brainstem cavernous malformations: surgical indications based on natural history and surgical outcomes. World Neurosurg. 2018; 110:55–63

[34] Awad I, Jabbour P. Cerebral cavernous malformations and epilepsy. Neurosurg Focus. 2006; 21(1):e7

[35] Awad IA, Robinson JR. Cavernous malformations and epilepsy. In: Awad IA, Barrow DL, eds. Cavernous Malformation. park Ridge, IL: American Association of Neurological Surgeons; 1993

[36] Awad IA, Rosenfeld J, Ahl J, Hahn JF, Lüders H. Intractable epilepsy and structural lesions of the brain: mapping, resection strategies, and seizure outcome. Epilepsia. 1991; 32(2):179–186

[37] Cohen DS, Zubay GP, Goodman RR. Seizure outcome after lesionectomy for cavernous malformations. J Neurosurg. 1995; 83(2):237–242

[38] McCormick WF. Pathology of vascular malformations of the brain. In: Wilson CB, Steihn BM, eds. Intracranial Arteriovenous Malformations. Baltimore, MD: Williams & Wilkins; 1984

[39] Josephson CB, Leach JP, Duncan R, Roberts RC, Counsell CE, Al-Shahi Salman R, Scottish Audit of Intracranial Vascular Malformations (SAIVMs) steering committee and collaborators. Seizure risk from cavernous or arteriovenous malformations: prospective population-based study. Neurology. 2011; 76 (18):1548–1554

[40] Morris Z, Whiteley WN, Longstreth WT, Jr, et al. Incidental findings on brain magnetic resonance imaging: systematic review and meta-analysis. BMJ. 2009; 339:b3016

[41] Porter PJ, Willinsky RA, Harper W, Wallace MC. Cerebral cavernous malformations: natural history and prognosis after clinical deterioration with or without hemorrhage. J Neurosurg. 1997; 87(2):190–197

[42] Taslimi S, Modabbernia A, Amin-Hanjani S, Barker FG, II, Macdonald RL. Natural history of cavernous malformation: Systematic review and meta-analysis of 25 studies. Neurology. 2016; 86(21):1984–1991

[43] Abdulrauf SI, Kaynar MY, Awad IA. A comparison of the clinical profile of cavernous malformations with and without associated venous malformations. Neurosurgery. 1999; 44(1):41–46, discussion 46–47

[44] Washington CW, McCoy KE, Zipfel GJ. Update on the natural history of cavernous malformations and factors predicting aggressive clinical presentation. Neurosurg Focus. 2010; 29(3):E7

[45] Cakirer S. De novo formation of a cavernous malformation of the brain in the presence of a developmental venous anomaly. Clin Radiol. 2003; 58(3):251–256

[46] Campeau NG, Lane JI. De novo development of a lesion with the appearance of a cavernous malformation adjacent to an existing developmental venous anomaly. AJNR Am J Neuroradiol. 2005; 26(1):156–159

[47] Desal HA, Lee SK, Kim BS, Raoul S, Tymianski M, TerBrugge KG. Multiple de novo vascular malformations in relation to diffuse venous occlusive disease: a case report. Neuroradiology. 2005; 47(1):38–42

[48] Brinjikji W, El-Masri AE, Wald JT, Flemming KD, Lanzino G. Prevalence of cerebral cavernous malformations associated with developmental venous anomalies increases with age. Childs Nerv Syst. 2017; 33(9):1539–1543

[49] Hong YJ, Chung TS, Suh SH, et al. The angioarchitectural factors of the cerebral developmental venous anomaly; can they be the causes of concurrent sporadic cavernous malformation? Neuroradiology. 2010; 52(10): 883–891

[50] Kivelev J, Laakso A, Niemelä M, Hernesniemi J. A proposed grading system of brain and spinal cavernomas. Neurosurgery. 2011; 69(4):807–813, discussion 813–814

[51] Baumann CR, Schuknecht B, Lo Russo G, et al. Seizure outcome after resection of cavernous malformations is better when surrounding hemosiderin-stained brain also is removed. Epilepsia. 2006; 47(3):563–566

[52] Hammen T, Romstöck J, Dörfler A, Kerling F, Buchfelder M, Stefan H. Prediction of postoperative outcome with special respect to removal of hemosiderin fringe: a study in patients with cavernous haemangiomas associated with symptomatic epilepsy. Seizure. 2007; 16(3):248–253

[53] Gross BA, Batjer HH, Awad IA, Bendok BR. Brainstem cavernous malformations. Neurosurgery. 2009; 64(5):E805–E818, discussion E818

[54] Hsu FP, Rigamonti D, Huhn SL. Epidemiology of cavernous malformations. In: Awad I, Barrow DL, eds. Cavernous Malformations. Park Ridge, IL: American Association of Neurological Surgeons; 1993:18

19 Natural History and Management Options of Skull Base Chordoma

Vinayak Narayan, Fareed Jumah, Bharath Raju, and Anil Nanda

The good physician treats the disease; the great physician treats the patient who has the disease.

–Sir William Osler

Abstract

Chordomas, constituting 1 to 4% of primary brain tumors, are slow growing extra-axial tumors arising from the ectopic remnants of embryonal notochord cells along the craniospinal axis, presenting with the characteristic features of local invasiveness and clinical malignancy. The clinical characteristics depend on the anatomic location of the tumor. The optimum standard of care for patients with skull base chordoma (SBC) comprises proper clinical and radiological assessment, adequate presurgical planning, ideal surgical approach selection, careful preservation of neurovascular structures, and safe maximal cytoreductive surgical resection. Adjuvant treatment comprises various modalities like proton-beam radiation, photon-based radiation, conventional RT, stereotactic radiosurgery, and charged ion therapy, and most studies report the best results with the proton beam radiation. The overall 5-year survival rate of SBC is around 67% and the overall 10-year survival rate is around 39%. The size of tumor, location, and extent of surgical resection influence long-term local control, overall survival, and recurrence free survival. Older age and greater tumor size were found to be associated with inferior survival.

Keywords: skull base, chordoma, natural history, treatment, outcome

19.1 Introduction

Chordomas are rare slow-growing extra-axial tumors arising from the ectopic remnants of embryonal notochord cells along the craniospinal axis, presenting with the characteristic features of local invasiveness and clinical malignancy.[2,3] Within the clivus, the notochord follows a sinuous course. It explains the diverse origin and projections of cranial base chordomas (▶ Fig. 19.1).[4] Virchow described for the first time "chordomas" as small nodules along the clivus in 1846 and named them "ecchondrosis physaliphora" in 1857.[1] Tumor recurrence is frequent; therefore, their clinical progression leads to their categorization among the malignant types of tumors.[5,6,7,8]

Chordoma constitutes around 1 to 4% of primary brain tumors with an age-adjusted incidence rate of 0.08 per 100,000 patient-years.[10] It accounts for 1.4% of all primary malignant bone tumors, 0.4% of all intracranial tumors, 0.2% of skull base tumors, and 17% of primary bone tumors of the spine, most commonly at the C1–C2 level.[11,12,13,14]

The peak age of incidence is between 50 and 60 years (range: 3–95 years), with a male preponderance.[7,9] There is a five-time increased incidence in the white population and chordoma is uncommon among African Americans. Its anatomic distribution varies and is commonly seen in the spine (32.8%), the spheno-occipital region (32%), and the sacrum (29.2%).[9] Skull base chordoma (SBC) is found more frequently among female patients (39%). Patients with SBC are younger than those with sacral and mobile spine chordomas (49 vs. 69 years).[15]

These tumors are relatively insensitive to both radiotherapy and chemotherapy. Although surgery is the primary treatment of choice, the attempt to achieve maximal resection should be weighed against the potential surgical morbidity. The advancements in surgical technique, radiotherapy, and chemotherapy may further improve the overall survival (OS) outcome. In the era of evidence-based medicine, although randomized controlled trials remain the current gold standard for high-quality data pertaining to the natural history and treatment outcome, the relative rarity of SBCs makes the implementation of such a trial logistically challenging.

19.2 Selected Papers on the Natural History of Skull Base Chordoma

- Walcott BP, Nahed BV, Mohyeldin A, Coumans JV, Kahle KT, Ferreira MJ. Chordoma: current concepts, management, and future directions. Lancet Oncol 2012;13(2):e69–e76

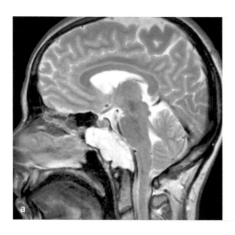
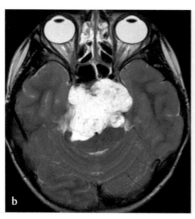

Fig. 19.1 Magnetic resonance imaging of clival chordoma. **(a)** T2-weighted (T2W) sagittal image and **(b)** T2 W axial image demonstrating hyperintense lesion originating from the clival region.

- McMaster ML, Goldstein AM, Bromley CM, Ishibe N, Parry DM. Chordoma: incidence and survival patterns in the United States, 1973–1995. Cancer Causes Control 2001;12(1):1–11
- Lanzino G, Dumont AS, Lopes MB, Laws ER Jr. Skull base chordomas: overview of disease, management options, and outcome. Neurosurg Focus 2001;10(3):E12

19.3 Natural History of Skull Base Chordoma

Chordomas are slow-growing, expansile, locally infiltrating tumors arising from the most rostral notochord extension in the dorsum sella and present as sellar or parasellar tumors. Those arising from the most ventral aspect of the clivus can present as nasopharyngeal chordomas, whereas those associated with the body and dorsal aspect of the clivus manifest as spheno-occipital or petrosal lesions. Chordomas related to the lower clivus will present at the ventral portion of the foramen magnum. Lateral growth of these neoplasms from their midline origin frequently results in invasion of the cavernous sinus, which can be demonstrated radiologically in 54 to 75% of cases.[4] Sellar chordomas are rare and may constitute around 0.5 to 2% of sellar lesions.[16,17] However, among the skull base locations, the clivus constitutes the maximum for SBCs (▶ Fig. 19.2).

The mean growth rate of chordoma is 8 ± 9% per month and the mean growth volume is 0.8 ± 0.7 cm³ per month.[18] Higher growth rate of SBC is commonly seen in female population, endophytic tumors, absent duramater breakthrough, soft textured and small lesions. The growth rate of SBC may slow as the volume increases.[18] The spread of tumor usually happens in varying stages. Expansive destruction of bone at the site of origin is the initial stage; this is followed by subsequent infiltration and transgression of the dura, eventual widespread intracranial extension, and encasement of cranial nerves, brainstem, and vascular structures followed by metastasis to distant locations.[4] Direct dural invasion, however, is the most likely pattern responsible for extension into the posterior fossa. The intradural chordoma usually remains in the subdural plane, and the true subarachnoid or pia mater infiltrations are rare and commonly seen at times of recurrence.

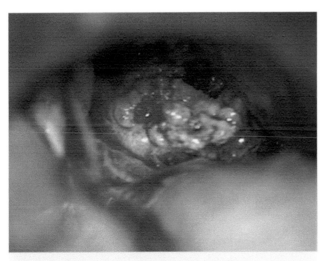

Fig. 19.2 Intraoperative image showing clival chordoma.

The clinical characteristics depend on the anatomic location of the tumor. Patients with cranial chordomas may present with headache, neck pain, cranial neuropathies, and even endocrine abnormalities. The symptoms usually worsen when the tumor breaks through the dura mater.[18] Deficits of cranial nerves III and VI, hydrocephalus, and sensorimotor problems are the most common initial symptoms in patients with SBC.[19] Volpe et al reported on 48 patients with SBC, 52% of whom were initially seen with ocular symptoms such as diplopia, visual impairment as a result of visual field defects, or deterioration of visual acuity.[20,21] The diplopia was initially intermittent and associated with cranial nerve VI palsy, but it continued to be progressive in the majority of patients. Patients with spinal chordomas have back pain, pathologic fractures, myelopathy, and radiculopathy. Sacral chordomas tend to be quite large at the time of diagnosis because of the insidious onset of symptoms such as pain and bowel or bladder dysfunction.[22]

Although SBCs are indolent, slow growing, and histologically benign tumors, their natural history can be clinically aggressive. They have the potential to be locally invasive and destructive, with high rates of recurrence and a predilection to seed any contaminated area of the operative field.[23,24] Much of the morbidity and mortality of SBC are attributable to the local disease.[7] The survival rate of SBC varies. The 5-year OS is around 67% and the 10-year OS rate is around 39% for SBC. Though distant metastasis to the lung, liver, and bone may occur with such tumors, it usually happens in the late stage of the disease process. However, local recurrence could be considered as one of the major predictors of mortality in chordomas.[9] The factors related to recurrence include female gender, older age, larger tumor size, increasing extent of tumor invasion, incomplete resection, presence of metastasis, higher Ki-67 index, and dedifferentiated histologic type.[18] The summary of the natural history of SBCs reported in selected studies is provided in ▶ Table 19.1.[13,16,25,26,27,28,29,30,31,32,33,34,35,36,37,38,39,40,41,42,43,44,45,46,47,48,49,50,51,52,53,54,55,56,57,58,59,60,61,62,63,64,65,66,67,68,69,70,71,72,73,74,75,76,77,78,79,80,81,82,83,84,85,86,87,88,89]

19.4 Selected Papers on the Treatment Outcomes of Skull Base Chordoma

- Hulou MM, Garcia CR, Slone SA, et al. Comprehensive review of cranial chordomas using national databases in the USA. Clin Oncol (R Coll Radiol) 2019;31(9):e149–e159
- Tzortzidis F, Elahi F, Wright D, Natarajan SK, Sekhar LN. Patient outcome at long-term follow-up after aggressive microsurgical resection of cranial base chordomas. Neurosurgery 2006;59(2):230–237, discussion 230–237
- Amichetti M, Cianchetti M, Amelio D, Enrici RM, Minniti G. Proton therapy in chordoma of the base of the skull: a systematic review. Neurosurg Rev 2009;32(4):403–416

19.5 Treatment Options and Surgical Outcome

The large tumor burden of chordomas upon presentation and their intimate association with critical neurological and vascular structures make the treatment of chordomas, especially in the skull base, challenging.[7,43,90] Treatment options for SBCs are

Table 19.1 Summary of the natural history of SBC reported in selected studies

Variable	Clival chordoma: 766 patients from 37 studies		Sellar chordoma: 80 patients from 30 studies
	Microsurgical series (n = 639)	Endoscopic series (n = 127)	
Study period	1950–2010	1950–2010	1960–2017
Mean patient age (y)	43	44	55.7
Male (%)	56	44	M:F = 1:1.16
Mean tumor volume (cm^3)	57.9	30.5	N/A
Mean tumor diameter (cm)	4.7	3.7	N/A
Extent of resection Gross total	48	61	7.5
Subtotal	48.4	27.3	58.8
Follow up in months (mean)	59.7	18.5	54
Local recurrence (mo)	40	16.8	N/A
Mean overall survival (3 y) in months	72.7	N/A	N/A
Mean overall survival (5 y) in months	65.7	N/A	60
Adjuvant treatment (%) EBRT	42.7	49.1	42.5
Proton beam	15.5	14.3	N/A
Radiosurgery	10.5	1.3	N/A
Complications (%) CN deficit	24.2	1.3	7.5
Meningitis	5.9	0.9	
CSF leak	10.7	5	
Mortality	21.6	4.7	

Abbreviations: CN, cranial nerve; CSF, cerebrospinal fluid; EBRT, external beam radiation therapy; SBC, skull base chordomas.

surgical resection, proton beam therapy, conventional radiotherapy, stereotactic fractionated radiation therapy, radiosurgery, and ion therapy. Maximal safe surgical resection, when feasible, predicts improved OS. However, for SBCs, this goal can be difficult to achieve.[4,91] Proton radiotherapy combined with radical resection offers superior results.[92] SBCs are usually rare in pediatric patients; however, they do have a better prognosis than their adult counterparts.[88,93] There are many reports that mention the optimal treatment for SBC as maximal surgical resection, followed by high dose targeted radiation therapy, particularly proton beam radiation therapy.[89,94,95]

Classically, the local treatment of SBC is surgery aimed primarily to assess the pathological diagnosis and to remove the tumor as much as possible. But the major limitation of surgery is to achieve a complete resection owing to the critical location and the infiltrative characteristics.[96] The option of postoperative radiotherapy is gaining importance for the treatment of residual disease; however, the need for increased dose of radiation (range of 70 Gy) may affect the adjacent critical neurovascular structures. Charged particles such as protons have consequentially been used in addition or instead of photons for their distinct advantage over conventional external beam radiation therapy (EBRT) because of the superior dose distribution due to the rapid radiation falloff beyond the target.[96] In addition, proton beams have a finite penetration range, that is, no exit dose, and produce a dose distribution that increases with depth until the distal edge of the Bragg peak.[97] Amichetti et al report negligible acute toxicity and 5 to 17% late toxicity with a few cases of grade 4 side effects.[96] They report an average 5-year local control (LC) of 69.2% and 5-year OS of 79.8%. Munzenrider et al reported their 10-year experience with proton therapy of 54% OS and LC.[98]

In a systematic review with a total of 191 patients, the median total radiation dose to the SBC was 52.7 (22.9–69.3) Gy.[96]

The 5- and 10-year OS rates were 53.5 and 50.3%. Tumor controls at 5 and 10 years were 36 and 23.8%, respectively. A reasonable level of LC was achieved only in the cases where doses higher than 50 Gy were employed.[99] The complication rate of 0 to 5% was reported in the study. Debus et al reports the 5-year OS and LC of 82 and 50%, respectively, with stereotactic fractionated radiation therapy with permanent complication rate of 2.2%.[100] Amichetti et al reports the 5-year OS and LC of 75 and 56%, respectively, after radiosurgery for SBC, whereas the 5-year OS and LC were 79.9 and 64%, respectively, with ion therapy.[96] The median OS reported for intrasellar chordoma is 90 months and the 5-year OS is around 60.7%.[72]

Regarding the surgical approach, both open and endoscopic approaches have been proved excellent in SBC management. A comparison of both in terms of short- and long-term outcome is provided in ▶ Table 19.1. A recently published meta-analysis by Amit et al shows the added advantages of endoscopic surgery over conventional open surgery. The authors report that the 5-year OS was 96% for patients who underwent open surgery for clival chordoma compared with 76% for those who underwent endoscopic surgery.[101] The 5-year progression-free survival (PFS) for patients who underwent open surgery and endoscopic surgery was 94 and 79%, respectively. The 5-year OS of patients treated with surgery followed by adjuvant radiation was 87% compared with 69% of those treated by surgery alone. The summary of the treatment modalities and outcome reported in various studies including the National Cancer Database (NCDB) and the Surveillance, Epidemiology, and End Results (SEER) database of SBC are provided in ▶ Table 19.2 and ▶ Table 19.3.[28,45,84,89,93,94,95,98,99,100,101,102,103,104,105,106,107,108,109,110,111,112,113,114,115,116,117,118,119,120,121,122,123,124,125,126,127,128,129,130,131,132,133,134,135,136,137,138]

Table 19.2 Summary of the treatment modalities and outcome of SBC reported in selected studies

Variables	Treatment modality			
	Proton/proton and photon (study, n = 15)	Conventional RT (study, n = 16)	Radiosurgery/fractionated SRT (study, n = 12)	Charged particle (ions) (study, n = 5)
Study period	1975–2017	1952–2017	1987–2018	1977–2016
Mean age (y)	58 [9.7–61]	46.4 [2–79]	46 [10–81]	48 [9–71]
Mean tumor volume (cm³)	27.8	N/A	20.2	N/A
Male-to-female ratio	1.1:1	2.1:1	1.8:1	2:1
Follow-up in months (median)	37	68.4	48	54
3-y local control rate (%)	84	N/A	N/A	N/A
5-y local control rate (%)	69.4	36.4	58	64
5-y OS rate (%)	78.4	54.6	77.3	78
Complication (%)	8	9	4.5	10

Abbreviations: OS, overall survival; RT, radiotherapy; SBC, skull base chordomas; SRT, stereotactic radiation therapy.

Table 19.3 Summary of the treatment modalities and outcome of SBC reported in NCDB and the SEER database

Variable	Subcategory	NCDB (n = 936), %	SEER (n = 405), %
Age (y)	0–20	10.3	8.4
	21–59	62.9	63.2
	60 +	26.8	28.4
Gender	Male	56.2	54.8
	Female	43.8	45.2
Ethnicity	Caucasian	80.9	83.2
	African American	8.9	5.7
Tumor size (cm)	0–2	70.9	73.8
	2–5	1.4	0.7
	5 +	0.1	0.3
Surgery	Yes	83.4	87.2
	No	11.4	13.6
Radiation	Yes	46.8	45.4
	No	51.4	54.6
Radiation type	Proton	15.1	N/A
	Photon	11.1	
	IMRT	10.6	
	SRS	9.3	
Chemotherapy	Yes	1.6	97.5
	No	93.9	2.5
Combination treatment	RT + CT + Sx	0.3	1.7
	RT + CT	0.2	0
	RT + Sx	41.8	43.7
	CT + Sx	0.6	0.5
	Sx	41.1	40.2
	RT	3	0
	CT	0.1	0.2
Overall survival		79.8	76.9
Age and 5-y survival	0–20	87.4	74.6
	21–59	84.5	85
	60 +	65.8	61.5

(Continued)

Table 19.3 *(Continued)* Summary of the treatment modalities and outcome of SBC reported in NCDB and the SEER database

Variable	Subcategory	NCDB (n = 936), %	SEER (n = 405), %
Gender and 5-y survival	Male	78.6	75.4
	Female	81.3	78.9
Race and 5-y survival	African American	81.5	95
	Other	85.1	78.1
Chemotherapy and 5-y survival	Yes	83.1	48
	No	80	77.8
Treatment combination and 5-y survival	Surgery	80.2	78.9
	Radiation	48.9	N/A
	Surgery and radiation	84.8	83.4
	None	61.1	54.5

Abbreviations: CT, chemotherapy; NCDB, National Cancer Database; RT, radiotherapy; SBC, skull base chordomas; SEER, Surveillance, Epidemiology, and End Results; Sx, surgery.

On the basis of the available literature, superiority in terms of LC proton therapy has been demonstrated in terms of treatment planning and delivery with respect to other modalities mainly in larger lesions in proximity to normal critical structures and in irregularly shaped tumors.

19.6 Authors' Recommendations

- The optimum standard of care for patients with SBC comprises adequate presurgical planning, ideal surgical approach selection, careful preservation of neurovascular structures, and safe maximal cytoreductive surgical resection (resection of the tumor and drilling the adjacent bone).
- Although the primary goal of surgery is tumor resection, preservation of neurological function and minimizing postoperative morbidity are also key considerations.
- Cranial neuropathies, cerebrospinal fluid leakage, and cerebrovascular injuries are the common devastating complications of SBC surgery.

- Tumor size, location, and extent of surgical resection affect long-term LC, OS, and recurrence-free survival.
- Older age and greater tumor size were found to be associated with inferior survival in patients with SBC.
- Reoperation in SBC carries a far higher risk for neurologic morbidity than the primary surgery as the tumor tends to be more invasive and infiltrative at the region of recurrence.
- Adjuvant treatment of SBC comprises various modalities like proton beam radiation, photon-based radiation, conventional radiotherapy, stereotactic radiosurgery, and charged ion therapy, and most studies report the best results with proton beam radiation.

References

[1] Bailey P, Bagdasar D. Intracranial chordoblastoma. Am J Pathol. 1929; 5(5):439–450, 5

[2] Eriksson B, Gunterberg B, Kindblom LG. Chordoma. A clinicopathologic and prognostic study of a Swedish national series. Acta Orthop Scand. 1981; 52(1):49–58

[3] Stacchiotti S, Sommer J, Chordoma Global Consensus Group. Building a global consensus approach to chordoma: a position paper from the medical and patient community. Lancet Oncol. 2015; 16(2):e71–e83

[4] Lanzino G, Dumont AS, Lopes MB, Laws ER, Jr. Skull base chordomas: overview of disease, management options, and outcome. Neurosurg Focus. 2001; 10(3):E12

[5] Abdulrauf SI. Decision-making process for the treatment of intracranial chordomas. World Neurosurg. 2014; 82(5):612–613

[6] Bergh P, Kindblom LG, Gunterberg B, Remotti F, Ryd W, Meis-Kindblom JM. Prognostic factors in chordoma of the sacrum and mobile spine: a study of 39 patients. Lancet Oncol. 2000; 88(9):2122–2134

[7] Walcott BP, Nahed BV, Mohyeldin A, Coumans JV, Kahle KT, Ferreira MJ. Chordoma: current concepts, management, and future directions. Lancet Oncol. 2012; 13(2):e69–e76

[8] Schwab JH, Boland PJ, Agaram NP, et al. Chordoma and chondrosarcoma gene profile: implications for immunotherapy. Cancer Immunol Immunother. 2009; 58(3):339–349

[9] McMaster ML, Goldstein AM, Bromley CM, Ishibe N, Parry DM. Chordoma: incidence and survival patterns in the United States, 1973–1995. Cancer Causes Control. 2001; 12(1):1–11

[10] Chugh R, Tawbi H, Lucas DR, Biermann JS, Schuetze SM, Baker LH. Chordoma: the nonsarcoma primary bone tumor. Oncologist. 2007; 12(11):1344–1350

[11] Dahlin DC, MacCarty CS. Chordoma. Cancer. 1952; 5(6):1170–1178

[12] Healey JH, Lane JM. Chordoma: a critical review of diagnosis and treatment. Orthop Clin North Am. 1989; 20(3):417–426

[13] Samii A, Gerganov VM, Herold C, et al. Chordomas of the skull base: surgical management and outcome. J Neurosurg. 2007; 107(2):319–324

[14] Fuentes JM, Benezech J. Strategy of the surgical treatment of primary tumors of the spine. Neurochirurgie. 1989; 35(5):323–327, 352

[15] George B, Bresson D, Herman P, Froelich S. Chordomas: a review. Neurosurg Clin N Am. 2015; 26(3):437–452

[16] Fatemi N, Dusick JR, de Paiva Neto MA, Kelly DF. The endonasal microscopic approach for pituitary adenomas and other parasellar tumors: a 10-year experience. Neurosurgery. 2008; 63(4) Suppl 2:244–256, discussion 256

[17] Saeger W, Lüdecke DK, Buchfelder M, Fahlbusch R, Quabbe HJ, Petersenn S. Pathohistological classification of pituitary tumors: 10 years of experience with the German Pituitary Tumor Registry. Eur J Endocrinol. 2007; 156(2):203–216

[18] Wang K, Xie SN, Wang L, et al. Natural growth dynamics of untreated skull base chordomas in vivo. World Neurosurg. 2020; 136:e310–e321

[19] Noël G, Habrand J-L, Jauffret E, et al. Radiation therapy for chordoma and chondrosarcoma of the skull base and the cervical spine. Prognostic factors and patterns of failure. Strahlenther Onkol. 2003; 179(4):241–248

[20] Volpe NJ, Lessell S. Remitting sixth nerve palsy in skull base tumors. Arch Ophthalmol. 1993; 111(10):1391–1395

[21] Volpe NJ, Liebsch NJ, Munzenrider JE, Lessell S. Neuro-ophthalmologic findings in chordoma and chondrosarcoma of the skull base. Am J Ophthalmol. 1993; 115(1):97–104

[22] Muro K, Das S, Raizer JJ. Chordomas of the craniospinal axis: multimodality surgical, radiation and medical management strategies. Expert Rev Neurother. 2007; 7(10):1295–1312

[23] Chambers KJ, Lin DT, Meier J, Remenschneider A, Herr M, Gray ST. Incidence and survival patterns of cranial chordoma in the United States. Laryngoscope. 2014; 124(5):1097–1102

[24] Arnautović KI, Al-Mefty O. Surgical seeding of chordomas. Neurosurg Focus. 2001; 10(3):E7

[25] Sekhar LN, Schramm VL, Jr, Jones NF. Subtemporal-preauricular infratemporal fossa approach to large lateral and posterior cranial base neoplasms. J Neurosurg. 1987; 67(4):488–499

[26] Uttley D, Moore A, Archer DJ. Surgical management of midline skull-base tumors: a new approach. J Neurosurg. 1989; 71(5, Pt 1):705–710

[27] Keisch ME, Garcia DM, Shibuya RB. Retrospective long-term follow-up analysis in 21 patients with chordomas of various sites treated at a single institution. J Neurosurg. 1991; 75(3):374–377

[28] Watkins L, Khudados ES, Kaleoglu M, Revesz T, Sacares P, Crockard HA. Skull base chordomas: a review of 38 patients, 1958–88. Br J Neurosurg. 1993; 7(3):241–248

[29] Blevins NH, Jackler RK, Kaplan MJ, Gutin PH. Combined transpetrosal-subtemporal craniotomy for clival tumors with extension into the posterior fossa. Laryngoscope. 1995; 105(9, Pt 1):975–982

[30] Gay E, Sekhar LN, Rubinstein E, et al. Chordomas and chondrosarcomas of the cranial base: results and follow-up of 60 patients. Neurosurgery. 1995; 36(5):887–896, discussion 896–897

[31] Goel A. Extended middle fossa approach for petroclival lesions. Acta Neurochir (Wien). 1995; 135(1–2):78–83

[32] Mizerny BR, Kost KM. Chordoma of the cranial base: the McGill experience. J Otolaryngol. 1995; 24(1):14–19

[33] Maira G, Pallini R, Anile C, et al. Surgical treatment of clival chordomas: the transsphenoidal approach revisited. J Neurosurg. 1996; 85(5):784–792

[34] Menezes AH, Gantz BJ, Traynelis VC, McCulloch TM. Cranial base chordomas. Clin Neurosurg. 1997; 44:491–509

[35] Colli B, Al-Mefty O. Chordomas of the craniocervical junction: follow-up review and prognostic factors. J Neurosurg. 2001; 95(6):933–943

[36] Sekhar LN, Pranatartiharan R, Chanda A, Wright DC. Chordomas and chondrosarcomas of the skull base: results and complications of surgical management. Neurosurg Focus. 2001; 10(3):E2

[37] Sen C, Triana A. Cranial chordomas: results of radical excision. Neurosurg Focus. 2001; 10(3):E3

[38] Mortini P, Mandelli C, Franzin A, Giugni E, Giovanelli M. Surgical excision of clival tumors via the enlarged transcochlear approach. Indications and results. J Neurosurg Sci. 2001; 45(3):127–139, discussion 140

[39] Tamaki N, Nagashima T, Ehara K, Motooka Y, Barua KK. Surgical approaches and strategies for skull base chordomas. Neurosurg Focus. 2001; 10(3):E9

[40] Kyoshima K, Oikawa S, Kanaji M, et al. Repeat operations in the management of clival chordomas: palliative surgery. J Clin Neurosci. 2003; 10(5):571–578

[41] Pallini R, Maira G, Pierconti F, et al. Chordoma of the skull base: predictors of tumor recurrence. J Neurosurg. 2003; 98(4):812–822

[42] Stüer C, Schramm J, Schaller C. Skull base chordomas: management and results. Neurol Med Chir (Tokyo). 2006; 46(3):118–124, discussion 124–125

[43] Tzortzidis F, Elahi F, Wright D, Natarajan SK, Sekhar LN. Patient outcome at long-term follow-up after aggressive microsurgical resection of cranial base chordomas. Neurosurgery. 2006; 59(2):230–237, discussion 230–237

[44] Khaoroptham S, Jittapiromsak P, Siwanuwatn R, Chantra K. The outcome of surgical treatment for tumors of the craniocervical junction. J Med Assoc Thai. 2007; 90(7):1450–1457

[45] Cho YH, Kim JH, Khang SK, Lee J-K, Kim CJ. Chordomas and chondrosarcomas of the skull base: comparative analysis of clinical results in 30 patients. Neurosurg Rev. 2008; 31(1):35–43, discussion 43

[46] Komotar RJ, Starke RM, Raper DMS, Anand VK, Schwartz TH. Endoscopic endonasal versus open transcranial resection of anterior midline skull base meningiomas. World Neurosurg. 2012; 77(5–6):713–724

[47] Yoneoka Y, Tsumanuma I, Fukuda M, et al. Cranial base chordoma–long term outcome and review of the literature. Acta Neurochir (Wien). 2008; 150(8):773–778, discussion 778

[48] Takahashi S, Kawase T, Yoshida K, Hasegawa A, Mizoe JE. Skull base chordomas: efficacy of surgery followed by carbon ion radiotherapy. Acta Neurochir (Wien). 2009; 151(7):759–769

[49] Choi D, Melcher R, Harms J, Crockard A. Outcome of 132 operations in 97 patients with chordomas of the craniocervical junction and upper cervical spine. Neurosurgery. 2010; 66(1):59–65, discussion 65

[50] Ito E, Saito K, Okada T, Nagatani T, Nagasaka T. Long-term control of clival chordoma with initial aggressive surgical resection and gamma knife radiosurgery for recurrence. Acta Neurochir (Wien). 2010; 152(1):57–67, discussion 67

[51] de Divitiis E, Cappabianca P, Cavallo LM. Endoscopic transsphenoidal approach: adaptability of the procedure to different sellar lesions. Neurosurgery. 2002; 51(3):699–705, discussion 705–707

[52] Clifford SC, Lusher ME, Lindsey JC, et al. Wnt/Wingless pathway activation and chromosome 6 loss characterize a distinct molecular sub-group of medulloblastomas associated with a favorable prognosis. Cell Cycle. 2006; 5 (22):2666–2670

[53] Frank G, Sciarretta V, Calbucci F, Farneti G, Mazzatenta D, Pasquini E. The endoscopic transnasal transsphenoidal approach for the treatment of cranial base chordomas and chondrosarcomas. Neurosurgery. 2006; 59(1) Suppl 1: ONS50–ONS57, discussion ONS50–ONS57

[54] Al-Mefty O, Kadri PAS, Hasan DM, Isolan GR, Pravdenkova S. Anterior clivectomy: surgical technique and clinical applications. J Neurosurg. 2008; 109(5):783–793

[55] Dehdashti AR, Karabatsou K, Ganna A, Witterick I, Gentili F. Expanded endoscopic endonasal approach for treatment of clival chordomas: early results in 12 patients. Neurosurgery. 2008; 63(2):299–307, discussion 307–309

[56] Fatemi N, Dusick JR, Gorgulho AA, et al. Endonasal microscopic removal of clival chordomas. Surg Neurol. 2008; 69(4):331–338

[57] Zhang Q, Kong F, Yan B, Ni Z, Liu H. Endoscopic endonasal surgery for clival chordoma and chondrosarcoma. ORL J Otorhinolaryngol Relat Spec. 2008; 70(2):124–129

[58] Arbolay OL, González JG, González RH, Gálvez YH. Extended endoscopic endonasal approach to the skull base. Minim Invasive Neurosurg. 2009; 52 (3):114–118

[59] Ceylan S, Koc K, Anik I. Extended endoscopic approaches for midline skull-base lesions. Neurosurg Rev. 2009; 32(3):309–319, discussion 318–319

[60] Fraser JF, Nyquist GG, Moore N, Anand VK, Schwartz TH. Endoscopic endonasal transclival resection of chordomas: operative technique, clinical outcome, and review of the literature. J Neurosurg. 2010; 112(5): 1061–1069

[61] Hong Jiang W, Ping Zhao S, Hai Xie Z, Zhang H, Zhang J, Yun Xiao J. Endoscopic resection of chordomas in different clival regions. Acta Otolaryngol. 2009; 129(1):71–83

[62] Stippler M, Gardner PA, Snyderman CH, Carrau RL, Prevedello DM, Kassam AB. Endoscopic endonasal approach for clival chordomas. Neurosurgery. 2009; 64(2):268–277, discussion 277–278

[63] Solares CA, Grindler D, Luong A, et al. Endoscopic management of sphenoclival neoplasms: anatomical correlates and patient outcomes. Otolaryngol Head Neck Surg. 2010; 142(3):315–321

[64] Navas M, Martinez P, Shakur SF, et al. Intrasellar chordoma associated with a primitive persistent trigeminal artery. Turk Neurosurg. 2015; 25 (1):146–153

[65] Karamchandani J, Wu MY, Das S, et al. Highly proliferative sellar chordoma with unusually rapid recurrence. Neuropathology. 2013; 33(4):424–430

[66] Koutourousiou M, Kontogeorgos G, Seretis A. Non-adenomatous sellar lesions: experience of a single centre and review of the literature. Neurosurg Rev. 2010; 33(4):465–476

[67] Werner A. On 2 cases of intrasellar chordomas. Acta Neurochir (Wien). 1960; 8:436–443

[68] Arnold H, Herrmann H-D. Skull base chordoma with cavernous sinus involvement. Partial or radical tumour-removal? Acta Neurochir (Wien). 1986; 83(1–2):31–37

[69] Belza J. Double midline intracranial tumors of vestigial origin: contiguous intrasellar chordoma and suprasellar craniopharyngioma. Case report. J Neurosurg. 1966; 25(2):199–204

[70] Chadduck WM. Unusual lesions involving the sella turcica. South Med J. 1973; 66(8):948–955

[71] de Cremoux P, Turpin G, Hamon P, de Gennes JL. Intrasellar chordoma (author's transl). Sem Hop. 1980; 56(43–44):1769–1773

[72] Ahmed AK, Dawood HY, Arnaout OM, Laws ER, Jr, Smith TR. Presentation, treatment, and long-term outcome of intrasellar chordoma: a pooled analysis of institutional, SEER (Surveillance Epidemiology and End Results), and published data. World Neurosurg. 2018; 109:e676–e683

[73] Falconer MA, Bailey IC, Duchen LW. Surgical treatment of chordoma and chondroma of the skull base. J Neurosurg. 1968; 29(3):261–275

[74] Haridas A, Ansari S, Afshar F. Chordoma presenting as pseudoprolactinoma. Br J Neurosurg. 2003; 17(3):260–262

[75] Hattori Y, Tahara S, Nakakuki T, et al. Sellar chondroma with endocrine dysfunction that resolved after surgery: case report. J Nippon Med Sch. 2015; 82(3):146–150

[76] Kagawa T, Takamura M, Moritake K, Tsutsumi A, Yamasaki T. A case of sellar chordoma mimicking a non-functioning pituitary adenoma with survival of more than 10 years. Noshuyo Byori. 1993; 10(2):103–106

[77] Kakuno Y, Yamada T, Hirano H, Mori H, Narabayashi I. Chordoma in the sella turcica. Neurol Med Chir (Tokyo). 2002; 42(7):305–308

[78] Khaled A, Joarder A, Chandy M, Nasir T. Chordoma in the sella turcica. Pulse. 2009; 3:33–34

[79] Kikuchi K, Watanabe K. Huge sellar chordoma: CT demonstration. Comput Med Imaging Graph. 1994; 18(5):385–390

[80] Kumar P, Kumar P, Singh S, Kumari N, Datta NR. Chordoma with increased prolactin levels (pseudoprolactinoma) mimicking pituitary adenoma: a case report with review of the literature. J Cancer Res Ther. 2009; 5(4):309–311

[81] Mathews W, Wilson CB. Ectopic intrasellar chordoma. Case report. J Neurosurg. 1974; 40(2):260–263

[82] Mohammed AR, Amin P. An unusual cause of a sellar mass. BMJ Case Rep. 2010; 2010:2010

[83] Pluot M, Bernard MH, Rousseaux P, Scherpereel B, Roth A, Caulet T. Two cases of sellar chordomas. Ultrastructural and histochemical study (author's transl). Arch Anat Cytol Pathol. 1980; 28(4):230–236

[84] Raffel C, Wright DC, Gutin PH, Wilson CB. Cranial chordomas: clinical presentation and results of operative and radiation therapy in twenty-six patients. Neurosurgery. 1985; 17(5):703–710

[85] Takahashi T, Kuwayama A, Kobayashi T, Watanabe M, Katoh T, Kageyama N. Transsphenoidal microsurgery of sellar-parasellar chordomas (author's transl). Neurol Med Chir (Tokyo). 1982; 22(2):141–146

[86] Thodou E, Kontogeorgos G, Scheithauer BW, et al. Intrasellar chordomas mimicking pituitary adenoma. J Neurosurg. 2000; 92(6):976–982

[87] Wang H-F, Ma H-X, Ma C-Y, Luo Y-N, Ge P-F. Sellar chordoma presenting as pseudo-macroprolactinoma with unilateral third cranial nerve palsy. Chin J Cancer Res. 2012; 24(2):167–170

[88] Wold LE, Laws ER, Jr. Cranial chordomas in children and young adults. J Neurosurg. 1983; 59(6):1043–1047

[89] Forsyth PA, Cascino TL, Shaw EG, et al. Intracranial chordomas: a clinicopathological and prognostic study of 51 cases. J Neurosurg. 1993; 78 (5):741–747

[90] Bohman LE, Koch M, Bailey RL, Alonso-Basanta M, Lee JYK. Skull base chordoma and chondrosarcoma: influence of clinical and demographic factors on prognosis: a SEER analysis. World Neurosurg. 2014; 82(5): 806–814

[91] al-Mefty O, Borba LA. Skull base chordomas: a management challenge. J Neurosurg. 1997; 86(2):182–189

[92] Erdem E, Angtuaco EC, Van Hemert R, Park JS, Al-Mefty O. Comprehensive review of intracranial chordoma. Radiographics. 2003; 23(4):995–1009

[93] Hoch BL, Nielsen GP, Liebsch NJ, Rosenberg AE. Base of skull chordomas in children and adolescents: a clinicopathologic study of 73 cases. Am J Surg Pathol. 2006; 30(7):811–818

[94] Alonso-Basanta M, Lustig RA, Kennedy DW. Proton beam therapy in skull base pathology. Otolaryngol Clin North Am. 2011; 44(5):1173–1183

[95] Igaki H, Tokuuye K, Okumura T, et al. Clinical results of proton beam therapy for skull base chordoma. Int J Radiat Oncol Biol Phys. 2004; 60(4): 1120–1126

[96] Amichetti M, Cianchetti M, Amelio D, Enrici RM, Minniti G. Proton therapy in chordoma of the base of the skull: a systematic review. Neurosurg Rev. 2009; 32(4):403–416

[97] Blanco Kiely JP, White BM. Dosimetric feasibility of single-energy proton modulated arc therapy for treatment of chordoma at the skull base. Acta Oncol. 2016; 55(9–10):1243–1245

[98] Munzenrider JE, Liebsch NJ. Proton therapy for tumors of the skull base. Strahlenther Onkol. 1999; 175 Suppl 2:57–63

[99] Catton C, O'Sullivan B, Bell R, et al. Chordoma: long-term follow-up after radical photon irradiation. Radiother Oncol. 1996; 41(1):67–72

[100] Debus J, Schulz-Ertner D, Schad L, et al. Stereotactic fractionated radiotherapy for chordomas and chondrosarcomas of the skull base. Int J Radiat Oncol Biol Phys. 2000; 47(3):591–596

[101] Amit M, Na'ara S, Binenbaum Y, et al. Treatment and outcome of patients with skull base chordoma: a meta-analysis. J Neurol Surg B Skull Base. 2014; 75(6):383–390

[102] Hulou MM, Garcia CR, Slone SA, et al. Comprehensive review of cranial chordomas using national databases in the USA. Clin Oncol (R Coll Radiol). 2019; 31(9):e149–e159

[103] Terahara A, Niemierko A, Goitein M, et al. Analysis of the relationship between tumor dose inhomogeneity and local control in patients with skull base chordoma. Int J Radiat Oncol Biol Phys. 1999; 45(2):351–358

[104] Deraniyagala RL, Yeung D, Mendenhall WM, et al. Proton therapy for skull base chordomas: an outcome study from the university of Florida proton therapy institute. J Neurol Surg B Skull Base. 2014; 75(1):53–57

[105] Grosshans DR, Zhu XR, Melancon A, et al. Spot scanning proton therapy for malignancies of the base of skull: treatment planning, acute toxicities, and preliminary clinical outcomes. Int J Radiat Oncol Biol Phys. 2014; 90(3):540–546

[106] Weber DC, Malyapa R, Albertini F, et al. Long term outcomes of patients with skull-base low-grade chondrosarcoma and chordoma patients treated with pencil beam scanning proton therapy. Radiother Oncol. 2016; 120(1):169–174

[107] McDonald MW, Linton OR, Moore MG, Ting JY, Cohen-Gadol AA, Shah MV. Influence of residual tumor volume and radiation dose coverage in outcomes for clival chordoma. Int J Radiat Oncol Biol Phys. 2016; 95(1):304–311

[108] Förander P, Bartek J, Jr, Fagerlund M, et al. Multidisciplinary management of clival chordomas; long-term clinical outcome in a single-institution consecutive series. Acta Neurochir (Wien). 2017; 159(10):1857–1868

[109] Jägersberg M, El Rahal A, Dammann P, Merkler D, Weber DC, Schaller K. Clival chordoma: a single-centre outcome analysis. Acta Neurochir (Wien). 2017; 159(10):1815–1823

[110] Sen CN, Sekhar LN, Schramm VL, Janecka IP. Chordoma and chondrosarcoma of the cranial base: an 8-year experience. Neurosurgery. 1989; 25(6):931–940, discussion 940–941

[111] Hug EB, Sweeney RA, Nurre PM, Holloway KC, Slater JD, Munzenrider JE. Proton radiotherapy in management of pediatric base of skull tumors. Int J Radiat Oncol Biol Phys. 2002; 52(4):1017–1024

[112] Hug EB, Loredo LN, Slater JD, et al. Proton radiation therapy for chordomas and chondrosarcomas of the skull base. J Neurosurg. 1999; 91(3):432–439

[113] Weber DC, Rutz HP, Pedroni ES, et al. Results of spot-scanning proton radiation therapy for chordoma and chondrosarcoma of the skull base: the Paul Scherrer Institut experience. Int J Radiat Oncol Biol Phys. 2005; 63(2):401–409

[114] Noël G, Feuvret L, Calugaru V, et al. Chordomas of the base of the skull and upper cervical spine. One hundred patients irradiated by a 3D conformal technique combining photon and proton beams. Acta Oncol. 2005; 44(7):700–708

[115] Fuller DB, Bloom JG. Radiotherapy for chordoma. Int J Radiat Oncol Biol Phys. 1988; 15(2):331–339

[116] Zorlu F, Gürkaynak M, Yildiz F, Oge K, Atahan IL. Conventional external radiotherapy in the management of clivus chordomas with overt residual disease. Neurol Sci. 2000; 21(4):203–207

[117] Cummings BJ, Hodson DI, Bush RS. Chordoma: the results of megavoltage radiation therapy. Int J Radiat Oncol Biol Phys. 1983; 9(5):633–642

[118] Amendola BE, Amendola MA, Oliver E, McClatchey KD. Chordoma: role of radiation therapy. Radiology. 1986; 158(3):839–843

[119] Chetiyawardana AD. Chordoma: results of treatment. Clin Radiol. 1984; 35(2):159–161

[120] Krishnan S, Foote RL, Brown PD, Pollock BE, Link MJ, Garces YI. Radiosurgery for cranial base chordomas and chondrosarcomas. Neurosurgery. 2005; 56(4):777–784, discussion 777–784

[121] Martin JJ, Niranjan A, Kondziolka D, Flickinger JC, Lozanne KA, Lunsford LD. Radiosurgery for chordomas and chondrosarcomas of the skull base. J Neurosurg. 2007; 107(4):758–764

[122] Chang SD, Martin DP, Lee E, Adler JR, Jr. Stereotactic radiosurgery and hypofractionated stereotactic radiotherapy for residual or recurrent cranial base and cervical chordomas. Neurosurg Focus. 2001; 10(3):E5

[123] Crockard A, Macaulay E, Plowman PN. Stereotactic radiosurgery. VI. Posterior displacement of the brainstem facilitates safer high dose radiosurgery for clival chordoma. Br J Neurosurg. 1999; 13(1):65–70

[124] Hasegawa T, Ishii D, Kida Y, Yoshimoto M, Koike J, Iizuka H. Gamma Knife surgery for skull base chordomas and chondrosarcomas. J Neurosurg. 2007; 107(4):752–757

[125] Berson AM, Castro JR, Petti P, et al. Charged particle irradiation of chordoma and chondrosarcoma of the base of skull and cervical spine: the Lawrence Berkeley Laboratory experience. Int J Radiat Oncol Biol Phys. 1988; 15(3):559–565

[126] Castro JR, Linstadt DE, Bahary J-P, et al. Experience in charged particle irradiation of tumors of the skull base: 1977–1992. Int J Radiat Oncol Biol Phys. 1994; 29(4):647–655

[127] Schulz-Ertner D, Karger CP, Feuerhake A, et al. Effectiveness of carbon ion radiotherapy in the treatment of skull-base chordomas. Int J Radiat Oncol Biol Phys. 2007; 68(2):449–457

[128] Tsujii H, Mizoe J, Kamada T, et al. Clinical results of carbon ion radiotherapy at NIRS. J Radiat Res (Tokyo). 2007; 48 Suppl A:A1–A13

[129] Kano H, Niranjan A, Lunsford LD. Radiosurgery for chordoma and chondrosarcoma. Prog Neurol Surg. 2019; 34:207–214

[130] Kano H, Lunsford LD. Stereotactic radiosurgery of intracranial chordomas, chondrosarcomas, and glomus tumors. Neurosurg Clin N Am. 2013; 24(4):553–560

[131] Buizza G, Molinelli S, D'Ippolito E, et al. MRI-based tumour control probability in skull-base chordomas treated with carbon-ion therapy. Radiother Oncol. 2019; 137:32–37

[132] Erazo IS, Galvis CF, Aguirre LE, Iglesias R, Abarca LC. Clival chondroid chordoma: a case report and review of the literature. Cureus. 2018; 10(9):e3381

[133] Alahmari M, Temel Y. Skull base chordoma treated with proton therapy: a systematic review. Surg Neurol Int. 2019; 10:96

[134] Slater JM, Slater JD, Archambeau JO. Proton therapy for cranial base tumors. J Craniofac Surg. 1995; 6(1):24–26

[135] Tewfik HH, McGinnis WL, Nordstrom DG, Latourette HB. Chordoma: evaluation of clinical behavior and treatment modalities. Int J Radiat Oncol Biol Phys. 1977; 2(9–10):959–962

[136] Romero J, Cardenes H, la Torre A, et al. Chordoma: results of radiation therapy in eighteen patients. Radiother Oncol. 1993; 29(1):27–32

[137] Zhou Y, Hu B, Wu Z, Cheng H, Dai M, Zhang B. The clinical outcomes for chordomas in the cranial base and spine: a single center experience. Medicine (Baltimore). 2019; 98(23):e15980

[138] Zakaria WK, Hafez RF, Taha AN. Gamma Knife management of skull base chordomas: is it a choice? Asian J Neurosurg. 2018; 13(4):1037–1041

20 Natural History and Management Options of Chiari 1 Malformation

Samuel Wreghitt, Bryden H. Dawes, and Augusto Gonzalvo

Abstract

This chapter explores the evidence related to the pathophysiology and management of Chiari malformation type 1 (CM-1). It reviews the natural history of both symptomatic and asymptomatic CM-1 patients and collates the available evidence to aid with management decisions. It examines the efficacy and complication rate of the various surgical techniques used to treat the condition.

Keywords: Chiari malformation, syringomyelia, syrinx, posterior fossa decompression, duroplasty

20.1 Introduction

Chiari malformation type 1 (CM-1) is a structural abnormality at the craniocervical junction, which involves the descent of the cerebellar tonsils through the foramen magnum affecting the dynamic flow of the cerebrospinal fluid (CSF). It is important to understand that normal craniocervical anatomy can include the cerebellar tonsils lying up to 3 to 5 mm below the rim of the foramen magnum in adults and up to 6 mm in infants.[1]

The presentation of patients with a CM-1 is variable and the indication for surgical management has always been controversial. While various Chiari malformations have been described, the focus of this chapter is on CM-1 (▶ Fig. 20.1).

CM-1 presents in a variety of ways and, in most cases, symptoms start at the end of adolescence. They are generally related to raised intracranial pressure, cerebellar deficit, or associated spinal cord syrinx.

The most common presenting symptom in adults is an occipital headache worsened by coughing (cough headache) or Valsalva maneuvers, which typically last less than 5 minutes. However, many studies show that the type of headache can vary greatly, as shown in ▶ Table 20.1.[2] The International Headache Society has defined Chiari headaches under its own definition in an attempt to differentiate them from a primary cough headache—which is similar but generally can last longer (up to 2 h). Patients initially diagnosed with a primary cough headache require neuroimaging, as 40% of cases have an associated CM-1.[3]

In addition, various other symptoms can be associated with a CM-1, as shown in ▶ Table 20.2.[2] Descent of the cerebellar tonsils can lead to central nystagmus, scanning speech, and truncal ataxia. Compression of the brainstem can present with hoarseness, dysarthria, palatal weakness, tongue atrophy, and sleep-related breathing disorders.

20.1.1 CM-1-Associated Syringomyelia

CM-1 may be associated with syrinx in 30% of cases. The size of the CM-1-associated syringomyelia is noticeably wider (7–8 mm) in comparison to idiopathic forms of syringomyelia (3–4 mm). CM-1-associated syrinx is also more likely to have cranial extent into the cervical spine.[4] It is also important to be aware that 25% of Charcot joints in the upper limbs are associated with syringomyelia.[5]

In contrast to type 2 malformations, there are generally no associated brain abnormalities to the cerebellar tonsillar descent. There are, however, a number of osseous abnormalities that include shortened clivus, underdeveloped posterior cranial fossa, basilar invagination, platybasia, pro-atlantal remnants, Klippel–Feil anomaly, atlantoaxial assimilation, odontoid retroflexion, and scoliosis.[6]

20.1.2 Pathophysiology of Chiari Malformation Type 1

CM-1 encompasses a heterogeneous and complex entity and may be idiopathic or acquired. Idiopathic CM-1 is associated with many congenital conditions. The abnormality results in crowding at the foramen magnum and impaction of the cerebellar tonsils. When compared with controls, patients with CM-1 have a smaller posterior fossa,[7,8,9] shallow basiocciputs, and a disproportionate cerebellum-to-posterior fossa volume. In some cases, this correlates with the degree of cerebellar ectopia. It is proposed that this results from an underdevelopment of the occipital endochondrium during embryology.[10,11] However, this is not true for all patients with CM-1 and other factors are likely to contribute to the pathogenesis of the disease.

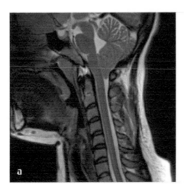
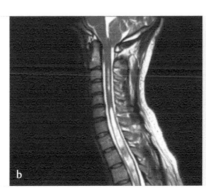

Fig. 20.1 **(a)** T2 sagittal magnetic resonance imaging (MRI) of craniocervical junction demonstrating a Chiari malformation type 1 (CM-1). **(b)** T2 sagittal MRI of the cervicothoracic spine showing CM-1-associated syringomyelia.

Table 20.1 Types of headache associated with Chiari malformation type 1 (CM-1)

Headache	Incidence (%)
Worsened by Valsalva maneuver	87
Tension type	67
Long-lasting (from 3 h to 3 d)	41
Migraine type	29
Continuous	16
Headache only precipitated by Valsalva maneuver	13

Source: Adapted from Curone et al.[2]

Table 20.2 Symptoms associated with Chiari malformation type 1 (CM-1)

Symptom	Incidence (%)
Headache of any type	74
Paresthesia	35
Cough headache only	34
Cerebellar symptoms	23
Migraine headache only	21
Both cough and migraine headaches	22
Dysphagia	21
Cranial nerve dysfunction	15
Nausea	13
Dysphagia or apnea	9

Source: Adapted from Curone et al.[2]

Table 20.3 Studies included in qualitative synthesis

Studies	Adult/pediatrics	n	Type	Focus
Killeen et al[27]	Both: mainly adult	68	Retrospective cohort study	Nonoperative outcomes
Chavez et al[28]	Both: mainly adult	177	Cohort study	Comparison of operative and nonoperative outcomes
Leon et al[30]	Peds	427	Retrospective cohort study	Conservatively managed patients who later required surgery
Klekamp et al[31]	Adult	1	Case report and lit review	Spontaneous resolution of CM-1
Massimi et al[32]	Both	3	Case reports	Sudden onset of symptoms in CM-1 patients
Langridge et al[26]	Both	n/a	Systematic review	Systematic review of natural history and conservative management
Nishizawa et al[33]	Adult	10	Retrospective cohort study	Follow-up of incidentally identified syringomyelia associated with CM-1
Strahle et al[38]	Peds	147	Retrospective cohort study	Natural history of conservatively managed patients
Bindal et al[29]	Adult	27	Retrospective cohort study	Proposed classification system for CM-1 management

Abbreviation: CM-1, Chiari malformation type 1.

In addition to a reduced posterior fossa volume, patients with CM-1 have abnormal craniocervical junction CSF dynamics,[12] hyperdynamic motion of the craniocervical junction neural structures,[13,14,15] and a reduced intracranial CSF compliance.

The pathophysiology of the cough headache typically associated with CM-1 is not known. Various mechanisms have been proposed, including compression of the upper cervical nerve roots by the descending tonsils,[16,17] transient craniospinal pressure dissociation,[18,19] strain of the cerebellar tonsils,[13] increased CSF pressure,[20] and reduced CSF compliance of the posterior fossa.[21] However, these theories fail to describe the spectrum of clinical and radiological presentation.

Similarly, the pathogenesis of CM-1-associated syringomyelia is not well understood. The classic theories include the hydrodynamic theory,[22] the craniospinal dissociation theory,[23] and the ball valve (or ball-in-cone) theory.[24] Current theories propose that alternate CSF dynamics result in the transportation of fluid into the cord parenchyma via perivascular and extracellular spaces.[25]

20.2 Selected Papers on the Natural History of Chiari Malformation Type 1

- Langridge B, Phillips E, Choi D. Chiari malformation type 1: a systematic review of natural history and conservative management. World Neurosurg 2017;104:213–219

- Killeen A, Roguski M, Chavez A, Heilman C, Hwang S. Non-operative outcomes in Chiari I malformation patients. J Clin Neurosci 2015;22(1):133–138
- Chavez A, Roguski M, Killeen A, Heilman C, Hwang S. Comparison of operative and non-operative outcomes based on surgical selection criteria for patients with Chiari I malformations. J Clin Neurosci 2014;21(12):2201–2206

20.3 Natural History of Chiari Malformation Type 1

Patients presenting with CM-1 normally fall into one of the following scenarios:
- Incidental CM-1 (with or without associated syrinx).
- New diagnosed symptomatic CM-1 and decision to manage conservatively.
- Clinical progression of a previously asymptomatic or minimally symptomatic CM-1.

Due to the fact that the general treatment of CM-1 is biased toward surgical management,[29] there are only few studies presenting its natural history. Therefore, the evidence to support decision-making is limited. The majority of studies into the natural history of CM-1 are based on a pediatric population, but the evidence presented here is targeted to the natural history of the adult population (▶ Table 20.3).

20.3.1 Asymptomatic Chiari Malformation Type 1

CM-1 is a relatively slowly progressing disease. For this reason, many patients with CM-1 are diagnosed as incidental findings. This is confirmed by the fact that the diagnosis of CM-1 is relatively common upon the reviewing of imaging. Morris et al[35] collated several magnetic resonance imaging (MRI) studies of normal adults to show diagnoses of CM-1 in 71 of 15,559 (0.24%) cases. In comparison, Meadows et al[36] reviewed consecutive imaging performed at a single institution, which showed diagnoses of CM-1 in 175 of 22,591 (0.8%) patients.

Two large studies in the pediatric population revealed the slow progression toward symptoms. Benglis et al[37] managed 124 patients, ranging from 0.9 to 19.8 years (mean: 7 years), conservatively over approximately 3 years. On initial review, 43 were asymptomatic and 67 of the remaining 81 were deemed to have symptoms not related to their CM-1. Over this short period, none of the 124 patients had a progression of symptoms relating to their CM-1. Furthermore, in a larger study by Strahle et al[38] of 147 patients (mean: 7.7 years) over a longer follow-up of 4 years, 133 (90.5%) patients remained either asymptomatic or minimally symptomatic and not requiring surgical intervention.

An adult-based study by Nishizawa et al[33] followed 10 asymptomatic patients with incidentally identified syrinx associated with CM-1 for a period of 11 years. Only one patient required surgical intervention at the 7-year mark and, after surgical decompression, made a full recovery. Of note in this study is the fact that the imaging remained stable over the follow-up period. This selected evidence shows there is a benign nature to CM-1, with slow (if any) progression from either asymptomatic or minimally symptomatic patients.

Moriwaka et al[21,63] produced an epidemiological study in Japan of syringomyelia showing 1,243 cases, of which 684 (51.2%) related to CM-1. The follow-up of these 1,243 patients showed the clinical course was slowly progressive; 202 (17.9%) patients showed rather stable course including spontaneous resolution in 29 (2.3%) patients. These numbers include all pathologies with surgical and nonsurgical treatment but highlight that there is the option of a more conservative approach to managing the finding of a syrinx. In addition, there is also documented evidence of resolution of patients' syrinx and their symptoms. Klekamp et al[31] published a case report and literature review showing 10 patients (5 adults and 5 children) who experienced resolution of their CM-1-associated syrinx. Of the symptomatic patients, five showed improvement of their symptoms. This suggests that the common consensus of the presence of a syrinx associated with a CM-1 as a strong indication for surgical management is debatable.

20.3.2 Symptomatic Chiari Malformation Type 1

When providing medical advice to a patient with CM-1, it is imperative to know the natural history of this condition. Killeen et al[27] and Chavez et al[28] provide high-quality follow-up data of conservatively managed patients. Langridge et al have undertaken a detailed systematic review[26] that similarly shows, as in ▶ Table 20.4, the presenting symptoms of conservatively treated CM-1 patients.

▶ Table 20.5 highlights outcomes for both of these papers. When combined, one is able to follow 115 patients who were considered only mildly symptomatic and allocated for conservative management over 4.5 years. On careful follow-up, 47% of patient noted an overall improvement with only 20 to 25% reporting worsening symptoms. Of note, the typical cough headache associated with CM-1 remained either unchanged or improved in the majority of cases—with only 10% of patients showing worsening symptoms.

These studies show that the natural history of patients who are either asymptomatic or only mildly symptomatic from their CM-1 have an indolent course, with a significant proportion of patients experiencing improvement of the symptoms with conservative management. There have been a few cases reports of patients experiencing acute deterioration attributed to that CM-1, but these appear very infrequent.[32] The presence of an associated syringomyelia must be noted and carefully examined

Table 20.4 Presenting symptoms on diagnosis of CM-1

	Killeen et al[27]	Chavez et al[28]
n	n = 47	n = 68
Cough headaches only	9 (19.2%)	11 (21%)
Migraine headaches only	14 (29.8%)	20 (40%)
Both migraine and cough headaches	18 (38.3%)	19 (38%)
Nausea	7 (14.9%)	9 (13.2%)
Paresthesia	27 (57.5%)	31 (45.6%)
Ataxia	26 (55.3%)	28 (41.2%)
Abnormal reflexes	6 (12.8%)	9 (13.2%)
Dysphagia	10 (21.3%)	10 (14.7%)
Scoliosis	7 (14.9%)	13 (19.1%)
Syrinx	7 (14.9%)	12 (17.7%)

Note: Adapted from papers by Killeen et al[27] and Chavez et al.[28]

Table 20.5 Improvement of symptoms after conservative management

	Killeen et al[27]	Chavez et al[28]
Mean follow-up, mo (range)	56.1 (45.7–66.3)	57.9 (11.6–138.5)
Overall outcome	n = 47	n = 68
Improved	22 (46.8%)	32 (47.1%)
Unchanged	8 (17.0%)	18 (26.5%)
Worse	12 (25.5%)	13 (19.1%)
Both improvement and worsening	5 (10.6%)	5 (7.4%)
Cough headache	n = 27	n = 30
Improved	10 (37.0%)	12 (40%)
Unchanged	14 (51.9%)	15 (50%)
Worse	3 (11.1%)	3 (10%)
Migraine headache		n = 39
Improved		24 (61.5%)
Unchanged		13 (31.3%)
Worse		2 (5.1%)

Note: Adapted from papers by Killeen et al[27] and Chavez et al.[28]

for signs and symptoms, but, as Nishizawa et al[33] suggest, an asymptomatic syrinx can be monitored with a low chance of progression, which is then reversible after operative management.

Defining symptomatic CM-1 is challenging; patients with only headaches are considered symptomatic if the headaches are compatible with CM-1 (cough component, short duration) and lack of migraine-type headache features.[38]

Minimally symptomatic patients can also be managed conservatively, as only 10 to 25% of them report deterioration. In most cases, this deterioration is not severe and serious events are infrequent. Awaiting clinical deterioration does not seem to affect surgical outcomes, and most symptoms improve with surgery.[27]

Severely symptomatic patients (cerebellar, brainstem, or spinal cord signs) should be considered for surgical treatment at the time of diagnosis. Additionally, if there is no clinical improvement following a period of conservative measures and symptomatic treatment (usually 6–12 weeks), patients who are significantly debilitated by headaches are good surgical candidates.[28]

20.4 Selected Papers on the Management Options of Chiari Malformation Type 1

20.4.1 Adults

- Klekamp J. Surgical treatment of Chiari I malformation–analysis of intraoperative findings, complications, and outcome for 371 foramen magnum decompressions. Neurosurgery 2012;71(2):365–380, discussion 380

20.4.2 Pediatrics

- Tubbs RS, Beckman J, Naftel RP, et al. Institutional experience with 500 cases of surgically treated pediatric Chiari malformation type I. J Neurosurg Pediatr 2011;7(3):248–256
- Shweikeh F, Sunjaya D, Nuno M, Drazin D, Adamo MA. National trends, complications, and hospital charges in pediatric patients with Chiari malformation type I treated with posterior fossa decompression with and without duraplasty. Pediatr Neurosurg 2015;50(1):31–37

20.5 Management Options for Chiari Malformation Type 1

Management options for CM-1 include observation and surgery.

The goal of surgical intervention is to enlarge the volume of the posterior fossa and restore CSF flow at the craniocervical junction. This commonly consists of a suboccipital craniectomy (with or without resection of the posterior arch of C1). Various techniques, or combinations thereof, have been described including the following: bone-only posterior fossa decompression (PFD), opening of the outer layer of the dura, opening of the dura with duroplasty (various materials used), opening and division of the arachnoid, resection of tonsils, fourth ventricle shunting, and various syrinx shunt techniques (▶ Table 20.6).

The results of these various techniques have been subject to numerous systematic reviews.[58,59,60,61] A summary of the outcomes and the complication rate of the commonly used methods is provided in ▶ Table 20.7. Other surgical strategies not covered in the summary include durotomy without duraplasty[41] and occipitocervical fusion (OCF).[58,59]

Table 20.6 Literature summaries of included studies on the management of CM-1

Study	n	Mean age (y)	Technique	Duroplasty material
Aghakhani et al[2]	157	30.9	156 DAO, 1 VPS	Various techniques
Alfieri and Pinna[43]	109	45.9	DAO	Various techniques
Arruda et al[44]	60	35.6	TR	Unclear
Beretta et al[45]	132	40.6	DAI	Unclear
Bowers et al[34]	119	34.0	DAO	Various techniques
Chen et al[46]	103	40.6	33 BO, 70 DAI	Various techniques
Chotai and Medhkour[47]	41	33.8	29 BO, 12 TR	Various techniques
Deng et al[48]	152	39.2	DAI	Autologous: unclear
El-Ghandour[49]	46	37.4	14 DAI, 12 DAO, 14 4th VS, 6 SSS	Autologous graft: fascia lata
Guyotat et al[50]	75	38.0	42 DAO, 8 TR, 16 4th VS, 9 SSS	Various techniques
Klekamp[39]	326	40.0	DAO	Various techniques
Kotil et al[51]	61	34.4	BO	N/A
Krishna et al[52]	47	40.1	BO	N/A
Lee et al[53]	81	38.5	DAO	Various techniques
Sindou et al[54]	44	40	DAI	Autologous: pericranium
Thakar et al[55]	57	38.3	DAO	Various techniques
Yilmaz et al[56]	82	36.6	24 BO, 58 DAO	Various techniques
Zhang et al[57]	132	33	TR	Autologous: occipital muscle fascia

Abbreviations: BO, bone only decompression; DAI, duroplasty with arachnoid intact; DAO, duroplasty with arachnoid opened; TR, duroplasty and resection of cerebellar tonsils; VPS, ventriculoperitoneal shunt; VS, ventricle shunt; SSS, syringosubarachnoid shunt.

Table 20.7 Summary of management outcomes and complications[34,43,44,45,46,47,48,49,50,51,52,53,54,55,56,57]

	BO series (5 studies)	DAI series (5 studies)	DAO series (9 studies)	TR series (4 studies)	Shunt series (2 studies)
Study period	2011–2018	2002–2017	1998–2018	1998–2014	1998–2012
Patient no.	194	412	961	212	39
Patient age (median)	36.4	39.8	38	34	38.1
Mean follow-up (mo)	70.8	68.6	60.2	39.7	75.8
Syrinx					
Improved (%)	56.9	64.6	67.3	83.4	92.6*
Stabilized (%)	41.5	35.4	25.6	13.1	7.4*
Aggravated (%)	1.6	0	7	3.4	0*
Symptoms					
Improved (%)	82.1	84.6	69.6	80.7	56.4
Stabilized (%)	15.4	10.8	24.4	15.7	33.3
Aggravated (%)	2.4	4.6	6	3.6	15.4
Complications					
Meningitis (%)	1	6.3	3.5	4.4	5.1
CSF fistula (%)	1.5	3.2	5.9	11.3	11.3
Morbidity (%)	7.7	20.3	16.3	28.4	26.3
Mortality (%)	0	0	0.6	0	0
Reoperation (%)	7.7	0.4	6.3	7.3	7.4

Abbreviations: BO, bone-only decompression; DAI, duroplasty with arachnoid intact; DAO, duroplasty with arachnoid opened; TR, duroplasty and resection of cerebellar tonsils.
Note: * findings limited by small sample size.

Surgical indication should be individualized, as the natural history is unpredictable. Patients suffering from severe symptoms and those with progression over time benefit from early intervention. Asymptomatic and mildly symptomatic patients can safely be followed up over a period of time, and most of them will remain stable.

In general, patients with asymptomatic or incidental CM-1 (with or without syrinx) do not require surgery unless an associated condition—such as severe scoliosis requiring correction—triggers an intervention.

Headache-only patients represent the most challenging group in terms of decision-making. However, due to the slow progression of CM-1, a trial of conservative management for a period is a common practice. It is also important to point out that the outcome of surgery for CM-1-associated headaches is favorable. Therefore, low-surgical-risk patients should be considered for surgery early on in their treatment, if conservative management fails.

In patients with an established deficit of more than 24 months, intervention is unlikely to improve outcomes. On the contrary, progressive deficit of a few weeks' duration is likely to stop deterioration and may even improve.[62]

Patients with clinical progression—those that stop responding to conservative treatment (also an indication of deterioration)—present almost no controversy and should be considered for surgery.[28]

Patients with radiological progression of CM-1-associated syrinx also benefit from early surgery as there are no conservative treatment options. In most cases, the radiological progression is eventually associated with clinical progression. Additionally, symptoms from syringomyelia do not tend to improve with treatment.

Patients with neurological deficit (with or without headaches) should be offered surgical treatment as soon as a CM-1 diagnosis is reached. An exception to this approach would be patients with long-standing deficits that have not had progression in over 12 months and where surgical risk is significantly elevated by their comorbidities or the complexity of their disease.

For example, patients with associated basilar invagination and syringobulbia may have poor respiratory function beforehand. Consequently, these patients may require a tracheostomy prior to or following the decompression that may, in some cases, become permanent or take several months to be weaned off.

There is significant heterogeneity in the literature regarding the management options of CM-1. No randomized controlled trials comparing techniques have been performed. The evidence is limited to cohort studies and case series, which are subject to significant inherent bias. This is further complicated by the heterogeneity of the disease. Despite this, within the adult population, PFD with duroplasty (with or without opening of the arachnoid) provides superior outcomes when compared to other techniques.[49,50,51] However, the technique is associated with an increased complication rate when compared with bone-only decompression.

20.6 Authors' Recommendations

- Observation of patients with mild to moderate symptoms of CM-1-associated Valsalva (cough) headaches is reasonable.
- Asymptomatic syringomyelia may be treated conservatively. However, close clinical and radiological observation is warranted.

- PFD is warranted in patients with severe symptoms, symptom progression, and those with cough-associated headaches affecting their quality of life.
- In adult patients, PFD with duraplasty provides improved outcomes when compared with PFD alone.
- There is insufficient evidence to recommend a specific duroplasty graft. However, it is the authors' practice to utilize locally harvested autologous cervical fascia, or synthetic suturable dural graft when cervical fascia is not an option.
- There is insufficient evidence regarding the resection of the tonsils. Additionally, the unusual cases of severe morbidity and mortality with this operation have been associated with vascular events likely related to the dissection of the arachnoid around the PICA.[41]
- There is insufficient evidence to recommend OCF in the primary management of CM-1.
- Recurrent symptoms following PFD represent a challenging scenario. Altered CSF hydrodynamics usually play an important role in these cases.

References

[1] Elster AD, Chen MY. Chiari I malformations: clinical and radiologic reappraisal. Radiology. 1992; 183(2):347–353

[2] Curone M, Valentini LG, Vetrano I, et al. Chiari malformation type 1-related headache: the importance of a multidisciplinary study. Neurol Sci. 2017; 38 Suppl 1:91–93

[3] Headache Classification Committee of the International Headache Society (IHS) The International Classification of Headache Disorders. 3rd edition. Cephalalgia. 2018; 38(1):1–211

[4] Strahle J, Muraszko KM, Garton HJ, et al. Syrinx location and size according to etiology: identification of Chiari-associated syrinx. J Neurosurg Pediatr. 2015; 16(1):21–29

[5] Hatzis N, Kaar TK, Wirth MA, Toro F, Rockwood CA, Jr. Neuropathic arthropathy of the shoulder. J Bone Joint Surg Am. 1998; 80(9):1314–1319

[6] Cesmebasi A, Loukas M, Hogan E, Kralovic S, Tubbs RS, Cohen-Gadol AA. The Chiari malformations: a review with emphasis on anatomical traits. Clin Anat. 2015; 28(2):184–194

[7] Yan H, Han X, Jin M, et al. Morphometric features of posterior cranial fossa are different between Chiari I malformation with and without syringomyelia. Eur Spine J. 2016; 25(7):2202–2209

[8] Karagöz F, Izgi N, Kapíjcíjoğlu Sencer S. Morphometric measurements of the cranium in patients with Chiari type I malformation and comparison with the normal population. Acta Neurochir (Wien). 2002; 144(2):165–171, discussion 171

[9] Alperin N, Loftus JR, Oliu CJ, et al. Magnetic resonance imaging measures of posterior cranial fossa morphology and cerebrospinal fluid physiology in Chiari malformation type I. Neurosurgery. 2014; 75(5):515–522, discussion 522

[10] Nishikawa M, Sakamoto H, Hakuba A, Nakanishi N, Inoue Y. Pathogenesis of Chiari malformation: a morphometric study of the posterior cranial fossa. J Neurosurg. 1997; 86(1):40–47

[11] Marin-Padilla M, Marin-Padilla TM. Morphogenesis of experimentally induced Arnold: Chiari malformation. J Neurol Sci. 1981; 50(1):29–55

[12] Clarke EC, Fletcher DF, Stoodley MA, Bilston LE. Computational fluid dynamics modelling of cerebrospinal fluid pressure in Chiari malformation and syringomyelia. J Biomech. 2013; 46(11):1801–1809

[13] Leung V, Magnussen JS, Stoodley MA, Bilston LE. Cerebellar and hindbrain motion in Chiari malformation with and without syringomyelia. J Neurosurg Spine. 2016; 24(4):546–555

[14] Cousins J, Haughton V. Motion of the cerebellar tonsils in the foramen magnum during the cardiac cycle. AJNR Am J Neuroradiol. 2009; 30(8): 1587–1588

[15] Lawrence BJ, Luciano M, Tew J, et al. Cardiac-related spinal cord tissue motion at the foramen magnum is increased in patients with type I Chiari malformation and decreases postdecompression surgery. World Neurosurg. 2018; 116:e298–e307

[16] Pascual J, Oterino A, Berciano J. Headache in type I Chiari malformation. Neurology. 1992; 42(8):1519–1521

[17] Edmeads J. The cervical spine and headache. Neurology. 1988; 38(12): 1874–1878

[18] Williams B. Cough headache due to craniospinal pressure dissociation. Arch Neurol. 1980; 37(4):226–230

[19] Stovner LJ. Headache associated with the Chiari type I malformation. Headache. 1993; 33(4):175–181

[20] Sansur CA, Heiss JD, DeVroom HL, Eskioglu E, Ennis R, Oldfield EH. Pathophysiology of headache associated with cough in patients with Chiari I malformation. J Neurosurg. 2003; 98(3):453–458

[21] Milhorat TH, Chou MW, Trinidad EM, et al. Chiari I malformation redefined: clinical and radiographic findings for 364 symptomatic patients. Neurosurgery. 1999; 44(5):1005–1017

[22] Gardner WJ. Hydrodynamic mechanism of syringomyelia: its relationship to myelocele. J Neurol Neurosurg Psychiatry. 1965; 28:247–259

[23] Williams B. The distending force in the production of communicating syringomyelia. Lancet. 1969; 2(7622):696

[24] Oldfield EH, Muraszko K, Shawker TH, Patronas NJ. Pathophysiology of syringomyelia associated with Chiari I malformation of the cerebellar tonsils. Implications for diagnosis and treatment. J Neurosurg. 1994; 80(1):3–15

[25] Lloyd RA, Fletcher DF, Clarke EC, Bilston LE. Chiari malformation may increase perivascular cerebrospinal fluid flow into the spinal cord: a subject-specific computational modelling study. J Biomech. 2017; 65:185–193

[26] Langridge B, Phillips E, Choi D. Chiari malformation type 1: a systematic review of natural history and conservative management. World Neurosurg. 2017; 104:213–219

[27] Killeen A, Roguski M, Chavez A, Heilman C, Hwang S. Non-operative outcomes in Chiari I malformation patients. J Clin Neurosci. 2015; 22(1):133–138

[28] Chavez A, Roguski M, Killeen A, Heilman C, Hwang S. Comparison of operative and non-operative outcomes based on surgical selection criteria for patients with Chiari I malformations. J Clin Neurosci. 2014; 21(12):2201–2206

[29] Bindal AK, Dunsker SB, Tew JM, Jr. Chiari I malformation: classification and management. Neurosurgery. 1995; 37(6):1069–1074

[30] Leon TJ, Kuhn EN, Arynchyna AA, et al. Patients with "benign" Chiari I malformations require surgical decompression at a low rate. J Neurosurg Pediatr. 2019; 23(4):498–506

[31] Klekamp J, Iaconetta G, Samii M. Spontaneous resolution of Chiari I malformation and syringomyelia: case report and review of the literature. Neurosurgery. 2001; 48(3):664–667

[32] Massimi L, Della Pepa GM, Tamburrini G, Di Rocco C. Sudden onset of Chiari malformation type I in previously asymptomatic patients. J Neurosurg Pediatr. 2011; 8(5):438–442

[33] Nishizawa S, Yokoyama T, Yokota N, Tokuyama T, Ohta S. Incidentally identified syringomyelia associated with Chiari I malformations: is early interventional surgery necessary? Neurosurgery. 2001; 49(3):637–640, discussion 640–641

[34] Bowers CA, Brimley C, Cole C, Gluf W, Schmidt RH. AlloDerm for duraplasty in Chiari malformation: superior outcomes. Acta Neurochir (Wien). 2015; 157(3):507–511

[35] Morris Z, Whiteley WN, Longstreth WT, Jr, et al. Incidental findings on brain magnetic resonance imaging: systematic review and meta-analysis. BMJ. 2009; 339(1):b3016

[36] Meadows J, Kraut M, Guarnieri M, Haroun RI, Carson BS. Asymptomatic Chiari type I malformations identified on magnetic resonance imaging. J Neurosurg. 2000; 92(6):920–926

[37] Benglis D, Jr, Covington D, Bhatia R, et al. Outcomes in pediatric patients with Chiari malformation Type I followed up without surgery. J Neurosurg Pediatr. 2011; 7(4):375–379

[38] Strahle J, Muraszko KM, Kapurch J, Bapuraj JR, Garton HJ, Maher CO. Natural history of Chiari malformation Type I following decision for conservative treatment. J Neurosurg Pediatr. 2011; 8(2):214–221

[39] Klekamp J. Surgical treatment of Chiari I malformation–analysis of intraoperative findings, complications, and outcome for 371 foramen magnum decompressions. Neurosurgery. 2012; 71(2):365–380, discussion 380

[40] Tubbs RS, Beckman J, Naftel RP, et al. Institutional experience with 500 cases of surgically treated pediatric Chiari malformation type I. J Neurosurg Pediatr. 2011; 7(3):248–256

[41] Shweikeh F, Sunjaya D, Nuno M, Drazin D, Adamo MA. National trends, complications, and hospital charges in pediatric patients with Chiari malformation type I treated with posterior fossa decompression with and without duraplasty. Pediatr Neurosurg. 2015; 50(1):31–37

[42] Aghakhani N, Parker F, David P, et al. Long-term follow-up of Chiari-related syringomyelia in adults: analysis of 157 surgically treated cases. Neurosurgery. 2009; 64(2):308–315, discussion 315

[43] Alfieri A, Pinna G. Long-term results after posterior fossa decompression in syringomyelia with adult Chiari type I malformation. J Neurosurg Spine. 2012; 17(5):381–387

[44] Arruda JA, Costa CM, Tella OI, Jr. Results of the treatment of syringomyelia associated with Chiari malformation: analysis of 60 cases. Arq Neuropsiquiatr. 2004; 62 2A:237–244

[45] Beretta E, Vetrano IG, Curone M, et al. Chiari malformation-related headache: outcome after surgical treatment. Neurol Sci. 2017; 38 Suppl 1:95–98

[46] Chen J, Li Y, Wang T, et al. Comparison of posterior fossa decompression with and without duraplasty for the surgical treatment of Chiari malformation type I in adult patients: a retrospective analysis of 103 patients. Medicine (Baltimore). 2017; 96(4):e5945

[47] Chotai S, Medhkour A. Surgical outcomes after posterior fossa decompression with and without duraplasty in Chiari malformation-I. Clin Neurol Neurosurg. 2014; 125:182–188

[48] Deng X, Yang C, Gan J, et al. Long-term outcomes after small-bone-window posterior fossa decompression and duraplasty in adults with Chiari malformation type I. World Neurosurg. 2015; 84(4):998–1004

[49] El-Ghandour NM. Long-term outcome of surgical management of adult Chiari I malformation. Neurosurg Rev. 2012; 35(4):537–546, discussion 546–547

[50] Guyotat J, Bret P, Jouanneau E, Ricci AC, Lapras C. Syringomyelia associated with type I Chiari malformation. A 21-year retrospective study on 75 cases treated by foramen magnum decompression with a special emphasis on the value of tonsils resection. Acta Neurochir (Wien). 1998; 140(8):745–754

[51] Kotil K, Ozdogan S, Kayaci S, Duzkalir HG. Long-term outcomes of a new minimally invasive approach in Chiari type 1 and 1.5 malformations: technical note and preliminary results. World Neurosurg. 2018; 115:407–413

[52] Krishna V, McLawhorn M, Kosnik-Infinger L, Patel S. High long-term symptomatic recurrence rates after Chiari-1 decompression without dural opening: a single center experience. Clin Neurol Neurosurg. 2014; 118:53–58

[53] Lee CK, Mokhtari T, Connolly ID, et al. Comparison of porcine and bovine collagen dural substitutes in posterior fossa decompression for Chiari I malformation in adults. World Neurosurg. 2017; 108:33–40

[54] Sindou M, Chávez-Machuca J, Hashish H. Cranio-cervical decompression for Chiari type I-malformation, adding extreme lateral foramen magnum opening and expansile duroplasty with arachnoid preservation. Technique and long-term functional results in 44 consecutive adult cases: comparison with literature data. Acta Neurochir (Wien). 2002; 144(10):1005–1019

[55] Thakar S, Sivaraju L, Jacob KS, et al. A points-based algorithm for prognosticating clinical outcome of Chiari malformation Type I with syringomyelia: results from a predictive model analysis of 82 surgically managed adult patients. J Neurosurg Spine. 2018; 28(1):23–32

[56] Yilmaz A, Kanat A, Musluman AM, et al. When is duraplasty required in the surgical treatment of Chiari malformation type I based on tonsillar descending grading scale? World Neurosurg. 2011; 75(2):307–313

[57] Zhang Y, Zhang N, Qiu H, et al. An efficacy analysis of posterior fossa decompression techniques in the treatment of Chiari malformation with associated syringomyelia. J Clin Neurosci. 2011; 18(10):1346–1349

[58] Chai Z, Xue X, Fan H, et al. Efficacy of posterior fossa decompression with duraplasty for patients with Chiari malformation type I: a systematic review and meta-analysis. World Neurosurg. 2018; 113:357–365.e1

[59] de Oliveira Sousa U, de Oliveira MF, Heringer LC, Barcelos ACES, Botelho RV. The effect of posterior fossa decompression in adult Chiari malformation and basilar invagination: a systematic review and meta-analysis. Neurosurg Rev. 2018; 41(1):311–321

[60] Zhao JL, Li MH, Wang CL, Meng W. A systematic review of Chiari I malformation: techniques and outcomes. World Neurosurg. 2016; 88:7–14

[61] Lin W, Duan G, Xie J, Shao J, Wang Z, Jiao B. Comparison of results between posterior fossa decompression with and without duraplasty for the surgical treatment of Chiari malformation type I: a systematic review and meta-analysis. World Neurosurg. 2018; 110:460–474.e5

[62] Dyste GN, Menezes AH, VanGilder JC. Symptomatic Chiari malformations. An analysis of presentation, management, and long-term outcome. J Neurosurg. 1989; 71(2):159–168

[63] Moriwaka F, Tashiro K, Tachibana S, Yada K: Epidemiology of syringomyelia in Japan: the nationwide survey [in Japanese]. Rinsho Shinkeigaku. 1995; 35:1395–1397

21 Natural History and Management Options of Cranial Dural Arteriovenous Fistulas

Hugo Andrade-Barazarte, Felix Goehre, Behnam Rezai Jahromi, Zhao Tongyuan, Jiangyu Xue, Zhongcan Cheng, Ajmal Zemmar, Tianxiao Li, and Juha Hernesniemi

Abstract

Intracranial dural arteriovenous fistulas (DAVFs) are pathological anastomoses between meningeal arteries and dural venous sinuses or cortical veins. DAVFs are rare lesions having a documented incidence between 10 and 15% among all intracranial vascular malformations. DAVFs frequently affect patients in their middle-to-later years of life (e.g., 50–60 years of age) and tend to present with a wide variety of symptoms such as intolerable pulsatile tinnitus, exophthalmos and chemosis (when the fistula is in the cavernous sinus), progressive dementia, seizures, or neurological deficits often caused by intraparenchymal hemorrhage. Classification of DAVFs is based on their venous drainage and characteristics, as an attempt to predict their clinical behavior. One of the most important features among these classifications is the distinction (presence or absence) of cortical venous drainage (CVD). The natural history of DAVFs depends on their clinical presentation and the presence of CVD. Therefore, we subdivided the DAVFs in fistulas without CDV or low-grade, and fistulas with CVD or high-grade based on their angioarchitecture and clinical presentation. Low-grade fistulas have a reported annual rate of new neurological event from 0 to 0.6% and an annual mortality rate of 0%. High-grade fistulas have an aggressive natural history and a high risk of early rebleeding of about 35% within 2 weeks after the first hemorrhage with an annual mortality rate of 10.4%. The treatment strategy should be tailored individually to patients considering the anatomical features of the DAVF, the severity of symptoms, and the potential risk of intracranial hemorrhage.

Keywords: dural arteriovenous fistulas, DAVF, hemorrhage, neurological deficit, cortical venous drainage, venous ectasia

21.1 Introduction

Intracranial dural arteriovenous fistulas (DAVFs) are pathological anastomoses between meningeal arteries and dural venous sinuses or cortical veins.[42] They differentiate from brain arteriovenous malformations (AVMs) due to the lack of a parenchymal nidus and the arterial supply vessels only arise from arteries that typically perfuse the dura mater.[35] DAVFs are uncommon lesions having a reported incidence of between 10 and 15% among all intracranial vascular malformations (6% supratentorial and 35% infratentorial vascular malformations).[36] It has been suggested that there is a slightly higher incidence of DAVFS among Finnish and Japanese populations (incidence of 29–32%).[39,44] DAVFs frequently affect patients in their middle to later years of life (50–60 years),[6] and there is no clear sex predilection or genetic components associated with DAVFs.

Clinical presentation of DAVFs depends on the location of the fistula. Typically, patients may present with intolerable pulsatile tinnitus (transverse–sigmoid sinus junction), exophthalmos and chemosis (cavernous sinus [CS]), progressive dementia (superior sagittal sinus), seizures, or neurological deficits often caused by intraparenchymal hemorrhage.[29,39] DAVFs are frequently located at the transverse–sigmoid junction and also at the CS, superior sagittal sinus, anterior cranial fossa, and tentorium, among others.[29,35]

Various classification systems have been described to predict high-risk fistulas and to guide treatment decision-making. These classification systems are based on angiographic characteristics of the DAVF such as involvement of a venous sinus and presence or absence of retrograde cortical venous drainage (CVD), as well as clinical presentation (hemorrhagic vs. nonhemorrhagic neurological deficits [NHND]).[4,6,13,56]

21.1.1 Pathophysiology

The pathophysiological development of DAVFs remains unclear. It is generally accepted that DAVFs are acquired lesions, with a small subgroup that develops following direct trauma, infection, previous craniotomies, tumors, or venous sinus thrombosis.[5,7,54]

One accepted theory regarding DAVF formation is that these lesions arise from progressive stenosis or occlusion of a dural venous sinus. As venous pressure increases, meningeal arteries develop fistulous connections with the dural sinus or cortical veins, which may occur due to the presence of de novo fistulas based on neoangiogenesis or due to the enlargement of preexisting physiological shunts.[11,26,36] These result in a complex network of venous tributaries under arterial pressure with progressing sinus outflow obstruction and venous hypertension. Therefore, the regular and normal antegrade venous flow pattern is altered and reversed resulting in retrograde flow through cortical veins (CVD), which can cause venous hypertension within the surrounding brain.[11,26,36]

DAVF formation is a dynamic process since their hemodynamic may change over time due to the recanalization of the respective sinus or in contrary with the recruitment of more arterial feeders (with the possible progression from a low-risk DAVF to a higher grade). It is thought that intracerebral hemorrhage (ICH) occurs when fragile arterialized parenchymal veins rupture due to the presence of unrelenting venous reflux and cortical venous hypertension.[5,6,13,26,51]

Carotid cavernous fistulas (CCFs) involve an abnormal connection between the internal carotid artery (ICA), external carotid artery (ECA), and the CS. These fistulas comprise a particular subgroup among intracranial DAVFs.[3] CCFs are defined based on their pathogenesis (spontaneous vs. traumatic), angioarchitecture (direct shunt from the cavernous ICA or its branches, shunt from branches of the ECA, or a combination of both), and hemodynamics (high vs. low flow).[3] Commonly, direct CCFs occur as a result of trauma (skull base fracture or iatrogenic) involving the vessel wall at the horizontal segment

Table 21.1 Different dural arteriovenous classifications with their respective characteristics, natural history, and management

Borden–Shucart type	Cognard type	Zipfel type	Venous drainage	Presence of CVD	Cortical venous hypertension	Clinical presentation (ICH or NHND)	Risk of ICH (%)	Mortality risk	Management
I	I, IIa	1	Dural sinus	No	No	No	0	0	Conservative
II	IIb, IIa + IIb	2A	Dural sinus	Yes	No	No	1.4–1.5	0	Elective treatment to eliminate risks
II	IIb, IIa + IIb	2S	Dural sinus	Yes	Yes	Yes	7.4–7.6	3.8%	Early treatment
III	III–V	3A	Cortical vein	Yes	No	No	1.4–1.5	0	Elective treatment to eliminate risks
III	III–V	3S	Cortical vein	Yes	Yes	Yes	7.4–7.6	3.8%	Early treatment

Abbreviations: CVD, cortical venous drainage; ICH, intracerebral hemorrhage; NHND, nonhemorrhagic neurological deficit.

of the cavernous ICA or because of rupture of an aneurysm at the cavernous ICA, which results in a high-flow fistula between the ICA and the CS.[3,10]

Indirect CCFs are normally associated with medical comorbidities such as diabetes mellitus, hypertension, collagen vascular disease, and pregnancy, among others. These fistula subtypes are typically low-flow lesions that occur spontaneously.[3]

Due to the specific characteristics and venous drainage, CCFs have been considered a different pathological entity as DAVFs. Accordingly, their natural history and treatment options are not discussed.

21.1.2 Classification

Classification of DAVFs is based on venous drainage patterns. The most commonly used classifications are the Borden–Shucart and Cognard classifications.[4,12] One of the most important features among these classifications is the distinction (presence or absence) of CVD.

Borden–Shucart classification: Type I fistula is characterized by the absence of CVD; this type harbors dural arteries that drain exclusively into a dural sinus with antegrade venous flow. Type II and III fistulas are characterized by the presence of CVD. Type II fistulas drain into a dural sinus with venous flow that is both antegrade into the dural sinus and retrograde into the cortical veins, whereas type III fistulas drain exclusively into cortical veins in a retrograde fashion.[4]

Cognard classification: This classification is based on venous drainage characteristics, shunt location, and venous outflow.[4] The Cognard classification includes five subtypes of DAVF. type I and IIa DAVFs are similar to Borden–Shucart type I (absence of CVD) DAVFs, where type I lesions drain antegrade into a dural sinus and type II lesions drain retrograde into a venous sinus. Type IIb fistulas drain antegrade into a venous sinus and show cortical venous reflux (presence of CVD). Type IIa + IIb DAVFs drain retrograde into a venous sinus and have cortical venous reflux. Type III fistulas drain directly into a cortical veins and type IV fistulas besides draining into cortical veins also show signs of venous ectasia. Type V DAVFs drain directly and exclusively into spinal perimedullary veins.

From these two previous classifications, Borden–Shucart type II and III and Cognard type IIb to V DAVFs are considered high-grade fistulas with a more aggressive natural history due to the presence of CVD.

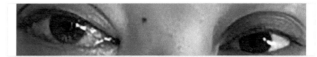

Fig. 21.1 Right eye unilateral exophthalmos and chemosis in a patient with caroticocavernous fistula (CCF).

Additionally, Zipfel et al in 2009 proposed a modified classification based on the Borden–Shucart classification.[56] This new modification includes clinical data regarding the presentation of the DAVF (asymptomatic, hemorrhage, or NHNDs) besides well-identified angiographic parameters. This simple classification system accurately predicts the risks of hemorrhagic and nonhemorrhagic events. Therefore, it is extremely important for risk stratification to guide further management and treatment.[56] ▶ Table 21.1 summarizes the classifications mentioned earlier.

21.1.3 Clinical Presentation and Imaging Evaluation

DAVF patients can present with pulsatile tinnitus, exophthalmos, and chemosis among other symptoms due to increased sinus drainage, which may occur in any kind of DAVF with venous sinus drainage (▶ Fig. 21.1). Moreover, patients can present with more aggressive symptoms such as seizures, strong headaches, or decreased conscious level related to the presence of ICH or NHND caused by cortical venous hypertension, which only develops in a DAVF with CVD.[29,39] Hemorrhagic symptoms occur acutely, whereas NHNDs are gradually developed over days to weeks as the product of focal or global cortical venous hypertension that causes different degrees of cerebral ischemia.[23,27]

Regarding the initial imaging evaluation, computed tomography (CT) can detect DAVF-related ICH and vasogenic edema caused by cortical venous hypertension. Often, venous varices are the cause of hemorrhage, and these can be located distally from the actual DAVF.[15] Magnetic resonance imaging (MRI) is helpful to identify the anatomy of the DAVF and its location in relation to the brain. On T2-weighted images, it is possible to identify the presence of flow voids from large arterialized draining veins and varices (▶ Fig. 21.2a). Additionally,

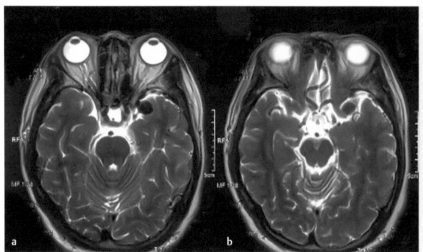

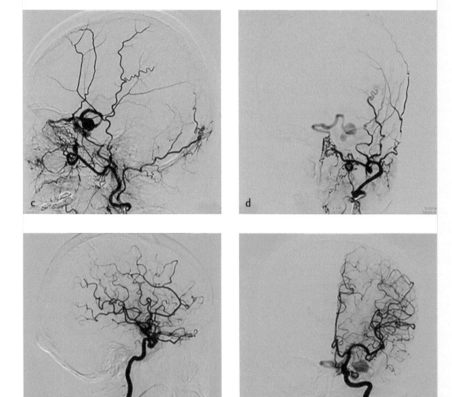

Fig. 21.2 (a, b) Axial sections of T2-weighted magnetic resonance imaging study showing large vascular flow voids near the left anterior fossa floor and left Sylvian fissure. Digital subtraction angiography on (c) lateral and (d) anteroposterior views after a left external carotid artery contrast injection showing a Borden–Shucart type III intracranial dural arteriovenous fistula draining into a cortical frontal vein causing venous ectasia and a large venous varix. Digital subtraction angiography on (e) lateral and (f) anteroposterior views after a left internal carotid artery contrast injection showing a Borden–Shucart type III intracranial dural arteriovenous fistula feed by ethmoidal branches of a hypertrophic ophthalmic artery.

postcontrast T1-weighted images can show dilated leptomeningeal and medullary vessels, venous ectasia, parenchymal enhancement, and venous sinus occlusion or thrombosis.[31] Digital subtraction angiography (DSA) still remains the gold standard for diagnosis and it is essential to identify the presence of the fistula, location, angioarchitecture, anatomy of the ECA and its branches, degree of dural sinus stenosis or occlusion, venous ectasia, and presence of CVD (▶ Fig. 21.2b–e). Additionally, it can provide information regarding venous congestion not only by the presence of CVD but also by the presence of a pseudophlebitic pattern (tortuous engorged leptomeningeal veins) in the venous phase.[53]

21.2 Selected Papers on the Natural History of Cranial Dural Arteriovenous Fistula

- Gross BA, Du R. The natural history of cerebral dural arteriovenous fistulae. Neurosurgery 2012;71(3):594–602, discussion 602–603
- Satomi J, van Dijk JM, Terbrugge KG, Willinsky RA, Wallace MC. Benign cranial dural arteriovenous fistulas: outcome of conservative management based on the natural history of the lesion. J Neurosurg 2002;97(4):767–770

- Shah MN, Botros JA, Pilgram TK, et al. Borden–Shucart type I dural arteriovenous fistulas: clinical course including risk of conversion to higher-grade fistulas. J Neurosurg 2012;117(3):539–545

21.3 Natural History of DAVFs

One important parameter when considering the risks of hemorrhage and further treatment decisions is the presence of CVD and the clinical presentation of the patient. Therefore, we subdivided the DAVFs into fistulas without CVD (low grade) and fistulas with CVD (high grade) based on their angioarchitecture and clinical presentation.

21.3.1 Natural History of Low-Grade DAVFs

DAVFs without CVD (Borden–Shucart type I, Zipfel type I, and Cognard types I and IIa) are considered to have a benign natural history and rarely cause ICH or NHND.[16,20,45,46] Based on follow-up studies of patients treated conservatively or through endovascular palliative methods (without complete obliteration of the DAVF), these lesions have a reported annual rate of new neurological event from 0 to 0.6% and an annual mortality rate of 0%.[16,20,45,46]

DAVFs are dynamic lesions that can evolve to become aggressive over time (DAVF with CVD). It is thought that this is due to progressive stenosis or thrombosis of venous outlets, increased arterial flow, or recruitment or extension of the fistulous connections.[20,43,45]

Benign DAVFs have in general a reported conversion rate or risk of developing CVD of about 0.8 to 2%, thus mandating for clinical follow-up review in such cases and the need for new radiological evaluation in the presence of new or modification (improvement or worsening) of previous neurological symptoms.[45,46]

21.3.2 Natural History of High-Grade DAVFs

DAVFs with CVD (Borden–Shucart types II and III; Zipfel types 2A, 2S, 3A, and 3S; and Cognard types IIb, IIa +b, and III–V) have an aggressive natural history and can frequently cause ICH or NHND.[6,15,17,20,42,49,51,56] The aggressive nature of these lesions was first reported by Duffau et al[18] in 1999. The authors analyzed 20 patients with Borden–Shucart type II and III DAVFs, and identified a 35% risk of early rebleeding within 2 weeks following the first hemorrhage.[18] Additionally, van Dijk et al retrospectively identified in a subcohort of 20 patients that the presence of cerebral venous reflux (CVR) in cranial DAVFs yields an annual mortality rate of 10.4%.[50] Also, in this series the annual risk for hemorrhage or NHND during follow-up was 8.1 and 6.9%, respectively, resulting in an annual event rate of 15.0%. ▶ Table 21.2 summarizes the risks of high-grade DAVFs.[50] Based on these reports, it became clear that DAVFs with CVD are at risk of ICH, NHND, or even death; therefore, in the majority of these patients, treatment should be considered to eliminate those risks.

Clinical presentation plays an important role in DAVFs with CVD since some patients present with aggressive symptoms such as ICH or NHND and others develop benign symptoms

Table 21.2 Natural history of high-grade DAVFs (Borden–Shucart types II and III; Zipfel types 2A, 2S, 3A, and 3S; and Cognard types IIb, IIa + b, and III–V)

	Risk (%)	Mortality risk (%)
Early rebleeding (within 2 wk from first hemorrhage)[18]	35%	
Presence of cerebral venous reflux [50]		10.4%.
Annual risk of hemorrhage [50]	8.1%	
Annual risk of neurological deficit [50]	6.9%	

Abbreviation: DAVFs, dural arteriovenous fistulas.

such as tinnitus. Söderman et al observed a significant difference in the annual rate of new neurological events between patients presenting with ICH as compared to those without ICH (7.4 vs. 1.5%, respectively).[49] Additionally, Gross and Du reported a significant difference in the annual rate of ICH in patients presenting with ICH versus those presenting with NHND versus those presenting incidentally or with more benign symptoms of increased sinus drainage (46 vs. 10 vs. 2%, respectively).[20] Based on these reports, it can be concluded that a relevant association exists between clinical presentation and natural history of DAVFs with CVD.

Moreover, venous ectasia has been demonstrated to impact the natural history of DAVFs with CVD.[20] Bulters et al noted a statistically significant increase in annual risk of hemorrhage between patients with DAVFs having venous ectasia and those with DAVFs without venous ectasia (19.0 vs. 1.4%, respectively).[7]

21.4 Selected Papers on Treatment Outcomes of DAVFs

- Kakarla UK, Deshmukh VR, Zabramski JM, Albuquerque FC, McDougall CG, Spetzler RF. Surgical treatment of high-risk intracranial dural arteriovenous fistulae: clinical outcomes and avoidance of complications. Neurosurgery 2007;61(3):447–457, discussion 457–459
- Piippo A, Niemelä M, van Popta J, et al. Characteristics and long-term outcome of 251 patients with dural arteriovenous fistulas in a defined population. J Neurosurg 2013;118(5):923–934
- Rangel-Castilla L, Barber SM, Klucznik R, Diaz O. Mid and long term outcomes of dural arteriovenous fistula endovascular management with Onyx. Experience of a single tertiary center. J Neurointerv Surg 2014;6(8):607–613
- Satomi J, van Dijk JM, Terbrugge KG, Willinsky RA, Wallace MC. Benign cranial dural arteriovenous fistulas: outcome of conservative management based on the natural history of the lesion. J Neurosurg 2002;97(4):767–770
- Söderman M, Edner G, Ericson K, et al. Gamma knife surgery for dural arteriovenous shunts: 25 years of experience. J Neurosurg 2006;104(6):867–875

21.5 Treatment Strategy

In general, treatment options for DAVFs include conservative management, endovascular embolization, microsurgical disconnection, stereotactic radiosurgery (SRS), or a combination of any of these methods.[8,20,37,39,47,48,50] However, most DAVFs can be at least partially treated by endovascular methods, which should be the first-line approach to obtain complete occlusion.[40] If complete occlusion is not possible, the patient can undergo SRS or microsurgery depending on the clinical context. Endovascular treatment can also be used as a complementary treatment if there is residual filling after microsurgery or vice versa. ▸ Table 21.3 summarizes the treatment options and their respective risks and outcomes.

The treatment strategy should be tailored individually to patients considering the anatomical features of the DAVF, the severity of symptoms, and the potential risk of intracranial hemorrhage. ▸ Fig. 21.3 summarizes the treatment algorithm for cranial DAVFs.

DAVFs with CVD and presenting with aggressive symptoms such as ICH or NHND (annual rate of ICH and NHND of 7.4–19% and mortality of 3.8%) require urgent treatment of the lesion by modalities that can eliminate the risks immediately (endovascular, microsurgery, or a combination of both).[24,28,41]

DAVFs with CVD incidentally found or with more benign symptoms such as tinnitus or ophthalmological phenomena (annual rate of ICH and NHND 1.4–1.5% and mortality rate of 0%) require treatment in properly selected patients (e.g., patients without major comorbidities and prolonged life expectancy); however, in these cases, treatment can be offered in a more elective setting and treatment modalities can include SRS (1–3 years to achieve complete obliteration).[24,25,28,41,48]

DAVFs without CVD carry a very low risk of ICH and NHND (annual rate of 0–0.6% and mortality rate of 0%); therefore, these patients should be treated according to the severity of their symptoms. Benign DAVFs without CVD and incidentally found should be managed conservatively with repeated vascular imaging studies performed if new symptoms appear (e.g., tinnitus, seizures, ophthalmologic symptoms, etc.), based on the risk of upgrade of the fistula to a higher type with CVD and more aggressive behavior. However, those patients presenting with symptoms of tinnitus or ophthalmologic phenomena should be treated regarding the severity of their symptoms and the impact of these symptoms in their quality of life.[5,16,39]

21.6 Therapeutic Options

21.6.1 Endovascular Treatment

With the improvement of microcatheters and liquid embolic agents, endovascular treatment is often considered the first-line treatment modality of intracranial DAVFs.[40] The goals of this therapeutic option depend on the DAVF characteristics such as location, angioarchitecture, and mode of presentation.

Table 21.3 Treatment options and respective outcomes

Treatment modality	Angiographic obliteration rate (%)	Complication risk (%)
Endovascular series[8,19,22]	65–95	2
Microsurgery series[1,21,24,32]	92–100	7.1–17
Stereotactic radiosurgery series[9,38,48]	68–90	Low complication rate

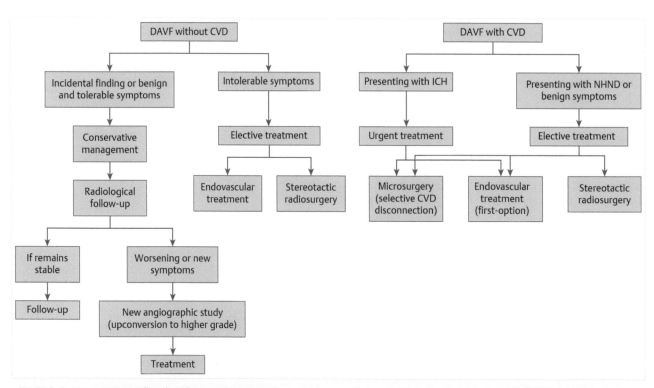

Fig. 21.3 Treatment strategy flowchart for cranial DAVFs (CVD, cortical venous drainage; DAVFs, dural arteriovenous fistulas; ICH, intracerebral hemorrhage; NHND, nonhemorrhagic neurological deficit).

High-grade DAVFs presenting with ICH or NHND require rapid resolution of the fistula through occlusion of the proximal segment of the draining vein to eliminate the risk of rebleeding or further NHND. For high-grade DAVFs presenting with more benign symptoms such as tinnitus, the treatment to cure the fistula can be initiated in a more elective manner, given the less aggressive behavior observed in these patients. Moreover, for low-grade DAVF presenting with intolerable symptoms such as tinnitus, the main goal is the palliation of the symptoms due to the relative benign natural history associated with these particular lesions. This palliation can be achieved either by complete occlusion and cure of the fistula or by partial embolization and flow reduction without complete radiographic resolution. Additionally, endovascular treatment can be used to reduce the DAVF flow for further microsurgical disconnection or in association with radiosurgical treatment.

Endovascular treatment can be performed through either transarterial embolization or transvenous embolization or a combination of both. The main goal to achieve protection against future ICH or NHND is to completely obliterate the proximal portion of the draining vein. Technically, the transarterial embolization includes distal microcatheterization of arterial feeders and embolization with liquid embolic agents. The transvenous approach includes distal microcatheterization of the proximal draining vein or the involved dural sinus and embolization with liquid agents or coils.

21.6.2 Endovascular Outcomes

With the refinement on microcatheters and the incorporation of new embolic agents, the endovascular occlusion rate of DAVF has increased. Gross et al, in a large retrospective study comprising 260 DAVFs, reported an increasing angiographic occlusion rate from 60% before the use of onyx to 76 to 80% thereafter.[19] Additionally, Chandra et al reported an angiographic occlusion rate of 95% and a complication rate of 2% in 41 DAVFs treated using a single-agent onyx embolization.[8] Moreover, a large retrospective multicenter observational study that included 1,940 embolizations of DAVFs reported an overall complication rate of 7.7% and a 30-day morbidity and mortality of 2.8 and 0.6%, respectively.[22] Based on this, it appears that endovascular treatment provides good rates of angiographic obliteration, carries a low risk of related complications, and is effective to improve DAVF-related symptoms. (▶ Table 21.3 summarizes endovascular outcomes and complication rates.)

21.6.3 Microsurgical Treatment

Microsurgery is now generally reserved for those lesions that are unable to be treated successfully or safely through endovascular procedures and it remains the preferred treatment modality for anterior fossa floor DAVFs.[34]

Historically, surgical treatment of DAVFs included ligation of the feeders and arterialized veins, complete resection of the fistula and the dura incorporated, resection, packing, or occlusion of the compromised sinus, which were associated with a higher rate of complication.[33] Currently, the microsurgical treatment of DAVF includes a more targeted approach to selectively disconnect the CVD by occluding the arterialized vein(s) as close as possible to the DAVF.[14] The primary goal is to eliminate the risk of further bleeding or NHND by disconnecting the most dangerous part of the DAVF (the CVD). During the exposure, encountered feeding dural arteries are as well coagulated and divided; however, nonarterialized cortical veins close to the fistula should be preserved to avoid the risk of venous infarction.

21.6.4 Microsurgical Outcomes

The safety and long-term efficacy of this treatment modality have been demonstrated by multiple single-institution case series.[14,30,52] Surgical treatment is associated with an angiographic obliteration rate of 92 to 100% and a morbidity rate of 4 to 17%.[1,21,24,32] It is important to mention that with the advancement of microsurgical techniques and targeted approaches, the selective surgical disconnection of DAVF CVD is associated with lower morbidity (< 7%).[1,52,55] Van Dijk et al published a surgical series of 70 DAVFs with CVD and compared the outcomes of those treated by selective CVD disconnection (n = 52) versus those treated with complete DAVF resection (n = 18). They reported that both groups had similar angiographic and clinical outcomes; however, the selective CVD disconnection group suffered fewer perioperative complications (5.8 vs. 55.6%).[52] Additionally, Al-Mahfoudh et al, in a surgical series of 25 high-grade DAVFs treated only by selective CVD disconnection, reported an angiographic obliteration rate of 100% and a temporary perioperative morbidity of 4%.[1]

These surgical series demonstrate that high-grade DAVFs can be treated by microsurgery with high rates of angiographic obliteration and CVD disconnection but with significant rate of morbidity. Additionally, it also suggests that surgical treatment by direct selective disconnection of the CVD offers protection against future bleeding or NHND with less risk of perioperative complications as compared to more aggressive surgical modalities.

21.6.5 Radiosurgical Treatment

SRS for DAVFs was initially described by Barcia-Salorio et al in 1982.[2] SRS is a feasible treatment modality for carefully selected DAVFs, especially those with low flow and located in the CS and the transverse/sigmoid sinuses. Technically, a dose of 20 to 30 Gy is given to the DAVF at the 50% isodose line with dynamic planning to avoid affecting sensitive neural structures. SRS has a delayed effect on DAVFs, which constitutes a major disadvantage of the procedure. On the one hand, this latency period can be well tolerated for benign fistulas, but on the other hand, high-grade fistulas with CVD are at higher risk of hemorrhage, making radiosurgery problematic as a first-line therapy. Therefore, SRS is amenable for those situations where the lesion is not feasible for endovascular/microsurgical treatment or in patients with severe comorbidities.[48] Additionally, good candidates for SRS are those patients harboring DAVFs without CVD and with intolerable or progressive symptoms of increased sinus drainage (e.g., tinnitus), since symptom resolution would be expected to occur within 1 to 3 years after treatment. It is important to mention that patients harboring high-grade DAVFs and presenting with aggressive symptoms such as ICH or NHND are not good candidates for SRS due to the latency period required for fistula obliteration and the unacceptably high risk of possible ICH and NHND during that period.

21.6.6 Radiosurgical Outcomes

A recent meta-analysis and extensive 25-year experience on DAVF treated by SRS reported an obliteration rate of 68% over an overall mean follow-up period of 28.9 months.[9,38,48] Additionally, the authors noted a flow reduction in another 24% of cases; based on that, they suggested that SRS is an effective therapy for selected DAVF with low risk of complications. Recently, Park et al reported their experience in 20 patients with DAVF (8 without CVD and with intolerable symptoms and 12 with CVD and without ICH or NHND) treated only by SRS. In their series, they achieved a complete angiographic cure in 90% of cases and subtotal cure in 10%. Among this cohort, all symptomatic patients experienced complete resolution of their initial symptoms and one patient had a transient complication after the procedure.[37] This confirms that SRS is most appropriate for selected DAVFs without CVD with intolerable clinical symptoms, but likely not for high-grade DAVFs.

21.7 Authors' Recommendations

- DAVFs are dynamic lesions and can be classified as low- and high-grade DAVFs associated with the absence or presence of CVD.
- Most frequently used classifications for DAVFs are the Borden–Shucart, Cognard, and Zipfel classifications. These classifications were created to stratify and simplify the natural history and management of DAVFs based on radiological characteristics and clinical presentation.
- Low-grade DAVFs or DAVFs without CVD (Borden–Shucart type I, Cognard types I and IIa, and Zipfel type I) have a benign natural history and an annual rate of ICH or NHND of 0 to 0.6% and mortality rate of 0%.
- High-grade DAVFs or DAVFs with CVD (Borden–Shucart types II and III; Zipfel types 2A, 2S, 3A, and 3S; and Cognard types IIb, IIa + b, and III–V) have an aggressive natural history (annual rate of ICH and NHND of 7.4–19% and mortality of 3.8%).
- DAVFs without CVD and incidentally found should be managed conservatively with repeated vascular imaging studies performed if new symptoms appear due to the possible risk of upconversion.
- DAVFs without CVD presenting with tinnitus and ophthalmologic phenomena should be treated according to the severity of the symptoms and patient's quality of life.
- DAVFs with CVD presenting with aggressive symptoms caused by ICH or NHND should be treated urgently by modalities that can immediately eliminate the risks.
- DAVFs with CVD presenting with less aggressive symptoms such as tinnitus and ophthalmologic phenomena should be treated in properly selected patients; however, the treatment can be scheduled in a more elective manner and the modalities considered can include radiosurgery.
- The treatment strategy should be tailored individually to patients considering the anatomical features of the DAVF, the severity of symptoms, and the potential risk of intracranial hemorrhage.

References

[1] Al-Mahfoudh R, Kirollos R, Mitchell P, Lee M, Nahser H, Javadpour M. Surgical disconnection of the cortical venous reflux for high-grade intracranial dural arteriovenous fistulas. World Neurosurg. 2015; 83(4):652–656

[2] Barcia-Salorio JL, Herandez G, Broseta J, Gonzalez-Darder J, Ciudad J. Radiosurgical treatment of carotid-cavernous fistula. Appl Neurophysiol. 1982; 45(4–5):520–522

[3] Barrow DL, Spector RH, Braun IF, Landman JA, Tindall SC, Tindall GT. Classification and treatment of spontaneous carotid-cavernous sinus fistulas. J Neurosurg. 1985; 62(2):248–256

[4] Borden JA, Wu JK, Shucart WA. A proposed classification for spinal and cranial dural arteriovenous fistulous malformations and implications for treatment. J Neurosurg. 1995; 82(2):166–179

[5] Brown RD, Jr, Flemming KD, Meyer FB, Cloft HJ, Pollock BE, Link ML. Natural history, evaluation, and management of intracranial vascular malformations. Mayo Clin Proc. 2005; 80(2):269–281

[6] Brown RD, Jr, Wiebers DO, Nichols DA. Intracranial dural arteriovenous fistulae: angiographic predictors of intracranial hemorrhage and clinical outcome in nonsurgical patients. J Neurosurg. 1994; 81(4):531–538

[7] Bulters DO, Mathad N, Culliford D, Millar J, Sparrow OC. The natural history of cranial dural arteriovenous fistulae with cortical venous reflux: the significance of venous ectasia. Neurosurgery. 2012; 70(2):312–318, discussion 318–319

[8] Chandra RV, Leslie-Mazwi TM, Mehta BP, et al. Transarterial onyx embolization of cranial dural arteriovenous fistulas: long-term follow-up. AJNR Am J Neuroradiol. 2014; 35(9):1793–1797

[9] Chen CJ, Lee CC, Ding D, et al. Stereotactic radiosurgery for intracranial dural arteriovenous fistulas: a systematic review. J Neurosurg. 2015; 122 (2):353–362

[10] Chi CT, Nguyen D, Duc VT, Chau HH, Son VT. Direct traumatic carotid cavernous fistula: angiographic classification and treatment strategies. Study of 172 cases. Interv Neuroradiol. 2014; 20(4):461–475

[11] Chung SJ, Kim JS, Kim JC, et al. Intracranial dural arteriovenous fistulas: analysis of 60 patients. Cerebrovasc Dis. 2002; 13(2):79–88

[12] Cognard C, Gobin YP, Pierot L, et al. Cerebral dural arteriovenous fistulas: clinical and angiographic correlation with a revised classification of venous drainage. Radiology. 1995; 194(3):671–680

[13] Cognard C, Houdart E, Casasco A, Gabrillargues J, Chiras J, Merland JJ. Long-term changes in intracranial dural arteriovenous fistulae leading to worsening in the type of venous drainage. Neuroradiology. 1997; 39(1): 59–66

[14] Collice M, D'Aliberti G, Talamonti G, et al. Surgical interruption of leptomeningeal drainage as treatment for intracranial dural arteriovenous fistulas without dural sinus drainage. J Neurosurg. 1996; 84(5):810–817

[15] Daniels DJ, Vellimana AK, Zipfel GJ, Lanzino G. Intracranial hemorrhage from dural arteriovenous fistulas: clinical features and outcome. Neurosurg Focus. 2013; 34(5):E15

[16] Davies MA, Saleh J, Ter Brugge K, Willinsky R, Wallace MC. The natural history and management of intracranial dural arteriovenous fistulae. Part 1: benign lesions. Interv Neuroradiol. 1997; 3(4):295–302

[17] Davies MA, Ter Brugge K, Willinsky R, Wallace MC. The natural history and management of intracranial dural arteriovenous fistulae. Part 2: aggressive lesions. Interv Neuroradiol. 1997; 3(4):303–311

[18] Duffau H, Lopes M, Janosevic V, et al. Early rebleeding from intracranial dural arteriovenous fistulas: report of 20 cases and review of the literature. J Neurosurg. 1999; 90(1):78–84

[19] Gross BA, Albuquerque FC, Moon K, McDougall CG. Evolution of treatment and a detailed analysis of occlusion, recurrence, and clinical outcomes in an endovascular library of 260 dural arteriovenous fistulas. J Neurosurg. 2017; 126(6):1884–1893

[20] Gross BA, Du R. The natural history of cerebral dural arteriovenous fistulae. Neurosurgery. 2012; 71(3):594–602, discussion 602–603

[21] Gross BA, Du R. Surgical treatment of high grade dural arteriovenous fistulae. J Clin Neurosci. 2013; 20(11):1527–1532

[22] Hiramatsu M, Sugiu K, Hishikawa T, et al. Results of 1940 embolizations for dural arteriovenous fistulas: Japanese Registry of Neuroendovascular Therapy (JR-NET3). J Neurosurg. 2019; 33:166–173

[23] Iwama T, Hashimoto N, Takagi Y, et al. Hemodynamic and metabolic disturbances in patients with intracranial dural arteriovenous fistulas: positron emission tomography evaluation before and after treatment. J Neurosurg. 1997; 86(5):806–811

[24] Kakarla UK, Deshmukh VR, Zabramski JM, Albuquerque FC, McDougall CG, Spetzler RF. Surgical treatment of high-risk intracranial dural arteriovenous fistulae: clinical outcomes and avoidance of complications. Neurosurgery. 2007; 61(3):447–457, discussion 457–459

[25] Kirsch M, Liebig T, Kühne D, Henkes H. Endovascular management of dural arteriovenous fistulas of the transverse and sigmoid sinus in 150 patients. Neuroradiology. 2009; 51(7):477–483

[26] Kojima T, Miyachi S, Sahara Y, et al. The relationship between venous hypertension and expression of vascular endothelial growth factor: hemodynamic and immunohistochemical examinations in a rat venous hypertension model. Surg Neurol. 2007; 68(3):277–284, discussion 284

[27] Kuroda S, Furukawa K, Shiga T, et al. Pretreatment and posttreatment evaluation of hemodynamic and metabolic parameters in intracranial dural arteriovenous fistulae with cortical venous reflux. Neurosurgery. 2004; 54(3):585–591, discussion 591–592

[28] Kuwayama N, Kubo M, Yamamoto H, et al. Combined surgical and endovascular treatment of high-risk intracranial dural arteriovenous fistulas. J Clin Neurosci. 2002; 9 Suppl 1:11–15

[29] Lasjaunias P, Chiu M, ter Brugge K, Tolia A, Hurth M, Bernstein M. Neurological manifestations of intracranial dural arteriovenous malformations. J Neurosurg. 1986; 64(5):724–730

[30] Lawton MT, Chun J, Wilson CB, Halbach VV. Ethmoidal dural arteriovenous fistulae: an assessment of surgical and endovascular management. Neurosurgery. 1999; 45(4):805–810, discussion 810–811

[31] Letourneau-Guillon L, Cruz JP, Krings T. CT and MR imaging of non-cavernous cranial dural arteriovenous fistulas: findings associated with cortical venous reflux. Eur J Radiol. 2015; 84(8):1555–1563

[32] Liu JK, Dogan A, Ellegala DB, et al. The role of surgery for high-grade intracranial dural arteriovenous fistulas: importance of obliteration of venous outflow. J Neurosurg. 2009; 110(5):913–920

[33] Lucas CP, Zabramski JM, Spetzler RF, Jacobowitz R. Treatment for intracranial dural arteriovenous malformations: a meta-analysis from the English language literature. Neurosurgery. 1997; 40(6):1119–1130, discussion 1130–1132

[34] McConnell KA, Tjoumakaris SI, Allen J, et al. Neuroendovascular management of dural arteriovenous malformations. Neurosurg Clin N Am. 2009; 20(4):431–439

[35] Mossa-Basha M, Chen J, Gandhi D. Imaging of cerebral arteriovenous malformations and dural arteriovenous fistulas. Neurosurg Clin N Am. 2012; 23(1):27–42

[36] Newton TH, Cronqvist S. Involvement of dural arteries in intracranial arteriovenous malformations. Radiology. 1969; 93(5):1071–1078

[37] Park KS, Kang DH, Park SH, Kim YS. The efficacy of gamma knife radiosurgery alone as a primary treatment for intracranial dural arteriovenous fistulas. Acta Neurochir (Wien). 2016; 158(4):821–828

[38] Park SH, Park KS, Kang DH, Hwang JH, Hwang SK. Stereotactic radiosurgery for intracranial dural arteriovenous fistulas: its clinical and angiographic perspectives. Acta Neurochir (Wien). 2017; 159(6):1093–1103

[39] Piippo A, Niemelä M, van Popta J, et al. Characteristics and long-term outcome of 251 patients with dural arteriovenous fistulas in a defined population. J Neurosurg. 2013; 118(5):923–934

[40] Rammos S, Bortolotti C, Lanzino G. Endovascular management of intracranial dural arteriovenous fistulae. Neurosurg Clin N Am. 2014; 25(3):539–549

[41] Rangel-Castilla L, Barber SM, Klucznik R, Diaz O. Mid and long term outcomes of dural arteriovenous fistula endovascular management with Onyx. Experience of a single tertiary center. J Neurointerv Surg. 2014; 6(8):607–613

[42] Reynolds MR, Lanzino G, Zipfel GJ. Intracranial dural arteriovenous fistulae. Stroke. 2017; 48(5):1424–1431

[43] Satomi J, Ghaibeh AA, Moriguchi H, Nagahiro S. Predictability of the future development of aggressive behavior of cranial dural arteriovenous fistulas based on decision tree analysis. J Neurosurg. 2015; 123(1):86–90

[44] Satomi J, Satoh K. Epidemiology and etiology of dural arteriovenous fistula. Brain Nerve. 2008; 60(8):883–886

[45] Satomi J, van Dijk JM, Terbrugge KG, Willinsky RA, Wallace MC. Benign cranial dural arteriovenous fistulas: outcome of conservative management based on the natural history of the lesion. J Neurosurg. 2002; 97(4):767–770

[46] Shah MN, Botros JA, Pilgram TK, et al. Borden-Shucart type I dural arteriovenous fistulas: clinical course including risk of conversion to higher-grade fistulas. J Neurosurg. 2012; 117(3):539–545

[47] Signorelli F, Della Pepa GM, Sabatino G, et al. Diagnosis and management of dural arteriovenous fistulas: a 10 years single-center experience. Clin Neurol Neurosurg. 2015; 128:123–129

[48] Söderman M, Edner G, Ericson K, et al. Gamma knife surgery for dural arteriovenous shunts: 25 years of experience. J Neurosurg. 2006; 104(6):867–875

[49] Söderman M, Pavic L, Edner G, Holmin S, Andersson T. Natural history of dural arteriovenous shunts. Stroke. 2008; 39(6):1735–1739

[50] van Dijk JM, terBrugge KG, Willinsky RA, Wallace MC. Clinical course of cranial dural arteriovenous fistulas with long-term persistent cortical venous reflux. Stroke. 2002; 33(5):1233–1236

[51] van Dijk JM, Terbrugge KG, Willinsky RA, Wallace MC. The natural history of dural arteriovenous shunts: the toronto experience. Stroke. 2009; 40(5):e412–, author reply e413–e414

[52] van Dijk JM, TerBrugge KG, Willinsky RA, Wallace MC. Selective disconnection of cortical venous reflux as treatment for cranial dural arteriovenous fistulas. J Neurosurg. 2004; 101(1):31–35

[53] van Rooij WJ, Sluzewski M, Beute GN. Intracranial dural fistulas with exclusive perimedullary drainage: the need for complete cerebral angiography for diagnosis and treatment planning. AJNR Am J Neuroradiol. 2007; 28(2):348–351

[54] Vellimana AK, Daniels DJ, Shah MN, Zipfel GJ, Lanzino G. Dural arteriovenous fistulas associated with benign meningeal tumors. Acta Neurochir (Wien). 2014; 156(3):535–544

[55] Wachter D, Hans F, Psychogios MN, Knauth M, Rohde V. Microsurgery can cure most intracranial dural arteriovenous fistulae of the sinus and non-sinus type. Neurosurg Rev. 2011; 34(3):337–345, discussion 345

[56] Zipfel GJ, Shah MN, Refai D, Dacey RG, Jr, Derdeyn CP. Cranial dural arteriovenous fistulas: modification of angiographic classification scales based on new natural history data. Neurosurg Focus. 2009; 26(5):E14

22 Natural History and Management Options of Cerebral Metastases

Anthea H. O'Neill, Mendel Castle-Kirszbaum, Cristian Gragnaniello, and Leon T. Lai

Abstract

Cerebral metastases are the most commonly encountered brain tumors in clinical practice. The majority of patients have a known primary malignancy at presentation, and 70% have multiple cerebral metastases. The natural history of untreated cerebral metastases is dismal, and thus treatment should be offered to all but the most severely ill patients. Treatment modality is determined by surgical aims (such as acute relief of mass effect or need for tissue diagnosis), functional status, and patient wishes. Patients with radiosensitive histology, a large burden of intracranial disease, or those with poor functional status are treated with radiotherapy. Solitary, surgically accessible metastases should be offered microsurgical resection with adjuvant radiotherapy to the tumor bed. Treatment is associated with a significant survival benefit, particularly in patients with lung, breast, or renal primary. The management of patients with cerebral metastases is complex and evolving, and is best executed by an experienced multidisciplinary team of surgeons, medical and radiation oncologists, and palliative care physicians.

Keywords: metastases, brain, radiotherapy, radiosurgery, microsurgery, biopsy, natural history

22.1 Introduction

Cerebral metastases are the most encountered brain tumor in clinical practice, comprising up to 50% of cerebral malignancies. An aging population, improved treatment for primary disease, and increasing surveillance of individuals with cancer have seen cerebral metastases increasingly outnumber primary brain tumors in recent years.[1] In decreasing order of frequency, lung, breast, melanoma, renal, and colorectal cancers account for the majority of brain metastases.[2] This list reflects not only the prevalence of the primary malignancy but also its propensity for metastatic spread, tropism for the brain, and ability to establish a metastatic seed in the cerebral microenvironment.

Melanoma appears particularly trophic to brain tissue, with nearly half of all patients developing brain metastases. In approximately 15% of all cases, symptomatic cerebral metastasis is the first indication of malignancy, and by the time cerebral metastases become symptomatic, approximately 70% of patients will have multiple cerebral lesions.[3]

Carcinomatous malignancies are a disease of older age, and it should come as no surprise that the incidence of brain metastases peaks in the 5th to 7th decades.[4] A much smaller spike in incidence occurs in the first decade of life, where leukemia, lymphoma, sarcoma, and germ cell tumors are the most common primary cancer. Brain metastases occur with equal prevalence in both sexes; however, the type of primary cancer responsible differs somewhat, with lung cancer more common in males and breast cancer in females.[5]

The distribution of brain metastases corresponds to the relative volume and blood flow of different parts of the brain,[6] with the exception that the region supplied by the terminal branches of the middle cerebral artery is more greatly affected, presumably as embolic tumor aggregates follow the center of the blood flow column. Clinical studies show that 80% of solitary metastases are in the cerebral hemispheres (▶ Fig. 22.1), while 16% are situated in the cerebellum. Intracranial metastases cause symptoms due to the mass effect of the tumor itself, or the intense vasogenic edema they induce. Symptoms thus depend on the location and eloquence of their bed. Rarely, hormonal dysfunction can occur from metastases to the sella.[7] Symptoms of increased intracranial pressure may develop from obstructive hydrocephalus, large tumor burden, or lesional hemorrhage. In most series, headache is the most common symptom; however, altered cognition, weakness, and seizures all occur in greater than 20% of cases.[8] The latter may be especially common in melanoma given its propensity to involve the cortex and to hemorrhage.

Magnetic resonance imaging (MRI) with gadolinium is the gold standard imaging technique to assess brain metastases.[9] Multiplicity, mass effect, marked vasogenic edema, and contrast enhancement are typical of cerebral metastases, with the addition of gadolinium increasing the sensitivity for detection of small lesions (▶ Fig. 22.2).[10] Metastases are usually iso- or hypointense on T1 and hyperintense on T2; however, the

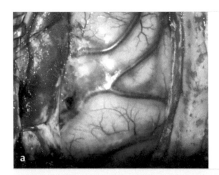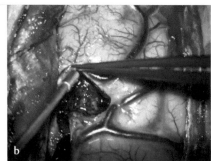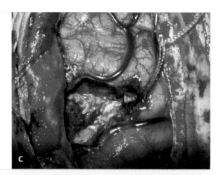

Fig. 22.1 Intraoperative images demonstrating **(a)** a preresection view of a metastatic melanoma involving the cerebral cortex, **(b)** dissection of the tumor, and **(c)** posttumor resection cavity.

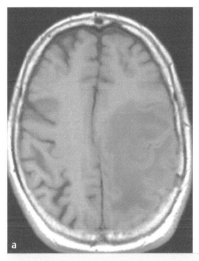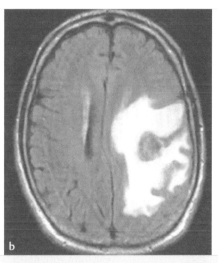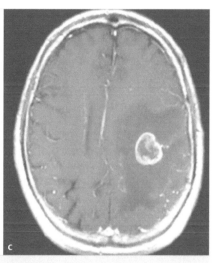

Fig. 22.2 Cerebral metastasis. **(a)** Axial T1 non–contrast-enhanced, **(b)** axial fluid-attenuated inversion recovery (FLAIR), and **(c)** axial T1-weighted contrast-enhanced magnetic resonance images demonstrating a rim-enhancing lesion with surrounding edema.

paramagnetic effects of melanin in melanoma and iron in hemorrhagic lesions may cause intrinsic T1 hyperintensity.

Diffusion-weighted imaging is helpful in the differential diagnosis of brain metastases. The nonenhancing T2 hyperintense area surrounding a metastasis represents vasogenic edema, whereas in high-grade glioma, it may additionally represent tumor invasion, and thus peritumoral apparent diffusion coefficient (ADC) values are typically higher in metastases. Cerebral abscess, another differential, generally demonstrated markedly restricted diffusion in their central necrotic (nonenhancing) region.[11]

22.2 Selected Papers on the Natural History of Cerebral Metastases

- Mulvenna P, Nankivell M, Barton R, et al. Dexamethasone and supportive care with or without whole brain radiotherapy in treating patients with non-small cell lung cancer with brain metastases unsuitable for resection or stereotactic radiotherapy (QUARTZ): results from a phase 3, non-inferiority, randomised trial. Lancet 2016;388(10055):2004–2014
- Fife KM, Colman MH, Stevens GN, et al. Determinants of outcome in melanoma patients with cerebral metastases. J Clin Oncol 2004;22(7):1293–1300

22.3 Natural History of Cerebral Metastases

The natural history of cerebral metastases is difficult to elucidate as most patients in the modern era, even those with poor functional status, will receive some form of therapy. The overall prognosis, in general, is poor and brain metastases are generally the harbinger to end-stage metastatic disease. An overview of currently published case series regarding the survival and cause of death in patients with cerebral metastases is presented in ▶ Table 22.1.[12,13,14,15,16,17,18,19,20,21,22,23,24,25,26,27,28,29,30,31] Based

on our pooled analysis of 1,724 patients over 20 studies, the median survival time of untreated cerebral metastases, or those managed with best supportive care only, is guarded (5.9 weeks from diagnosis; 95% confidence interval [95%CI]: 2.0–8.0). Most patients (72.7%) die from neurological causes, whereas the remaining minority (18.2%) die due to complications of their systemic disease.

Prognostic factors include performance status (e.g., high Karnofsky performance scale), number of brain metastases, number of systemic metastases, control of primary tumor, and age,[32] the former likely being the most important factor.[33]

22.4 Selected Papers on the Treatment Outcomes of Cerebral Metastases

- Patel KR, Burri SH, Boselli D, et al. Comparing pre-operative stereotactic radiosurgery (SRS) to post-operative whole brain radiation therapy (WBRT) for resectable brain metastases: a multi-institutional analysis. J Neurooncol 2017;131(3):611–618
- Yoshida S, Morii K. The role of surgery in the treatment of brain metastasis: a retrospective review. Acta Neurochirurgica 2004;146(8):767–770[34]
- Bowden G, Kano H, Caparosa E, et al. Gamma Knife radiosurgery for the management of cerebral metastases from non-small cell lung cancer. J Neurosurg 2015;122(4):766–772
- Jeene PM, de Vries KC, van Nes JGH, et al. Survival after whole brain radiotherapy for brain metastases from lung cancer and breast cancer is poor in 6325 Dutch patients treated between 2000 and 2014. Acta Oncol 2018;57(5):637–643

22.5 Treatment Options for Cerebral Metastases

Management options for cerebral metastases include supportive care, microsurgical resection, stereotactic radiosurgery (SRS),

Table 22.1 Natural history of cerebral metastases

Studies	Patients	Primary malignancy, n (%)						Median survival, wk (range)	Cause of death			
		Lung	Breast	Melanoma	Renal	GIT	Other		Neurological, n (%; 95%CI)	Systemic, n (%; 95%CI)	Unknown, n (%; 95%CI)	Other, n (%; 95%CI)
Madajewicz et al[24]	15	0	0	15	0	0	0	3.0 (0–12.0)	ne	ne	ne	ne
Pladdet et al[29]	107	ne	ne	ne	ne	ne	ne	11.0 (ne)	ne	ne	ne	ne
Gambardella et al[16]	13	0	0	0	0	0	13	8.0 (ne)	ne	ne	ne	ne
Cormio et al[13]	6	0	0	0	0	0	6	4.0 (4.0–8.0)	ne	ne	ne	ne
Farnell et al[14]	17	0	0	0	0	17	0	2.0 (0–7.8)	ne	ne	ne	ne
Lagerwaard et al[20]	118	0	0	0	0	0	118	5.2 (ne)	ne	ne	ne	ne
Tremont-Lukats et al[30]	68	0	0	0	0	0	61	4.0 (ne)	ne	ne	ne	ne
Fife et al[15]	327	0	0	327	0	0	0	6.8 (ne)	ne	ne	ne	ne
	210	0	0	210	0	0	0	8.4 (ne)	ne	ne	ne	ne
Choi et al[12]	25	0	0	0	0	0	25	2.0 (1.6–2.4)	21	4	0	0
Lee et al[21]	9	0	9	0	0	0	0	8.4 (ne)	ne	ne	ne	ne
Nieder et al[26]	7	4	0	2	1	0	0	5.7 (1.7–12.3)	2	0	2	3
Jung et al[18]	20	0	0	0	0	20	0	1.5 (ne)	ne	ne	ne	ne
Jiang et al[17]	23	0	0	0	0	0	23	1.5 (ne)	17	6	0	0
Langley et al[92]	76	76	0	0	0	0	0	7.3 (ne)	ne	ne	ne	ne
Nieder et al[27]	41	23	2	9	2	3	2	6.8 (ne)	ne	ne	ne	ne
	17	17	0	0	0	0	0	7.6 (ne)	ne	ne	ne	ne
Lim and Lin[22]	41	0	0	0	0	0	41	2.0 (1.6–2.4)	ne	ne	ne	ne
Ostheimer et al[28]	16	0	16	0	0	0	0	6.0 (ne)	ne	ne	ne	ne
Lin et al[23]	38	0	0	0	0	38	0	1.2 (ne)	ne	ne	ne	ne
Mulvenna et al[25]	269	269	0	0	0	0	0	8.5 (ne)	ne	ne	ne	ne
Ryoo et al[31]	261	261	0	0	0	0	0	9.9 (ne)	ne	ne	ne	ne
	1,724	650 (37.7)	27 (1.6)	563 (32.7)	3 (0.2)	78 (4.5)	289 (16.8)	5.9 (95%CI: 2.0–8.0) (0–12.3)	40 (72.7; 95%CI: 59.7–82.7)	10 (18.2; 95% CI: 10.2–30.3)	2 (3.6; 95% CI: 1.0–12.3)	3 (5.5; 95%CI: 1.9–14.9)

Abbreviations: CI, confidence interval; GIT, gastrointestinal tract; ne, not extractable.

Table 22.2 Summary of the literature regarding the management of cerebral metastases according to primary malignancy

	Lung (56 studies)	Breast (37 studies)	Melanoma (25 studies)	Renal (14 studies)	GIT (12 studies)
Study period	1974–2015	1970–2014	1952–2015	1974–2014	1974–2012
No. of patients (n)	19,020	7,523	7,874	1,225	1,229
Treatment modality[a]					
Surgery (%)	2.8	4.5	5.2	4.1	5.0
Surgery + radiotherapy (%)	0.8	1.8	10.3	1.7	9.4
Surgery + systemic (%)	0.0	0.0	0.0	0.0	0.0
Systemic (%)	11.8	26.9	22.1	39.8	0.5
Systemic + radiotherapy (%)	6.9	5.3	1.4	3.3	4.1
SRS (%)	29.2	24.0	43.3	45.0	41.7
WBRT (%)	46.5	66.2	27.1	15.2	33.7
SRS + WBRT (%)	4.2	1.8	5.3	4.3	3.2
Other radiotherapy (%)	4.5	0.0	0.0	0.0	0.0
Median OS, mo (95%CI) (range)	10.7 (95%CI: 8.5–13.0) (0–175.0)	11.3 (95%CI: 9.0–13.8) (0–126.0)	7.0 (95%CI: 6.4–8.9) (0–114.3)	10.8 (95%CI: 8.1–12.9) (ne)	6.8 (95%CI: 4.9–9.8) (ne)
Mean 12-mo actuarial survival (%)	44.9 (95%CI: 37.6–52.3)	38.0 (95%CI: 29.9–36.1)	15.9 (95%CI: 3.1–26.7)	40.5 (95%CI: –57.8 to 135.8)	9.6 (95%CI: –111.8 to 130.9)
Median PFS, % (95%CI) (range)	7.2 (95%CI: 5.7–11.6) (0–85.0)	5.5 (95%CI: 2.4–7.4) (ne)	2.8 (95%CI: 1.1–4.3) (0–10.9)	5.6 (na) (ne)	Ne

Abbreviations: CI, confidence interval; GIT, gastrointestinal tract; na, not applicable; ne, not extractable; OS, overall survival; PFS, progression-free survival; SRS, stereotactic radiosurgery; WBRT, whole brain radiation therapy.
[a]Some patients underwent treatment with multiple therapies.

whole brain radiotherapy (WBRT), systemic treatments, or a combination thereof. The results of a literature review performed of the available treatment options published between 1952 and 2018 are presented in ▶ Table 22.2 and ▶ Table 22.3.[14,15,18,20,21,25,27,31,35,36,37,38,39,40,41,42,43,44,45,46,47,48,49, 50,51,52,53,54,55,56,57,58,59,60,61,62,63,64,65,66,67,68,69,70,71,72,73,74,75,76,77,78,79,80, 81,82,83,84,85,86,87,88,89,90,91,92,93,94,95,96,97,98,99,100,101,102,103,104,105,106,107, 108,109,110,111,112,113,114,115,116,117,118,119,120,121,122,123,124,125,126,127,128,129, 130,131,132,133,134,135,136,137,138,139,140,141,142,143,144,145,146,147,148,149,150,151, 152,153,154,155,156,157,158,159,160,161,162,163,164,165,166,167,168,169,170,171,172,173, 174,175,176,177,178,179,180,181,182,183,184]

Treatment recommendations should be offered in the view to improve the quality and quantity of the patient's remaining life. The selection of treatment modality must be tailored to the individual, considering factors such as the type of primary malignancy, their functional status, the size, multiplicity, and location of metastases, but most importantly the patient's and family's attitudes and wishes.

Our recommended management plan for cerebral metastases is outlined in ▶ Fig. 22.3.[185] For those patients who present without a known primary malignancy, histological diagnosis is therefore required in addition to whole body imaging and pathology workup. In these circumstances, surgical resection or stereotactic biopsy should be offered to obtain tissue, which is important to confirm the diagnosis of metastatic disease, for selection of subsequent therapy, and prognostication. For patients who present in extremis due to severe raised intracranial pressure from hemorrhage, obstructive hydrocephalus, or herniation, emergency surgery may be performed prior to extensive investigations of the systemic oncological burden.

22.5.1 Supportive

Corticosteroids provide temporary symptomatic relief of symptoms related to peritumoral vasogenic edema.[186,187] Side effects are dose and duration dependent, and thus the lowest dose at which the patient remains asymptomatic should be used. Steroids have been shown to reduce vasogenic edema radiologically,[188] and should be considered in all patients with symptomatic metastases. Dexamethasone is commonly used, due to its lack of mineralocorticoid activity and long half-life.

The literature does not support routine use of prophylactic antiepileptic medications for those with cerebral metastases[189]; however, data are scant and mostly predate the availability of novel agents with less morbid side effect profiles. Such agents (e.g., levetiracetam) have shifted the point of clinical equipoise such that many patients are prescribed prophylaxis.

22.5.2 Surgery

In appropriately selected patients, with suitable lesions, treatment with microsurgical resection followed by either SRS or WBRT is recommended to maximize overall survival and decrease rates of local recurrence.[190] Conversely, there is lack of sufficient data to recommend surgery in patients with unfavorable prognostic factors such as poor performance status, advanced systemic disease, or large intracranial burden of disease. The caveat is patients with large lesions with symptomatic mass effect, where surgical decompression is necessary.

Table 22.3 Summary of the literature regarding the management of cerebral metastases according to treatment modality

	Surgery (21 studies)	Surgery + radiotherapy (29 studies)	SRS (70 studies)	WBRT (53 studies)	SRS + WBRT (7 studies)	Systemic (20 studies)	All treatments (166 studies)
Study period	1952–2016	1952–2016	1975–2016	1952–2016	1985–2015	1970–2015	1952–2016
No. of patients (n)	2,782	2,817	29,411	17,537	1,984	2,775	63,553
Primary cancer							
Lung (%)	34.8	19.6	54.2	52.7	53.0	44.5	50.1
Breast (%)	9.8	9.9	14.3	24.6	10.5	16.0	17.7
Melanoma (%)	14.2	24.4	11.7	6.9	15.7	24.2	12.7
Renal (%)	2.1	2.8	5.8	0.8	3.5	15.3	4.2
GIT (%)	8.3	5.4	7.1	2.1	2.9	0.0	4.9
Other (%)	9.1	9.5	5.2	1.6	4.0	0.0	4.0
Combined (%)	21.7	28.9	2.2	11.3	10.8	0.0	6.4
Median OS (mo) (95%CI) (range)	8.5 (95%CI: 7.2–11.3) (0.1–116.0)	12.7 (95%CI: 11.0–13.8) (0.6–114.0)	9.2 (95%CI: 8.3–10.4) (0.1–175.0)	4.4 (95%CI: 3.7–5.8) (0–86.0)	9.0 (95%CI: 7.1–14.0) (0.2–64.8)	9.2 (95%CI: 5.7–13.9) (0–98.0)	8.9 (95%CI: 8.3–10.0) (0–175.0)
Mean 12-mo actuarial survival (%) (95%CI)	44.7 (95%CI: 29.4–60.0)	57.6 (95%CI: 54.0–61.2)	42.1 (95%CI: 36.7–47.6)	27.2 (95%CI: 20.2–34.1)	48.9 (95%CI: 33.3–64.4)	34.5 (95%CI: 17.7–51.4)	39.4 (95%CI: 36.0–42.9)
Response rate							
Complete response (%)	na	83.3*	20.4	9.0	30.5	4.6	16.7
Partial response (%)	na	na	36.4	30.1	31.8	25.0	31.3
Stable disease (%)	na	0.0	18.8	21.8	24.5	31.9	22.6
Progression (%)	na	16.7	14.0	34.1	8.9	33.5	21.4
Degree of resection							
Gross total resection (%)	61.2	81.5	na	na	na	na	72.4
Subtotal resection (%)	38.8	18.5	na	na	na	na	27.6
Median PFS, % (95%CI) (range)	6.5 (95%CI: 3.6–8.1) (ne)	10.4 (95%CI: 6.0–27.5) (3.0–17.0)	8.5 (95%CI: 5.3–12.4) (6.0–42.0)	6.9 (95%CI: 4.8–11.3) (0–85.0)	8.1 (na) (ne)	5.2 (95%CI 3.1–8.6) (0–10.9)	6.0 (95%CI 5.2–8.0) (0–85.0)

Abbreviations: CI, confidence interval; GIT, gastrointestinal tract; na, not applicable; ne, not extractable; OS, overall survival; PFS, progression-free survival; SRS, stereotactic radiosurgery; WBRT, whole brain radiation therapy.

22.5.3 Whole Brain Radiotherapy

WBRT is a simple and widely used method for treating brain metastasis and is the method of choice for treating patients with many lesions, poor functional status, advanced systemic disease, or radiosensitive histologies (lymphoma, small cell lung carcinoma). Moreover, it is often utilized as an adjuvant to SRS or surgery to decrease rates of local and distant recurrence. The neurocognitive consequences of WBRT include extreme lethargy in the immediate posttreatment period and increased risk of significant neurocognitive decline, which may present as early as 3 months after treatment and persist lifelong. Hippocampal sparing WBRT and the addition of the NMDA antagonist memantine have both been demonstrated to reduce the risk of delayed neurocognitive toxicity.[191,192]

Compared to SRS or surgery alone, the addition of WBRT improves intracranial progression-free survival, and local and distant recurrence, but not overall survival.[193,194] There are no prospective randomized controlled trials in patients with more than 4 brain lesions; however, data from class III studies demonstrate the addition of WBRT to surgery or SRS does not improve survival in patients with more than 4 lesions unless the summative volume exceeds 7 mL or there are more than 15 metastases.[195] Interestingly, human epidermal growth factor receptor 2 (HER-2) positive status in breast carcinoma and epidermal growth factor receptor (EGFR) mutation in non-small-cell lung carcinoma (NSCLC) predict a beneficial response to WBRT.

22.5.4 Stereotactic Radiosurgery

SRS utilizes well-collimated, noncoplanar beams of ionizing radiation to provide focused, high-dose radiation to a small target volume.[196] It can be thought of as an alternative to conventional surgery, with the benefits of being less invasive, and conferring a lower risk of hemorrhage, infection, and tumor seeding. However, mass effect and edema are not immediately relieved as with surgery and no tissue is procured for diagnosis.

SRS is a valid alternative to surgery where surgery is likely to induce new, debilitating neurological deficits and tumor volume and location are protective for radiation-induced injury to surrounding structures.[197] Generally, an upper limit for lesion diameter of 3 cm is given to avoid radiation-induced injury, though hypofractionated SRS can be offered in larger lesions.

SRS may be used as the primary treatment for small, inaccessible, or multiple lesions, and additionally as an adjunct to surgery to decrease the risk of local recurrence in the tumor bed, but not overall survival. In patients with multiple lesions, SRS

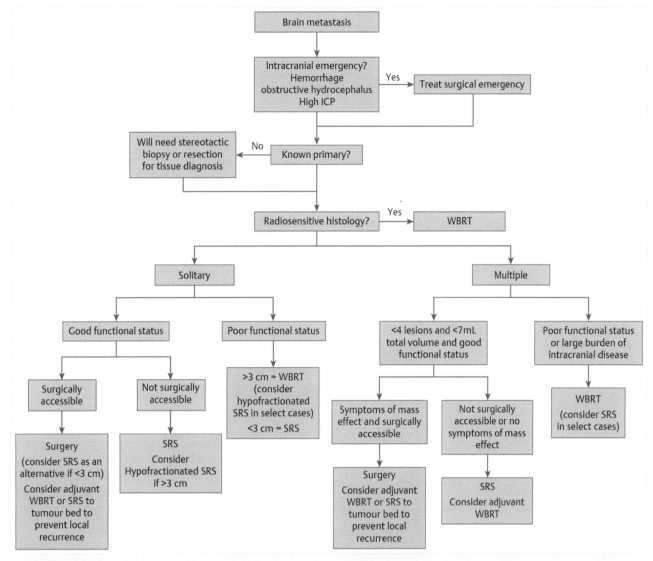

Fig. 22.3 Simplified recommended treatment algorithm for management of patients with new brain metastases (ICP, intracranial pressure; SRS, stereotactic radiosurgery; WBRT, whole brain radiation therapy).

alone is appropriate when total tumor volume is less than 7 mL and there are no debilitating symptoms of mass effect.[197]

22.5.5 Chemotherapy and Novel Agents

Routine cytotoxic chemotherapy alone for brain metastases has not been shown to increase overall survival. Several reasons may account for this ineffectiveness, including the presence of the blood–brain barrier and the fact that cerebral metastases are often seen in patients who have already failed chemotherapy and thus selection for chemoresistant tumor clones has already occurred. Small cell lung, germ cell, and breast carcinomas appear to be the few chemoresponsive metastases.[2]

Immune checkpoint inhibitors, monoclonal antibodies to cytotoxic T-lymphocyte-associated protein 4 (CTLA-4), programmed cell death protein 1 (PD-1), and programmed death-ligand 1 (PD-L1), are novel agents with substantial efficacy in certain tumor types, including melanoma and NSCLC. Early trials of checkpoint inhibitors have shown intracranial

activity, but further trials are needed to establish their role in the treatment of brain metastases.[198]

22.5.6 Treatment Outcomes by Primary Malignancy

Most cases of cerebral metastases from primary lung cancer and breast cancer are treated with WBRT (46.5 and 66.2%, respectively). Melanoma metastases are most likely to undergo SRS (43.3%) or surgery with adjuvant radiotherapy (10.3%). Patients with renal cell carcinoma are frequently treated with systemic therapies (39.8%) or SRS (45.0%). Radiosurgery is also commonly used to treat metastases from gastrointestinal tract (GIT) malignancies (41.7%).

Patients with cerebral metastases from lung, breast, and renal cell carcinoma are most likely to experience a significant survival benefit following treatment, with a median overall survival of 10.7, 11.3, and 10.8 months, and a 12-month survival rate of 44.9,

38.0, and 40.5%, respectively. However, patients with melanoma and GIT metastases do not respond as readily, with a median survival of just 7.0 and 6.8 months, and a 12-month survival of 15.9 and 9.6%, respectively.

Currently published literature demonstrates that the greatest survival benefit in patients with cerebral metastases is to be gained via treatment with a combination of microsurgical excision and radiotherapy (SRS or WBRT), with a median survival of 12.7 months, and a 12-month actuarial survival of 57.6% following therapy. Microsurgery, SRS, SRS combined with WBRT, and systemic therapies exhibit similar efficacy, with a median survival of 8.5, 9.2, 9.0, and 9.2%, respectively, and approximately 40% of patients surviving to 12 months. However, the efficacy of WBRT alone appears diminished in comparison, with patients managed with this modality surviving only a median 4.4 months following treatment, and only 27.2% surviving for 12 months.

Overall, patients with a cerebral metastasis treated with any methodology have a median survival of 8.9 months, and 39.4% can be expected to live longer than 12 months following treatment.

22.6 Authors' Recommendations

- Our recommended treatment strategy is summarized in ▸ Fig. 22.3.
- Quality of life, as well as overall survival, should be a key consideration in decision-making regarding treatment modality.
- Treatment modality should be a highly individualized decision based on both patient factors (functional status, primary cancer) and tumor factors (size, multiplicity, location).
- In all but the most severely ill patients, treatment of cerebral metastases should be offered, given the overall survival benefit associated with intervention.
- Patients with primary malignancies arising from the lung, breast, or kidneys are most likely to receive significant benefit from treatment of their cerebral metastases.
- In appropriately selected patients, with suitable lesions, treatment with microsurgical resection followed by either SRS to the tumor bed or WBRT is recommended to maximize overall survival and decrease the risk of local recurrence.
- Microsurgery alone, SRS, targeted systemic treatments, or a combination of SRS and WBRT may also be utilized in the treatment of cerebral metastases in appropriate cases. All have similar efficacy, and thus decision-making should be based on individual patient factors.
- WBRT as a stand-alone treatment should be reserved for patients in whom the above-mentioned therapies are inappropriate.

References

[1] Dolgushin M, Kornienko V, Pronin I. Prevalence of brain metastases. In: Brain Metastases. Cham: Springer International Publishing; 2018:3–8

[2] Kaye AH, Laws ER, eds. Brain Tumors: An Encyclopedic Approach. 3rd ed. New York, NY: Saunders/Elsevier; 2012

[3] Cagney DN, Martin AM, Catalano PJ, et al. Incidence and prognosis of patients with brain metastases at diagnosis of systemic malignancy: a population-based study. Neuro-oncol. 2017; 19(11):1511–1521

[4] Takakura K, ed. Metastatic Tumors of the Central Nervous System. 1st ed. Tokyo: Igaku-Shoin; 1982

[5] Walker AE, Robins M, Weinfeld FD. Epidemiology of brain tumors: the national survey of intracranial neoplasms. Neurology. 1985; 35(2):219–226

[6] Delattre JY, Krol G, Thaler HT, Posner JB. Distribution of brain metastases. Arch Neurol. 1988; 45(7):741–744

[7] Castle-Kirszbaum M, Goldschlager T, Ho B, Wang YY, King J. Twelve cases of pituitary metastasis: a case series and review of the literature. Pituitary. 2018; 21(5):463–473

[8] Lassman AB, DeAngelis LM. Brain metastases. Neurol Clin. 2003; 21(1):1–23, vii

[9] Davis PC, Hudgins PA, Peterman SB, Hoffman JC, Jr. Diagnosis of cerebral metastases: double-dose delayed CT vs contrast-enhanced MR imaging. AJNR Am J Neuroradiol. 1991; 12(2):293–300

[10] Balériaux D, Colosimo C, Ruscalleda J, et al. Magnetic resonance imaging of metastatic disease to the brain with gadobenate dimeglumine. Neuroradiology. 2002; 44(3):191–203

[11] Fink KR, Fink JR. Imaging of brain metastases. Surg Neurol Int. 2013; 4 Suppl 4:S209–S219

[12] Choi HJ, Cho BC, Sohn JH, et al. Brain metastases from hepatocellular carcinoma: prognostic factors and outcome—brain metastasis from HCC. J Neurooncol. 2009; 91(3):307–313

[13] Cormio G, Lissoni A, Losa G, Zanetta G, Pellegrino A, Mangioni C. Brain metastases from endometrial carcinoma. Gynecol Oncol. 1996; 61(1):40–43

[14] Farnell GF, Buckner JC, Cascino TL, O'Connell MJ, Schomberg PJ, Suman V. Brain metastases from colorectal carcinoma. The long term survivors. Cancer. 1996; 78(4):711–716

[15] Fife KM, Colman MH, Stevens GN, et al. Determinants of outcome in melanoma patients with cerebral metastases. J Clin Oncol. 2004; 22(7):1293–1300

[16] Gambardella G, Santamaria LB, Toscano SG, et al. Brain metastases: surgical versus conservative treatment. J Neurosurg Sci. 1990; 34(3–4):309–314

[17] Jiang XS, Xiao JP, Zhang Y, et al. Hypofractionated stereotactic radiotherapy for brain metastases larger than three centimeters. Radiat Oncol. 2012; 7(1):36

[18] Jung M, Ahn JB, Chang JH, et al. Brain metastases from colorectal carcinoma: prognostic factors and outcome. J Neurooncol. 2011; 101(1):49–55

[19] Langley RR, Fidler IJ. The biology of brain metastasis. Clin Chem. 2013; 59(1):180–189

[20] Lagerwaard FJ, Levendag PC, Nowak PJ, Eijkenboom WM, Hanssens PE, Schmitz PI. Identification of prognostic factors in patients with brain metastases: a review of 1292 patients. Int J Radiat Oncol Biol Phys. 1999; 43(4):795–803

[21] Lee SS, Ahn J-H, Kim MK, et al. Brain metastases in breast cancer: prognostic factors and management. Breast Cancer Res Treat. 2008; 111(3):523–530

[22] Lim E, Lin NU. Updates on the management of breast cancer brain metastases. Oncology (Williston Park). 2014; 28(7):572–578

[23] Lin L, Zhao C-H, Ge F-J, et al. Patients with brain metastases derived from gastrointestinal cancer: clinical characteristics and prognostic factors. Clin Transl Oncol. 2016; 18(1):93–98

[24] Madajewicz S, Karakousis C, West CR, Caracandas J, Avellanosa AM. Malignant melanoma brain metastases. Review of Roswell Park Memorial Institute experience. Cancer. 1984; 53(11):2550–2552

[25] Mulvenna P, Nankivell M, Barton R, et al. Dexamethasone and supportive care with or without whole brain radiotherapy in treating patients with non-small cell lung cancer with brain metastases unsuitable for resection or stereotactic radiotherapy (QUARTZ): results from a phase 3, non-inferiority, randomised trial. Lancet. 2016; 388(10055):2004–2014

[26] Nieder C, Spanne O, Mehta MP, Grosu AL, Geinitz H. Presentation, patterns of care, and survival in patients with brain metastases: what has changed in the last 20 years? Cancer. 2011; 117(11):2505–2512

[27] Nieder C, Norum J, Dalhaug A, Aandahl G, Pawinski A. Radiotherapy versus best supportive care in patients with brain metastases and adverse prognostic factors. Clin Exp Metastasis. 2013; 30(6):723–729

[28] Ostheimer C, Bormann C, Fiedler E, Marsch W, Vordermark D. Malignant melanoma brain metastases: treatment results and prognostic factors—a single-center retrospective study. Int J Oncol. 2015; 46(6):2439–2448

[29] Pladdet I, Boven E, Nauta J, Pinedo HM. Palliative care for brain metastases of solid tumour types. Neth J Med. 1989; 34(1–2):10–21

[30] Tremont-Lukats IW, Bobustuc G, Lagos GK, Lolas K, Kyritsis AP, Puduvalli VK. Brain metastasis from prostate carcinoma: the M. D. Anderson Cancer Center experience. Cancer. 2003; 98(2):363–368

[31] Ryoo JJ, Batech M, Zheng C, et al. Radiotherapy for brain metastases near the end of life in an integrated health care system. Ann Palliat Med. 2017; 6 Suppl 1:S28–S38

[32] Dorai Z, Sawaya R, Alfred Yung WK. Brain metastasis. In: Tonn J-C, Grossman SA, Rutka JT, Westphal M, eds. Neuro-Oncology of CNS Tumors. Berlin: Springer-Verlag; 2006:303–323

[33] Gaspar L, Scott C, Rotman M, et al. Recursive partitioning analysis (RPA) of prognostic factors in three Radiation Therapy Oncology Group (RTOG) brain metastases trials. Int J Radiat Oncol Biol Phys. 1997; 37(4):745–751

[34] Yoshida S, Morii K. The role of surgery in the treatment of brain metastasis: a retrospective review. Acta Neurochir (Wien). 2004; 146(8):767–770

[35] Agarwala SS, Kirkwood JM, Gore M, et al. Temozolomide for the treatment of brain metastases associated with metastatic melanoma: a phase II study. J Clin Oncol. 2004; 22(11):2101–2107

[36] Amsbaugh MJ, Yusuf MB, Gaskins J, et al. A dose-volume response model for brain metastases treated with frameless single-fraction robotic radiosurgery: seeking to better predict response to treatment. Technol Cancer Res Treat. 2017; 16(3):344–351

[37] Andrews DW, Scott CB, Sperduto PW, et al. Whole brain radiation therapy with or without stereotactic radiosurgery boost for patients with one to three brain metastases: phase III results of the RTOG 9508 randomised trial. Lancet. 2004; 363(9422):1665–1672

[38] Aoyama H, Shirato H, Tago M, et al. Stereotactic radiosurgery plus whole-brain radiation therapy vs stereotactic radiosurgery alone for treatment of brain metastases: a randomized controlled trial. JAMA. 2006; 295(21):2483–2491

[39] Arita H, Narita Y, Miyakita Y, Ohno M, Sumi M, Shibui S. Risk factors for early death after surgery in patients with brain metastases: reevaluation of the indications for and role of surgery. J Neurooncol. 2014; 116(1):145–152

[40] Aydemir F, Tufan K, Cekinmez M, et al. Prognostic impact of histologic subtype in non-small cell lung cancer patients treated with gamma knife radiosurgery: retrospective analysis of 104 patients. Turk Neurosurg. 2017; 27(1):14–21

[41] Baek JY, Kang MH, Hong YS, et al. Characteristics and prognosis of patients with colorectal cancer-associated brain metastases in the era of modern systemic chemotherapy. J Neurooncol. 2011; 104(3):745–753

[42] Bernhardt D, Adeberg S, Bozorgmehr F, et al. Outcome and prognostic factors in patients with brain metastases from small-cell lung cancer treated with whole brain radiotherapy. J Neurooncol. 2017; 134(1):205–212

[43] Bougie E, Masson-Côté L, Mathieu D. Comparison between surgical resection and stereotactic radiosurgery in patients with a single brain metastasis from non-small cell lung cancer. World Neurosurg. 2015; 83(6):900–906

[44] Bowden G, Kano H, Caparosa E, et al. Gamma Knife radiosurgery for the management of cerebral metastases from non-small cell lung cancer. J Neurosurg. 2015; 122(4):766–772

[45] Braccini AL, Azria D, Thezenas S, Romieu G, Ferrero JM, Jacot W. Prognostic factors of brain metastases from breast cancer: impact of targeted therapies. Breast. 2013; 22(5):993–998

[46] Brown PD, Ballman KV, Cerhan JH, et al. Postoperative stereotactic radiosurgery compared with whole brain radiotherapy for resected metastatic brain disease (NCCTG N107C/CEC·3): a multicentre, randomised, controlled, phase 3 trial. Lancet Oncol. 2017; 18(8):1049–1060

[47] Brown PD, Jaeckle K, Ballman KV, et al. Effect of radiosurgery alone vs radiosurgery with whole brain radiation therapy on cognitive function in patients with 1 to 3 brain metastases: a randomized clinical trial. JAMA. 2016; 316(4):401–409

[48] Buglione M, Pedretti S, Gipponi S, et al. Neuro-Oncology Group, Spedali Civili Hospital and Brescia University. The treatment of patients with 1–3 brain metastases: is there a place for whole brain radiotherapy alone, yet? A retrospective analysis. Radiol Med (Torino). 2015; 120(12):1146–1152

[49] Cai Y, Wang J-Y, Liu H. Clinical observation of whole brain radiotherapy concomitant with targeted therapy for brain metastasis in non-small cell lung cancer patients with chemotherapy failure. Asian Pac J Cancer Prev. 2013; 14(10):5699–5703

[50] Cairncross JG, Kim JH, Posner JB. Radiation therapy for brain metastases. Ann Neurol. 1980; 7(6):529–541

[51] Cao KI, Lebas N, Gerber S, et al. Phase II randomized study of whole-brain radiation therapy with or without concurrent temozolomide for brain metastases from breast cancer. Ann Oncol. 2015; 26(1):89–94

[52] Chabot P, Hsia T-C, Ryu J-S, et al. Veliparib in combination with whole-brain radiation therapy for patients with brain metastases from non-small cell lung cancer: results of a randomized, global, placebo-controlled study. J Neurooncol. 2017; 131(1):105–115

[53] Chan S, Rowbottom L, McDonald R, et al. Could time of whole brain radiotherapy delivery impact overall survival in patients with multiple brain metastases? Ann Palliat Med. 2016; 5(4):267–279

[54] Chang WS, Kim HY, Chang JW, Park YG, Chang JH. Analysis of radiosurgical results in patients with brain metastases according to the number of brain lesions: is stereotactic radiosurgery effective for multiple brain metastases? J Neurosurg. 2010; 113 Suppl:73–78

[55] Chen JCT, Petrovich Z, O'Day S, et al. Stereotactic radiosurgery in the treatment of metastatic disease to the brain. Neurosurgery. 2000; 47(2):268–279, discussion 279–281

[56] Chen Y, Yang J, Li X, et al. First-line epidermal growth factor receptor (EGFR)-tyrosine kinase inhibitor alone or with whole-brain radiotherapy for brain metastases in patients with EGFR-mutated lung adenocarcinoma. Cancer Sci. 2016; 107(12):1800–1805

[57] Choi KN, Withers HR, Rotman M. Metastatic melanoma in brain. Rapid treatment or large dose fractions. Cancer. 1985; 56(1):10–15

[58] Choi CYH, Chang SD, Gibbs IC, et al. What is the optimal treatment of large brain metastases? An argument for a multidisciplinary approach. Int J Radiat Oncol Biol Phys. 2012; 84(3):688–693

[59] Combs SE, Schulz-Ertner D, Thilmann C, Edler L, Debus J. Treatment of cerebral metastases from breast cancer with stereotactic radiosurgery. Strahlenther Onkol. 2004; 180(9):590–596

[60] Dawood S, Gonzalez-Angulo AM, Albarracin C, et al. Prognostic factors of survival in the trastuzumab era among women with breast cancer and brain metastases who receive whole brain radiotherapy: a single-institution review. Cancer. 2010; 116(13):3084–3092

[61] Deinsberger R, Tidstrand J. LINAC radiosurgery as single treatment in cerebral metastases. J Neurooncol. 2006; 76(1):77–83

[62] D'Elia F, Bonucci I, Biti GP, Pirtoli L. Different fractionation schedules in radiation treatment of cerebral metastases. Acta Radiol Oncol. 1986; 25(3):181–184

[63] DiLuna ML, King JT, Jr, Knisely JPS, Chiang VL. Prognostic factors for survival after stereotactic radiosurgery vary with the number of cerebral metastases. Cancer. 2007; 109(1):135–145

[64] Doherty MK, Korpanty GJ, Tomasini P, et al. Treatment options for patients with brain metastases from EGFR/ALK-driven lung cancer. Radiother Oncol. 2017; 123(2):195–202

[65] Dyer MA, Arvold ND, Chen Y-H, et al. The role of whole brain radiation therapy in the management of melanoma brain metastases. Radiat Oncol. 2014; 9(1):143

[66] Edelman MJ, Belani CP, Socinski MA, et al. Alpha Oncology Research Network. Outcomes associated with brain metastases in a three-arm phase III trial of gemcitabine-containing regimens versus paclitaxel plus carboplatin for advanced non-small cell lung cancer. J Thorac Oncol. 2010; 5(1):110–116

[67] Emery A, Trifiletti DM, Romano KD, Patel N, Smolkin ME, Sheehan JP. More than just the number of brain metastases: evaluating the impact of brain metastasis location and relative volume on overall survival after stereotactic radiosurgery. World Neurosurg. 2017; 99:111–117

[68] Feigl GC, Horstmann GA. Volumetric follow up of brain metastases: a useful method to evaluate treatment outcome and predict survival after Gamma Knife surgery? J Neurosurg. 2006; 105 Suppl:91–98

[69] Fleckenstein K, Hof H, Lohr F, Wenz F, Wannenmacher M. Prognostic factors for brain metastases after whole brain radiotherapy. Data from a single institution. Strahlenther Onkol. 2004; 180(5):268–273

[70] Franciosi V, Cocconi G, Michiara M, et al. Front-line chemotherapy with cisplatin and etoposide for patients with brain metastases from breast carcinoma, nonsmall cell lung carcinoma, or malignant melanoma: a prospective study. Cancer. 1999; 85(7):1599–1605

[71] Gaudy-Marqueste C, Dussouil AS, Carron R, et al. Survival of melanoma patients treated with targeted therapy and immunotherapy after systematic upfront control of brain metastases by radiosurgery. Eur J Cancer. 2017; 84:44–54

[72] Gerber NK, Yamada Y, Rimner A, et al. Erlotinib versus radiation therapy for brain metastases in patients with EGFR-mutant lung adenocarcinoma. Int J Radiat Oncol Biol Phys. 2014; 89(2):322–329

[73] Golden DW, Lamborn KR, McDermott MW, et al. Prognostic factors and grading systems for overall survival in patients treated with radiosurgery for brain metastases: variation by primary site. J Neurosurg. 2008; 109 Suppl:77–86

[74] Gonda DD, Kim TE, Goetsch SJ, et al. Prognostic factors for stereotactic radiosurgery-treated patients with cerebral metastasis: implications on randomised control trial design and inter-institutional collaboration. Eur J Cancer. 2014; 50(6):1148–1158

[75] Gore ME, Szczylik C, Porta C, et al. Safety and efficacy of sunitinib for metastatic renal-cell carcinoma: an expanded-access trial. Lancet Oncol. 2009; 10(8):757–763

[76] Graham PH, Bucci J, Browne L. Randomized comparison of whole brain radiotherapy, 20 Gy in four daily fractions versus 40 Gy in 20 twice-daily fractions, for brain metastases. Int J Radiat Oncol Biol Phys. 2010; 77(3):648–654

[77] Grønberg BH, Ciuleanu T, Fløtten Ø, et al. A placebo-controlled, randomized phase II study of maintenance enzastaurin following whole brain radiation therapy in the treatment of brain metastases from lung cancer. Lung Cancer. 2012; 78(1):63–69

[78] Harris KB, Corbett MR, Mascarenhas H, et al. A single-institution analysis of 126 patients treated with stereotactic radiosurgery for brain metastases. Front Oncol. 2017; 7:90

[79] Hashimoto K, Narita Y, Miyakita Y, et al. Comparison of clinical outcomes of surgery followed by local brain radiotherapy and surgery followed by whole brain radiotherapy in patients with single brain metastasis: single-center retrospective analysis. Int J Radiat Oncol Biol Phys. 2011; 81(4):e475–e480

[80] Iorio-Morin C, Masson-Côté L, Ezahr Y, Blanchard J, Ebacher A, Mathieu D. Early Gamma Knife stereotactic radiosurgery to the tumor bed of resected brain metastasis for improved local control. J Neurosurg. 2014; 121 Suppl:69–74

[81] Jeene PM, de Vries KC, van Nes JGH, et al. Survival after whole brain radiotherapy for brain metastases from lung cancer and breast cancer is poor in 6325 Dutch patients treated between 2000 and 2014. Acta Oncol. 2018; 57(5):637–643

[82] Jiang T, Su C, Li X, et al. EGFR TKIs plus WBRT demonstrated no survival benefit other than that of TKIs alone in patients with NSCLC and EGFR mutation and brain metastases. J Thorac Oncol. 2016; 11(10):1718–1728

[83] Karam I, Hamilton S, Nichol A, et al. Population-based outcomes after brain radiotherapy in patients with brain metastases from breast cancer in the Pre-Trastuzumab and Trastuzumab eras. Radiat Oncol. 2013; 8(1):12

[84] Karlsson B, Hanssens P, Wolff R, Söderman M, Lindquist C, Beute G. Thirty years' experience with Gamma Knife surgery for metastases to the brain. J Neurosurg. 2009; 111(3):449–457

[85] Keller A, Doré M, Cebula H, et al. Hypofractionated stereotactic radiation therapy to the resection bed for intracranial metastases. Int J Radiat Oncol Biol Phys. 2017; 99(5):1179–1189

[86] Kepka L, Cieslak E, Bujko K, Fijuth J, Wierzchowski M. Results of the whole-brain radiotherapy for patients with brain metastases from lung cancer: the RTOG RPA intra-classes analysis. Acta Oncol. 2005; 44(4):389–398

[87] Kerschbaumer J, Bauer M, Popovscaia M, Grams AE, Thomé C, Freyschlag CF. Correlation of tumor and peritumoral edema volumes with survival in patients with cerebral metastases. Anticancer Res. 2017; 37(2):871–875

[88] Kim KH, Lee J, Lee J-I, et al. Can upfront systemic chemotherapy replace stereotactic radiosurgery or whole brain radiotherapy in the treatment of non-small cell lung cancer patients with asymptomatic brain metastases? Lung Cancer. 2010; 68(2):258–263

[89] Knisely JPS, Berkey B, Chakravarti A, et al. A phase III study of conventional radiation therapy plus thalidomide versus conventional radiation therapy for multiple brain metastases (RTOG 0118). Int J Radiat Oncol Biol Phys. 2008; 71(1):79–86

[90] Kondziolka D, Kano H, Harrison GL, et al. Stereotactic radiosurgery as primary and salvage treatment for brain metastases from breast cancer. Clinical article. J Neurosurg. 2011; 114(3):792–800

[91] Laakmann E, Riecke K, Goy Y, et al. Comparison of nine prognostic scores in patients with brain metastases of breast cancer receiving radiotherapy of the brain. J Cancer Res Clin Oncol. 2016; 142(1):325–332

[92] Langley RE, Stephens RJ, Nankivell M, et al. QUARTZ Investigators. Interim data from the Medical Research Council QUARTZ Trial: does whole brain radiotherapy affect the survival and quality of life of patients with brain metastases from non-small cell lung cancer? Clin Oncol (R Coll Radiol). 2013; 25(3):e23–e30

[93] Le Scodan R, Massard C, Jouanneau L, et al. Brain metastases from breast cancer: proposition of new prognostic score including molecular subtypes and treatment. J Neurooncol. 2012; 106(1):169–176

[94] Lee SM, Lewanski CR, Counsell N, et al. Randomized trial of erlotinib plus whole-brain radiotherapy for NSCLC patients with multiple brain metastases. J Natl Cancer Inst. 2014; 106(7):dju151

[95] Lee MH, Kong D-S, Seol HJ, Nam D-H, Lee J-I. The influence of biomarker mutations and systemic treatment on cerebral metastases from NSCLC treated with radiosurgery. J Korean Neurosurg Soc. 2017; 60(1):21–29

[96] Leth T, von Oettingen G, Lassen-Ramshad YA, Lukacova S, Høyer M. Survival and prognostic factors in patients treated with stereotactic radiotherapy for brain metastases. Acta Oncol. 2015; 54(1):107–114

[97] Likhacheva A, Pinnix CC, Parikh NR, et al. Predictors of survival in contemporary practice after initial radiosurgery for brain metastases. Int J Radiat Oncol Biol Phys. 2013; 85(3):656–661

[98] Lin NU, Diéras V, Paul D, et al. Multicenter phase II study of lapatinib in patients with brain metastases from HER2-positive breast cancer. Clin Cancer Res. 2009; 15(4):1452–1459

[99] Lindvall P, Bergström P, Löfroth P-O, Tommy Bergenheim A. A comparison between surgical resection in combination with WBRT or hypofractionated stereotactic irradiation in the treatment of solitary brain metastasis. Acta Neurochir (Wien). 2009; 151(9):1053–1059

[100] Liu Y, Deng L, Zhou X, et al. Concurrent brain radiotherapy and EGFR-TKI may improve intracranial metastases control in non-small cell lung cancer and have survival benefit in patients with low DS-GPA score. Oncotarget. 2017; 8(67):111309–111317

[101] Lutterbach J, Cyron D, Henne K, Ostertag CB. Radiosurgery followed by planned observation in patients with one to three brain metastases. Neurosurgery. 2003; 52(5):1066–1073, discussion 1073–1074

[102] Ma L-H, Li G, Zhang H-W, et al. Hypofractionated stereotactic radiotherapy with or without whole-brain radiotherapy for patients with newly diagnosed brain metastases from non-small cell lung cancer. J Neurosurg. 2012; 117 Suppl:49–56

[103] Magnuson WJ, Lester-Coll NH, Wu AJ, et al. Management of brain metastases in tyrosine kinase inhibitor-naïve epidermal growth factor receptor-mutant non-small-cell lung cancer: a retrospective multi-institutional analysis. J Clin Oncol. 2017; 35(10):1070–1077

[104] Mahajan A, Ahmed S, McAleer MF, et al. Post-operative stereotactic radiosurgery versus observation for completely resected brain metastases: a single-centre, randomised, controlled, phase 3 trial. Lancet Oncol. 2017; 18(8):1040–1048

[105] Marcus DM, Lowe M, Khan MK, et al. Prognostic factors for overall survival after radiosurgery for brain metastases from melanoma. Am J Clin Oncol. 2014; 37(6):580–584

[106] Marshall DC, Marcus LP, Kim TE, et al. Management patterns of patients with cerebral metastases who underwent multiple stereotactic radiosurgeries. J Neurooncol. 2016; 128(1):119–128

[107] Mathieu D, Kondziolka D, Cooper PB, et al. Gamma knife radiosurgery in the management of malignant melanoma brain metastases. Neurosurgery. 2007; 60(3):471–481, discussion 481–482

[108] Matsunaga S, Shuto T, Kawahara N, Suenaga J, Inomori S, Fujino H. Gamma Knife surgery for metastatic brain tumors from primary breast cancer: treatment indication based on number of tumors and breast cancer phenotype. J Neurosurg. 2010; 113 Suppl:65–72

[109] Matsuyama T, Kogo K, Oya N. Clinical outcomes of biological effective dose-based fractionated stereotactic radiation therapy for metastatic brain tumors from non-small cell lung cancer. Int J Radiat Oncol Biol Phys. 2013; 85(4):984–990

[110] Miller JA, Kotecha R, Ahluwalia MS, et al. Overall survival and the response to radiotherapy among molecular subtypes of breast cancer brain metastases treated with targeted therapies. Cancer. 2017; 123(12):2283–2293

[111] Minniti G, Esposito V, Clarke E, et al. Multidose stereotactic radiosurgery (9 Gy ×3) of the postoperative resection cavity for treatment of large brain metastases. Int J Radiat Oncol Biol Phys. 2013; 86(4):623–629

[112] Minniti G, D'Angelillo RM, Scaringi C, et al. Fractionated stereotactic radiosurgery for patients with brain metastases. J Neurooncol. 2014; 117(2):295–301

[113] Minniti G, Scaringi C, Paolini S, et al. Repeated stereotactic radiosurgery for patients with progressive brain metastases. J Neurooncol. 2016; 126(1):91–97

[114] Miyazawa K, Shikama N, Okazaki S, Koyama T, Takahashi T, Kato S. Predicting prognosis of short survival time after palliative whole-brain radiotherapy. J Radiat Res (Tokyo). 2018; 59(1):43–49

[115] Mohammadi AM, Schroeder JL, Angelov L, et al. Impact of the radiosurgery prescription dose on the local control of small (2 cm or smaller) brain metastases. J Neurosurg. 2017; 126(3):735–743

[116] Moro-Sibilot D, Smit E, de Castro Carpeño J, et al. Non-small cell lung cancer patients with brain metastases treated with first-line platinum-doublet chemotherapy: analysis from the European FRAME study. Lung Cancer. 2015; 90(3):427–432

[117] Motta M, del Vecchio A, Attuati L, et al. Gamma knife radiosurgery for treatment of cerebral metastases from non-small-cell lung cancer. Int J Radiat Oncol Biol Phys. 2011; 81(4):e463–e468

[118] Muacevic A, Kreth FW, Horstmann GA, et al. Surgery and radiotherapy compared with gamma knife radiosurgery in the treatment of solitary cerebral metastases of small diameter. J Neurosurg. 1999; 91(1):35–43

[119] Muacevic A, Kreth FW, Mack A, Tonn J-C, Wowra B. Stereotactic radiosurgery without radiation therapy providing high local tumor control of multiple brain metastases from renal cell carcinoma. Minim Invasive Neurosurg. 2004; 47(4):203–208

[120] Muacevic A, Kufeld M, Wowra B, Kreth F-W, Tonn J-C. Feasibility, safety, and outcome of frameless image-guided robotic radiosurgery for brain metastases. J Neurooncol. 2010; 97(2):267–274

[121] Nam T-K, Lee J-I, Jung Y-J, et al. Gamma knife surgery for brain metastases in patients harboring four or more lesions: survival and prognostic factors. J Neurosurg. 2005; 102 Suppl:147–150

[122] Obermueller T, Schaeffner M, Gerhardt J, Meyer B, Ringel F, Krieg SM. Risks of postoperative paresis in motor eloquently and non-eloquently located brain metastases. BMC Cancer. 2014; 14:21

[123] Pan H-C, Sheehan J, Stroila M, Steiner M, Steiner L. Gamma knife surgery for brain metastases from lung cancer. J Neurosurg. 2005; 102 Suppl: 128–133

[124] Park YH, Park MJ, Ji SH, et al. Trastuzumab treatment improves brain metastasis outcomes through control and durable prolongation of systemic extracranial disease in HER2-overexpressing breast cancer patients. Br J Cancer. 2009; 100(6):894–900

[125] Park Y, Kim KS, Kim K, et al. Nomogram prediction of survival in patients with brain metastases from hepatocellular carcinoma treated with whole-brain radiotherapy: a multicenter retrospective study. J Neurooncol. 2015; 125(2):377–383

[126] Patel KR, Burri SH, Boselli D, et al. Comparing pre-operative stereotactic radiosurgery (SRS) to post-operative whole brain radiation therapy (WBRT) for resectable brain metastases: a multi-institutional analysis. J Neurooncol. 2017; 131(3):611–618

[127] Patel KR, Burri SH, Asher AL, et al. Comparing preoperative with postoperative stereotactic radiosurgery for resectable brain metastases: a multi-institutional analysis. Neurosurgery. 2016; 79(2):279–285

[128] Patel KR, Prabhu RS, Kandula S, et al. Intracranial control and radiographic changes with adjuvant radiation therapy for resected brain metastases: whole brain radiotherapy versus stereotactic radiosurgery alone. J Neurooncol. 2014; 120(3):657–663

[129] Postmus PE, Haaxma-Reiche H, Smit EF, et al. Treatment of brain metastases of small-cell lung cancer: comparing teniposide and teniposide with whole-brain radiotherapy: a phase III study of the European Organization for the Research and Treatment of Cancer Lung Cancer Cooperative Group. J Clin Oncol. 2000; 18(19):3400–3408

[130] Queirolo P, Spagnolo F, Ascierto PA, et al. Efficacy and safety of ipilimumab in patients with advanced melanoma and brain metastases. J Neurooncol. 2014; 118(1):109–116

[131] Rades D, Dziggel L, Nagy V, et al. A new survival score for patients with brain metastases who received whole-brain radiotherapy (WBRT) alone. Radiother Oncol. 2013; 108(1):123–127

[132] Rades D, Panzner A, Dziggel L, Haatanen T, Lohynska R, Schild SE. Dose-escalation of whole-brain radiotherapy for brain metastasis in patients with a favorable survival prognosis. Cancer. 2012; 118(15):3852–3859

[133] Rades D, Raabe A, Bajrovic A, Alberti W. Treatment of solitary brain metastasis. Resection followed by whole brain radiation therapy (WBRT) and a radiation boost to the metastatic site. Strahlenther Onkol. 2004; 180 (3):144–147

[134] Rades D, Janssen S, Dziggel L, et al. A matched-pair study comparing whole-brain irradiation alone to radiosurgery or fractionated stereotactic radiotherapy alone in patients irradiated for up to three brain metastases. BMC Cancer. 2017; 17(1):30

[135] Robinet G, Thomas P, Breton JL, et al. Results of a phase III study of early versus delayed whole brain radiotherapy with concurrent cisplatin and vinorelbine combination in inoperable brain metastasis of non-small-cell lung cancer: Groupe Français de Pneumo-Cancérologie (GFPC) Protocol 95–1. Ann Oncol. 2001; 12(1):59–67

[136] Romano KD, Trifiletti DM, Garda A, et al. Choosing a prescription isodose in stereotactic radiosurgery for brain metastases: implications for local control. World Neurosurg. 2017; 98:761–767.e1

[137] Rosner D, Nemoto T, Lane WW. Chemotherapy induces regression of brain metastases in breast carcinoma. Cancer. 1986; 58(4):832–839

[138] Ruge MI, Suchorska B, Maarouf M, et al. Stereotactic 125iodine brachytherapy for the treatment of singular brain metastasis: closing a gap? Neurosurgery. 2011; 68(5):1209–1218, discussion 1218–1219

[139] Rush S, Elliott RE, Morsi A, et al. Incidence, timing, and treatment of new brain metastases after Gamma Knife surgery for limited brain disease: the case for reducing the use of whole-brain radiation therapy. J Neurosurg. 2011; 115(1):37–48

[140] Saito EY, Viani GA, Ferrigno R, et al. Whole brain radiation therapy in management of brain metastasis: results and prognostic factors. Radiat Oncol. 2006; 1:20

[141] Sampson JH, Carter JH, Jr, Friedman AH, Seigler HF. Demographics, prognosis, and therapy in 702 patients with brain metastases from malignant melanoma. J Neurosurg. 1998; 88(1):11–20

[142] Sanghavi SN, Miranpuri SS, Chappell R, et al. Radiosurgery for patients with brain metastases: a multi-institutional analysis, stratified by the RTOG recursive partitioning analysis method. Int J Radiat Oncol Biol Phys. 2001; 51 (2):426–434

[143] Schackert G, Steinmetz A, Meier U, Sobottka SB. Surgical management of single and multiple brain metastases: results of a retrospective study. Onkologie. 2001; 24(3):246–255

[144] Schackert G, Lindner C, Petschke S, Leimert M, Kirsch M. Retrospective study of 127 surgically treated patients with multiple brain metastases: indication, prognostic factors, and outcome. Acta Neurochir (Wien). 2013; 155(3):379–387

[145] Shuch B, La Rochelle JC, Klatte T, et al. Brain metastasis from renal cell carcinoma: presentation, recurrence, and survival. Cancer. 2008; 113(7): 1641–1648

[146] Schüttrumpf LH, Niyazi M, Nachbichler SB, et al. Prognostic factors for survival and radiation necrosis after stereotactic radiosurgery alone or in combination with whole brain radiation therapy for 1–3 cerebral metastases. Radiat Oncol. 2014; 9:105

[147] Scott C, Suh J, Stea B, Nabid A, Hackman J. Improved survival, quality of life, and quality-adjusted survival in breast cancer patients treated with efaproxiral (Efaproxyn) plus whole-brain radiation therapy for brain metastases. Am J Clin Oncol. 2007; 30(6):580–587

[148] Sekine A, Satoh H, Iwasawa T, et al. Prognostic factors for brain metastases from non-small cell lung cancer with EGFR mutation: influence of stable extracranial disease and erlotinib therapy. Med Oncol. 2014; 31(10):228

[149] Serizawa T, Yamamoto M, Nagano O, et al. Gamma Knife surgery for metastatic brain tumors. J Neurosurg. 2008; 109 Suppl:118–121

[150] Serizawa T, Hirai T, Nagano O, et al. Gamma knife surgery for 1–10 brain metastases without prophylactic whole-brain radiation therapy: analysis of cases meeting the Japanese prospective multi-institute study (JLGK0901) inclusion criteria. J Neurooncol. 2010; 98(2):163–167

[151] Serizawa T, Higuchi Y, Nagano O, et al. Testing different brain metastasis grading systems in stereotactic radiosurgery: Radiation Therapy Oncology Group's RPA, SIR, BSBM, GPA, and modified RPA. J Neurosurg. 2012; 117 Suppl:31–37

[152] Serizawa T, Higuchi Y, Nagano O, et al. A new grading system focusing on neurological outcomes for brain metastases treated with stereotactic radiosurgery: the modified Basic Score for Brain Metastases. J Neurosurg. 2014; 121(2) Suppl:35–43

[153] Shen CJ, Kummerlowe MN, Redmond KJ, Rigamonti D, Lim MK, Kleinberg LR. stereotactic radiosurgery: treatment of brain metastasis without interruption of systemic therapy. Int J Radiat Oncol Biol Phys. 2016; 95(2):735–742

[154] Siena S, Crinò L, Danova M, et al. Dose-dense temozolomide regimen for the treatment of brain metastases from melanoma, breast cancer, or lung cancer not amenable to surgery or radiosurgery: a multicenter phase II study. Ann Oncol. 2010; 21(3):655–661

[155] Sneed PK, Mendez J, Vemer-van den Hoek JGM, et al. Adverse radiation effect after stereotactic radiosurgery for brain metastases: incidence, time course, and risk factors. J Neurosurg. 2015; 123(2):373–386

[156] Song T-W, Kim I-Y, Jung S, Jung T-Y, Moon K-S, Jang W-Y. Resection and observation for brain metastasis without prompt postoperative radiation therapy. J Korean Neurosurg Soc. 2017; 60(6):667–675

[157] Sperduto PW, Chao ST, Sneed PK, et al. Diagnosis-specific prognostic factors, indexes, and treatment outcomes for patients with newly diagnosed brain metastases: a multi-institutional analysis of 4,259 patients. Int J Radiat Oncol Biol Phys. 2010; 77(3):655–661

[158] Sperduto PW, Wang M, Robins HI, et al. A phase 3 trial of whole brain radiation therapy and stereotactic radiosurgery alone versus WBRT and SRS with temozolomide or erlotinib for non-small cell lung cancer and 1 to 3

brain metastases: Radiation Therapy Oncology Group 0320. Int J Radiat Oncol Biol Phys. 2013; 85(5):1312–1318

[159] Sperduto PW, Shanley R, Luo X, et al. Secondary analysis of RTOG 9508, a phase 3 randomized trial of whole-brain radiation therapy versus WBRT plus stereotactic radiosurgery in patients with 1–3 brain metastases; poststratified by the graded prognostic assessment (GPA). Int J Radiat Oncol Biol Phys. 2014; 90(3):526–531

[160] Sperduto PW, Yang TJ, Beal K, et al. Estimating survival in patients with lung cancer and brain metastases: an update of the graded prognostic assessment for lung cancer using molecular markers (Lung-molGPA). JAMA Oncol. 2017; 3(6):827–831

[161] Sperduto PW, Jiang W, Brown PD, et al. Estimating survival in melanoma patients with brain metastases: an update of the graded prognostic assessment for melanoma using molecular markers (Melanoma-molGPA). Int J Radiat Oncol Biol Phys. 2017; 99(4):812–816

[162] Stark AM, Tscheslog H, Buhl R, Held-Feindt J, Mehdorn HM. Surgical treatment for brain metastases: prognostic factors and survival in 177 patients. Neurosurg Rev. 2005; 28(2):115–119

[163] Stokes WA, Binder DC, Jones BL, et al. Impact of immunotherapy among patients with melanoma brain metastases managed with radiotherapy. J Neuroimmunol. 2017; 313:118–122

[164] Tang N, Guo J, Zhang Q, Wang Y, Wang Z. Greater efficacy of chemotherapy plus bevacizumab compared to chemo- and targeted therapy alone on non-small cell lung cancer patients with brain metastasis. Oncotarget. 2016; 7 (3):3635–3644

[165] Trifiletti DM, Hill C, Cohen-Inbar O, Xu Z, Sheehan JP. Stereotactic radiosurgery for small brain metastases and implications regarding management with systemic therapy alone. J Neurooncol. 2017; 134(2):289–296

[166] Ulm AJ, Friedman WA, Bova FJ, Bradshaw P, Amdur RJ, Mendenhall WM. Linear accelerator radiosurgery in the treatment of brain metastases. Neurosurgery. 2004; 55(5):1076–1085

[167] Viani GA, da Silva LGB, Stefano EJ. Prognostic indexes for brain metastases: which is the most powerful? Int J Radiat Oncol Biol Phys. 2012; 83(3):e325–e330

[168] Viani GA, Castilho MS, Salvajoli JV, et al. Whole brain radiotherapy for brain metastases from breast cancer: estimation of survival using two stratification systems. BMC Cancer. 2007; 7:53

[169] Vickers MM, Al-Harbi H, Choueiri TK, et al. Prognostic factors of survival for patients with metastatic renal cell carcinoma with brain metastases treated with targeted therapy: results from the international metastatic renal cell carcinoma database consortium. Clin Genitourin Cancer. 2013; 11(3):311–315

[170] Videtic GMM, Adelstein DJ, Mekhail TM, et al. Validation of the RTOG recursive partitioning analysis (RPA) classification for small-cell lung cancer-only brain metastases. Int J Radiat Oncol Biol Phys. 2007; 67(1):240–243

[171] Vuong DA, Rades D, van Eck ATC, Horstmann GA, Busse R. Comparing the cost-effectiveness of two brain metastasis treatment modalities from a payer's perspective: stereotactic radiosurgery versus surgical resection. Clin Neurol Neurosurg. 2013; 115(3):276–284

[172] Willfurth P, Mayer R, Stranzl H, Prettenhofer U, Genser B, Arnulf H. Dividing patients with brain metastases into classes derived from the RTOG recursive partitioning analysis (RPA) with emphasis on prognostic poorer patient groups. Radiol Oncol. 2001; 35(2):127–131

[173] Williams BJ, Suki D, Fox BD, et al. Stereotactic radiosurgery for metastatic brain tumors: a comprehensive review of complications. J Neurosurg. 2009; 111(3):439–448

[174] Wowra B, Muacevic A, Tonn J-C. Quality of radiosurgery for single brain metastases with respect to treatment technology: a matched-pair analysis. J Neurooncol. 2009; 94(1):69–77

[175] Wroński M, Arbit E, Burt M, Galicich JH. Survival after surgical treatment of brain metastases from lung cancer: a follow-up study of 231 patients treated between 1976 and 1991. J Neurosurg. 1995; 83(4):605–616

[176] Yamamoto M, Serizawa T, Shuto T, et al. Stereotactic radiosurgery for patients with multiple brain metastases (JLGK0901): a multi-institutional prospective observational study. Lancet Oncol. 2014; 15(4):387–395

[177] Yamamoto M, Serizawa T, Higuchi Y, et al. A multi-institutional prospective observational study of stereotactic radiosurgery for patients with multiple brain metastases (JLGK0901 Study Update): irradiation-related complications and long-term maintenance of mini-mental state examination scores. Int J Radiat Oncol Biol Phys. 2017; 99(1):31–40

[178] Yang TJ, Oh JH, Folkert MR, et al. Outcomes and prognostic factors in women with 1 to 3 breast cancer brain metastases treated with definitive stereotactic radiosurgery. Int J Radiat Oncol Biol Phys. 2014; 90(3):518–525

[179] Yang J-J, Zhou C, Huang Y, et al. Icotinib versus whole-brain irradiation in patients with EGFR-mutant non-small-cell lung cancer and multiple brain metastases (BRAIN): a multicentre, phase 3, open-label, parallel, randomised controlled trial. Lancet Respir Med. 2017; 5(9):707–716

[180] Yoshida S, Takahashi H. Cerebellar metastases in patients with cancer. Surg Neurol. 2009; 71(2):184–187, discussion 187

[181] Zacest AC, Besser M, Stevens G, Thompson JF, McCarthy WH, Culjak G. Surgical management of cerebral metastases from melanoma: outcome in 147 patients treated at a single institution over two decades. J Neurosurg. 2002; 96(3):552–558

[182] Zimm S, Wampler GL, Stablein D, Hazra T, Young HF. Intracerebral metastases in solid-tumor patients: natural history and results of treatment. Cancer. 1981; 48(2):384–394

[183] Zindler JD, Bruynzeel AME, Eekers DBP, Hurkmans CW, Swinnen A, Lambin P. Whole brain radiotherapy versus stereotactic radiosurgery for 4–10 brain metastases: a phase III randomised multicentre trial. BMC Cancer. 2017; 17 (1):500

[184] Zindler JD, Slotman BJ, Lagerwaard FJ. Patterns of distant brain recurrences after radiosurgery alone for newly diagnosed brain metastases: implications for salvage therapy. Radiother Oncol. 2014; 112(2):212–216

[185] Hatiboglu MA, Akdur K, Sawaya R. Neurosurgical management of patients with brain metastasis. Neurosurg Rev. 2020; 43(2):483–495

[186] Vecht CJ, Hovestadt A, Verbiest HB, van Vliet JJ, van Putten WL. Dose-effect relationship of dexamethasone on Karnofsky performance in metastatic brain tumors: a randomized study of doses of 4, 8, and 16 mg per day. Neurology. 1994; 44(4):675–680

[187] Wolfson AH, Snodgrass SM, Schwade JG, et al. The role of steroids in the management of metastatic carcinoma to the brain. A pilot prospective trial. Am J Clin Oncol. 1994; 17(3):234–238

[188] Andersen C, Astrup J, Gyldensted C. Quantitation of peritumoural oedema and the effect of steroids using NMR-relaxation time imaging and blood-brain barrier analysis. Acta Neurochir Suppl (Wien). 1994; 60:413–415

[189] Chen CC, Rennert RC, Olson JJ. Congress of neurological surgeons systematic review and evidence-based guidelines on the role of prophylactic anticonvulsants in the treatment of adults with metastatic brain tumors. Neurosurgery. 2019; 84(3):E195–E197

[190] Nahed BV, Alvarez-Breckenridge C, Brastianos PK, et al. Congress of neurological surgeons systematic review and evidence-based guidelines on the role of surgery in the management of adults with metastatic brain tumors. Neurosurgery. 2019; 84(3):E152–E155

[191] Brown PD, Pugh S, Laack NN, et al. Radiation Therapy Oncology Group (RTOG). Memantine for the prevention of cognitive dysfunction in patients receiving whole-brain radiotherapy: a randomized, double-blind, placebo-controlled trial. Neuro Oncol. 2013 Oct;15(10):1429-1437. doi: 10.1093/neuonc/not114. Epub 2013 Aug 16. PMID: 23956241; PMCID: PMC3779047

[192] Brown PD, Gondi V, Pugh S, et al. For NRG oncology. Hippocampal avoidance during whole-brain radiotherapy plus memantine for patients with brain metastases: phase III trial NRG oncology CC001. J Clin Oncol. 2020 Apr 1;38(10):1019-1029. doi: 10.1200/JCO.19.02767. Epub 2020 Feb 14. PMID: 32058845; PMCID: PMC7106984

[193] Sahgal A, Aoyama H, Kocher M, et al. Phase 3 trials of stereotactic radiosurgery with or without whole-brain radiation therapy for 1 to 4 brain metastases: individual patient data meta-analysis. Int J Radiat Oncol Biol Phys. 2015; 91(4):710–717

[194] Kocher M, Soffietti R, Abacioglu U, et al. Adjuvant whole-brain radiotherapy versus observation after radiosurgery or surgical resection of one to three cerebral metastases: results of the EORTC 22952–26001 study. J Clin Oncol. 2011; 29(2):134–141

[195] Gaspar LE, Prabhu RS, Hdeib A, et al. Congress of neurological surgeons systematic review and evidence-based guidelines on the role of whole brain radiation therapy in adults with newly diagnosed metastatic brain tumors. Neurosurgery. 2019; 84(3):E159–E162

[196] Winn HR. Youmans and Winn Neurological Surgery. New York, NY: Elsevier Health Sciences; 2016

[197] Graber JJ, Cobbs CS, Olson JJ. Congress of neurological surgeons systematic review and evidence-based guidelines on the use of stereotactic radiosurgery in the treatment of adults with metastatic brain tumors. Neurosurgery. 2019; 84(3):E168–E170

[198] Berghoff AS, Venur VA, Preusser M, Ahluwalia MS. Immune checkpoint inhibitors in brain metastases: from biology to treatment. Am Soc Clin Oncol Educ Book. 2016; 35(36):e116–e122

23 Natural History and Management Options of Convexity Meningioma

Chien Yew Kow and Arnold Bok

Abstract

The management of convexity meningiomas remains controversial and usually depends on the preference of the neurosurgeon who manages the patient. The size, location, vascularity, and growth rate of a meningioma play a role, as do the preference of the patient and the opinion and experience of the treating neurosurgeon. Weighing up the natural history of these lesions against the treatment injury risks remains key to successful management. In this chapter, we present the natural history and management options for convexity meningiomas.

Keywords: convexity meningioma, natural history, risk factors, management options

23.1 Introduction

Meningiomas are benign extra-axial growths that arise from the arachnoid cap cells present in the arachnoid granulations along the dura. They account for 36.4% of overall primary central nervous system (CNS) tumors and 53.4% of nonmalignant primary CNS tumors.[1] The overall incidence is estimated at 7.75 per 100,000 population,[1] and this has increased over time due to the growing availability of neuroimaging. In general, meningiomas are more common among females, and the incidence increases with advancing age.[1,2] Uncommon malignant meningioma tend to be more prevalent among men.[1,2]

Convexity meningiomas are lesions that arise along the perimeter of the cranial vault with dural attachments not involving dural venous sinuses, the falx, or the skull base. Approximately 90% of all meningiomas are supratentorial, with 15 to 19% located along the convexity.[3,4] Convexity meningiomas have the greatest potential for cure as they lend themselves to total resection, including removal of the involved dura. The results of surgery for convexity meningiomas are generally better compared to other anatomical locations (1.7–9.4% morbidity and 0% 30-day mortality).[24,25]

Convexity meningiomas have traditionally been classified into several subtypes based on anatomic location: precoronal, coronal, postcoronal, paracentral, parietal, temporal, and occipital.[5] Most convexity meningiomas are located with a component of the tumor anterior to the central sulcus as there is an increased density of arachnoid granulations anterior and adjacent to the coronal suture. In addition, convexity meningiomas can be morphologically classified as globoid (spherical, lobulated mass) or en plaque (flatter, carpetlike appearance infiltrating the dura).

Most convexity meningiomas are asymptomatic and are incidentally detected following radiological investigation for other unrelated clinical presentations. In symptomatic patients, headache is the most common complaint (39–48% of patients).[24,25] Convexity lesions around the precentral cortical area may cause contralateral weakness and focal motor seizures (▶ Fig. 23.1),

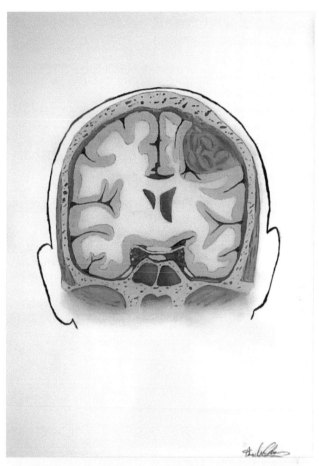

Fig. 23.1 Convexity meningioma over the left motor cortex region.

whereas tumors of the postcentral area may cause sensory deficits. Speech disturbance may arise from tumors compressing Broca's or Wernicke's area on the dominant hemisphere. Visual deficits may result from lesions overlying the temporal or occipital lobes. Up to 40% of patients with convexity meningiomas experience seizures preoperatively.

With greater availability of neuroimaging, incidental convexity meningiomas are becoming more prevalent. This leads to the management dilemma for asymptomatic patients. This chapter discusses the natural history and management options for convexity meningiomas.

23.2 Selected Papers on the Natural History of Convexity Meningioma

- Hashimoto N, Rabo CS, Okita Y, et al. Slower growth of skull base meningiomas compared with non-skull base meningiomas based on volumetric and biological studies. J Neurosurg 2012;116(3):574–580

- Lee EJ, Park JH, Park ES, Kim JH. "Wait-and-see" strategies for newly diagnosed intracranial meningiomas based on the risk of future observation failure. World Neurosurg 2017;107:604–611
- Oya S, Kim SH, Sade B, Lee JH. The natural history of intracranial meningiomas. J Neurosurg 2011;114(5):1250–1256
- Nakamura M, Roser F, Michel J, Jacobs C, Samii M. The natural history of incidental meningiomas. Neurosurgery 2003;53(1):62–70, discussion 70–71
- Yano S, Kuratsu J; Kumamoto Brain Tumor Research Group. Indications for surgery in patients with asymptomatic meningiomas based on an extensive experience. J Neurosurg 2006;105(4):538–543

23.3 Natural History of Incidental Convexity Meningioma

The natural history of untreated meningioma is not clear. In the past, most patients with meningioma presented with neurological symptoms due to large tumors causing mass effect. Recent advances in neuroimaging and its wide availability have led to increased detection of small incidental lesions and the inherent dilemma in recommending treatment options for asymptomatic patients. Understanding the natural history of meningioma is critical, as it forms the basis for treatment.

▶ Table 23.1[6,7,8,9,10,11,12,13,14,15,16,17,18,19,20] summarizes the published studies on the natural history of convexity meningioma and the salient features associated with growth.

23.3.1 Size

Tumor size affects treatment recommendation. Larger tumor sizes are more likely to cause symptoms and, therefore, early surgical intervention.[19] A review of the published series identified that larger initial tumor size predicts subsequent growth and the potential for treatment recommendation. Lee et al[12] found that meningiomas larger than 4 cm are likely to eventually cause neurological symptoms, with 65% of patients with a meningioma greater than 4 cm in their cohort developing new, or an aggravation of, neurological symptoms. Asymptomatic tumors less than 3 cm may be closely observed with regular radiological surveillance.

23.3.2 Growth Rate and Tumor Doubling Time

Studies of the natural history of meningiomas have found that most tumors grow very slowly. These were conducted on

Table 23.1 Published studies on the natural history of convexity meningiomas

Study	n	Proportion with growth (%)	Growth rate (mm/y)	Relative growth rate (%/y)	Absolute growth rate (cm³/y)	Doubling time (y)	Factors a/w growth	Factors a/w nongrowth
Firsching et al[7]	17	–	–	3.6	–	–	–	–
Olivero et al[15]	57	22.0	2.4	–	–	–	–	–
Kuratsu et al[11]	63	31.7	–	–	–	–	–	Calcification and MRI T2 isointensity
Niiro et al[14]	40	35.0	–	–	–	–	–	–
Yoneoka et al[20]	37	24.3a	–	–	–	–	Younger age, larger initial tumor size	–
Nakamura et al[13]	47	33.0	–	14.6	0.80	21.6	–	Calcification and MRI T2 iso- or hypointensity
Herscovici et al[9]	44	37.0	4.0	–	–	–	–	–
Yano and Kuratsu[19]	351	37.3	1.9	–	–	–	MRI T2 hyperintensity	Calcification
Oya et al[16]	273	74.0a	–	–	0.68	–	MRI T2 hyperintensity, age <60 y, peritumoral edema, initial tumor size >25 mm	Calcification
Rubin et al[18]	63	38.0	4.0	–	–	–	–	–
Chang et al[6]	31	84.0a	0.7	15.2	–	13.4	–	–
Hashimoto et al[8]	113	75.0a	–	13.8	1.15	9.3	MRI T2 hyperintensity	Calcification
Jadid et al[10]	65	35.4	–	–	–	–	–	–
Lee et al[12]	232	–	–	20.4	2.20	18.0	peritumoral edema	Calcification and MRI T2 hypointensity
Romani et al[17]	136	–	–	–	–	–	Peritumoral edema	Calcification

Abbreviations: a/w, associated with; MRI, magnetic resonance imaging; –, not available.
aProgression measured using volumetric measurements

patients with incidental tumors with many remaining asymptomatic during the follow-up period. Based on our literature review, meningiomas have an annual growth rate of 0.7 to 4 mm per year and increase 3.6 to 20.4% per year in volumetric measures. This amounts to a tumor doubling time of 9.3 to 21.6 years. Growth rate for multiple meningiomas does not appear to be significantly different from solitary meningiomas.[21] During a surveillance period, a 22 to 38% proportion of meningiomas demonstrated growth on linear measurement, and the proportion increased to 74 to 84% when volumetric measurements were utilized. However, inherent limitations of these natural history studies are characterized by a selection biased toward elderly patients subjected to observation and short follow-up period, ranging between 29 and 67 months.

Although most meningiomas are slow growing, some show aggressive or malignant biological behavior. Mean tumor doubling time was found to vary according to the World Health Organization (WHO) histological grading: 425 days (range: 138–1045 days) for grade I, 178 days (range: 34–551 days) for grade II, and 205 days (range: 30–472 days) for grade III.[27]

23.4 Risk Factors That Predict Tumor Growth

Identifying the risk factors that predict tumor growth is important for planning therapeutic strategies. The following factors are associated with tumor growth over time[13]:
- Presence of intratumoral T2 hyperintensity.
- Peritumoral cerebral edema.
- Larger tumor size (> 25 mm) at initial diagnosis.
- Younger patient age (< 60).
- Sphenoid ridge location.

In contrast, tumors with calcification (demonstrated on computed tomography [CT] and/or hypointensity on T2-weighted magnetic resonance imaging [MRI]) are associated with a slower growth rate.[11,13]

Furthermore, meningiomas are known to become larger during pregnancy and during the luteal phase of the menstrual cycle, suggesting that their growth may be related to female hormones. Furthermore, Ki-67 expression was found to be inversely correlated with progesterone receptor concentration, both in paraffin tissues and in cell culture. Most malignant meningiomas are PR negative, suggesting a loss of PR during tumor progression.

23.5 Recurrence

Tumor recurrence depends on the extent of surgical resection, histopathological grading, and the biological potential (▶ Table 23.2).

Tumor location dictates the surgical resectability, which in turn affects the risk of recurrence. In 1957, Donald Simpson[26] introduced a five-grade classification of surgical removal of meningiomas, which correlated well with tumor recurrence. Convexity meningiomas are mostly amenable to optimal surgical resection and are associated with a low recurrence/progression rate.

The WHO classifies meningiomas into three histological grades based on (1) hypercellularity, (2) mitotic figures, and (3) presence of necrosis. Higher WHO grades are associated with a greater risk for recurrence and/or aggressive clinical behavior following surgical resection. Therefore, atypical or malignant meningiomas need to be closely followed up during the postoperative period.

In addition, high mitotic index is a significant predictor for shorter progression-free interval.

23.6 Selected Papers on the Treatment Options for Convexity Meningioma

- Alvernia JE, Dang ND, Sindou MP. Convexity meningiomas: study of recurrence factors with special emphasis on the cleavage plane in a series of 100 consecutive patients. J Neurosurg 2011;115(3):491–498
- Hasseleid BF, Meling TR, Rønning P, Scheie D, Helseth E. Surgery for convexity meningioma: Simpson Grade I resection as the goal—clinical article. J Neurosurg 2012;117(6):999–1006
- Morokoff AP, Zauberman J, Black PM. Surgery for convexity meningiomas. Neurosurgery 2008;63(3):427–433, discussion 433–434

Table 23.2 Predictors of tumor recurrence following surgical resection

	Grades			5-y recurrence
EOR (Simpson grading)	1		Tumor completely resected; dural base removed; any abnormal bone removed; venous sinus resected if involved	9%
	2		Tumor completely resected; dural base not removed but diathermied	19%
	3		Tumor completely resected; dural base left alone	29%
	4		Subtotal resection	39%
	5		Decompression, with or without biopsy	100%
WHO grading	1		Tumor lacks atypical or malignant features or brain invasion	5%
	2		Tumors require ≥ 4 mitotic figures per 10 HPF or ≥ 3 of 5 features (sheetlike growth, spontaneous necrosis, hypercellularity, prominent nucleoli, and presence of small cells with high N/C ratio)	40%
	3		Tumors require ≥ 20 mitotic figures per 10 HPF or frank anaplasia with histology resembling carcinoma, melanoma, or sarcoma	80%

Abbreviations: EOR, extent of resection; HPF, high power fields; N/C, nuclear-to-cytoplasmic; WHO, World Health Organization.

• Kaur G, Sayegh ET, Larson A, et al. Adjuvant radiotherapy for atypical and malignant meningiomas: a systematic review. Neuro-oncol 2014;16(5):628–636

23.7 Treatment Options for Convexity Meningioma

Management of asymptomatic convexity meningiomas depends on their natural history, growth, and the assessment of the potential postoperative complications. In general, treatment options include observation, surgical resection, and radiotherapy. To rationalize treatment, management recommendation must consider tumor size, location, associated edema, patient's age, and medical comorbidities.

23.8 Observation

Given the slow growth rate of convexity meningiomas, asymptomatic tumors should be observed with regular radiological surveillance. It should be noted that a small proportion of patients may become symptomatic during the observational period, ranging from 0 to 6.4%.[15,19,20] For elderly patients, meningiomas often demonstrate a slower growth pattern, which, in conjunction with increased operative morbidity, may necessitate a more conservative approach in this cohort. For younger patients, asymptomatic tumors (< 3 cm) may be observed with regular radiological surveillance. Consideration for observation also needs to consider the potential higher-grade meningiomas, in which subsequent delay in intervention may result in potentially higher operative morbidity and impacting on long-term outcome.

23.9 Surgery

As good dural margin resection can often be achieved, surgical resection remains an effective curative treatment for convexity meningioma. The ease of resection depends on various factors, including location, size, blood supply, and involvement of critical structures. A Simpson grade 0 or 1 resection can be achieved in 80 to 95% of patients, as shown in ▶ Table 23.3.[22,23,24,25] This is generally associated with low retreatment risk, with rates between 2 and 10%, in line with previous findings by Simpson[26] and Jääskeläinen et al,[27] especially if the histology is benign. Extensive resection (Simpson grade 0) proposed by Kinjo et al[28] is likely to offer further protection against recurrence. For cases with bony invasion, we attempt to curet or drill out the tumor from the craniotomy bone flap prior to replacement, although a customized acrylic cranioplasty flap can also be used as an alternative in cases with extensive invasion.

Contemporary surgical series (▶ Table 23.3) demonstrate an overall lower procedural morbidity and higher complete resection rate with comparable retreatment risks. Prognosis for convexity meningiomas is excellent given its accessible location, which allows for total resection. Complete resection, even if there is en plaque growth, almost always excludes recurrence. In addition, when comparing patients of different age groups, Yano and Kuratsu[19] found that 9.3% of patients who were older than 70 years suffered from persistent morbidity 3 months postoperation, compared to 4.4% of their younger counterparts. This series included resection of skull base meningiomas, which are usually more difficult to remove, and where surgery has a higher postoperative morbidity. Nonetheless, it remains important to be mindful of the risk of complications in the elderly.

The rationale of preoperative embolization is to facilitate surgical resection by minimizing perioperative surgical blood loss and softening the tumor. Existing data derived from several low-quality studies suggest that embolization decreases blood loss, but not operative time. Surgical complications may be reduced with preoperative embolization, but the available evidence is not clear. Meningiomas selected to embolization are subjected to inherent biases toward those judged to be more likely to benefit.[29,30] Therefore, in carefully selected patients with large convexity meningiomas undergoing surgery, preoperative embolization may be considered.

23.10 Radiotherapy

Radiotherapy has not traditionally been considered a primary treatment modality for convexity meningiomas. However, as the indication and utilization of radiosurgery expanded over the last few decades, radiosurgery has been considered a potential form of primary treatment for convexity meningiomas. Kondziolka et al[31] published their experience of treating convexity meningiomas less than 3.5 cm in size using the Leksell Gamma Knife in patients who refused other treatment options, and in patients with concomitant medical illness or of advanced age, and also in patients with symptomatic lesions located in areas of higher surgical risk. They reported a tumor control rate of 92% for their cohort who had primary radiosurgery, with a 6.2% incidence of morbidity. The effectiveness and risk of radiosurgery is therefore similar to the efficacy and morbidity of surgical resection and should be considered for patients who present with a meningioma that is increasing in size and who refuse surgery or are medically unfit for surgery.

In a review by Kaur et al,[32] adjuvant radiotherapy was found to improve progression-free survival and overall survival for anaplastic meningiomas, but not atypical meningiomas where a good surgical resection had been achieved. Postoperative

Table 23.3 Surgical outcomes of convexity meningiomas in recently published studies

Study	n	SG 1 resection achieved (%)	Morbidity (%)	30-d mortality (%)	Retreatment rate (%) based on SG resection				
					Overall	Grade 1	Grade 2	Grade 3	Grade 4
Morokoff et al[24]	163	95.0	9.4	0	4.3	–	–	–	–
Sanai et al[25]	141	87.0	10.0	0	2.0	–	–	–	–
Alvernia et al[22]	100	91.0	8.0	0	4.4	2.2	–	22.0	–
Hasseleid et al[23]	391	80.6%	–	1.5	10.0	3.2	15.2	12.5	50.0

Abbreviation: SG, Simpson grade.

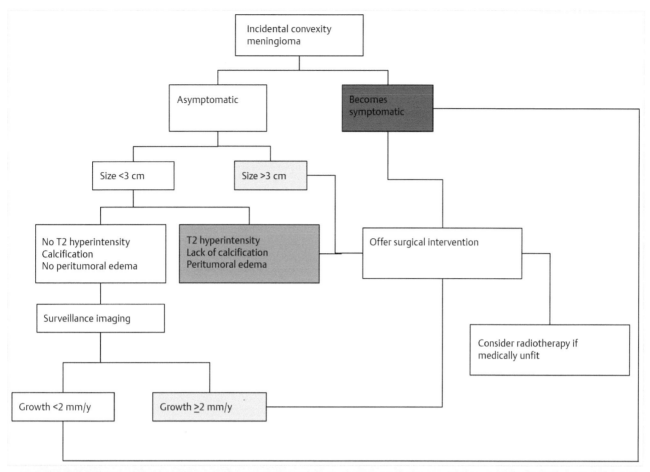

Fig. 23.2 Proposed color-coded treatment algorithm for incidental meningioma, with *red* being a strong indication for surgical intervention, *yellow* being a moderate indication for surgical intervention, and *green* being a weak indication.

radiotherapy may be considered for atypical meningioma with subtotal resection.

23.11 Authors' Recommendations

Based on the available data, we propose a simplified treatment algorithm for incidental convexity meningiomas as shown in ▶ Fig. 23.2. The patient's comorbidity and functional capacity should always be taken into consideration.

- Meningiomas that are greater than 3 cm in size should be considered for surgical excision, as they are likely to become symptomatic as they enlarge.
- Lesions that demonstrate T2 hyperintensity on MRI, lack of calcification on imaging, and lesions that are associated with surrounding cerebral edema could be considered for surgery, although observation with surveillance MRI at shorter intervals is an alternative, especially if the lesion is small (<2 cm).
- Meningiomas that demonstrate a high growth rate (≥2 mm/ y) on serial imaging should be considered for surgical excision, especially in younger patients in good health.
- Meningiomas that become symptomatic at any point during the follow-up period should be considered for surgical intervention.

- Postoperative radiotherapy should be considered for patients with subtotal resection of WHO grade II, and all WHO grade III meningiomas.

References

[1] Ostrom QT, Gittleman H, Fulop J, et al. CBTRUS statistical report: primary brain and central nervous system tumors diagnosed in the United States in 2008–2012. Neuro-oncol. 2015; 17 Suppl 4:iv1–iv62

[2] Ambe SN, Lyon KA, Nizamutdinov D, Fonkem E. Incidence trends, rates, and ethnic variations of primary CNS tumors in Texas from 1995 to 2013. Neurooncol Pract. 2018; 5(3):154–160

[3] Maxwell R, Chou S. Convexity meningiomas and general principles of meningioma surgery. In: Schmidek H, Sweet W, eds. Operative Neurosurgical Techniques, Indications and Methods. New York, NY: Grune & Stratton; 1982:491–501

[4] Giombini S, Solero CL, Morello G. Late outcome of operations for supratentorial convexity meningiomas. Report on 207 cases. Surg Neurol. 1984; 22(6):588–594

[5] Hofmann B, Fahlbusch R. Surgical Management of convexity, parasagittal, and falx meningiomas. In: Schmidek H, Roberts D, eds. Operative Neurosurgical Techniques: Indications, Methods, and Results. Philadelphia, PA: Elsevier Inc.; 2006:721–38

[6] Chang V, Narang J, Schultz L, et al. Computer-aided volumetric analysis as a sensitive tool for the management of incidental meningiomas. Acta Neurochir (Wien). 2012; 154(4):589–597, discussion 597

[7] Firsching RP, Fischer A, Peters R, Thun F, Klug N. Growth rate of incidental meningiomas. J Neurosurg. 1990; 73(4):545–547

[8] Hashimoto N, Rabo CS, Okita Y, et al. Slower growth of skull base meningiomas compared with non-skull base meningiomas based on volumetric and biological studies. J Neurosurg. 2012; 116(3):574–580

[9] Herscovici Z, Rappaport Z, Sulkes J, Danaila L, Rubin G. Natural history of conservatively treated meningiomas. Neurology. 2004; 63(6):1133–1134

[10] Jadid KD, Feychting M, Höijer J, Hylin S, Kihlström L, Mathiesen T. Long-term follow-up of incidentally discovered meningiomas. Acta Neurochir (Wien). 2015; 157(2):225–230, discussion 230

[11] Kuratsu J, Kochi M, Ushio Y. Incidence and clinical features of asymptomatic meningiomas. J Neurosurg. 2000; 92(5):766–770

[12] Lee EJ, Park JH, Park ES, Kim JH. "Wait-and-see" strategies for newly diagnosed intracranial meningiomas based on the risk of future observation failure. World Neurosurg. 2017; 107:604–611

[13] Nakamura M, Roser F, Michel J, Jacobs C, Samii M. The natural history of incidental meningiomas. Neurosurgery. 2003; 53(1):62–70, discussion 70–71

[14] Niiro M, Yatsushiro K, Nakamura K, Kawahara Y, Kuratsu J. Natural history of elderly patients with asymptomatic meningiomas. J Neurol Neurosurg Psychiatry. 2000; 68(1):25–28

[15] Olivero WC, Lister JR, Elwood PW. The natural history and growth rate of asymptomatic meningiomas: a review of 60 patients. J Neurosurg. 1995; 83(2):222–224

[16] Oya S, Kim SH, Sade B, Lee JH. The natural history of intracranial meningiomas. J Neurosurg. 2011; 114(5):1250–1256

[17] Romani R, Ryan G, Benner C, Pollock J. Non-operative meningiomas: long-term follow-up of 136 patients. Acta Neurochir (Wien). 2018; 160(8):1547–1553

[18] Rubin G, Herscovici Z, Laviv Y, Jackson S, Rappaport ZH. Outcome of untreated meningiomas. Isr Med Assoc J. 2011; 13(3):157–160

[19] Yano S, Kuratsu J, Kumamoto Brain Tumor Research Group. Indications for surgery in patients with asymptomatic meningiomas based on an extensive experience. J Neurosurg. 2006; 105(4):538–543

[20] Yoneoka Y, Fujii Y, Tanaka R. Growth of incidental meningiomas. Acta Neurochir (Wien). 2000; 142(5):507–511

[21] Wong RH, Wong AK, Vick N, Farhat HI. Natural history of multiple meningiomas. Surg Neurol Int. 2013; 4:71

[22] Alvernia JE, Dang ND, Sindou MP. Convexity meningiomas: study of recurrence factors with special emphasis on the cleavage plane in a series of 100 consecutive patients. J Neurosurg. 2011; 115(3):491–498

[23] Hasseleid BF, Meling TR, Rønning P, Scheie D, Helseth E. Surgery for convexity meningioma: Simpson Grade I resection as the goal—clinical article. J Neurosurg. 2012; 117(6):999–1006

[24] Morokoff AP, Zauberman J, Black PM. Surgery for convexity meningiomas. Neurosurgery. 2008; 63(3):427–433, discussion 433–434

[25] Sanai N, Sughrue ME, Shangari G, Chung K, Berger MS, McDermott MW. Risk profile associated with convexity meningioma resection in the modern neurosurgical era. J Neurosurg. 2010; 112(5):913–919

[26] Simpson D. The recurrence of intracranial meningiomas after surgical treatment. J Neurol Neurosurg Psychiatry. 1957; 20(1):22–39

[27] Jääskeläinen J, Haltia M, Servo A. Atypical and anaplastic meningiomas: radiology, surgery, radiotherapy, and outcome. Surg Neurol. 1986; 25(3):233–242

[28] Kinjo T, al-Mefty O, Kanaan I. Grade zero removal of supratentorial convexity meningiomas. Neurosurgery. 1993; 33(3):394–399, discussion 399

[29] Bendszus M, Rao G, Burger R, et al. Is there a benefit of preoperative meningioma embolization? Neurosurgery. 2000; 47(6):1306–1311, discussion 1311–1312

[30] Raper DM, Starke RM, Henderson F, Jr, et al. Preoperative embolization of intracranial meningiomas: efficacy, technical considerations, and complications. AJNR Am J Neuroradiol. 2014; 35(9):1798–1804

[31] Kondziolka D, Madhok R, Lunsford LD, et al. Stereotactic radiosurgery for convexity meningiomas. J Neurosurg. 2009; 111(3):458–463

[32] Kaur G, Sayegh ET, Larson A, et al. Adjuvant radiotherapy for atypical and malignant meningiomas: a systematic review. Neuro-oncol. 2014; 16(5):628–636

24 Natural History and Management Options of Ruptured Brain Arteriovenous Malformation

Darius Tan, Helen Huang, and Leon T. Lai

Abstract

Ruptured bAVM have an increased risk of rerupture. Various other factors such as location, associated aneurysm, and drainage may also affect rerupture risk. Intervention options include surgery, stereotactic radiosurgery, endovascular embolization, or combinations of the above with the goals to obviate further rupture risk. Each of these modalities have associated benefits and risks that clinicians need to weigh carefully in decision making in order to provide the patient with the best available treatment. This chapter aims to review the current evidence in relation to the natural history and treatment options in ruptured brain arteriovenous malformations.

Keywords: brain arteriovenous malformation, subarachnoid hemorrhage, intracerebral hemorrhage, natural history, microsurgery, stereotactic radiosurgery, embolization, endovascular treatment

24.1 Introduction

Ruptured brain arteriovenous malformations (bAVMs) are relatively uncommon with reported incidence between 0.4 and 3.5 per 100,000 person-years.[1,2,3,4,5] Approximately 1.4% of strokes can be attributed to ruptured bAVM.[6] In young patients (≤ 40 years), ruptured bAVM accounts for approximately 33% of intracerebral hemorrhages (ICHs)[7] and represents a major cause of morbidity and mortality.[8,9,10,11,12,13] The prevalence of incidental bAVM is estimated to be approximately 45 per 100,000 persons.[14] However, this may be an overestimate, and to date, there are no studies to determine an accurate prevalence of bAVMs.[15,16,17] The mean age at presentation is around 33.7 years (95% confidence interval [CI]: 31.1–36.2), with no significant differences in gender predilection (females: 45%; 95% CI: 42–49%).[13] The risk of rupture is cumulative over a lifetime, with the overall risk potentially affected by age; however, there has been suggestions that pediatric bAVM may have a greater propensity for rupture.[18,19,20,21]

Although there are individuals with a clear genetic predisposition, for example, hereditary hemorrhagic telangiectasia, most bAVMs are sporadic.[22] Molecular association with bAVMs has been increasingly studied such as matrix metalloproteinases, ApoE ε2, interleukin-1α, and interleukin-6.[23] These have been found to be in greater expression in individuals with ruptured bAVMs and observational studies have shown an increased risk of hemorrhage in the affected individuals.[24,25,26,27,28,29,30,31] Single nucleotide polymorphisms in proinflammatory molecules such as interleukin-1 lead to increased inflammation of vasculature that has been associated with increased bAVM rupture risk and may contribute to the natural history of bAVM rupture.[24]

Understanding the natural clinical sequelae following bAVM rupture is important to guide clinical practice. Few studies in the literature have captured the natural history of ruptured bAVM due to selection bias, retrospective analysis, short follow-up, and/or partial or complete treatment. This chapter aims to summarize the natural history and treatment options for ruptured bAVMs.

24.2 Selected Papers on the Natural History of Ruptured bAVMs

- Stapf C, Mast H, Sciacca RR, et al. Predictors of hemorrhage in patients with untreated brain arteriovenous malformation. Neurology 2006;66(9):1350–1355
- Yamada S, Takagi Y, Nozaki K, Kikuta K, Hashimoto N. Risk factors for subsequent hemorrhage in patients with cerebral arteriovenous malformations. J Neurosurg 2007;107(5):965–972
- Kim H, Al-Shahi Salman R, McCulloch CE, Stapf C, Young WL; MARS Coinvestigators. Untreated brain arteriovenous malformation: patient-level meta-analysis of hemorrhage predictors. Neurology 2014;83(7):590–597
- da Costa L, Wallace MC, Ter Brugge KG, O'Kelly C, Willinsky RA, Tymianski M. The natural history and predictive features of hemorrhage from brain arteriovenous malformations. Stroke 2009;40(1):100–105

24.3 Natural History of Ruptured bAVM

To date, there are no specific studies that examine the natural history of ruptured bAVM. Most literature data were discussed in conjunction with unruptured cases. Ruptured bAVMs may lead to variable clinical presentation depending on hemorrhage location, degree of raised intracranial pressure (ICP), and possible associated hydrocephalus from intraventricular hemorrhage. Typically, grading scales for subarachnoid hemorrhage have been used for clinical assessment following rupture. In addition, novel grading scales (► Table 24.1 and ► Table 24.2) have been developed to correlate with outcomes.[32,33]

Compared to spontaneous/primary ICH, ruptured bAVM is generally associated with a more favorable clinical outcome.[9,34,35] Younger patients (20–40 years) have a lower risk of death and are more likely to be discharged home.[35] However, outcomes are generally worse for ICH, when compared to subarachnoid hemorrhage or intraventricular hemorrhage.[34] Whereas studies have a heterogenous classification of morbidity, approximately 60% of patients with ruptured bAVMs will have a modified Rankin Scale (mRS) score of 1 to 2 at 1 year postrupture.[9] Comparison of outcomes for ICH due to bAVM versus non-bAVM-related cases are summarized in ► Table 24.3.

Morgan et al reported that for ruptured bAVMs that are untreated, subsequent hemorrhage has a cumulative 70% risk of new permanent neurological deficit or death and a 42% risk of death.[10] Choi et al suggested recurrent AVM hemorrhage does not convey much additional mortality risk. Recurrent hemorrhage only resulted in a slightly greater morbidity than initial hemorrhage (mean National Institute of Health Stroke Scale [NIHSS]: 5.7 ± 8.4 compared to 3.6 ± 6.2).[36] This has also been shown in other smaller studies.[37,38] These studies are limited to retrospective, relatively small-sized studies, or databases with methodological limitations, which limits generalization of results and the quantification of effect. Nonetheless, it is accepted that the risk of recurrent hemorrhage following bAVM rupture is initially higher.[38]

24.4 Risk of Recurrent Hemorrhage

Once a bAVM has ruptured, its behavior is altered and the risk of rehemorrhage increases. Rate of rerupture is between 6.2 and 15.4% in the first year,[19] and gradually returning to the baseline in the following years. Key studies are summarized in ▶ Table 24.4 and ▶ Fig. 24.1 (as graphical representation). A meta-analysis including 16,978 patients-years calculated an annual rerupture rate of 4.5% (range: 3.7–5.5%) compared to 2.2% in unruptured bAVM (range: 1.7–2.7%) and the risk of hemorrhage

following rupture of bAVM was HR 3.2 (95% CI 2.1–4.3) compared to unruptured bAVM.[13] A recent review by Morgan et al demonstrated in survival curves for cumulative risk of rupture based on studies with substantial sample sizes and follow-up an estimated risk of rerupture of 4.8% in the first 8 years that subsequently decreased to 1.8% per year.[10] In all studies, due to relatively short length of follow-up, it is difficult to predict rupture risk beyond 10 years.[10]

24.5 Other Factors

A recent meta-analysis demonstrated prior hemorrhage to infer the greater risk for subsequent rupture (hazard ratio [HR]: 3.2;

Table 24.1 Ruptured arteriovenous malformation grading scale[33]

Variable	Value	Points
Hunt and Hess score	1–5	1–5
Age (y)	<35	0
	35–70	1
	>70	2
Deep venous drainage	No	0
	Yes	1
Eloquent area	No	0
	Yes	1
Total score		1–9

Note: A lower score indicates a more favorable prognosis.

Table 24.2 Arteriovenous malformation–related intracerebral hemorrhage (AVICH) score[32]

Variable	Value	Points
Size (cm³)	<3	1
	3–6	2
	>6	3
Deep venous drainage	No	0
	Yes	1
Eloquent area	No	0
	Yes	1
Age (y)	<20	1
	20–40	2
	>40	3
Diffuse nidus	No	0
	Yes	1
Glasgow Coma Scale score	13–15	0
	5–12	1
	3–4	2
Intracerebral hemorrhage volume (cm³)	<30	0
	≥30	1
Intraventricular hemorrhage	No	0
	Yes	1
Total		2–13

Note: A lower score indicates a more favorable prognosis.

Table 24.3 Comparison of outcomes for intracranial hemorrhage due to bAVM versus non-bAVM related

Studies	Databases	Patients (no.)	Morbidity	Mortality
Choi et al[34]	Columbia AVM database, NOMAS	198	3.9 ± 6.2 vs. 13.6 ± 9.5, p <0.001[a]	NR
Murthy et al[35]	NIS, CAESAR	NIS = 619,167 CAESAR = 342	NIS: OR: 2.03 (95% CI: 1.38–2.98), p <0.001[b] CAESAR: OR: 4.39 (95% CI: 1.47–13.06), p = 0.008[b]	NIS: 12.9 vs. 29.5%; OR: 0.53 (95% CI: 0.40–0.71), p <0.001 CAESAR: 13.3 vs. 25.0%; OR: 0.85 (95% CI: 0.19–7.82), p = 0.625
Van Beijnum et al[9]	OXVASC, SIVMS	OXVASC = 90 SIVMS = 60	40 vs. 83%, OR: 7.5 (95% CI: 3.0–19)[c]	11 vs. 50%, OR: 8.0 (95% CI: 3.5–18)

Abbreviations: bAVM, brain arteriovenous malformation; CAESAR, Cornell Acute stroke Academic Registry; ICH, intracranial hemorrhage; IPH, intraparenchymal hemorrhage; OR, odds ratio; mRS, modified Rankin Scale; NIHSS, National Institute of Health Stroke Scale; NIS, Nationwide Inpatient Sample; NOMAS, Northern Manhattan Study; NR, not reported; OXVASC, Oxford Vascular Study; SD, standard deviation; SIVMS, Scottish Intracranial Vascular Malformation Study.
[a]Morbidity measured by median NIHSS score ≤30 days after hemorrhage.
[b]Morbidity measured by discharge home.
[c]mRS ≥3 at 12 months.

Table 24.4 Rehemorrhage rates following ruptured bAVM

Studies	No. of patients	Risk of rehemorrhage, % (95% CI)	Follow-up, median (range)
Crawford et al[51]	140	3.6 at 0–10 y 1.7 at ≥20 y	9.0 (1–35) y
Yamada et al[19]	159	15.42 at 1 y 5.32 at 2–5 y 1.72 at >5 y	4.1 mo (1 d–314 mo)
Hernesniemi et al 2008[40]	139	6.2 at 0–5 y 2.8 overall	5.0 (0.1–41.8) y
Stapf et al[42]	282	5.9 (3.8–8.6)	65.0 (NR) d
Da Costa et al[39]	258	9.65 at 1 y 6.30 at 2–5 y 3.67 at ≥5 y 7.48 overall	2.9 (NR) y
Kim et al[21] (UCSF, COL, SIVMS and KPNC databases)	389	9.76 (7.16–13.31) at 1 y 10.73 (8.06–14.29) at 2 y 5.85 (4.61–7.42) at 5 y 4.8 (3.88–5.94) at 10 y	NR (up to 10 y)

Abbreviations: bAVM, brain arteriovenous malformation; CI, confidence interval; COL, Columbia; HR, hazards ratio; KPNC, Kaiser Permanente of Northern California; RR, relative risk; SIVMS, Scottish Intracranial Vascular Malformation Study; UCSF, University of California San Francisco.

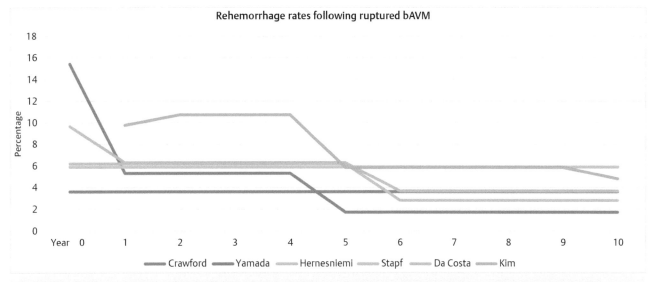

Fig. 24.1 Graphical representation of key studies on the rehemorrhage rates following ruptured brain arteriovenous malformation (bAVM). Note: Hemorrhage rate averaged across several years and therefore yearly variation may not be accounted for in the data. Kim et al[21] provided hemorrhage rates at points 1, 2, 5, and 10 years.

95% CI: 2.1–4.1), followed by deep nidal location (HR: 2.4; 95% CI: 1.4–3.4), exclusively deep venous drainage (HR: 2.4; 95% CI: 1.1–3.8), and associated aneurysm (HR: 1.8; 95% CI: 1.6–2.0).[13] Female gender, age, and size were shown to have no significant relationship to hemorrhage.[13] Age was shown to be a significant factor for rupture in the Multicenter AVM Research Study (MARS), which was in concordance with Stapf et al.[42] However, multiple other studies have not confirmed this relationship.[21,39,40,41] It has been suggested that lack of treatment in the older population, or increased formation with age of associated AVM aneurysm may confound the results.[10] Other factors that are thought to influence the rate of hemorrhage in ruptured bAVM include associated intranidal/perinidal aneurysms, location, deep venous drainage, pregnancy, and size. Importantly, these risk factors can change with hemorrhage,

which may reflect alteration of physiology and flow dynamics of the bAVM following rupture.[19,42] Therefore, these risk factors are not static and need to be taken into consideration with other factors when discerning the natural history between an already ruptured bAVM compared to an unruptured bAVM (▶ Table 24.5).

24.6 Associated Aneurysms

Associated aneurysms are found in approximately 20% of bAVMs and can be classified according to location and whether it is within the nidus, distant from the nidus, or flow related (saccular aneurysm from artery feeding the nidus).[13,43] Flow-related aneurysms can be further divided into whether they stem from a major proximal artery (i.e., internal carotid artery, circle of

Table 24.5 Key factors associated with risk of rehemorrhage following ruptured bAVM

Risk factor	Hazard ratio (95% CI)	p-value
Age	1.05 (1.03–1.07)	<0.0001
Deep nidal location	3.52 (1.66–7.47)	0.001
Deep venous drainage only	3.10 (1.58–6.08)	0.001
Associated aneurysm (intranidal and feeding artery aneurysm)	1.83 (0.95–3.50)	0.07

Abbreviations: bAVM, brain arteriovenous malformation; CI, confidence interval.
Source: Adapted from Stapf et al.[42]

Willis, anterior cerebral artery up to the anterior communicating artery, vertebrobasilar trunk, and middle cerebral artery) or distal to the aforementioned. A large, pooled analysis of bAVM-associated aneurysms showed flow-related aneurysms account for approximately 71% (proximal 47%, distal 25%), intranidal aneurysm account for 25%, and unrelated aneurysms account for 4%.[43] In this study of 10,093 ruptured bAVMs (first and/or subsequent), the source of bleed was from the aneurysm in 49% of cases and the nidus in 45% of cases.[43] There are limited studies to adequately assess the natural history of subsequent rupture, but there may be a trend for increased bAVM rupture if there is an associated aneurysm.[42,44] One study showed associated aneurysms (either intranidal or feeding artery aneurysms) had an odds ratio of 2.27 (95% CI: 1.55–3.34; $p < 0.0001$) of rupture at initial presentation, but this effect was not significant when analyzing those that already ruptured with an HR of 1.83 (95% CI: 0.95–3.5; $p = 0.07$).[42] In contrast, in a study of ruptured pediatric bAVMs, there was a relative risk of 2.68 ($p = 0.04$) of subsequent rupture with associated aneurysms.[44]

24.7 Infratentorial Brain Arteriovenous Malformations

Few studies have explored the relation between infratentorial bAVM and rupture. Although it is thought that the initial risk of rupture from an infratentorial bAVM is higher than that of a supratentorial bAVM with odds of rupture up to 3.89 (95% CI: 1.10–13.72; $p = 0.0092$),[40,42,45] this effect may be different with subsequent rupture. Stapf et al comprehensively studied risk factors at initial presentation, and then on subsequent hemorrhage, and found the risk profile altered.[42] For instance, infratentorial AVM location had an initial hemorrhage odds ratio of 3.27 (95% CI: 1.93–5.53; $p < 0.0001$), whereas posthemorrhage, the HR of rupture was 0.68 (95% CI: 0.16–2.82; $p = 0.59$). These effect differences may have treatment bias due to small numbers or confounding factors. Small sample size in analyzing risk factors in the hemorrhagic group may also be due to treatment bias as infratentorial bAVMs may be treated more expediently due to poorer outcomes in infratentorial bAVMs,[38,46] whereas poor outcome in this group may reduce numbers for further analysis in the subsequent hemorrhage cohort. Therefore, these challenges must be kept in mind when interpreting the risk factors associated with subsequent bAVM rupture.

24.8 Deep Venous Drainage

Deep venous drainage is defined as venous drainage into deep veins that include the internal cerebral veins, basal veins, or precentral cerebral veins. Within the posterior fossa, drainage to locations other than the straight sinus, torcula, or transverse sinus is considered deep.[47] Drainage to the deep venous drainage is associated with increased risk of rupture (HR: 1.3; 95% CI: 0.9–1.75; $p > 0.05$), and this risk is further increased with solely deep venous drainage (HR: 2.4; 95% CI: 1.1–3.8; $p < 0.05$).[13,21,42,48] This has been postulated to be secondary to increased pressure in the deep venous system that translates to increased pressures across the nidus, thereby increasing the risk of hemorrhage.[13] There are few studies that determine the nature of a bAVM following rupture.[42,49] However, once a bAVM with solely deep venous drainage has ruptured, the risk for further rupture remains increased, albeit slightly less than if unruptured (HR: 3.39–3.1; $p < 0.05$).[42]

24.9 Selected Papers on the Treatment of Ruptured bAVMs

- Lawton MT, Du R, Tran MN, et al. Effect of presenting hemorrhage on outcome after microsurgical resection of brain arteriovenous malformations. Neurosurgery 2005;56(3):485–493, discussion 485–493
- Aboukaïs R, Marinho P, Baroncini M, et al. Ruptured cerebral arteriovenous malformations: outcomes analysis after microsurgery. Clin Neurol Neurosurg 2015;138:137–142
- Ding D, Yen CP, Starke RM, Xu Z, Sheehan JP. Radiosurgery for ruptured intracranial arteriovenous malformations. J Neurosurg 2014;121(2):470–481

24.10 Treatment Options for Ruptured bAVM

Much of the initial management following ruptured bAVM stems from ICH management studies, which includes ICP control, blood pressure management to less than 140 mm Hg, external ventricular drainage for management of hydrocephalus/monitoring of ICP, reversal of coagulopathy, and monitoring in a neurological intensive care setting.[52,53,54] Whether aggressive blood pressure targets are beneficial in ICH is debatable and several studies have shown varying results with no significant differences in mortality but potentially some benefit with functional outcomes.[53,55,56,57] Following initial diagnosis and management, subsequent goals are to decide on whether the bAVM is treatable and then the optimal timing for definitive treatment of the bAVM. Treatment options include conservative management, endovascular embolization, radiosurgery, microsurgery, or a combination of these strategies.

24.11 Surgery

Surgical treatment should be carried out for ruptured bAVMs in accordance with initial management of ICP and where large supratentorial hematoma (> 30 mL) or infratentorial hematoma

(> 10 mL) is present, these should be evacuated initially with or without bAVM removal.[58] Risk of rerupture, while initially increased following rupture, is still relatively low enough to delay treatment by several weeks or months. Irrespective of timing, surgery is dependent on previously described surgical grading systems, which are used for risk stratification following treatment. These help the neurosurgeon decide which ruptured bAVMs are suitable from a risk–benefit point of view for surgical resection. Grading systems include the Spetzler–Martin (SM), Spetzler–Ponce classification (SPC), and Lawton–Young (LY) supplementary grading systems.[47,59,60,61,62] The SM and SPC gradings include size, venous drainage, and eloquent cortex involvement as proven predictors for operative outcome. The LY supplementary grading added on compactness, age, and rupture status. With rupture, the hematoma creates corridors that previously would require transection of cerebral tissue and therefore can improve surgical access to the bAVM.[63] In patients with already ruptured bAVMs and presurgery neurological deficits, patients have a decreased chance of developing new deficits. Comparing surgical resection in those who had ruptured bAVMs and nonruptured bAVMs in 232 patients, there were no significant differences in improved/unchanged outcomes (compared to preoperation) with surgery.[64]

The initial study by Lawton et al also evaluated deep perforating artery supply, but this was not significantly related to outcome; however, a subsequent study with a greater number of surgically treated SM IV to V has suggested this may be a significant predictor.[59,63] The SM scale has traditionally been the major scale utilized as a guide for treatment/outcomes and is validated in multiple studies.[60,67,68] A meta-analysis by Spetzler and Ponce (mix of ruptured/unruptured data) showed good concordance with grading among the SM and SPC gradings.[61] Unfavorable outcomes were the following: SM I to II, 4 to 10% compared to SPC A, 8%; SM III, 18% compared to SPC B 18%; and SM IV to V, 31 to 37% compared to SPC C, 32%.[61] Although these studies are heterogenous in the definition of negative outcomes, subject to inclusion bias, and have varying adjuvant treatment, generally, SM grades I to II (SPC A) are considered favorable for microsurgical operative management, SM III (SPC B) typically require multimodal therapy, and SM IV to V (SPC C) are generally for conservative treatment.[61] An LY grading of ≤6 correlated to a morbidity of ≤24%, which has been suggested to be the cutoff for resection and provides an acceptable risk of morbidity. Whereas all these studies did not exclusively analyze ruptured bAVMs, a large study (n = 529) showed concordant outcomes despite approximately 50% of cases presenting as ruptured bAVMs.[68]

Although the literature suggests that resection of higher-grade AVMs is associated with poor outcomes, it is difficult to quantify these due to small numbers partly fueled by inherent selection bias and clinical trends to no longer treat higher-grade bAVMs. For instance, in 1986 when Spetzler initially described the grading system, 16% of patients operated on were SM V AVMs. In a similar time, Heros operated on 14% of these; comparing these with a cohort in the 2000s, Lawton only operated on 1% of these.[61] Based on current evidence, it appears that for low-grade bAVMs, the "gold standard" should be surgery regardless of whether it is ruptured or unruptured as it provides high cure rates (up to 98.5%), and low unfavorable outcomes (2.2% morbidity and 0.3% mortality).[10,61,64,68,69,70] Surgery for

moderate-grade (SM III) AVMs also has high obliteration rates of approximately 97% with acceptable postoperative outcomes for ruptured bAVM (~13% worse mRS compared to preoperative state).[65,70,71] In contrast, microsurgery on ruptured SM IV or V bAVMs has significantly poorer outcomes compared to unruptured bAVMs. Deterioration and death compared to preoperative mRS scores were 40 and 100%, respectively.[70] This is consistent with other studies that examined solely ruptured bAVMs as well as mixed ruptured/unruptured bAVMs.[47,61,68,72] Older age, higher World Federation of Neurosurgical Societies (WFNS) grades, higher SM grading, or presence of hydrocephalus are predictive factors for poor outcome following microsurgery.[72] These predictive factors are factored into the AVM-related ICH (AVICH) and ruptured AVM Grading Scale (RAGS) scores.

24.11.1 Timing of Intervention

Evidence on the optimal timing of intervention following ruptured bAVM is not well defined. Available data have been mostly historical or anecdotal. It has been hypothesized that early surgery may be negatively impacted by brain edema, which may lead to difficulty in hemostasis, increased risk of iatrogenic injury, and poor visualization of the AVM due to distortion by the hematoma.[58,73,74] Therefore, surgery was typically performed several weeks later to allow liquefaction of the hematoma, allowing for better visualization and dissection plane.[74] The exceptions to this may be with superficial small AVM nidus with easy access or those ruptured cases with large hematoma causing severe mass effect. Some authors may carry out decompressive craniectomy with little or no evacuation of hematoma.[75,76] As the rehemorrhage rate for ruptured bAVM is increased, the rationale and timing for delay must be weighed up with risk of rehemorrhage. In the acute period, an approximation of 1% rerupture risk per month (based on natural history and delayed treatment studies) is probably a safe estimate.[19,73] However, early resection prevents rerupture, decreases medical expenses, decreases potential reappearance of neurological deficits (that may have improved with rehab), and allows early rehabilitation.[77] It has been suggested that early surgery may also facilitate recovery from neurological damage carried out by compressive hematoma, allow recovery from hemorrhage and AVM simultaneously, and allow better dissection compared to when the hematoma forms chronic gliosis.[78,79] Nonetheless, there are few studies to suggest that early surgery may in fact be beneficial for AVMs with varying conclusions.[77,78,79,80] Key studies on the timing and surgical outcomes for ruptured bAVMs are summarized in ▶ Table 24.6.

There are no specific studies that evaluate timing of surgery for posterior fossa bAVMs. Many clinicians anecdotally condone delayed resection for these.[81,82,83,84] In any case, posterior fossa AVMs have a higher risk of rupture/poor outcomes (mRS >2 in ~90% of patients) and this needs to be considered when selecting the timing and modality of treatment.[40,42,46] As the posterior fossa is a "tighter" space with important structures such as the brainstem and the fourth ventricle located within, evacuation of hematoma with or without AVM resection should be considered. Deep brainstem/cerebellar AVMs are thought to be best suited for multimodal treatment or radiosurgery.[81,85] In Drake et al's study,[86] only 2/15 brainstem AVMs could be safely surgically resected without major improvement from

Table 24.6 Selected studies on early and delayed microsurgical treatment of ruptured bAVM

Study	No. of patients	Study type	Timing of treatment	SM/SPC grades	Obliteration rate	Clinical outcome measures	Study conclusion
Kuhmonen et al[80]	49	Retrospective	Within 4 d	SM I/II: 59% SM III: 27% SM IV/V: 14%	98%	Good outcome (GOS ≥4): 55.1%	Good outcomes with earlier surgery (no comparison)
Bir et al[116]	78	Retrospective	<24 h, 24–48 h, >48 h	SM I: 24.4% SM II: 37% SM III: 32% SM IV: 6.5% SM V: 0%	NR	Good outcome: mRS ≤2[a]	Improved outcome with earlier treatment
Hafez et al[77]	59	Retrospective	Median: 2 d (range: 0–360 d)	SM I/II: 53% SM III: 27% SM IV/V: 20%	NR	Good outcome (GOS ≥4) (overall) at 2–4 mo: 73% At 12 mo: 75%	No significant difference between timing and outcome
Beecher et al[73]	102	Retrospective	Mean: 6.1 mo	NR	NR	Good outcome (GOS ≥4) On discharge: 90.7% At 6 mo: 92.3%	Improved outcome with delayed treatment (no comparison)
Barone et al[76]	21	Prospective	Early (within 24 h)	SPC A: 61.9% SPC B: 23.8% SPB C: 14.3%	SPC A: 92% SPC B: 100% SPC C: 100%	Good outcome (mRS ≤2): SPC A: 69% SPC B: 20% SPB C: 33%	Improved outcome with delayed treatment
	44		Delayed (median: 12 d; IQR: 8–17 d)	SPC A: 75% SPC B: 20.5% SPB C: 4.5%	SPC A: 97% SPC B: 100% SPC C: 50%	Good outcome mRS ≤2: SPC A: 94% SPC B: 89% SPB C: 50%	

Abbreviations: bAVM, brain arteriovenous malformation; GOS, Glasgow Outcome Score; IQR, interquartile range; mRS, modified Rankin Scale; NR, not reported; OR, odds ratio; SM, Spetzler–Martin; SPC, Spetzler–Ponce classification.
[a]Mean mRS after surgery: <24 hours—0.84; 24–48 hours—0.73; >48 hours—2.06.

pretreatment. In this series of posterior fossa AVMs, 51/66 had attempted surgery with complete resection in 92% of patients, 73% of patients had a good outcome following excision of AVM, and 16% died following this.

24.12 Stereotactic Radiosurgery

Stereotactic radiosurgery (SRS) may be considered for ruptured high-grade bAVMs, small deep nidal lesions, or those located in eloquent regions. The effect is achieved by progressive intimal hyperplasia causing eventual thrombosis of vessels and thereby exclusion of the nidus from the circulation. However, SRS is not without risk and may cause radiation-induced changes (RICs) and risk of hemorrhage even with obliteration of the nidus.[87] The effects of SRS on obliteration of bAVM require time, and there is a period of latency where the AVM is not fully obliterated and still carries a risk of repeat hemorrhage. Post-SRS, the risk of hemorrhage does decrease but is not completely nullified until the bAVM is completely obliterated.[88,89,90,91] There are limited numbers of studies that evaluate SRS in ruptured bAVMs, and most studies include both ruptured and unruptured bAVMs. Nonetheless, it appears that SRS is effective in ruptured cases with early decreases in rupture risk.[88,91,92] Maruyama et al showed an 8% hemorrhage rate prior to SRS, which decreased to 5% following SRS until obliteration and 2% postobliteration.[88] Compared with the pre-SRS period, they calculated a 54%

decreased risk of hemorrhage (HR: 0.46; 95% CI: 0.26–0.80; $p = 0.006$) during the latency period between SRS and bAVM obliteration, and a 88%. Decreased risk following obliteration (HR: 0.26; 95% CI: 0.10–0.68; $p = 0.006$). This has also been demonstrated by Yen et al in patients with previous ruptured AVMs, with a 10.4% diagnosis-SRS hemorrhage rate that decreased to 2.8% during the latent period.[90] One study showed an adjusted HR of 0.34 (95% CI: 0.19–0.62; $p < 0.001$) for subsequent hemorrhage in ruptured bAVM patients treated with gamma knife SRS compared to those treated conservatively.[91] Factors that influenced the success (lack of hemorrhage or obliteration) of treatment include smaller size, presence of a single venous drainage, lower Virginia radiosurgery-based AVM score/ SM grading, absence of pre-embolization, and increased prescription dose.[90,92]

Although microsurgery is the "gold standard" for low-grade bAVMs,[64] SRS should be considered in patients who have higher-grade bAVMs, unsuitable operative candidates due to surgical, anesthesiological challenges or patient's preferences. Ding et al showed that in SRS for ruptured and unruptured bAVMs, there were no significant differences with similar obliteration and complication rates (~60 and 45% of hemorrhage and RIC mortality, respectively).[93] Although the complication rate may seem high when closely examined, approximately 30% of these were due to radiological RIC and when evaluating symptomatic RIC, this was approximately 9%, which were mainly transient. Permanent RIC in this cohort was approximately 2%.

Post-SRS rehemorrhage was 8% in the ruptured bAVM cohort and mortality was roughly 8%.[93] Factors that influence optimal outcomes for ruptured bAVMs are similar to unruptured bAVMs. Particularly, higher doses (≥ 20 Gy) were more effective at obliteration and were also associated with reduced post-SRS hemorrhage.[92,93,94] Adjuvant embolization of bAVM prior to SRS leads to lower obliteration rates, but may have a place in treatment of bAVM-related aneurysm (which are associated with higher hemorrhage rates).[92,93,95,96]

There is currently no series that evaluates SRS on solely ruptured high-grade bAVM. However, mixed ruptured and unruptured studies report obliteration rates of between 35.6 and 43.6% and morbidity of 10.0 to 11.6%.[97,98] Although the combined neurological morbidity and mortality may not be as high as that from surgical series, it is important to consider the lower obliteration rate from SRS in treatment decision.[61,66,67,68,99] An emerging strategy is combining volume-staged SRS with surgery, with the aim of SRS to downgrade the AVM to a more "favorable" surgical lesion.[100,101] In doing so, this can lead to improved outcomes, shorter operative times, decreased blood loss, and decreased length of hospital stay.[100]

24.12.1 Timing of Radiosurgery

Timing of SRS is likely to be more beneficial within 6 months of rupture as initial risks of rerupture are higher in the first year.[102] SRS is rarely used in the acute setting and it has been proposed that it should be carried out after 6 to 12 weeks post-rupture.[92] One study grouped the treatment into 0 to 3, 3 to 6, and greater than 6 months, and found that 25% of patients who waited more than 6 months had a recurrent hemorrhage.[102]

24.13 Embolization

The role of endovascular embolization for ruptured bAVMs continues to evolve rapidly. Although this modality was previously reserved for unruptured cases, or as adjunct therapy to microsurgical excision and SRS in ruptured lesions, growing experience with endovascular techniques, the introduction of nonadhesive, embolic, ethylene vinyl alcohol polymers, and the development of transvenous techniques have fundamentally altered ruptured bAVM treatment. In selected cases with favorable angioarchitecture, in opportune patients, performed in centers with endovascular expertise, embolization of ruptured bAVMs may be considered a safe and feasible pursuit.[103,104,105]

For ruptured bAVMs, the materials, equipment, and techniques employed are similar to those used to treat unruptured bAVMs (e.g., adhesive glues, liquid embolic agents, platinum coils). However, ruptured and unruptured bAVMs are clinically distinct entities with divergent natural history. The current literature largely pertains to either unruptured cohorts or heterogenous populations with a mixture of ruptured and unruptured bAVMs. There is a lack of data pertaining to embolization of bAVMs in purely ruptured cohorts, and current literature is largely limited to small, retrospective case series.

24.13.1 Role of Embolization

Given that the risk of subsequent hemorrhage is higher for previously ruptured bAVMs,[41] the aim of embolization, at least in the acute phase, should be to reduce the risk of rebleeding and to improve the subsequent natural history of these lesions, especially to avoid further insult and early rebleeding in acutely unwell patients.

In current practice, proponents of endovascular treatment have advocated for the role of targeted embolization of specific, "weak" structures, as an acute, temporizing measure prior to definitive treatment. These features include structures such as arterial flow aneurysms, venous outflow stenosis, varices, ectasias, and arteriovenous fistulas, within ruptured bAVMs. If thought to be the source of hemorrhage, the presence of these features presents a higher risk of rerupture, and their specific elimination is thought to reduce the risk of rebleeding and improve the overall outcome. This can be achieved without significantly altering hemodynamics within the bAVM, which may predispose to further rupture. However, there has been little evidence in literature to support the reduction of future rehemorrhage risk or a protective role for this approach.[103,106,107,108,109] Nonetheless, it has been reported that the annual rehemorrhage rate following targeted culprit aneurysm embolization is between 3.1 and 3.4%, which is similar to the baseline risk of hemorrhage in unruptured lesions.[106,108]

There has also been an emergence of curative approaches to endovascular embolization of bAVMs, even during the acute phase of rupture. This has been largely attempted in low-grade lesions (usually grade I–III), with small, compact nidi and relatively simple angioarchitecture.[103,110] In a small retrospective case series by van Rooij et al,[105] 23 ruptured bAVMs were embolized within the acute phase, post ictus, with 57% of cases achieving complete obliteration and with comparable rates of morbidity and mortality compared with other studies. Although the authors did not report the SM grade of the studied bAVMs, they were mostly small, supratentorial lesions with any complicating hydrocephalus or SAH. Overall, there are few reports of acute endovascular embolization of higher-grade bAVMs, with or without curative intent, which is often considered a challenging and treacherous task.[103]

24.13.2 Timing of Embolization

Optimal timing of treatment, especially of endovascular embolization, for ruptured bAVMs remains controversial. In a small case series by Signorelli et al,[108] 25 patients with ruptured aneurysms associated with bAVMs were embolized within days of ictus. The authors were able to achieve 100.0% occlusion rates of the culprit aneurysm with minimal morbidity and mortality risks. However, their subsequent occlusion rate of the remaining nidus, which was performed in a traditionally delayed fashion in 32% of patients, at a mean of 4.2 months post ictus (range: 1–10 months), was lower than other studies. In another two, small series by van Rooij et al[105] and Stemer et al[107] where embolization (of the aneurysm for the latter) was initiated acutely, within days of ictus, the occlusion, morbidity, and mortality rates were relatively similar in the two series (▶ Table 24.7). In comparison, both He et al[112] and Sun et al[106] reported relatively delayed median time to initial treatment, without any apparent improvement in outcome. Although it is difficult to compare such heterogenous studies, within the limitation of the literature, there is no clear consensus or trend for the optimal timing of endovascular intervention for ruptured bAVMs.

Table 24.7 Selected studies reporting single modality, endovascular treatment of ruptured bAVMs

Study	No. of patients	SM grade (%)	Timing of treatment	Obliteration rate (%)	Morbidity (%)	Annual rehemorrhage rate (%)	Mortality (%)
Andreou et al[114]	25	NR (Micro-AVM, nidus <1 cm)	Median: 2 wk; range: 1–28	84.6 (immediate) 77.0 (at 6 mo)	4.0 (mRS > 2)	0	4.0
Van Rooij et al[105]	23	NR	Within 10 d	57	13.0: classified by functional independence at most recent follow-up	0	4.3
Stemer et al[107]	21	I: 4.8 II: 28.6 III: 28.6 IV: 33.3 V: 0.0 VI: 4.8	Mean: 5.8 d; range: 0–19 Subsequent sessions at 4–6 wk	52.4	9.5: defined by discharge destination to long-term care facility	0	4.8
Signorelli et al[108]	25	I: 12.0 II: 44.0 III: 28.0 IV: 16.0 V: 0.0	Aneurysm: acute presentation (mean: 30.1 h), delayed presentation (mean: 17 d) Nidus: mean: 4.2 mo; range: 1–10	100.0 (aneurysm) 20.0 (nidus)	4%: defined as procedural morbidity	3.4	0.0
Iosif et al[113]	20	I: 0.0 II: 10.0 III: 50.0 IV: 30.0 V: 10.0	NR	95.0	5.0: classified by functional independence at 6 mo	0	5.0
Sun et al[106]	129	I–II: 58.2 III–IV: 41.1 V: 0.8	Aneurysm: median: 42 d; range: 1–160 Nidus: 2–6 wk	17.8	8.0: defined by mRS ≥ 3	3.1	0.9
He et al[112]	21	I: 14.3 II: 19.0 III: 52.4 IV: 14.3 V: 0.0	Median: 47 d; range: 9–164	76.2	4.8: mRS ≥ 3 at latest follow-up	0	4.8

Abbreviations: AVM, arteriovenous malformation; bAVMs, brain arteriovenous malformations; mRS, modified Rankin Scale; NR, not reported; SM, Spetzler–Martin.

24.13.3 Outcomes of Embolization

The relative disadvantage and criticism often leveled toward endovascular embolization is the relative lack of durability of this modality, lending itself to higher rates of recanalization and thus subsequent rebleeding. Moreover, embolization tends to require multiple treatments before complete obliteration can be achieved.[107] In purely ruptured cohorts, the reported complete obliteration rate of bAVMs ranges from 17.8 to 95.0% (▶ Table 24.7). In particular, novel endovascular transvenous embolization methods have garnered interest and have been readily studied. Both He et al[112] and Iosif et al[113] performed embolization of ruptured bAVMs exclusively using these techniques and found occlusion rates of 76.2 and 95.0%, respectively, which are significantly higher than occlusion rates using traditional arterial methods. In the study performed by Iosif et al,[113] the authors were able to achieve these occlusion rates in a single session.

Recurrence or recanalization rates have not been well studied, but even in bAVMs, with small nidus (<1 cm), 7.6% of previously completely occluded bAVMs demonstrated recurrence on follow-up angiography within 6 months.[114] No other recurrences were reported in these publications; however, it is important to take into account the differences in follow-up periods and reporting, as not all centers perform gold standard digital subtraction angiography to confirm bAVM occlusion with follow-up, which may account for the lack of reportable recurrences in the available literature.

Within the limited and heterogenous available data, the morbidity and mortality rates associated with endovascular embolization of ruptured bAVMs range between 4.0 and 13.0%, and 0 and 4.8%, respectively (▶ Table 24.7). Though limited by small-volume, heterogenous case series, the current literature suggests that endovascular embolization of ruptured bAVMs is a reasonable consideration in a select cohort of patients and may have acceptable results compared with alternative treatment. However, it is imperative that thorough radiological workup is undertaken to identify amenable lesions, in appropriate patients, being performed in tertiary centers with adequate neurovascular expertise.

24.14 Authors' Recommendations

- The risk of recurrent hemorrhage is increased in the first 12 months (between 6.2 and 15.4%), gradually returning to the baseline in the following years.
- Initial management of ruptured bAVMs should focus on optimization of raised ICP, which may include surgery to evacuate the hematoma, decompressive craniectomy, placement of an external ventricular drain, and aggressive medical management.
- Surgical resection should be considered for low-grade (SM 1–3) bAVMs in the cases where ICP has been optimized.
- For ruptured bAVMs with compact and deep located nidi, consideration may be given to alternative management strategies such as radiosurgery or targeted endovascular embolization of "weak" structures (e.g., arterial flow aneurysms, venous varices, ectasias, or arteriovenous fistulas) within the ruptured bAVMs.
- bAVMs that will remain unresectable even following adjuvant treatment should be discussed in multidisciplinary meetings as optimal treatment to date is still yet to be discerned.

References

[1] Kim T, Kwon O-K, Bang JS, et al. Epidemiology of ruptured brain arteriovenous malformation: a National Cohort Study in Korea. J Neurosurg. 2018; 130(6):1–6

[2] Gabriel RA, Kim H, Sidney S, et al. Ten-year detection rate of brain arteriovenous malformations in a large, multiethnic, defined population. Stroke. 2010; 41(1):21–26

[3] Al-Shahi R, Bhattacharya JJ, Currie DG, et al. Scottish Intracranial Vascular Malformation Study Collaborators. Prospective, population-based detection of intracranial vascular malformations in adults: the Scottish Intracranial Vascular Malformation Study (SIVMS). Stroke. 2003; 34(5):1163–1169

[4] Stapf C, Mohr JP, Pile-Spellman J, Solomon RA, Sacco RL, Connolly ES, Jr. Epidemiology and natural history of arteriovenous malformations. Neurosurg Focus. 2001; 11(5):e1

[5] Brown RD, Jr, Wiebers DO, Torner JC, O'Fallon WM. Incidence and prevalence of intracranial vascular malformations in Olmsted County, Minnesota, 1965 to 1992. Neurology. 1996; 46(4):949–952

[6] Bogousslavsky J, Van Melle G, Regli F. The Lausanne Stroke Registry: analysis of 1,000 consecutive patients with first stroke. Stroke. 1988; 19(9):1083–1092

[7] Ruíz-Sandoval JL, Cantú C, Barinagarrementeria F. Intracerebral hemorrhage in young people: analysis of risk factors, location, causes, and prognosis. Stroke. 1999; 30(3):537–541

[8] Fukuda K, Majumdar M, Masoud H, et al. Multicenter assessment of morbidity associated with cerebral arteriovenous malformation hemorrhages. J Neurointerv Surg. 2017; 9(7):664–668

[9] van Beijnum J, Lovelock CE, Cordonnier C, Rothwell PM, Klijn CJ, Al-Shahi Salman R, SIVMS Steering Committee and the Oxford Vascular Study. Outcome after spontaneous and arteriovenous malformation-related intracerebral haemorrhage: population-based studies. Brain. 2009; 132(Pt 2):537–543

[10] Morgan MK, Davidson AS, Assaad NNA, Stoodley MA. Critical review of brain AVM surgery, surgical results and natural history in 2017. Acta Neurochir (Wien). 2017; 159(8):1457–1478

[11] Majumdar M, Tan LA, Chen M. Critical assessment of the morbidity associated with ruptured cerebral arteriovenous malformations. J Neurointerv Surg. 2016; 8(2):163–167

[12] Abecassis IJ, Xu DS, Batjer HH, Bendok BR. Natural history of brain arteriovenous malformations: a systematic review. Neurosurg Focus. 2014; 37(3):E7

[13] Gross BA, Du R. Natural history of cerebral arteriovenous malformations: a meta-analysis. J Neurosurg. 2013; 118(2):437–443

[14] Morris Z, Whiteley WN, Longstreth WT, Jr, et al. Incidental findings on brain magnetic resonance imaging: systematic review and meta-analysis. BMJ. 2009; 339:b3016

[15] Berman MF, Sciacca RR, Pile-Spellman J, et al. The epidemiology of brain arteriovenous malformations. Neurosurgery. 2000; 47(2):389–396, discussion 397

[16] ApSimon HT, Reef H, Phadke RV, Popovic EA. A population-based study of brain arteriovenous malformation: long-term treatment outcomes. Stroke. 2002; 33(12):2794–2800

[17] Al-Shahi R, Fang JSY, Lewis SC, Warlow CP. Prevalence of adults with brain arteriovenous malformations: a community based study in Scotland using capture-recapture analysis. J Neurol Neurosurg Psychiatry. 2002; 73(5):547–551

[18] El-Ghanem M, Kass-Hout T, Kass-Hout O, et al. Arteriovenous Malformations in the Pediatric Population: Review of the Existing Literature. Intervent Neurol. 2016; 5(3–4):218–225

[19] Yamada S, Takagi Y, Nozaki K, Kikuta K, Hashimoto N. Risk factors for subsequent hemorrhage in patients with cerebral arteriovenous malformations. J Neurosurg. 2007; 107(5):965–972

[20] Goldberg J, Raabe A, Bervini D. Natural history of brain arteriovenous malformations: systematic review. J Neurosurg Sci. 2018; 62(4):437–443

[21] Kim H, Al-Shahi Salman R, McCulloch CE, Stapf C, Young WL, MARS Coinvestigators. Untreated brain arteriovenous malformation: patient-level meta-analysis of hemorrhage predictors. Neurology. 2014; 83(7):590–597

[22] Lawton MT, Rutledge WC, Kim H, et al. Brain arteriovenous malformations. Nat Rev Dis Primers. 2015; 1:15008

[23] Rangel-Castilla L, Russin JJ, Martinez-Del-Campo E, Soriano-Baron H, Spetzler RF, Nakaji P. Molecular and cellular biology of cerebral arteriovenous malformations: a review of current concepts and future trends in treatment. Neurosurg Focus. 2014; 37(3):E1

[24] Kim H, Hysi PG, Pawlikowska L, et al. Common variants in interleukin-1-Beta gene are associated with intracranial hemorrhage and susceptibility to brain arteriovenous malformation. Cerebrovasc Dis. 2009; 27(2):176–182

[25] Kim H, Pawlikowska L, Chen Y, Su H, Yang GY, Young WL. Brain arteriovenous malformation biology relevant to hemorrhage and implication for therapeutic development. Stroke. 2009; 40(3) Suppl:S95–S97

[26] Pawlikowska L, Poon KY, Achrol AS, et al. Apolipoprotein E epsilon 2 is associated with new hemorrhage risk in brain arteriovenous malformations. Neurosurgery. 2006; 58(5):838–843, discussion 838–843

[27] Pawlikowska L, Tran MN, Achrol AS, et al. UCSF BAVM Study Project. Polymorphisms in genes involved in inflammatory and angiogenic pathways and the risk of hemorrhagic presentation of brain arteriovenous malformations. Stroke. 2004; 35(10):2294–2300

[28] Weinsheimer S, Kim H, Pawlikowska L, et al. EPHB4 gene polymorphisms and risk of intracranial hemorrhage in patients with brain arteriovenous malformations. Circ Cardiovasc Genet. 2009; 2(5):476–482

[29] Wei T, Zhang H, Cetin N, et al. Elevated expression of matrix metalloproteinase-9 not matrix metalloproteinase-2 contributes to progression of extracranial arteriovenous malformation. Sci Rep. 2016; 6(1):24378

[30] Ota T, Komiyama M. Pathogenesis of non-hereditary brain arteriovenous malformation and therapeutic implications. Interv Neuroradiol. 2020; 26 (3):244–253

[31] Hashimoto T, Wen G, Lawton MT, et al. University of California, San Francisco BAVM Study Group. Abnormal expression of matrix metalloproteinases and tissue inhibitors of metalloproteinases in brain arteriovenous malformations. Stroke. 2003; 34(4):925–931

[32] Neidert MC, Lawton MT, Mader M, et al. The AVICH score: a novel grading system to predict clinical outcome in arteriovenous malformation-related intracerebral hemorrhage. World Neurosurg. 2016; 92:292–297

[33] Silva MA, Lai PMR, Du R, Aziz-Sultan MA, Patel NJ. The Ruptured Arteriovenous Malformation Grading Scale (RAGS): an extension of the Hunt and Hess scale to predict clinical outcome for patients with ruptured brain arteriovenous malformations. Neurosurgery. 2020; 87(2):193–199

[34] Choi JH, Mast H, Sciacca RR, et al. Clinical outcome after first and recurrent hemorrhage in patients with untreated brain arteriovenous malformation. Stroke. 2006; 37(5):1243–1247

[35] Murthy SB, Merkler AE, Omran SS, et al. Outcomes after intracerebral hemorrhage from arteriovenous malformations. Neurology. 2017; 88(20):1882–1888

[36] Choi JH, Mast H, Sciacca RR, et al. Clinical outcome after first and recurrent hemorrhage in patients with untreated brain arteriovenous malformation. Stroke. 2006; 37(5):1243–1247

[37] Itoyama Y, Uemura S, Ushio Y, et al. Natural course of unoperated intracranial arteriovenous malformations: study of 50 cases. J Neurosurg. 1989; 71(6):805–809

[38] Fults D, Kelly DL, Jr. Natural history of arteriovenous malformations of the brain: a clinical study. Neurosurgery. 1984; 15(5):658–662

[39] da Costa L, Wallace MC, Ter Brugge KG, O'Kelly C, Willinsky RA, Tymianski M. The natural history and predictive features of hemorrhage from brain arteriovenous malformations. Stroke. 2009; 40(1):100–105

[40] Hernesniemi JA, Dashti R, Juvela S, Väärt K, Niemelä M, Laakso A. Natural history of brain arteriovenous malformations: a long-term follow-up study of risk of hemorrhage in 238 patients. Neurosurgery. 2008; 63(5):823–829, discussion 829–831

[41] Halim AX, Johnston SC, Singh V, et al. Longitudinal risk of intracranial hemorrhage in patients with arteriovenous malformation of the brain within a defined population. Stroke. 2004; 35(7):1697–1702

[42] Stapf C, Mast H, Sciacca RR, et al. Predictors of hemorrhage in patients with untreated brain arteriovenous malformation. Neurology. 2006; 66 (9):1350–1355

[43] Cagnazzo F, Brinjikji W, Lanzino G. Arterial aneurysms associated with arteriovenous malformations of the brain: classification, incidence, risk of hemorrhage, and treatment—a systematic review. Acta Neurochir (Wien). 2016; 158(11):2095–2104

[44] Blauwblomme T, Bourgeois M, Meyer P, et al. Long-term outcome of 106 consecutive pediatric ruptured brain arteriovenous malformations after combined treatment. Stroke. 2014; 45(6):1664–1671

[45] Mine S, Hirai S, Ono J, Yamaura A. Risk factors for poor outcome of untreated arteriovenous malformation. J Clin Neurosci. 2000; 7(6):503–506

[46] Abla AA, Nelson J, Rutledge WC, Young WL, Kim H, Lawton MT. The natural history of AVM hemorrhage in the posterior fossa: comparison of hematoma volumes and neurological outcomes in patients with ruptured infra- and supratentorial AVMs. Neurosurg Focus. 2014; 37(3):E6

[47] Spetzler RF, Martin NA. A proposed grading system for arteriovenous malformations. J Neurosurg. 1986; 65(4):476–483

[48] Feghali J, Yang W, Xu R, et al. R2eD AVM score. Stroke. 2019; 50(7): 1703–1710

[49] Tong X, Wu J, Lin F, et al. Risk factors for subsequent hemorrhage in patients with cerebellar arteriovenous malformations. World Neurosurg. 2016; 92: 47–57

[50] Lv X, Wu Z, Jiang C, et al. Angioarchitectural characteristics of brain arteriovenous malformations with and without hemorrhage. World Neurosurg. 2011; 76(1–2):95–99

[51] Crawford PM, West CR, Chadwick DW, Shaw MD. Arteriovenous malformations of the brain: natural history in unoperated patients. J Neurol Neurosurg Psychiatry. 1986; 49(1):1–10

[52] Derdeyn CP, Zipfel GJ, Albuquerque FC, et al. American Heart Association Stroke Council. Management of brain arteriovenous malformations: a scientific statement for healthcare professionals from the American Heart Association/American Stroke Association. Stroke. 2017; 48(8):e200–e224

[53] Hemphill JC, III, Greenberg SM, Anderson CS, et al. American Heart Association Stroke Council, Council on Cardiovascular and Stroke Nursing, Council on Clinical Cardiology. Guidelines for the management of spontaneous intracerebral hemorrhage: a guideline for healthcare professionals from the American Heart Association/American Stroke Association. Stroke. 2015; 46(7): 2032–2060

[54] Diringer MN, Edwards DF. Admission to a neurologic/neurosurgical intensive care unit is associated with reduced mortality rate after intracerebral hemorrhage. Crit Care Med. 2001; 29(3):635–640

[55] Qureshi AI, Palesch YY, Barsan WG, et al. ATACH-2 Trial Investigators and the Neurological Emergency Treatment Trials Network. Intensive blood-pressure lowering in patients with acute cerebral hemorrhage. N Engl J Med. 2016; 375(11):1033–1043

[56] Anderson CS, Heeley E, Huang Y, et al. INTERACT2 Investigators. Rapid blood-pressure lowering in patients with acute intracerebral hemorrhage. N Engl J Med. 2013; 368(25):2355–2365

[57] Arima H, Heeley E, Delcourt C, et al. INTERACT2 Investigators, INTERACT2 Investigators. Optimal achieved blood pressure in acute intracerebral hemorrhage: INTERACT2. Neurology. 2015; 84(5):464–471

[58] Gao C, Xu B. Surgical technique and nuances in ruptured versus unruptured arteriovenous malformation surgery. J Neurosurg Sci. 2018; 62(4):478–483

[59] Lawton MT, Kim H, McCulloch CE, Mikhak B, Young WL. A supplementary grading scale for selecting patients with brain arteriovenous malformations for surgery. Neurosurgery. 2010; 66(4):702–713, discussion 713

[60] Hamilton MG, Spetzler RF. The prospective application of a grading system for arteriovenous malformations. Neurosurgery. 1994; 34(1):2–6, discussion 6–7

[61] Spetzler RF, Ponce FA. A 3-tier classification of cerebral arteriovenous malformations. Clinical article. J Neurosurg. 2011; 114(3):842–849

[62] Kim H, Pourmohamad T, Westbroek EM, McCulloch CE, Lawton MT, Young WL. Evaluating performance of the Spetzler-Martin supplemented model in selecting patients with brain arteriovenous malformation for surgery. Stroke. 2012; 43(9):2497–2499

[63] Hafez A, Koroknay-Pál P, Oulasvirta E, et al. The application of the novel grading scale (Lawton-Young Grading System) to predict the outcome of brain arteriovenous malformation. Neurosurgery. 2019; 84(2):529–536

[64] Potts MB, Lau D, Abla AA, Kim H, Young WL, Lawton MT, UCSF Brain AVM Study Project. Current surgical results with low-grade brain arteriovenous malformations. J Neurosurg. 2015; 122(4):912–920

[65] Lawton MT, UCSF Brain Arteriovenous Malformation Study Project. Spetzler-Martin grade III arteriovenous malformations: surgical results and a modification of the grading scale. Neurosurgery. 2003; 52(4):740–748, discussion 748–749

[66] Heros RC. Spetzler-Martin grades IV and V arteriovenous malformations. J Neurosurg. 2003; 98(1):1–2, discussion 2

[67] Heros RC, Korosue K, Diebold PM. Surgical excision of cerebral arteriovenous malformations: late results. Neurosurgery. 1990; 26(4):570–577, discussion 577–578

[68] Davidson AS, Morgan MK. How safe is arteriovenous malformation surgery? A prospective, observational study of surgery as first-line treatment for brain arteriovenous malformations. Neurosurgery. 2010; 66(3):498–504, discussion 504–505

[69] Kim H, Abla AA, Nelson J, et al. Validation of the supplemented Spetzler-Martin grading system for brain arteriovenous malformations in a multicenter cohort of 1009 surgical patients. Neurosurgery. 2015; 76(1):25–31, discussion 31–32, quiz 32–33

[70] Lawton MT, Du R, Tran MN, et al. Effect of presenting hemorrhage on outcome after microsurgical resection of brain arteriovenous malformations. Neurosurgery. 2005; 56(3):485–493, discussion 485–493

[71] Morgan MK, Assaad N, Korja M. Surgery for unruptured Spetzler-Martin grade 3 brain arteriovenous malformations: a prospective surgical cohort. Neurosurgery. 2015; 77(3):362–369, discussion 369–370

[72] Aboukaïs R, Marinho P, Baroncini M, et al. Ruptured cerebral arteriovenous malformations: outcomes analysis after microsurgery. Clin Neurol Neurosurg. 2015; 138:137–142

[73] Beecher JS, Lyon K, Ban VS, et al. Delayed treatment of ruptured brain AVMs: is it ok to wait? J Neurosurg. 2018; 128(4):999–1005

[74] Aoun SG, Bendok BR, Batjer HH. Acute management of ruptured arteriovenous malformations and dural arteriovenous fistulas. Neurosurg Clin N Am. 2012; 23(1):87–103

[75] Takeuchi S, Takasato Y, Masaoka H, et al. Decompressive craniectomy for arteriovenous malformation-related intracerebral hemorrhage. J Clin Neurosci. 2015; 22(3):483–487

[76] Barone DG, Marcus HJ, Guilfoyle MR, et al. Clinical experience and results of microsurgical resection of arterioveonous malformation in the presence of space-occupying intracerebral hematoma. Neurosurgery. 2017; 81(1):75–86

[77] Hafez A, Oulasvirta E, Koroknay-Pál P, Niemelä M, Hernesniemi J, Laakso A. Timing of surgery for ruptured supratentorial arteriovenous malformations. Acta Neurochir (Wien). 2017; 159(11):2103–2112

[78] Cohen-Gadol A. Challenging dogma in arteriovenous malformation surgery: personal reflections and lessons learned from 350 cases. World Neurosurg. 2020; 139:83–89

[79] Pavesi G, Rustemi O, Berlucchi S, Frigo AC, Gerunda V, Scienza R. Acute surgical removal of low-grade (Spetzler-Martin I-II) bleeding arteriovenous malformations. Surg Neurol. 2009; 72(6):662–667

[80] Kuhmonen J, Piippo A, Väärt K, et al. Early surgery for ruptured cerebral arteriovenous malformations. Acta Neurochir Suppl (Wien). 2005; 94: 111–114

[81] Sinclair J, Kelly ME, Steinberg GK. Surgical management of posterior fossa arteriovenous malformations. Neurosurgery. 2006; 58(4) Suppl 2:ONS-189–ONS-201, discussion ONS-201

[82] Batjer H, Samson D. Arteriovenous malformations of the posterior fossa. Clinical presentation, diagnostic evaluation, and surgical treatment. J Neurosurg. 1986; 64(6):849–856

[83] Samson D, Batjer H. Arteriovenous malformations of the cerebellar vermis. Neurosurgery. 1985; 16(3):341–349

[84] O'Shaughnessy BA, Getch CC, Bendok BR, Batjer HH. Microsurgical resection of infratentorial arteriovenous malformations. Neurosurg Focus. 2005; 19 (2):E5

[85] Kelly ME, Guzman R, Sinclair J, et al. Multimodality treatment of posterior fossa arteriovenous malformations. J Neurosurg. 2008; 108(6):1152–1161

[86] Drake CG, Friedman AH, Peerless SJ. Posterior fossa arteriovenous malformations. J Neurosurg. 1986; 64(1):1–10

[87] Shin M, Kawahara N, Maruyama K, Tago M, Ueki K, Kirino T. Risk of hemorrhage from an arteriovenous malformation confirmed to have been obliterated on angiography after stereotactic radiosurgery. J Neurosurg. 2005; 102(5):842–846

[88] Maruyama K, Kawahara N, Shin M, et al. The risk of hemorrhage after radiosurgery for cerebral arteriovenous malformations. N Engl J Med. 2005; 352(2):146–153

[89] Maruyama K, Shin M, Tago M, Kishimoto J, Morita A, Kawahara N. Radiosurgery to reduce the risk of first hemorrhage from brain arteriovenous malformations. Neurosurgery. 2007; 60(3):453–458, discussion 458–459

[90] Yen CP, Sheehan JP, Schwyzer L, Schlesinger D. Hemorrhage risk of cerebral arteriovenous malformations before and during the latency period after GAMMA knife radiosurgery. Stroke. 2011; 42(6):1691–1696

[91] Chye C-L, Wang K-W, Chen H-J, Yeh S-A, Tang JT, Liang C-L. Haemorrhage rates of ruptured and unruptured brain arteriovenous malformation after radiosurgery: a nationwide population-based cohort study. BMJ Open. 2020; 10(10):e036606

[92] Ding D, Yen CP, Starke RM, Xu Z, Sheehan JP. Radiosurgery for ruptured intracranial arteriovenous malformations. J Neurosurg. 2014; 121(2):470–481

[93] Ding D, Chen CJ, Starke RM, et al. Risk of brain arteriovenous malformation hemorrhage before and after stereotactic radiosurgery. Stroke. 2019; 50(6):1384–1391

[94] Ding D, Ilyas A, Sheehan JP. Contemporary management of high-grade brain arteriovenous malformations. Neurosurgery. 2018; 65 CN_suppl_1:24–33

[95] Sackey FNA, Pinsker NR, Baako BN. Highlights on cerebral arteriovenous malformation treatment using combined embolization and stereotactic radiosurgery: why outcomes are controversial? Cureus. 2017; 9(5):e1266

[96] Andrade-Souza YM, Ramani M, Scora D, Tsao MN, terBrugge K, Schwartz ML. Embolization before radiosurgery reduces the obliteration rate of arteriovenous malformations. Neurosurgery. 2007; 60(3):443–451, discussion 451–452

[97] Patibandla MR, Ding D, Kano H, et al. Stereotactic radiosurgery for Spetzler-Martin grade IV and V arteriovenous malformations: an international multicenter study. J Neurosurg. 2018; 129(2):498–507

[98] Ding D, Yen CP, Starke RM, Xu Z, Sun X, Sheehan JP. Outcomes following single-session radiosurgery for high-grade intracranial arteriovenous malformations. Br J Neurosurg. 2014; 28(5):666–674

[99] Han PP, Ponce FA, Spetzler RF. Intention-to-treat analysis of Spetzler-Martin grades IV and V arteriovenous malformations: natural history and treatment paradigm. J Neurosurg. 2003; 98(1):3–7

[100] Sanchez-Mejia RO, McDermott MW, Tan J, Kim H, Young WL, Lawton MT. Radiosurgery facilitates resection of brain arteriovenous malformations and reduces surgical morbidity. Neurosurgery. 2009; 64(2):231–238, discussion 238–240

[101] Abla AA, Rutledge WC, Seymour ZA, et al. A treatment paradigm for high-grade brain arteriovenous malformations: volume-staged radiosurgical downgrading followed by microsurgical resection. J Neurosurg. 2015; 122(2):419–432

[102] Maruyama K, Koga T, Shin M, Igaki H, Tago M, Saito N. Optimal timing for Gamma Knife surgery after hemorrhage from brain arteriovenous malformations. J Neurosurg. 2008; 109 Suppl:73–76

[103] Hou K, Xu K, Chen X, Ji T, Guo Y, Yu J. Targeted endovascular treatment for ruptured brain arteriovenous malformations. Neurosurg Rev. 2020; 43(6):1509–1518

[104] Zaki Ghali MG, Kan P, Britz GW. Curative embolization of arteriovenous malformations. World Neurosurg. 2019; 129:467–486

[105] van Rooij WJ, Jacobs S, Sluzewski M, Beute GN, van der Pol B. Endovascular treatment of ruptured brain AVMs in the acute phase of hemorrhage. AJNR Am J Neuroradiol. 2012; 33(6):1162–1166

[106] Sun Y, Jin H, Li Y, Tian Z. Target embolization of associated aneurysms in ruptured arteriovenous malformations. World Neurosurg. 2017; 101:26–32

[107] Stemer AB, Bank WO, Armonda RA, Liu AH, Herzig DW, Bell RS. Acute embolization of ruptured brain arteriovenous malformations. J Neurointerv Surg. 2013; 5(3):196–200

[108] Signorelli F, Gory B, Pelissou-Guyotat I, et al. Ruptured brain arteriovenous malformations associated with aneurysms: safety and efficacy of selective embolization in the acute phase of hemorrhage. Neuroradiology. 2014; 56(9):763–769

[109] Yu JL, Yang S, Luo Q, et al. Endovascular treatment of intracranial ruptured aneurysms associated with arteriovenous malformations: a clinical analysis of 14 hemorrhagic cases. Interv Neuroradiol. 2011; 17(1):78–86

[110] Gross BA, Moon K, Mcdougall CG. Endovascular management of arteriovenous malformations. Handb Clin Neurol. 2017; 143:59–68

[111] Zacharia BE, Vaughan KA, Jacoby A, Hickman ZL, Bodmer D, Connolly ES, Jr. Management of ruptured brain arteriovenous malformations. Curr Atheroscler Rep. 2012; 14(4):335–342

[112] He Y, Ding Y, Bai W, et al. Safety and efficacy of transvenous embolization of ruptured brain arteriovenous malformations as a last resort: a prospective single-arm study. AJNR Am J Neuroradiol. 2019; 40(10):1744–1751

[113] Iosif C, Mendes GA, Saleme S, et al. Endovascular transvenous cure for ruptured brain arteriovenous malformations in complex cases with high Spetzler-Martin grades. J Neurosurg. 2015; 122(5):1229–1238

[114] Andreou A, Ioannidis I, Lalloo S, Nickolaos N, Byrne JV. Endovascular treatment of intracranial microarteriovenous malformations. J Neurosurg. 2008; 109(6):1091–1097

[115] Valavanis A, Yasargil MG. The endovascular treatment of brain arteriovenous malformations. In: Cohadon F, Dolenc VV, Antunes JL, et al, eds. Advances and Technical Standards in Neurosurgery. Vienna: Springer Vienna; 1998:131–214

[116] Bir SC, Maiti TK, Konar S, Nanda A. Overall outcomes following early interventions for intracranial arteriovenous malformations with hematomas. Journal of Clinical Neuroscience. 2016; 23:95–100

25 Natural History and Management Options of Trigeminal Neuralgia

Adrian Praeger, Peter Teddy, Sarah Cain, Andranik Kahramanian, and Bhadrakant Kavar

Abstract

Trigeminal neuralgia is a challenging clinical problem for patient and clinician. An early multidisciplinary approach is vital. When medical therapies fail to obtain pain control, surgical options are available. When possible, the nerve preservation option of microvascular decompression should be considered in non-MS patient group. Alternatively, the ablative options of radiofrequency thermocoagulation, glycerol injection, ballon compression, or radiosurgery have a high but varing success rate.

Keywords: TN, trigeminal neuralgia, microvascular decompression, radiofrequency thermocoagulation, radiofreqency rhizotomy, glycerol injection, alcohol injection, balloon compression, radiosurgery, multiple sclerosis, MS

25.1 Introduction

Trigeminal neuralgia (TN), also known as *tic douloureux*, is a chronic debilitating neuropathic pain that affects the trigeminal nerve. Classically, it has been described as sudden, sharp, and lancinating unilateral facial pain that lasts from a few seconds to minutes per episode, followed by a refractory period. The pain may be triggered by light mechanical contact from a restricted site (trigger point or trigger zone). The attacks are paroxysmal and may occur at intervals, many times a day, or, in rare instances, follow one another almost continuously. Periodicity is characteristic, with episodes occurring for a few weeks to a month or two, followed by a pain-free interval of months or years and then recurrence of another bout of pain.[1]

TN incidence is estimated around 4.7/100,000 with a female preponderance (female-to-male ratio of 3:2). The maxillary (V2) and/or mandibular divisions (V3) are typically the most affected.[2] The peak age of incidence is between the sixth and eighth decades of life.[3] The most common cause of TN is a compressing loop of an artery (classically the superior cerebellar artery [SCA] but can be the anterior inferior cerebellar artery [AICA], a dolichoectatic vertebrobasilar complex, or a persistent fetal trigeminal artery).[4,5,6,7,8] Other causes include compression due to cerebellopontine angle (CPA) tumors or cysts, perineural tumor spread, multiple sclerosis, and demyelinating disease.[9,10]

Several classifications of facial pain have been proposed (▶ Table 25.1). The Burchiel classification[11] is comprehensive, widely used, and incorporates pathophysiology. Cruccu et al[12] provided a simpler classification that is also widely used. Typical TN, due to neurovascular conflict, is described as either TN type 1 (Burchiel) or classic TN (Cruccu, International Classification of Headache Disorders, 3rd edition [ICDH-3]). The diagnosis of TN is based on a patient's clinical history, and an imaging study is usually indicated to exclude posterior fossa pathologies (e.g., mass lesion in the CPA, demyelination). Vascular contact deforming the trigeminal nerve is seen in about 15% of cases.

25.2 Selected Papers on the Natural History of Trigeminal Neuralgia

- Burchiel KJ, Slavin KV. On the natural history of trigeminal neuralgia. Neurosurgery 2000;46(1):152–154, discussion 154–155
- Di Stefano G, La Cesa S, Truini A, Cruccu G. Natural history and outcome of 200 outpatients with classical trigeminal neuralgia treated with carbamazepine or oxcarbazepine in a tertiary centre for neuropathic pain. J Headache Pain 2014;15(1):34
- Taylor JC, Brauer S, Espir ML. Long-term treatment of trigeminal neuralgia with carbamazepine. Postgrad Med J 1981;57(663):16–18

25.3 Natural History of Trigeminal Neuralgia

The natural history of TN is not well defined. The initial presentation is often misdiagnosed, and the correct diagnosis is delayed for weeks to years. Attacks of pain present for weeks to

Table 25.1 Classifications of trigeminal neuralgia/facial pain

Burchiel[11]			ICDH-3[166]	Cruccu[12]	
Pain type	**Abb**	**History**			**Pathophysiology**
Trigeminal neuralgia	TN	Spontaneous onset			
Type 1 (mostly episodic pain)	TN1	>50% episodic pain	Classic TN	Classic TN	Neurovascular conflict
Type 2 (mostly constant pain)	TN2	<50% episodic pain			
Symptomatic TN	STN	Episodic, fluctuant	Painful trigeminal neuropathy	Secondary TN	Multiple sclerosis
Postherpetic neuralgia	PHN	Constant			Trigeminal herpes zoster
Trigeminal neuropathic pain	TNP	Constant, dysesthetic			Unintentional nerve injury
Trigeminal deafferentation pain	TDP	Constant, dysesthetic			Intentional nerve injury
Atypical facial pain[a]		Variable, fluctuant			Unknown etiology

Abbreviations: Abb, abbreviation; ICDH 3, International Classification of Headache Disorders.
[a]Cannot be a diagnosis by history alone.

Table 25.2 Characteristics of carbamazepine response and sides effects in 744 patients across 10 studies

Characteristics	
Patients	744 (10–143)
Initial control	79.5% (68–98%)
Follow-up	3–26.6 mo
Long-term control	66.3% (54–100%)
Relapse of pain	7.7–47.5%
Side effects	
Dizziness/ataxia	2.2–75%
Cognitive: drowsiness, confusion, mood	1.1–35.1%
Deranged liver function tests	2.3–7.5%
Hyponatremia	0–5.2%
Hematological	0–5%
Rash	2.1–11%

months with periods of remission lasting for months to years. Almost invariably, the pain recurs with increasing duration, frequency, and severity—mandating reevaluation of the initial diagnosis (if that of TN was not made), to the point where TN-specific treatment will be required.[13,14] Our systematic review of the literature identified no adequate study on the natural history of "untreated" TN or one that captures the patient population in which pain may resolve without treatment.

The initial response to treatment with carbamazepine is generally excellent. Even patients who have an unsatisfactory response to carbamazepine typically have an initial partial response, often within the first 48 hours.[15,16,17] This can be used to differentiate between typical TN and other causes of facial pain.[18] When the patient does not respond to carbamazepine, the diagnosis should be revisited.[19]

To assess the response to carbamazepine, we examined the literature and identified 744 patients in 10 studies (▶ Table 25.2).[15,17,18,20,21,22,23,24,25,26] Initial positive response rate is around 79.5% (range: 68–98%) with a declining control rate to 66.3% (range: 54–100%) over time. Studies with stricter inclusion criteria, that is, only type 1 TN (classic TN) without previous treatment generally reported better success rates. Di Stefano et al[20] reported 98% of 95 patients had an initial positive response. However, 27% of patients ceased taking carbamazepine because they had either a relapse of their pain or side effects, requiring a reduction of carbamazepine until it was no longer adequately controlling their pain.

The risk of side effects is low, particularly if carbamazepine is commenced at a low dose and increased slowly. Side effects can include cognitive side effects (drowsiness, confusion, and changes in mood), dizziness, ataxia, electrolyte, hematological, and liver function test (LFT) derangement. Rash is also common, with a significant potential for Stevens–Johnson syndrome in people with the allele HLA-B*1502, which is common in those of Han Chinese, Hong Kong Chinese, or Thai origin. Thus, these patients should be screened before the use of carbamazepine.[27]

25.4 Selected Papers on the Treatment of Trigeminal Neuralgia

- Bendtsen L, Zakrzewska JM, Abbott J, et al. European Academy of Neurology guideline on trigeminal neuralgia. Eur J Neurol 2019;26(6):831–849

- Gronseth G, Cruccu G, Alksne J, et al. Practice parameter: the diagnostic evaluation and treatment of trigeminal neuralgia (an evidence-based review): report of the Quality Standards Subcommittee of the American Academy of Neurology and the European Federation of Neurological Societies. Neurology 2008;71(15):1183–1190
- Holste K, Chan AY, Rolston JD, Englot DJ. Pain outcomes following microvascular decompression for drug-resistant trigeminal neuralgia: a systematic review and meta-analysis. Neurosurgery 2020;86(2):182–190
- Barker FG II, Jannetta PJ, Bissonette DJ, Larkins MV, Jho HD. The long-term outcome of microvascular decompression for trigeminal neuralgia. N Engl J Med 1996;334(17): 1077–1083

25.5 Treatment Options of Trigeminal Neuralgia

Optimal management for TN should include a multidisciplinary approach involving the neurologist, neurosurgeon, and pain management physician. Conservative management with medical therapy should be initially attempted in all patients. If this fails, the main treatment options are microvascular decompression (MVD), percutaneous ablative procedures (balloon microcompression, radiofrequency thermocoagulation, and glycerol injection), and stereotactic radiosurgery (SRS). Treatment recommendation should be based on the underlying etiology, radiological findings, patient symptoms and comorbidities, as well as the experience of the treating team.

25.5.1 Medical Therapy

Medical therapy is the mainstay of initial treatment, with literature evidence to support the use of either carbamazepine or oxcarbazepine as first-line therapy.[20,28,31] Di Stefano et al[20] reported 98% of patients had an initial response to carbamazepine, but 27% had to stop taking the drug due to side effects. In contrast, 94% of patients had initial control with oxcarbazepine, whereas 18% had to stop it due to side effects.

Other medical options to consider include baclofen, lamotrigine, gabapentin, botulinum toxin type A, pregabalin, and phenytoin. These can be prescribed in combination with or instead of carbamazepine or oxcarbazepine. Data to support the routine use of any of the second-line medical therapies is low (▶ Table 25.3).[16,18,19,20,21,24,28,29,32,33,34,35,36,37,38,39,40,41,42,43,44]

If a patient develops medically refractory pain or intolerable side effects to medication, they should progress to one of the more definitive treatments, either MVD or the percutaneous ablative techniques or SRS.[45]

25.5.2 Microvascular Decompression

MVD of the trigeminal nerve is generally the treatment of choice. MVD is generally recommended for patients with inadequate medical control, in whom a greater than 5-year survival is expected and who are medically fit.[46] In our analysis of the literature on the outcomes of MVDs, a total of 36 papers were included encompassing a total of 6,315 patients with an average age range of 41.6 to 79.4 years (▶ Table 25.4).[32,33,34,35,36,45,47,48,49,50,51,52,53,54,55,56,57,58,59,60,61,62,63,64,65,66,67,68,69,70,71,72,73,74,75,76] It should be noted, however, that there is wide variation in the

Table 25.3 Literature summary for medical management of trigeminal neuralgia

Medication	Initial control	Long-term control	Side effects	Evidence
Carbamazepine	79.5% (68–98%)	66.3% (54–100%)	Drowsiness, rash, Stevens–Johnson syndrome, relative leukopenia, hyponatremia	24,30,31,32,33, 34,35,36,37
Oxcarbazepine	Up to 94%	Needs further study	Teratogenic, drowsiness, hyponatremia	24
Baclofen	65%	Needs further study	Drowsiness, dizziness, fatigue, nausea	38
Lamotrigine	Better than placebo over 14 d	Needs further study	Rash, somnolence, dizziness, diplopia, Stevens–Johnson syndrome	39
Gabapentin	Needs further study	Needs further study	Vertigo, somnolence, dizziness, ataxia, fatigue	40
Botulinum	57–90%	Needs further study	Facial asymmetry (usually resolved by 12 wk) Hematoma at injection site	41,42

literature, with heterogeneity in patient population (pure typical TN vs. studies that mix typical TN and atypical TN), previous treatments, selection criteria for treatment, definition and documentation of retreatments, definition of treatment success, as well as wide variability in the documentation and nonuniform definition of complications. This makes it difficult to compare studies and explains some of the wide variability in the reported outcomes.

Initially, 87% (range: 67.3–100%) of patients were reported as being pain free and off medication. When patients reported as being pain free but still taking medication were included, this improved to 95% (range: 70.3–100%). Long term, with an average, follow-up of 6.9 years, 83% of patients were pain free. The reported recurrence rate varied between 6.1 and 29%, with some of the higher recurrence rates being reported in the earlier papers.

The above findings are supported by Barker et al[3] in their large study of 1,185 patients over 20 years with a mean follow-up of 6.2 years. Short-term outcome analysis revealed that 80% of patients had excellent results 1 year following MVD with an additional 8% achieving partial relief. Long-term data at 10 years after surgery demonstrated 70% with excellent results and 4% with partial relief. In total, 11% of patients required a second MVD, whereas 10% had a subsequent ablative procedure.

The postoperative complications following MVDs are summarized in ▶ Table 25.4. Mortality ranged from 0 to 2% but was 0.2 and 0.24% in the two largest series (▶ Table 25.4).[50,71] In the same two large series, hearing loss was 1.4 and 0.94%, whereas facial paralysis was 1.7%. Cerebrospinal fluid (CSF) leak was 1.6 and 0.47%. A permanent ocular palsy was recorded in 4.6% of patients. Anesthesia dolorosa was not recorded in any paper included in this systematic review; however, it is accepted that there is a low risk of it occurring post-MVD.[77]

Positive predictors of success of an MVD included disease duration less than 5 years, arterial compression, SCA involvement, and type 1 facial pain.[30] In addition, Barker et al's[3] retrospective study of 1,336 MVDs identified immediate postoperative relief, male sex, absence of venous compression, and less than 8 years of preoperative symptoms as positive predictors of success. These findings were reinforced by Panczykowski et al's[78] preoperative TN scoring system, which used classic TN, positive response to carbamazepine and/or oxcarbazepine, and the presence and nature of the neurovascular compression as the positive predictors. The nature and severity of the neurovascular conflict in a preoperative magnetic resonance imaging (MRI) appears to be related with outcome for MVD[79] and is included in another preoperative TN score, aimed at predicting the success of an MVD.[80]

Table 25.4 Systematic review on outcomes following MVD surgery

Demographic	
Patients (range)	6,315 (19–2,003)
Male (range)	2,667 (6–883)
Female (range)	3,849 (13–1,381)
Average age, range (y)	41.6–79.4
Length of disease, range (mo)	42–108
Clinical outcomes, % (range)	
Initial pain free without medication	87.0 (67.3–100.0)
Additional initial pain free with medication	2.0–26.4
Overall initial pain free	95.0 (70.3–100.0)
Pain free at last follow-up	83.0 (61.5–95.0)
Mean follow-up (mo)	86.0 (5.0–135.6)
Recurrence rate	6.1–29.0
Time to recurrence, range (mo)	6.1–29.0 mo
Repeat intervention rate	4.0–22.0
Complications (%)	
Mortality	0–2.0
Bacterial meningitis	0–7.8
Any hearing loss	0–16.0
Facial paralysis	0–8.3
Facial numbness	0–35.0
Ocular palsy/permanent diplopia	0–4.6
Post-op hematoma: subdural/cerebellar	0–4.2
Infarct	0–4.0
Cerebrospinal fluid leak	0–13.2
Wound infection	0–7.5
Anesthesia dolorosa	0
Loss of corneal reflex	0–5.7

Abbreviation: MVD, microvascular decompression.

Negative predictors of success include previous ablative procedures and patients with MS.[81]

25.5.3 Percutaneous Ablative Procedures

The three percutaneous ablative procedures (radiofrequency thermocoagulation, balloon compression [BC], and glycerol/alcohol injection) are used for patients who are a poor anesthetic risk, the elderly, patients with MS, and patients who decline an MVD.[79]

The most frequently used percutaneous technique is radiofrequency thermocoagulation (PRfT) for which the patient needs to

Table 25.5 Literature summary of outcomes following ablative procedures or SRS for trigeminal neuralgia

	PRfT, range (total)	Glycerol, range (total)	Balloon, range (total)	SRS, range (total)
Demographics				
Patients, total (range)	8,454 (154–1,600)	6,168 (53–4,012)	3,941 (47–496)	4,409 (99–870)
Procedures, total (range)	4,416 (280–2,138)	1,525 (69–544)	2,310 (56–531)	n/a
Male, total (range)	3,358 (54–766)	2,796 (21–1,807)	1,087 (19–279)	1,641 (33–334)
Female	3,607 (100–834)	3,269 (37–2,205)	1,193 (28–217)	2,297 (66–533)
Average age, range (y)	56.8–68 .0	52.0–72.1	53.0–85.6	48.2–69.0
Length of disease, range (mo)	86.7–96.0	32.4–121.0	60.0–133.3	48.7–132.0
Clinical outcomes				
Mean follow–up (mo)	22.6–111.6	12.0–72.0	12.0–226.8	1.0–106.0
Follow up range (mo)	3.0–300.0	0–300.0	1.0–202.7	1.0–168.0
Early failure (%)	3.2–6.0	5.0–20.0	6.2–14.8	n/a
Initial pain free (%)	91.0–100.0	73.0–97.1	61.6–98.6	1.0–90.7%
Recurrence rate, % (range)	19.8 (9.6–25.1)	17.7 (8–80.4)	5.2–77.4	19–43.7%
Mean time to recurrence (mo)	14.0–168.0	5.0–25.0	6.5–42.0	8.0–34.0
Pain free at last follow–up, % (range)	52.0–88.0	8.1–90.0	31.0–100.0	32.0–91.8
Complications (%)				
Hearing loss	0–0.52	0	0–10.2	0.5–3.0
Facial numbness initial	11.3–98.0	3.0–77.4	4.0–100	4.8–81.0
Facial numbness prolonged	9.0–15.2	1.8–44.0	4.6–44.0	10.0–72.0
Facial dysesthesia	1.8–8.6	1.0–40.0	0–10.0	10.0–15.0
Diplopia	0–2.0	0–1.2	0–8.0	0.5[a]
Herpes	0	2.0–37.6	0–48.1	NR
Masseter weakness initial	4.1–53.4	1.0–3.4	1.2–59.6	10.0%[a]
Masseter weakness prolonged	0–4.8	0	0–12.0	4.0[a]
Meningitis	0.3–0.4	0–2.7	0–1.4	NR
Mortality	0–0.3	0	0–1.5	NR
Keratitis	0.6–4.0	[b]	[b]	[b]
Diminished/absent corneal reflex	3.0–19.7	2.0–9.3	0–7.0[b]	6.0[a]

Abbreviations: PRfT, percutaneous radiofrequency thermocoagulation; SRS, stereotactic radiosurgery.
[a]Reported in one or two papers only.
[b]Keratitis was generally not reported in papers on balloon compression, glycerol injections, and SRS. In the papers that did report them, it was either zero or recorded as nonsignificant numbers. Diminished or absent corneal reflex was only recorded in half the papers on balloon compression. The rate was generally reported between 0 and 3% with one paper only reporting >3% (7%).

be sedated/awake/sedated to ensure accurate placement of the electrode.[82] Glycerol/alcohol injection into the Meckel s cave is performed under general anesthesia (GA) and thus avoids the awake phase of PRfT.[46,83] BC is also performed under GA with favorable results in most patients.[84,85,86] Literature review outcomes of the three percutaneous procedures are presented in detail in ► Table 25.5.

25.5.4 Percutaneous Radiofrequency Thermocoagulation

A total of 8,454 patients across 12 studies underwent PRfT.[36,82,87,88,89,90,91,92,93,94,95,96] The initial success rate ranged between 91 and 100%, with an early failure rate of 3.2 and 6.0% (often due to inability to cannulate the foramen ovale). The initial positive response typically declined over time, with the reported pain-free rate, with or without medication, diminishing to 52% at last follow-up (mean follow-up range: 22.6–111.6 months). Some patients may periodically require repeat procedures to maintain a good therapeutic response. The mean recurrence rate

was noted at 19.8% (range: 9.6–25.1%), with rates typically higher in patients who reported less hypoesthesia after the initial procedure. The overall initial facial numbness rate ranged from 11.3 to 98.0% of patients, whereas the range of prolonged/permanent facial numbness was between 9 and 15.2%.

While this procedure is generally well tolerated, complications can occur (► Table 25.4). These include a diminished or absent corneal reflex (3–19.7%), keratitis (0–6.4%), and anesthesia dolorosa (<2%; range: 0.2–8.9%). Mortality was low ranging from 0 to 0.3%.

25.5.5 Glycerol/Alcohol Injection

Glycerol/alcohol injection has several advantages including the ease and speed of the procedure, and the lack of requirement for GA with no awake phase and no stimulation. Sensory loss is variable and, if performed appropriately, should not result in corneal numbness secondary to V1 involvement. Meticulous positioning of the patient will minimize that risk, which was 2 to 9.3% in our literature review.

Excluding studies with less than 50 patients, 15 studies reported on outcomes for 6,168 patients.[97,98,99,100,101,102,103,104,105,106,107,108,109,110,111] The mean follow-up time varied between 12 and 72 months with a range of 0 to 300 months. Pain relief may be immediate or take 1 to 2 days to develop and rarely occurs after 2 weeks.[112] A repeat procedure can be considered if no relief is reported in 7 days following the index procedure.[113] The initial pain-free outcomes were noted in 73.0 to 97.1% of patients, with early failure rate noted in 5 to 20%. There was significant variability in the pain-free rates at last follow-up, with the range varying from 8.1 to 90%. The 8.1% appeared to be an outlier, with all other long-term rates being above 43%, and came from a study with significant loss to follow-up. The mean recurrence rate was 17.7% (range: 8–80%) with a mean time to recurrence of 5 to 25 months. Retreatments were documented by five studies and ranged between 15.7 and 45.9% of patients in those studies.

25.5.6 Balloon Compression

In total, 3,941 patients across 23 papers were included in the systematic review on BC, and the results are summarized in ▶ Table 25.5.[85,87,96,105,114,115,116,117,118,119,120,121,122,123,124,125,126,127,128,129,130,131,132] Initial control of pain varied from 61.6 to 98.6%. The recurrence rate varied between 5.2 and 77.4%. Patients pain free at last treatment varied widely from 31 to 100%. In terms of complications, prolonged facial numbness was seen in up to 44% of patients and diplopia in up to 8% of patients. Mortality ranged between 0 and 1.5%.

25.5.7 Stereotactic Radiosurgery

The mechanism of action is presumed to be axonal degeneration secondary to radiation as shown by Kondziolka et al on a primate model[133] and later confirmed histologically in a patient who had subsequent recurrent TN and underwent partial sectioning of the nerve.[134]

Although this was usually reserved for refractory TN and failure of other treatment options,[135] this practice is changing. It is the least invasive and ideal for patients with high morbidity or on antiplatelet or anticoagulants. In some series, the results are comparable to those of MVD.[136,137,138,139] In total, 4,409 patients were included in 15 studies in the systematic review (▶ Table 25.5).[64,123,140,141,142,143,144,145,146,147,148,149,150,151,152] Initially, up to 90.7% of patients were pain free, with the number of patients being pain free at last follow-up ranging from 32 to 91.8%. After SRS, there is a delay to treatment effect of weeks to months, and some patients may need to wait 12 months to be pain free.[145] The recurrence rate ranged from 19 to 43.7%.

Favorable prognostic factors for SRS include higher radiation dose (i.e., > 70 Gy),[153] previously unoperated patient, typical TN, and normal sensation pretreatment. The major complication is hyperesthesia in 20% after initial SRS and 32% after repeat treatment[154] and higher with higher radiation dose.[137] Patients with MS are less responsive than those without MS. SRS can be repeated with similar results as the initial SRS, but only 48 to 65% have good pain control.[155]

Maesawa et al found a higher rate of recurrence if patients had previously undergone an unsuccessful MVD with complete pain relief of 60% at 1 year, 53% at 2 years, and 33% at 5 years.[156]

25.6 Trigeminal Neuralgia in Multiple Sclerosis

TN is the most common pain syndrome in MS and MS-related TN (MS-TN) and represents 2 to 8% of all cases of TN.[157,158,159,160] Although the initial treatment should be medical, it is not unusual for patients to have medication-related side effects earlier, and/or exacerbation of their MS-related symptoms as a result of the medication. This often precipitates the need for consideration of surgical treatment; however, outcomes are less satisfactory in MS patients.

The mainstays of surgical management of MS-TN are the ablative procedures of PRfT, glycerol rhizolysis (GR), and BC. As the most likely cause for the pain is demyelination and not vascular compromise, there is generally no role for MVD in MS-TN.[161,162] However, MVD can be considered if there is evidence of vascular compromise and no evidence of demyelination in the pons or in the region of the trigeminal nerve.

All ablative procedures are reasonable treatment options for MS-TN. However, a recent retrospective analysis and review in the MS group of patients revealed 53.1% achieved excellent pain relief at 3 months, better for PRfT (55.2%) and BC (56.3%) than for GR (47.4%). Of note, the percentage of patients with ongoing severe pain was much higher after GR (21.1%) compared with PRfT (3.4%) or BC (6.3%).[157] Overall, several recent analyses confirm that the results of the ablative procedures are worse in the MS group of patients when compared to non-MS patients.[163,164]

SRS/Gamma Knife surgery (GKS) is rarely used due to delay in achieving short-term pain control. However, SRS/GKS should be considered if other modalities fail. In a recent retrospective commentary, Vulpe and Wang suggest that MS-TN patients are poorer responders to SRS, both after the primary treatment and repeat SRS.[165]

25.7 Authors' Recommendations

- Initial management is pharmacological, with carbamazepine having the best evidence. If there is no response to carbamazepine, the diagnosis should be reconsidered.
- A neurosurgical opinion regarding surgical options should be obtained early, with a prolonged disease course before surgical intervention associated with worse outcomes. Intervention should be offered to all patients failing medical management.
- MVD has low mortality and morbidity, and excellent initial control, with an approximately 10% reduction in that control over the first 10 years after MVD.
- The ablative procedures and SRS have a lower mortality rate, and a different morbidity profile when compared to an MVD. Overall, the initial results can be similar to an MVD; however, they all have a significant reduction in patients with control and a higher recurrence rate. As such, these procedures often have to be repeated.
- In patients without MS, MVD is the treatment of choice, unless the patient is medically unfit for the procedure, or prefers an alternative procedure.
- In patients with MS, the ablative treatments should be used, unless the MRI demonstrates neurovascular compression and no demyelination.
- Our recommendations for the treatment of TN follow the algorithm depicted in ▶ Fig. 25.1.

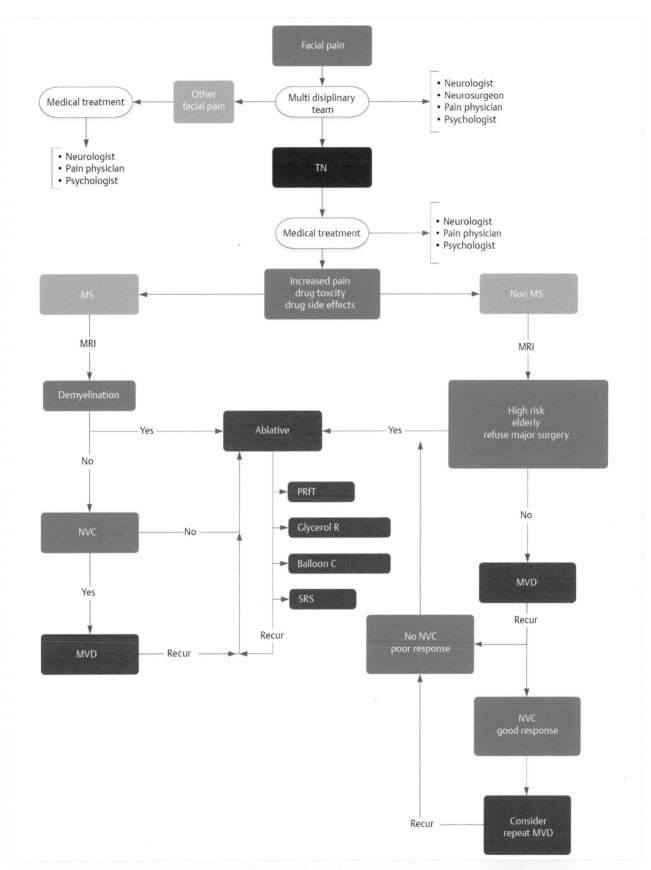

Fig. 25.1 Authors' recommended treatment algorithm for trigeminal neuralgia.

References

[1] Brisman R. Trigeminal neuralgia: diagnosis and treatment. World Neurosurg. 2011; 76(6):533–534

[2] Katusic S, Williams DB, Beard CM, Bergstralh EJ, Kurland LT. Epidemiology and clinical features of idiopathic trigeminal neuralgia and glossopharyngeal neuralgia: similarities and differences, Rochester, Minnesota, 1945–1984. Neuroepidemiology. 1991; 10(5–6):276–281

[3] Barker FG, II, Jannetta PJ, Bissonette DJ, Larkins MV, Jho HD. The long-term outcome of microvascular decompression for trigeminal neuralgia. N Engl J Med. 1996; 334(17):1077–1083

[4] Bahgat D, Ray DK, Raslan AM, McCartney S, Burchiel KJ. Trigeminal neuralgia in young adults. J Neurosurg. 2011; 114(5):1306–1311

[5] Bender MT, Pradilla G, James C, Raza S, Lim M, Carson BS. Surgical treatment of pediatric trigeminal neuralgia: case series and review of the literature. Childs Nerv Syst. 2011; 27(12):2123–2129

[6] Jannetta PJ. Observations on the etiology of trigeminal neuralgia, hemifacial spasm, acoustic nerve dysfunction and glossopharyngeal neuralgia. Definitive microsurgical treatment and results in 117 patients. Neurochirurgia (Stuttg). 1977; 20(5):145–154

[7] Jannetta PJ. Arterial compression of the trigeminal nerve at the pons in patients with trigeminal neuralgia. J Neurosurg. 1967; 26(1):159–162

[8] Inoue T, Hirai H, Shima A, Suzuki F, Fukushima T, Matsuda M. Diagnosis and management for trigeminal neuralgia caused solely by venous compression. Acta Neurochir (Wien). 2017; 159(4):681–688

[9] Solaro C, Brichetto G, Amato MP, et al. PaIMS Study Group. The prevalence of pain in multiple sclerosis: a multicenter cross-sectional study. Neurology. 2004; 63(5):919–921

[10] Putzki N, Pfriem A, Limmroth V, et al. Prevalence of migraine, tension-type headache and trigeminal neuralgia in multiple sclerosis. Eur J Neurol. 2009; 16(2):262–267

[11] Burchiel KJ. A new classification for facial pain. Neurosurgery. 2003; 53(5):1164–1166, discussion 1166–1167

[12] Cruccu G, Finnerup NB, Jensen TS, et al. Trigeminal neuralgia: new classification and diagnostic grading for practice and research. Neurology. 2016; 87(2):220–228

[13] Burchiel KJ, Slavin KV. On the natural history of trigeminal neuralgia. Neurosurgery. 2000; 46(1):152–154, discussion 154–155

[14] Patten J. Facial pain. In: Patten J, ed. Neurological Differential Diagnosis. 2nd Edition Springer 1996; 372–375

[15] Sturman RH, O'Brien FH. Non-surgical treatment of tic douloureux with carbamazepine (G32883). Headache. 1969; 9(1):88–91

[16] Rockliff BW, Davis EH. Controlled sequential trials of carbamazepine in trigeminal neuralgia. Arch Neurol. 1966; 15(2):129–136

[17] Marotta JT. A long term study in trigeminal neuralgia. Headache. 1969; 9(1):83–87

[18] Killian JM. Tegretol in trigeminal neuralgia with special reference to hematopoietic side effects. Headache. 1969; 9(1):58–63

[19] Sweet WH. The treatment of trigeminal neuralgia (tic douloureux). N Engl J Med. 1986; 315(3):174–177

[20] Di Stefano G, La Cesa S, Truini A, Cruccu G. Natural history and outcome of 200 outpatients with classical trigeminal neuralgia treated with carbamazepine or oxcarbazepine in a tertiary centre for neuropathic pain. J Headache Pain. 2014; 15(1):34

[21] Taylor JC, Brauer S, Espir ML. Long-term treatment of trigeminal neuralgia with carbamazepine. Postgrad Med J. 1981; 57(663):16–18

[22] Benoliel R, Zini A, Khan J, Almoznino G, Sharav Y, Haviv Y. Trigeminal neuralgia (part II): factors affecting early pharmacotherapeutic outcome. Cephalalgia. 2016; 36(8):747–759

[23] Davis EH. Clinical trials of Tegretol in trigeminal neuralgia. Headache. 1969; 9(1):77–82

[24] Rasmussen P, Riishede J. Facial pain treated with carbamazepin (Tegretol). Acta Neurol Scand. 1970; 46(4):385–408

[25] Graham JG, Zilkha KJ. Treatment of trigeminal neuralgia with carbamazepine: a follow-up study. BMJ. 1966; 1(5481):210–211

[26] Nicol CF. A four year double-blind study of Tegretol in facial pain. Headache. 1969; 9(1):54–57

[27] Ferrell PB, Jr, McLeod HL. Carbamazepine, HLA-B*1502 and risk of Stevens-Johnson syndrome and toxic epidermal necrolysis: US FDA recommendations. Pharmacogenomics. 2008; 9(10):1543–1546

[28] Bendtsen L, Zakrzewska JM, Abbott J, et al. European Academy of Neurology guideline on trigeminal neuralgia. Eur J Neurol. 2019; 26(6):831–849

[29] Gronseth G, Cruccu G, Alksne J, et al. Practice parameter: the diagnostic evaluation and treatment of trigeminal neuralgia (an evidence-based review): report of the Quality Standards Subcommittee of the American Academy of Neurology and the European Federation of Neurological Societies. Neurology. 2008; 71(15):1183–1190

[30] Holste K, Chan AY, Rolston JD, Englot DJ. Pain outcomes following microvascular decompression for drug-resistant trigeminal neuralgia: a systematic review and meta-analysis. Neurosurgery. 2020 Feb 1; 86(2):182–190

[31] Besi E, Boniface DR, Cregg R, Zakrzewska JM. Comparison of tolerability and adverse symptoms in oxcarbazepine and carbamazepine in the treatment of trigeminal neuralgia and neuralgiform headaches using the Liverpool Adverse Events Profile (AEP). J Headache Pain. 2015; 16:563

[32] Slettebø H, Eide PK. A prospective study of microvascular decompression for trigeminal neuralgia. Acta Neurochir (Wien). 1997; 139(5):421–425

[33] Sandel T, Eide PK. Long-term results of microvascular decompression for trigeminal neuralgia and hemifacial spasms according to preoperative symptomatology. Acta Neurochir (Wien). 2013; 155(9):1681–1692, discussion 1692

[34] Burchiel KJ, Steege TD, Howe JF, Loeser JD. Comparison of percutaneous radiofrequency gangliolysis and microvascular decompression for the surgical management of tic douloureux. Neurosurgery. 1981; 9(2):111–119

[35] Sindou M, Leston J, Howeidy T, Decullier E, Chapuis F. Micro-vascular decompression for primary trigeminal neuralgia (typical or atypical). Long-term effectiveness on pain; prospective study with survival analysis in a consecutive series of 362 patients. Acta Neurochir (Wien). 2006; 148(12):1235–1245, discussion 1245

[36] van Loveren H, Tew JM, Jr, Keller JT, Nurre MA. a 10-year experience in the treatment of trigeminal neuralgia. Comparison of percutaneous stereotaxic rhizotomy and posterior fossa exploration. J Neurosurg. 1982; 57(6):757–764

[37] Campbell FG, Graham JG, Zilkha KJ. Clinical trial of carbazepine (tegretol) in trigeminal neuralgia. J Neurol Neurosurg Psychiatry. 1966; 29(3):265–267

[38] Killian JM, Fromm GH. Carbamazepine in the treatment of neuralgia. Use of side effects. Arch Neurol. 1968; 19(2):129–136

[39] Fromm GH, Terrence CF, Chattha AS, Glass JD. Baclofen in trigeminal neuralgia: its effect on the spinal trigeminal nucleus: a pilot study. Arch Neurol. 1980; 37(12):768–771

[40] Fromm GH, Terrence CF, Chattha AS. Baclofen in the treatment of trigeminal neuralgia: double-blind study and long-term follow-up. Ann Neurol. 1984; 15(3):240–244

[41] Zakrzewska JM, Chaudhry Z, Nurmikko TJ, Patton DW, Mullens LE. Lamotrigine (Lamictal) in refractory trigeminal neuralgia: results from a double-blind placebo controlled crossover trial. Pain. 1997; 73(2):223–230

[42] Yuan M, Zhou HY, Xiao ZL, et al. Efficacy and safety of gabapentin vs. carbamazepine in the treatment of trigeminal neuralgia: a meta-analysis. Pain Pract. 2016; 16(8):1083–1091

[43] Morra ME, Elgebaly A, Elmaraezy A, et al. Therapeutic efficacy and safety of botulinum toxin A therapy in trigeminal neuralgia: a systematic review and meta-analysis of randomized controlled trials. J Headache Pain. 2016; 17(1):63

[44] Wu S, Lian Y, Zhang H, et al. Botulinum toxin type A for refractory trigeminal neuralgia in older patients: a better therapeutic effect. J Pain Res. 2019; 12:2177–2186

[45] Inoue T, Hirai H, Shima A, et al. Long-term outcomes of microvascular decompression and Gamma Knife surgery for trigeminal neuralgia: a retrospective comparison study. Acta Neurochir (Wien). 2017; 159(11):2127–2135

[46] Lunsford LD, Apfelbaum RI. Choice of surgical therapeutic modalities for treatment of trigeminal neuralgia: microvascular decompression, percutaneous retrogasserian thermal, or glycerol rhizotomy. Clin Neurosurg. 1985; 32:319–333

[47] Dai ZF, Huang QL, Liu HP, Zhang W. Efficacy of stereotactic Gamma Knife surgery and microvascular decompression in the treatment of primary trigeminal neuralgia: a retrospective study of 220 cases from a single center. J Pain Res. 2016; 9:535–542

[48] Shibahashi K, Morita A, Kimura T. Surgical results of microvascular decompression procedures and patient's postoperative quality of life: review of 139 cases. Neurol Med Chir (Tokyo). 2013; 53(6):360–364

[49] Jellish WS, Benedict W, Owen K, Anderson D, Fluder E, Shea JF. Perioperative and long-term operative outcomes after surgery for trigeminal neuralgia: microvascular decompression vs percutaneous balloon ablation. Head Face Med. 2008; 4:11

[50] Wei Y, Pu C, Li N, Cai Y, Shang H, Zhao W. Long-term therapeutic effect of microvascular decompression for trigeminal neuralgia: Kaplan-Meier analysis in a consecutive series of 425 patients. Turk Neurosurg. 2018; 28 (1):88–93

[51] Oh IH, Choi SK, Park BJ, Kim TS, Rhee BA, Lim YJ. The treatment outcome of elderly patients with idiopathic trigeminal neuralgia: micro-vascular decompression versus Gamma knife radiosurgery. J Korean Neurosurg Soc. 2008; 44(4):199–204

[52] Tucer B, Ekici MA, Demirel S, Başarslan SK, Koç RK, Güçlü B. Microvascular decompression for primary trigeminal neuralgia : short-term follow-up results and prognostic factors. J Korean Neurosurg Soc. 2012; 52(1):42–47

[53] Oesman C, Mooij JJA. Long-term follow-up of microvascular decompression for trigeminal neuralgia. Skull Base. 2011; 21(5):313–322

[54] Günther T, Gerganov VM, Stieglitz L, Ludemann W, Samii A, Samii M. Microvascular decompression for trigeminal neuralgia in the elderly: long-term treatment outcome and comparison with younger patients. Neurosurgery. 2009; 65(3):477–482, discussion 482

[55] Apfelbaum RI. A comparision of percutaneous radiofrequency trigeminal neurolysis and microvascular decompression of the trigeminal nerve for the treatment of tic douloureux. Neurosurgery. 1977; 1(1):16–21

[56] Sekula RF, Marchan EM, Fletcher LH, Casey KF, Jannetta PJ. Microvascular decompression for trigeminal neuralgia in elderly patients. J Neurosurg. 2008; 108(4):689–691

[57] Linskey ME, Ratanatharathorn V, Peñagaricano J. A prospective cohort study of microvascular decompression and Gamma Knife surgery in patients with trigeminal neuralgia. J Neurosurg. 2008; 109 Suppl:160–172

[58] Amagasaki K, Watanabe S, Naemura K, Shono N, Nakaguchi H. Safety of microvascular decompression for elderly patients with trigeminal neuralgia. Clin Neurol Neurosurg. 2016; 141:77–81

[59] Aryan HE, Nakaji P, Lu DC, Alksne JF. Multimodality treatment of trigeminal neuralgia: impact of radiosurgery and high resolution magnetic resonance imaging. J Clin Neurosci. 2006; 13(2):239–244

[60] Jo KW, Kong DS, Hong KS, Lee JA, Park K. Long-term prognostic factors for microvascular decompression for trigeminal neuralgia. J Clin Neurosci. 2013; 20(3):440–445

[61] Laghmari M, El Ouahabi A, Arkha Y, Derraz S, El Khamlichi A. Are the destructive neurosurgical techniques as effective as microvascular decompression in the management of trigeminal neuralgia? Surg Neurol. 2007; 68(5):505–512

[62] Nunta-Aree S, Patiwech K, Sitthinamsuwan B. Microvascular decompression for treatment of trigeminal neuralgia: factors that predict complete pain relief and study of efficacy and safety in older patients. World Neurosurg. 2018; 110:e979–e988

[63] Xiang H, Wu G, Ouyang J, Liu R. Prospective study of neuroendoscopy versus microscopy: 213 cases of microvascular decompression for trigeminal neuralgia performed by one neurosurgeon. World Neurosurg. 2018; 111: e335–e339

[64] Zeng YJ, Zhang H, Yu S, Zhang W, Sun XC. Efficacy and safety of microvascular decompression and Gamma Knife surgery treatments for patients with primary trigeminal neuralgia: a prospective study. World Neurosurg. 2018; 116:e113–e117

[65] Chen JF, Lee ST. Comparison of percutaneous trigeminal ganglion compression and microvascular decompression for the management of trigeminal neuralgia. Clin Neurol Neurosurg. 2003; 105(3):203–208

[66] Dahle L, von Essen C, Kourtopoulos H, Ridderheim PA, Vavruch L. Microvascular decompression for trigeminal neuralgia. Acta Neurochir (Wien). 1989; 99(3)(–)(4):109–112

[67] Ferguson GG, Brett DC, Peerless SJ, Barr HW, Girvin JP. Trigeminal neuralgia: a comparison of the results of percutaneous rhizotomy and microvascular decompression. Can J Neurol Sci. 1981; 8(3):207–214

[68] Huang C, Wan Z, Wan C, Li Y, Zhong R. Clinical factors and safety of microvascular decompression in the treatment of trigeminal neuralgia. Biomedical Research (India). 2018; 29(9):1845–1851

[69] Khan SA, Khan B, Khan AA, et al. Microvascular decompression for trigeminal neuralgia. JAMC. 2015; 27(3):539–542

[70] Mendoza N, Illingworth RD. Trigeminal neuralgia treated by microvascular decompression: a long-term follow-up study. Br J Neurosurg. 1995; 9(1): 13–19

[71] Tyler-Kabara EC, Kassam AB, Horowitz MH, et al. Predictors of outcome in surgically managed patients with typical and atypical trigeminal neuralgia: comparison of results following microvascular decompression. J Neurosurg. 2002; 96(3):527–531

[72] Walchenbach R, Voormolen JH, Hermans J. Microvascular decompression for trigeminal neuralgia: a critical reappraisal. Clin Neurol Neurosurg. 1994; 96 (4):290–295

[73] Zhao H, Tang Y, Zhang X, Li S. Microvascular decompression for idiopathic primary trigeminal neuralgia in patients over 75 years of age. J Craniofac Surg. 2016; 27(5):1295–1297

[74] Guo HC, Zhao C, Song G, Gu, o HT, Zhang Q, Bao Y. Main causes of trigeminal neuralgia and corresponding surgical strategies. Int J Clin Exp Med. 2016; 9 (11):22088–22092

[75] Broggi G, Ferroli P, Franzini A, Servello D, Dones I. Microvascular decompression for trigeminal neuralgia: comments on a series of 250 cases, including 10 patients with multiple sclerosis. J Neurol Neurosurg Psychiatry. 2000; 68(1):59–64

[76] Chen JCT. Microvascular decompression for trigeminal neuralgia in patients with and without prior stereotactic radiosurgery. World Neurosurg. 2012; 78(1)(–)(2):149–154

[77] Greenberg, M, ed. In: Handbook of Neurosurgery. 8th Edition. New York; Thieme Medical Publishers; 2016; 485–491

[78] Panczykowski DM, Jani RH, Hughes MA, Sekula RF. Development and evaluation of a preoperative trigeminal neuralgia scoring system to predict long-term outcome following microvascular decompression. Neurosurgery. 2020; 87(1):71–79

[79] Ruiz-Juretschke F, Guzmán-de-Villoria JG, García-Leal R, Sañudo JR. Predictive value of magnetic resonance for identifying neurovascular compressions in trigeminal neuralgia. Neurologia. 2019; 34(8):510–519

[80] Hardaway FA, Gustafsson HC, Holste K, Burchiel KJ, Raslan AM. A novel scoring system as a preoperative predictor for pain-free survival after microsurgery for trigeminal neuralgia. J Neurosurg. 20 20; 132(1):217–224

[81] Barba D, Alksne JF. Success of microvascular decompression with and without prior surgical therapy for trigeminal neuralgia. J Neurosurg. 1984; 60(1):104–107

[82] Sweet WH, Wepsic JG. Controlled thermocoagulation of trigeminal ganglion and rootlets for differential destruction of pain fibers. 1. Trigeminal neuralgia. J Neurosurg. 1974; 40(2):143–156

[83] Sweet WH, Poletti CE, Macon JB. Treatment of trigeminal neuralgia and other facial pains by retrogasserian injection of glycerol. Neurosurgery. 1981; 9(6):647–653

[84] Mullan S, Lichtor T. Percutaneous microcompression of the trigeminal ganglion for trigeminal neuralgia. J Neurosurg. 1983; 59(6):1007–1012

[85] Lichtor T, Mullan JF. A 10-year follow-up review of percutaneous microcompression of the trigeminal ganglion. J Neurosurg. 1990; 72(1):49–54

[86] Belber CJ, Rak RA. Balloon compression rhizolysis in the surgical management of trigeminal neuralgia. Neurosurgery. 1987; 20(6):908–913

[87] Fraioli B, Esposito V, Guidetti B, Cruccu G, Manfredi M. Treatment of trigeminal neuralgia by thermocoagulation, glycerolization, and percutaneous compression of the gasserian ganglion and/or retrogasserian rootlets: long-term results and therapeutic protocol. Neurosurgery. 1989; 24(2):239–245

[88] Kanpolat Y, Savas A, Bekar A, Berk C. Percutaneous controlled radiofrequency trigeminal rhizotomy for the treatment of idiopathic trigeminal neuralgia: 25-year experience with 1,600 patients. Neurosurgery. 2001; 48(3):524–532, discussion 532–534

[89] Taha JM, Tew JM, Jr. Comparison of surgical treatments for trigeminal neuralgia: reevaluation of radiofrequency rhizotomy. Neurosurgery. 1996; 38(5):865–871

[90] Taha JM, Tew JM, Jr, Buncher CR. A prospective 15-year follow up of 154 consecutive patients with trigeminal neuralgia treated by percutaneous stereotactic radiofrequency thermal rhizotomy. J Neurosurg. 1995; 83(6): 989–993

[91] Tang YZ, Wu BS, Yang LQ, et al. The long-term effective rate of different branches of idiopathic trigeminal neuralgia after single radiofrequency thermocoagulation: a cohort study. Medicine (Baltimore). 2015; 94(45):e1994

[92] Teixeira MJ, Siqueira SR, Almeida GM. Percutaneous radiofrequency rhizotomy and neurovascular decompression of the trigeminal nerve for the treatment of facial pain. Arq Neuropsiquiatr. 2006; 64(4):983–989

[93] Yao P, Deng YY, Hong T, et al. Radiofrequency thermocoagulation for V2/V3 idiopathic trigeminal neuralgia: effect of treatment temperatures on long-term clinical outcomes: A Cohort Study. Medicine (Baltimore). 2016; 95(26): e4019

[94] Broggi G, Franzini A, Lasio G, Giorgi C, Servello D. Long-term results of percutaneous retrogasserian thermorhizotomy for "essential" trigeminal neuralgia: considerations in 1000 consecutive patients. Neurosurgery. 1990; 26(5):783–786, discussion 786–787

[95] Mittal B, Thomas DG. Controlled thermocoagulation in trigeminal neuralgia. J Neurol Neurosurg Psychiatry. 1986; 49(8):932–936

[96] Frank F, Fabrizi AP. Percutaneous surgical treatment of trigeminal neuralgia. Acta Neurochir (Wien). 1989; 97(3)(–)(4):128–130

[97] Arias MJ. Percutaneous retrogasserian glycerol rhizotomy for trigeminal neuralgia. A prospective study of 100 cases. J Neurosurg. 1986; 65(1):32–36

[98] Bergenheim AT, Hariz MI. Influence of previous treatment on outcome after glycerol rhizotomy for trigeminal neuralgia. Neurosurgery. 1995; 36(2):303–309, discussion 309–310

[99] Burchiel KJ. Percutaneous retrogasserian glycerol rhizolysis in the management of trigeminal neuralgia. J Neurosurg. 1988; 69(3):361–366

[100] Chen L, Xu M, Zou Y. Treatment of trigeminal neuralgia with percutaneous glycerol injection into Meckel's cavity: experience in 4012 patients. Cell Biochem Biophys. 2010; 58(2):85–89

[101] Lunsford LD, Bennett MH. Percutaneous retrogasserian glycerol rhizotomy for tic douloureux: Part 1. Technique and results in 112 patients. Neurosurgery. 1984; 14(4):424–430

[102] Harries AM, Mitchell RD. Percutaneous glycerol rhizotomy for trigeminal neuralgia: safety and efficacy of repeat procedures. Br J Neurosurg. 2011; 25(2):268–272

[103] Jagia M, Bithal PK, Dash HH, Prabhakar H, Chaturvedi A, Chouhan RS. Effect of cerebrospinal fluid return on success rate of percutaneous retrogasserian glycerol rhizotomy. Reg Anesth Pain Med. 2004; 29(6):592–595

[104] Kodeeswaran M, Ramesh VG, Saravanan N, Udesh R. Percutaneous retrogasserian glycerol rhizotomy for trigeminal neuralgia: a simple, safe, cost-effective procedure. Neurol India. 2015; 63(6):889–894

[105] Kouzounias K, Lind G, Schechtmann G, Winter J, Linderoth B. Comparison of percutaneous balloon compression and glycerol rhizotomy for the treatment of trigeminal neuralgia. J Neurosurg. 2010; 113(3):486–492

[106] North RB, Kidd DH, Piantadosi S, Carson BS. Percutaneous retrogasserian glycerol rhizotomy. Predictors of success and failure in treatment of trigeminal neuralgia. J Neurosurg. 1990; 72(6):851–856

[107] Pickett GE, Bisnaire D, Ferguson GG. Percutaneous retrogasserian glycerol rhizotomy in the treatment of tic douloureux associated with multiple sclerosis. Neurosurgery. 2005; 56(3):537–545, discussion 537–545

[108] Pollock BE. Percutaneous retrogasserian glycerol rhizotomy for patients with idiopathic trigeminal neuralgia: a prospective analysis of factors related to pain relief. J Neurosurg. 2005; 102(2):223–228

[109] Saini SS. Reterogasserian anhydrous glycerol injection therapy in trigeminal neuralgia: observations in 552 patients. J Neurol Neurosurg Psychiatry. 1987; 50(11):1536–1538

[110] Young RF. Glycerol rhizolysis for treatment of trigeminal neuralgia. J Neurosurg. 1988; 69(1):39–45

[111] Bender M, Pradilla G, Batra S, et al. Effectiveness of repeat glycerol rhizotomy in treating recurrent trigeminal neuralgia. Neurosurgery. 2012; 70(5):1125–1133, discussion 1133–1134

[112] Jho HD, Lunsford LD. Percutaneous retrogasserian glycerol rhizotomy. Current technique and results. Neurosurg Clin N Am. 1997; 8(1):63–74

[113] Liu JK, Apfelbaum RI. Treatment of trigeminal neuralgia. Neurosurg Clin N Am. 2004; 15(3):319–334

[114] Abdennebi B, Guenane L. Technical considerations and outcome assessment in retrogasserian balloon compression for treatment of trigeminal neuralgia. Series of 901 patients. Surg Neurol Int. 2014; 5:118

[115] Asplund P, Blomstedt P, Bergenheim AT. Percutaneous balloon compression vs percutaneous retrogasserian glycerol rhizotomy for the primary treatment of trigeminal neuralgia. Neurosurgery. 2016; 78(3):421–428, discussion 428

[116] Grewal SS, Kerezoudis P, Garcia O, Quinones-Hinojosa A, Reimer R, Wharen RE. Results of percutaneous balloon compression in trigeminal pain syndromes. World Neurosurg. 2018; 114:e892–e899

[117] Du Y, Yang D, Dong X, Du Q, Wang H, Yu W. Percutaneous balloon compression (PBC) of trigeminal ganglion for recurrent trigeminal neuralgia after microvascular decompression (MVD). Ir J Med Sci. 2015; 184(4):745–751

[118] Martin S, Teo M, Suttner N. The effectiveness of percutaneous balloon compression in the treatment of trigeminal neuralgia in patients with multiple sclerosis. J Neurosurg. 2015; 123(6):1507–1511

[119] Park SS, Lee MK, Kim JW, Jung JY, Kim IS, Ghang CG. Percutaneous balloon compression of trigeminal ganglion for the treatment of idiopathic trigeminal neuralgia : experience in 50 patients. J Korean Neurosurg Soc. 2008; 43(4):186–189

[120] Skirving DJ, Dan NG. A 20-year review of percutaneous balloon compression of the trigeminal ganglion. J Neurosurg. 2001; 94(6):913–917

[121] Stomal-Słowińska M, Słowiński J, Lee TK, et al. Correlation of clinical findings and results of percutaneous balloon compression for patients with trigeminal neuralgia. Clin Neurol Neurosurg. 2011; 113(1):14–21

[122] Lobato RD, Rivas JJ, Sarabia R, Lamas E. Percutaneous microcompression of the gasserian ganglion for trigeminal neuralgia. J Neurosurg. 1990; 72(4):546–553

[123] Alvarez-Pinzon AM, Wolf AL, Swedberg HN, et al. Comparison of percutaneous retrogasserian balloon compression and Gamma Knife radiosurgery for the treatment of trigeminal neuralgia in multiple sclerosis. World Neurosurg. 2017; 97:590–594

[124] Brown JA, Pilitsis JG. Percutaneous balloon compression for the treatment of trigeminal neuralgia: results in 56 patients based on balloon compression pressure monitoring. Neurosurg Focus. 2005; 18(5):E10

[125] Baabor MG, Perez-Limonte L. Percutaneous balloon compression of the gasserian ganglion for the treatment of trigeminal neuralgia: personal experience of 206 patients. Acta Neurochir Suppl (Wien). 2011(108):251–254

[126] Corrêa CF, Teixeira MJ. Balloon compression of the Gasserian ganglion for the treatment of trigeminal neuralgia. Stereotact Funct Neurosurg. 1998; 71(2):83–89

[127] Chen JF, Tu PH, Lee ST. Long-term follow-up of patients treated with percutaneous balloon compression for trigeminal neuralgia in Taiwan. World Neurosurg. 2011; 76(6):586–591

[128] Ying X, Wang H, Deng S, Chen Y, Zhang J, Yu W. Long-term outcome of percutaneous balloon compression for trigeminal neuralgia patients elder than 80 years: a STROBE-compliant article. Medicine (Baltimore). 2017; 96(39):e8199

[129] Yadav S, Sonone RM, Jaiswara C, Bansal S, Singh D, Rathi VC. Long-term follow-up of trigeminal neuralgia patients treated with percutaneous balloon compression technique: a retrospective analysis. J Contemp Dent Pract. 2016; 17(3):263–266

[130] Meglio M, Cioni B. Percutaneous procedures for trigeminal neuralgia: microcompression versus radiofrequency thermocoagulation. Personal experience. Pain. 1989; 38(1):9–16

[131] Liu HB, Ma Y, Zou JJ, Li XG. Percutaneous microballoon compression for trigeminal neuralgia. Chin Med J (Engl). 2007; 120(3):228–230

[132] Noorani I, Lodge A, Vajramani G, Sparrow O. Comparing percutaneous treatments of trigeminal neuralgia: 19 years of experience in a single centre. Stereotact Funct Neurosurg. 2016; 94(2):75–85

[133] Kondziolka D, Lacomis D, Niranjan A, et al. Histological effects of trigeminal nerve radiosurgery in a primate model: implications for trigeminal neuralgia radiosurgery. Neurosurgery. 2000; 46(4):971–976, discussion 976–977

[134] Foy AB, Parisi JE, Pollock BE. Histologic analysis of a human trigeminal nerve after failed stereotactic radiosurgery: case report. Surg Neurol. 2007; 68(6):655–658

[135] Menzel J, Piotrowski W, Penzholz H. Long-term results of Gasserian ganglion electrocoagulation. J Neurosurg. 1975; 42(2):140–143

[136] Brisman R. Gamma Knife surgery with a dose of 75 to 76.8 Gray for trigeminal neuralgia. J Neurosurg. 2004; 100(5):848–854

[137] Pollock BE, Phuong LK, Foote RL, Stafford SL, Gorman DA. High-dose trigeminal neuralgia radiosurgery associated with increased risk of trigeminal nerve dysfunction. Neurosurgery. 2001; 49(1):58–62, discussion 62–64

[138] Kondziolka D, Lunsford LD, Flickinger JC. Stereotactic radiosurgery for the treatment of trigeminal neuralgia. Clin J Pain. 2002; 18(1):42–47

[139] Massager N, Lorenzoni J, Devriendt D, Desmedt F, Brotchi J, Levivier M. Gamma Knife surgery for idiopathic trigeminal neuralgia performed using a far-anterior cisternal target and a high dose of radiation. J Neurosurg. 2004; 100(4):597–605

[140] Zhao H, Shen Y, Yao D, Xiong N, Abdelmaksoud A, Wang H. Outcomes of Two-isocenter Gamma Knife radiosurgery for patients with typical trigeminal neuralgia: pain response and quality of life. World Neurosurg. 2018; 109:e531–e538

[141] Taich ZJ, Goetsch SJ, Monaco E, et al. Stereotactic radiosurgery treatment of trigeminal neuralgia: clinical outcomes and prognostic factors. World Neurosurg. 2016; 90:604–612.e11

[142] Kotecha R, Kotecha R, Modugula S, et al. trigeminal neuralgia treated with stereotactic radiosurgery: the effect of dose escalation on pain control and treatment outcomes. Int J Radiat Oncol Biol Phys. 2016; 96(1):142–148

[143] Lee CC, Chen CJ, Chong ST, et al. Early stereotactic radiosurgery for medically refractory trigeminal neuralgia. World Neurosurg. 2018; 112:e569–e575

[144] Lee JY, Sandhu S, Miller D, Solberg T, Dorsey JF, Alonso-Basanta M. Higher dose rate Gamma Knife radiosurgery may provide earlier and longer-lasting pain relief for patients with trigeminal neuralgia. J Neurosurg. 2015; 123(4): 961–968

[145] Wang Y, Zhang S, Wang W, et al. Gamma Knife surgery for recurrent trigeminal neuralgia in cases with previous microvascular decompression. World Neurosurg. 2018; 110:e593–e598

[146] Xu Z, Schlesinger D, Moldovan K, et al. Impact of target location on the response of trigeminal neuralgia to stereotactic radiosurgery. J Neurosurg. 2014; 120(3):716–724

[147] Martínez-Moreno NE, Martínez-Alvarez R, Rey-Portolés G, Gutiérrez-Sárraga J, Burzaco-Santurtún J, Bravo G. Gamma Knife radiosurgery treatment of trigeminal neuralgia and atypical facial pain. Rev Neurol. 2006; 42(4):195–201

[148] Niranjan A, Lunsford LD. Radiosurgery for the management of refractory trigeminal neuralgia. Neurol India. 2016; 64(4):624–629

[149] Régis J, Tuleasca C, Resseguier N, et al. Long-term safety and efficacy of Gamma Knife surgery in classical trigeminal neuralgia: a 497-patient historical cohort study. J Neurosurg. 2016; 124(4):1079–1087

[150] Romanelli P, Conti A, Bianchi L, Bergantin A, Martinotti A, Beltramo G. Image-guided robotic radiosurgery for trigeminal neuralgia. Neurosurgery. 2018; 83(5):1023–1030

[151] Chang CS, Huang CW, Chou HH, Lin LY, Huang CF. Outcome of Gamma Knife radiosurgery for trigeminal neuralgia associated with neurovascular compression. J Clin Neurosci. 2018; 47:174–177

[152] Debono B, Lotterie JA, Sol JC, et al. Dedicated linear accelerator radiosurgery for classic trigeminal neuralgia: a single-center experience with long-term follow-up. World Neurosurg. 2019; 121:e775–e785

[153] Kondziolka D, Flickinger JC, Lunsford LD, Habeck M. Trigeminal neuralgia radiosurgery: the University of Pittsburgh experience. Stereotact Funct Neurosurg. 1996; 66 Suppl 1:343–348

[154] Taha J. Trigeminal neuralgia: percutaneous procedures. Semin Neurosurg. 2004; 15(2–3):115–134

[155] Hasegawa T, Kondziolka D, Spiro R, Flickinger JC, Lunsford LD. Repeat radiosurgery for refractory trigeminal neuralgia. Neurosurgery. 2002; 50(3): 494–500, discussion 500–502

[156] Maesawa S, Salame C, Flickinger JC, Pirris S, Kondziolka D, Lunsford LD. Clinical outcomes after stereotactic radiosurgery for idiopathic trigeminal neuralgia. J Neurosurg. 2001; 94(1):14–20

[157] Noorani I, Lodge A, Vajramani G, Sparrow O. The effectiveness of percutaneous balloon compression, thermocoagulation, and glycerol rhizolysis for trigeminal neuralgia in multiple sclerosis. Neurosurgery. 2019; 85(4):E684–E692

[158] Chakravorty BG. Association of trigeminal neuralgia with multiple sclerosis. Arch Neurol. 1966; 14(1):95–99

[159] Jensen TS, Rasmussen P, Reske-Nielsen E. Association of trigeminal neuralgia with multiple sclerosis: clinical and pathological features. Acta Neurol Scand. 1982; 65(3):182–189

[160] Linderoth B, Håkanson S. Paroxysmal facial pain in disseminated sclerosis treated by retrogasserian glycerol injection. Acta Neurol Scand. 1989; 80(4): 341–346

[161] Meaney JF, Watt JW, Eldridge PR, Whitehouse GH, Wells JC, Miles JB. Association between trigeminal neuralgia and multiple sclerosis: role of magnetic resonance imaging. J Neurol Neurosurg Psychiatry. 1995; 59(3): 253–259

[162] Gass A, Kitchen N, MacManus DG, Moseley IF, Hennerici MG, Miller DH. Trigeminal neuralgia in patients with multiple sclerosis: lesion localization with magnetic resonance imaging. Neurology. 1997; 49(4):1142–1144

[163] Bender MT, Pradilla G, Batra S, et al. Glycerol rhizotomy and radiofrequency thermocoagulation for trigeminal neuralgia in multiple sclerosis. J Neurosurg. 2013; 118(2):329–336

[164] Zakrzewska JM, Wu J, Brathwaite TS-L. A systematic review of the management of trigeminal neuralgia in patients with multiple sclerosis. World Neurosurg. 2018; 111:291–306

[165] Vulpe H, Wang TJC. Commentary: Gamma Knife radiosurgery for multiple sclerosis-associated trigeminal neuralgia. Neurosurgery. 2019; 85(5): E940

[166] Headache Classification Committee of the International Headache Society (IHS). The International Classification of Headache Disorders, 3rd edition. Cephalalgia. 2018 Jan;38(1):1–211. doi: 10.1177/xxxxxxxxxxxxxxxx. PMID: 29368949

26 Natural History and Management Options of Cerebral Lymphoma

Jordan Elizabeth Cory and Mohammed Awad

Abstract

Cerebral lymphomas are relatively uncommon tumors that affect the lymph tissues of the brain. By definition, there is no coexisting systematic disease at the time of diagnosis. The natural history is difficult to assess due to evolving treatment over time, heterogeneity of patient population, and early intervention. Most cases require stereotactic brain biopsy for formal histopathological diagnosis prior to chemotherapy with either WBRT or autologous stem cell transplant. There is growing evidence to suggest survival benefit from cytoreductive surgery in carefully selected patients.

Keywords: lymphoma, cerebral lymphoma, primary CNS lymphoma

26.1 Introduction

Lymphomas are cancers that originate in the lymphatic system and are categorized into Hodgkin's and non-Hodgkin's lymphomas. Hodgkin's lymphomas are characterized by the presence of Reed–Sternberg cells, which are giant cells that can be observed on light microscopy in these lesions. Non-Hodgkin lymphomas originate mainly from lymphocytes.

The current (2016) World Health Organization (WHO) classification of central nervous system (CNS) tumors divides CNS lymphomas into a number of subtypes based on the cell of origin and histological features.[1] These include the following:

- Diffuse large B-cell lymphoma (DLBCL) of the CNS:
  - Primary CNS lymphoma (PCNSL).
  - Secondary CNS DLBCL.
- Immunodeficiency-associated CNS lymphomas:
  - Acquired immunodeficiency syndrome (AIDS) related DLBCL.
  - Epstein–Barr virus (EBV) positive DLBCL, not otherwise specified (NOS).
  - Lymphomatoid granulomatosis.
- Intravascular large B-cell lymphoma.
- Miscellaneous rare lymphomas:
  - Low-grade B-cell lymphomas.
  - T cell and natural killer (NK)/T-cell lymphomas.
  - Anaplastic large cell lymphoma.
- Mucosa-associated lymphoid tissue (MALT) lymphoma of the dura.

PCNSLs are patternless, highly cellular, DLBCLs isolated to the CNS. PCNSLs are mature B cells that are PAX5, CD19, C30, CD33, and CD79a positive, most expressing BCL6.[1] Whereas MALT lymphoma of the dura and miscellaneous rare lymphomas also present confined to the CNS, they are considered a different entity to PCNSL as per the 2016 WHO classification of CNS tumors.[1]

PCNSLs are a non-Hodgkin's lymphoma and account for 2.4 to 3% of all primary brain tumors, correlating to an incidence rate of 4.7 per million person-years.[1,2] PCNSLs comprise 4 to 6%

of extranodal lymphomas.[1] PCNSLs are most commonly associated with immunosuppression, either genetic (e.g., ataxia–telangiectasia, Wiskott–Aldrich syndrome, or IgA deficiency) or acquired (e.g., AIDS, post organ transplantation).[2] EBV exposure has been shown to be associated with PCNSLs in immunocompromised individuals.[1,3] Etiology in immunocompetent individuals remains to date unknown; genetic predisposition has not been described, and viruses, including EBV), have been shown to have no role.[1,2]

The characteristics and clinical presentation of PCNSL are summarized in ▶ Table 26.1. PCNSLs have a predominance in men, with a male-to-female ratio of 3:2.[1] The median age of diagnosis is 56 years for immunocompetent patients and younger in human immunodeficiency virus (HIV) associated PCNSLs at 37 years.[4,5] Typically, the duration of symptoms is short (at most a few months). In the recent years, there has been an increase in the incidence of sporadic, non-EBV-associated PCNSLs in immunocompetent individuals, which are particularly seen in older patients (50–80 years).[5,6] The rising incidence has been attributed by some to the increasing life expectancy and growing elderly population. Incidence rate in those older than 70 years is 10 times higher than in the general population.[7] Historically, the incidence of PCNSLs rose throughout the 1980s and 1990s, attributable at

Table 26.1 Characteristics and clinical presentation of PCNSL[1,2,9]

Number of lesions	Solitary (60–70%)
Location	Frontal lobe (15%) Posterior fossa (13%) Basal ganglia and periventricular parenchyma (10%)[a] Temporal lobe (8%) Parietal lobe (7%) Corpus callosum (5%)[a] Occipital lobe (3%) Spinal cord (1%)
Characteristic features	Uveocyclitis: • Coincident at diagnosis (8%) • Precedes diagnosis (11%) Subacute encephalitis with subependymal infiltration Glucocorticoid-induced remission (Steroid use is contraindicated) Leptomeningeal involvement (15–20%) (More common in PCNSL than in secondary CNS lymphoma)
Symptoms	Nonfocal symptoms (>50%): • Mental status change • Symptoms of increased intracranial pressure General seizures (<10%) Focal symptoms (30–42%): • Hemimotor or hemisensory symptoms • Cranial nerve deficits

Abbreviations: CNS, central nervous system; PCNSL, primary CNS lymphoma.
[a]Characteristic site.

least in part to the concurrent epidemic of AIDS and increasing use of immunosuppressant medications in patients.[8] The rising incidence not explained by the AIDS epidemic has been attributed by some to the increasing life expectancy and growing elderly population.[6]

26.2 Diagnosis and Evaluation

Comprehensive neurological, cognitive, and physical examination should be performed in all patients including careful examination of peripheral lymph nodes, and testes in men.[10] A guideline to diagnostic and prognostic investigations is summarized in ▶ Table 26.2. Age and performance status, Eastern Cooperative Oncology Group (ECOG) or Karnofsky Performance Status (KPS), should also be documented.

Cerebrospinal fluid (CSF) analysis is recommended for evaluation of extent of disease, rather than diagnosis.[9] Lumbar puncture should be performed in all patients, unless contraindicated, to assess for occult leptomeningeal disease. It is important to note CSF cytology has a low and variable sensitivity of 2 to 32%.[3] In a systematic review of 472 patients, preoperative lumbar puncture obviated diagnostic surgery in only 7.4% of patients.[11] However, during follow-up, this positive CSF increases to 14.9%, suggesting yield increases with number of lumbar punctures.[11] Sensitivity increases with CSF volume analyzed and cytology of at least 3 mL, ideally greater than 10 mL, should be performed. It is important to note that corticosteroid use has been postulated to decrease sensitivity of cytology.[3] However, one study showed no reduction in sensitivity with pretreatment with corticosteroids; however, this study was limited by a small noncorticosteroid cohort.[12] Including flow cytometry in addition to standard cytopathology has been suggested to increase sensitivity for occult leptomeningeal disease in the order of 43 to 50%.[13,14] Flow cytometry also limits false positives due to misinterpretation of reactive lymphocytes as malignant cells.[14] To avoid false positives, CSF should be sampled before or 1 week after brain biopsy.[9] Identification of lymphoma cells within CSF or vitreous fluid together only with high clinical and radiological suspicion for PCNSL can preclude the need for brain biopsy in high surgical risk patients.[15] As outlined, cytological diagnosis is often difficult, and review by a specialist pathologist is recommended.

A detailed ophthalmologic examination of all patients, including those without ocular symptoms, with suspected PCNSL is necessary. In the 15 to 25% of PCNSL patients with intraocular involvement, it is possible to make a diagnosis without brain biopsy.[3] The most common finding on examination and history is chronic posterior uveitis.[16] Vitreal biopsy, chorioretinal biopsy, or fine-needle aspiration of subretinal lesions can confirm the diagnosis.[16]

Given the aggressive nature of PCNSLs, prompt diagnosis to aid early treatment is critical to improving survival.[9] Significant diagnostic delay has been noted; PCNSLs compared with glioblastoma multiforme in one study noted mean time of 41.7 versus 16.2 days from initial neuroimaging to histologic diagnosis.[17] Navigation-guided or stereotactic brain biopsy is the gold standard of immunohistochemical diagnosis of lymphoma and lymphoma type.[2,10] PCNSL diagnosis is made much less frequently via CSF cytology and flow cytometry or vitrectomy/chorioretinal biopsy. Given that stereotactic biopsy is safe and the diagnostic yield of lumbar puncture is low, early stereotactic brain biopsy is preferred as it can avert diagnostic delay.[11]

26.2.1 Imaging

Imaging is not sufficient to differentiate PCNSL from other tumor types such as gliomas, space-occupying inflammatory lesions including tumefactive demyelination, acute disseminated encephalomyelitis and neurosarcoidosis, or more rarely infectious space-occupying lesions such as cerebral toxoplasmosis or abscess. Around 40 to 80% of PCNSLs initially treated with corticosteroids demonstrate radiological regression.[18,19] Magnetic resonance imaging (MRI) with gadolinium contrast is the most sensitive imaging modality in the diagnosis of PCNSL (▶ Fig. 26.1). Characteristic lesions demonstrate homogenous contrast enhancement with well-defined borders.[9] Radiologically, the MRI enhancement pattern is more variable in HIV-associated and immunosuppressed patients with ring enhancement in up to 75% of cases (vs. 0–13% in nonimmunosuppressed patients).[20] Multifocal disease is also more common in immunosuppressed patients.[12]

Vasogenic edema usually surrounds the lesion but is less prominent than in glioma or metastasis.[9,12] ▶ Fig. 26.1 demonstrates characteristic findings useful in differentiating PCNSLs from other lesions including a low signal on T2-weighted MRI and restricted diffusion on diffusion weighted imaging (DWI) MRI due to high nucleus-to-cytoplasm ratio and high cellular density.[9,21] Corticosteroid-induced radiological remission is common but is not diagnostic and does not rule out demyelinating or inflammatory diseases.[9,10] Rarely, PCNSLs can been

Table 26.2 Primary CNS lymphoma baseline diagnostic and prognostic evaluation[9]

Clinical evaluation

- Physical and neurological examination
- Age and performance status (ECOG or KPS)
- Cognitive function evaluation (MMSE at minimum)
- History of corticosteroid dosing

Laboratory evaluation

- Hepatic and renal function
- Serum LDH
- CD4 + T cell count
- HIV serologic testing

Extent of disease evaluation

- Gadolinium-enhanced brain MRI (or contrast-enhanced CT if MRI is contraindicated)
- CSF analysis, cytology, flow cytometry, cell counts, protein and glucose levels, B2-microglobulin, immunoglobulin heavy chain gene arrangement
- Ophthalmologic examination, including slit-lamp examination
- Gadolinium-enhanced whole-spine MRI (if suggestive symptoms of spinal involvement)
- PET or CT chest/abdomen/pelvis
- Bone marrow biopsy with aspirate
- Testicular ultrasound for men

Abbreviations: CNS, central nervous system; CSF, cerebrospinal fluid; CT, computed tomography; ECOG, Eastern Cooperative Oncology Group; HIV, human immunodeficiency virus; KPS, Karnofsky Performance Status; LDH, lactate dehydrogenase; MMSE, Mini-Mental State Examination; MRI, magnetic resonance imaging; PET, positron emission tomography.

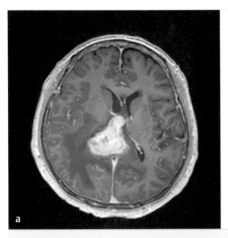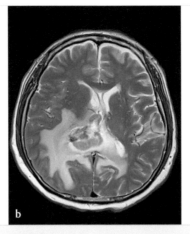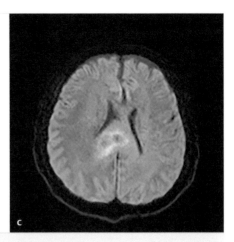

Fig. 26.1 Characteristic magnetic resonance imaging (MRI) findings. **(a)** T1-weighted sequence with gadolinium contrast enhancement. **(b)** T2-weighted sequence demonstrates low signal. **(c)** Diffusion weighted imaging (DWI) sequence demonstrates diffusion restriction.

seen as subtle focal abnormalities of cranial or radicular nerves or focal meningeal enhancement.[9,8] F-fluorodeoxyglucose (FDG) or ^{11}C-methionine positron emission tomography (PET) has been suggested to predict early response to therapy and early disease recurrence during posttreatment surveillance before it can be visualized on MRI; however, studies so far have been limited by small numbers.[22,23]

26.3 Selected Papers on Natural History of PCNSL

- Abrey LE, Ben-Porat L, Panageas KS, et al. Primary central nervous system lymphoma: the Memorial Sloan-Kettering Cancer Center prognostic model. J Clin Oncol 2006;24(36):5711–5715
- Ferreri AJ, Batchelor T, Zucca E, Cavalli F, Armitage J. International Collaborative Group against Primary CNS Lymphomas. J Clin Oncol 2003;21(8):1649–1650
- Mendez JS, Ostrom QT, Gittleman H, et al. The elderly left behind-changes in survival trends of primary central nervous system lymphoma over the past 4 decades. Neuro-oncol 2018;20(5):687–694

26.4 Natural History of PCNSL

The natural history of PCNSL is difficult to assess due to the literature being confounded by evolving and differing treatment regimens, as well as vastly different population characteristics.

PCNSL remains an aggressive disease with poor prognosis with age, performance status, and immune status universally accepted prognostic factors. PCNSL has a much poorer outcome than systemic DLBCL. The 5-year overall survival (OS) is 33% and if left untreated, the mean OS is 1.5 months.[9] This has been postulated to be due to evasion of the neoplastic B cells from T-cell lymphocyte surveillance via frequent loss of human leukocyte antigen (HLA) class I and/or class II seen in PCNS DLBCL.[9] Although similarly widely recognized to be a whole brain disease, unlike gliomas, when PCNSL relapses, it is often in a radiographic area remote to the primary site of disease suggesting

microscopic early evasion from the neurovascular unit.[24] Occasionally, PCNSL can metastasize outside the CNS.[2] Prognosis of PCNSL has improved significantly, with median OS improving from 2.5 months in the 1970s to 26 months in the 2010s.[7] This phenomenon likely represents natural history of untreated or poorly treated PCNSL in the early years with improving outcomes with modern treatment particularly increasing prevalence of high-dose methotrexate (HD-MTX) induction therapy. Interestingly, despite treatment advances, no improvement in median OS in those older than 70 years (OS: 6–7 months) has been observed in the same time period as seen in ▶ Fig. 26.2.[5,7] This is hypothesized to be due to deteriorating functional status and increasing comorbidities, particularly deteriorating renal function, limiting the use of HD-MTX induction therapy.

Age and performance status are universally accepted prognostic factors across the literature, independent of planned treatment regimen.[6,10] Two scoring systems have been described to predict prognosis of PCNSLs: Memorial Sloan Kettering Cancer Center (MSKCC) prognostic score and International Extranodal Lymphoma Study Group (IELSG) score.[25,26] These scoring systems are summarized in ▶ Table 26.3. Histology subtype, duration of symptoms, infratentorial localization, and bilateral brain involvement have not been found to be prognostic factors.[25,27]

26.5 AIDS-Associated PCNSL

AIDS-associated PCNSLs usually occur in a younger patient cohort.[5] HIV increases the risk of developing CNSL by 3,600-fold.[4] The majority of HIV-associated PCNSLs are EBV related due to ineffective immunoregulation of the virus, whereas there is no association with EBV in immunocompetent individuals.[1] Most patients with HIV and PCNSL have AIDS with a median CD4 count of 30 × 10[6]/L.[28] HIV-associated PCNSLs are more frequently multifocal and show larger areas of necrosis.[29] Differential diagnosis must include cerebral toxoplasmosis, which can also be concomitant with PCNSLs.[1] Clinically, PCNSLs and cerebral toxoplasmosis are nearly indistinguishable, with the exception of chorea, which is pathognomonic of cerebral toxoplasmosis.[30] Additional tests in a patient with HIV include EBV deoxyribonucleic acid (DNA) in CSF and toxoplasma gondii serology. As in

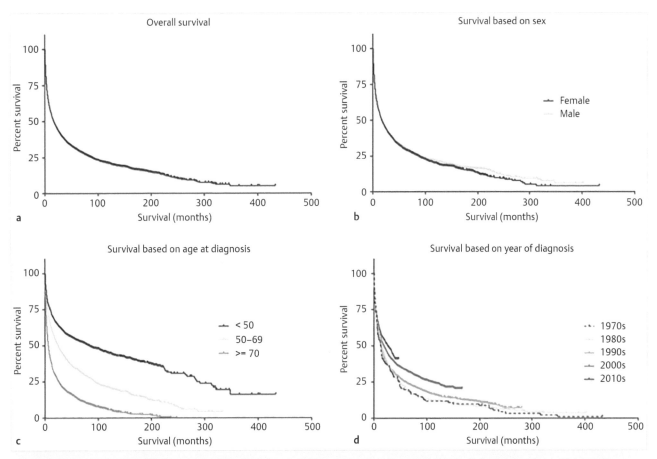

Fig. 26.2 Kaplan–Meier curves demonstrating clinical outcome in PCNSL; augmenting the natural history of disease over time with improving treatment options (SEER registries 1973–2013).[7] **(a)** Overall survival. **(b)** Survival based on sex. **(c)** Survival based on age at diagnosis. **(d)** Survival based on year of diagnosis. (Reprinted with permission from the Oxford University Press.[7])

Table 26.3 Primary CNS lymphoma prognostic scoring systems[25,26]

International Extranodal Lymphoma Study (IELS) group score			Memorial Sloan Kettering Cancer Center prognostic score		
Prognostic factor	Value	Points	Prognostic factor	Value	Class
Age	<60 y	0	Age	<50 y	Class I
	>60 y	1		>50 y	Proceed to KPS
ECOG performance status	0–1	0	Karnofsky performance status (KPS)	>70	Class II
	2–4	1		<70	Class III
Lactate dehydrogenase serum level	Normal	0			
	Elevated	1			
CSF protein concentration	Normal	0			
	Elevated	1			
Involvement of deep brain structures	No	0			
	Yes	1			
Maximum score		5	Maximum score	Class III	
Score	2-y overall survival rate		Score	Median survival (y)	
0–1	80%		Class I	8.5	
2–3	48%		Class II	3.2	
4–5	15%		Class III	1.1	

Abbreviations: CNS, central nervous system; CSF, cerebrospinal fluid; CT, computed tomography; ECOG, Eastern Cooperative Oncology Group.

Table 26.4 Disease course of PCNSL in HIV-negative compared to HIV-positive patients[31,32]

Study	Year of diagnosis	HIV negative				HIV positive				Hazard ratio (95% CI)
		n	Median age % male	Median PFS (mo)	Median OS (mo)	*n*	Median age % male	Median PFS (mo)	Median OS (mo)	
Norden et al[32]	1973–2003	1,732	63 y 55.3%	N/A	12	825	37 y 91.8%	N/A	2	4.55 (4.01–5.16)
Bayraktar et al[31]	1999–2008	45	59.8 y 49%	7.9	14.6	41	43.7 y 58%	3.4	4.0	1.99 (1.08–3.66)

Abbreviations: CI, confidence interval; HIV, human immunodeficiency virus; OS, overall survival; PCNSL, primary central nervous system lymphoma; PFS, progression-free survival.

immunocompetent individuals, confirmation via stereotactic biopsy remains the gold standard in diagnosis. Optimal combination antiretroviral therapy, in terms of compliance, side effects, and titration, is an important prognostic factor and treatment consideration in HIV-related PCNSLs.[31] Multiple studies demonstrate a significantly worse prognosis in HIV positive individuals compared to their immunocompetent counterparts as summarized in ▶ Table 26.4.[31,32]

26.6 Selected Papers on Treatment Outcomes of PCNSL

- Alnahhas I, Jawish M, Alsawas M, et al. Autologous stem-cell transplantation for primary central nervous system lymphoma: systematic review and meta-analysis. Clin Lymphoma Myeloma Leuk 2019;19(3):e129–e141
- Weller M, Martus P, Roth P, Thiel E, Korfel A; German PCNSL Study Group. Surgery for primary CNS lymphoma? Challenging a paradigm. Neuro-oncol 2012;14(12): 1481–1484
- Rae AI, Mehta A, Cloney M, et al. Craniotomy and survival for primary central nervous system lymphoma. Neurosurgery 2019;84(4):935–944

26.7 Treatment Outcomes of PCNSL

26.7.1 The Role of Steroids Prior to Biopsy

Historically, due to possible steroid-induced remission, corticosteroids have been avoided preoperatively if clinically feasible due to the possible increased risk of nondiagnostic yield.[15] In the case of steroid-induced remission or nondiagnostic biopsy yield as suggested by some early studies, close MRI follow-up is advised and stereotactic biopsy recommended if radiological tumor growth is observed.[15] However, a recent retrospective institutional review by Bullis et al joined a number of newer studies suggesting that this historical aversion should be challenged.[33,34,35] The study included 54 patients diagnosed with histological PCNSLs; 18 received preoperative dexamethasone, with doses ranging from 4 to 120 mg over a median of 2 days.[33] In all patients, tissue sampling was achieved via needle biopsy (46%), open biopsy (25%), and debulking surgery (28%).[33] The most obvious limitation in this study is the retrospective nature

as well as the exclusion of any patients not diagnosed with PCNSL, reliant on an assumption of accurate histological diagnosis. In summary, corticosteroids should be avoided preoperatively and surgery expedited where possible. Where steroids are unable to be avoided due to neurological deterioration, stereotactic brain biopsy should be imminently undertaken, as recent literature suggests that nondiagnostic yield is not as likely as historically suggested. However, further research is required to better define this controversy.

26.7.2 Induction Therapy

Chemotherapy

HD-MTX induction chemotherapy with the aim of complete radiological remission is the mainstay of first-line treatment regimen.[6] The increasing prevalence of HD-MTX induction therapy in the treatment of PCNSL is widely touted as being responsible for the improvement in prognosis in younger patients over the last 50 years. While PCNSL is initially responsive to the cyclophosphamide, doxorubicin, vincristine, prednisolone (CHOP) regimen widely used for non-Hodgkin's lymphomas, it does not induce a survival benefit when added to radiotherapy.[36] Typical chemotherapy regimens used for systemic non-Hodgkin's lymphomas do not readily cross the blood–brain barrier and so are ineffective in treating PCNSLs.[37] The optimal combination regimen is yet to be defined. Despite complete response rates as high as 65%, to initial HD-MTX treatment alone, more than half of the responders relapse, with a median progression-free survival (PFS) of 10 months, so consolidation therapy is imperative to treatment considerations.[38]

In two consecutive single-arm studies, intraventricular chemotherapy via reservoir in combination with HD-MTX achieved long-term (> 100 months) disease control in around half of the young patients (< 60 years), but has not been widely accepted as a treatment option due to high rates of intrathecal reservoir infections (19%) and conflicting evidence from multiple retrospective studies that showed no additional survival benefit when added to induction HD-MTX.[9,15,39,40]

26.7.3 Consolidation Therapy

Although PCNSL is typically responsive to inductive therapy, the high rate of relapse demands consolidative treatment. Consolidation chemotherapy is less defined, with regimens varying between centers. Historically, whole brain radiotherapy (WBRT) is utilized despite well-documented adverse side effects, most

Table 26.5 Summary of recent literature comparing consolidative WBRT and ASCT[46,47]

Study	Design	Arm		Intervals (y)				Interpretation
				1	2	3	5	
Ferreri et al[46]	Phase II randomized control trial	HD-CT + consolidative WBRT (n = 59)	PFS		80%			No significant difference in PFS or OS at 2 y (p = 0.17 and 0.91, respectively)
			OS		82%			
		HD-CT + consolidative ASCT (n = 59)	PFS		69%			
			OS		77%			
Alnahhas et al[47]	Systematic review and meta-analysis	HD-CT + consolidative ASCT (16 studies, n = 323)	PFS	79%	70%	64%	54%	Inclusive of and supporting of findings by Ferreri et al[46]
			OS	94%	86%	82%	72%	
		Salvage ASCT (4 studies, n = 75)	PFS	85%	62%	59%	54%	
			OS	75%	63%	56%	54%	

Abbreviations: ASCT, autologous stem cell transplant; HD-CT, high-dose chemotherapy; OS, overall survival; PFS, progression-free survival; WBRT, whole brain radiotherapy.

notably neurotoxicity. Increasing number of studies support autologous stem cell transplant (ASCT) with consolidative chemotherapy in suitable patients.

Radiation Therapy

Although PCNSL is responsive to radiation, it is not an effective treatment when used alone. So it became commonly used in conjunction with high-dose myeloablative chemotherapy. WBRT is complicated by delayed neurotoxicity, with the risk more than doubling in the elderly population.[9] In one study, 75% of patients older than 60 years who received WBRT developed neurotoxicity compared to 26% of those younger than 60 years.[41] Patients with radiotherapy-induced neurotoxicity clinically develop executive dysfunction, memory impairment, ataxia, psychomotor slowing, and incontinence, with radiological evaluation demonstrating diffuse white mater disease and cortical–subcortical atrophy.[42] At autopsy, radiotherapy-induced neurotoxicity is seen as white matter gliosis, thickening of small vessels, and demyelination.[42] While consolidation WBRT remains controversial, particularly in the elderly population, there is a growing evidence for consolidative reduced-dose WBRT (total dose: 23.4 Gy; 1.8 Gy × 13) with cytarabine. Early data showed that the 2-year PFS was 78% for those in the consolidative chemotherapy with reduced-dose radiotherapy arm compared to 54% who had consolidative chemotherapy alone.[43] Deferred and/or reduced-dose WBRT is commonly utilized as a salvage therapy in PCNSL.[15] Stereotactic radiosurgery is currently similarly reserved for treatment of PCNSL as an alternative to WBRT when the risks of neurotoxicity are determined too adverse or as a salvage therapy.[44]

Stem Cell Therapy

Another consolidative therapy utilized omits radiotherapy instead of autologous stem cell transplantation (ASCT) and typically a thiotepa-containing chemotherapy regimen following high-dose CNS-penetrant chemotherapy with methotrexate.[45] There have been an increasing number of studies suggesting the benefit of this rising practice.

The first international randomized trial addressing consolidative therapy in newly diagnosed PCNSLs was the 2017 International Extranodal Lymphoma Study Group-32 (IELSG32) study by Ferreri et al in which ASCT in combination with myeloablative

high-dose consolidative chemotherapy was shown to have equal efficacy to consolidation WBRT and with less neurotoxic adverse effects.[46] A systematic review and meta-analysis by Alnahhas et al summarized the most recent literature and suggested that 94% patients who underwent consolidative ASCT experienced or maintained their response (complete or partial).[47] A summary of their findings in relation to OS in consolidation and salvage therapy groups is provided in ▶ Table 26.5. They demonstrated that although relapses were higher in the salvage group than in the consolidative group (29 vs. 24%), both groups experienced less relapse than chemotherapy alone.[47]

Evidence for stem cell therapy remains limited as the highest level of studies at this time are open-label phase II studies, most on young patients without major comorbidities or stratified for performance status. ASCT also has complications such as immunosuppression, infections, mucositis, and mortality.[47]

26.7.4 Surgery

Stereotactic Biopsy

The role of surgery in treatment of PCNSLs has been historically largely limited to stereotactic biopsy, with retrospective studies demonstrating no survival benefit with partial tumor debulking or complete tumor resection.[6,48] Stereotactic brain biopsy, among HIV patients, has been demonstrated to be much riskier than that in non-HIV patients, with a 30-day morbidity of 8.4% and mortality of 2.9% (not attributable to disease progression) in a single-center retrospective study versus 2% morbidity and 0% mortality in the non-HIV population.[49]

Intraoperative rapid diagnosis with hematoxylin and eosin staining of frozen specimen can distort the cells and may lead to a misdiagnosis of malignant glioma.[50] Thus, if PCNSL is a differential diagnosis, awaiting formal histopathology is recommended before considering resection. Recent research from Japan suggests that intraoperative flow cytometry increases the specificity and sensitivity of intraoperative rapid diagnosis; this is awaiting prospective trials.[51]

Extent of Resection

The lack of efficacy of surgical resection has been previously hypothesized to be likely due to whole brain disease, or the microscopic infiltrative nature of PCNSL, evident in relapses often occurring in areas of the brain remote from the primary site.[15,24] The typical deep brain location of PCNSL also increases the risk of surgical complications such as intracranial hemorrhage and postoperative neurological deficits.[10] The early studies that advocated for stereotactic biopsy were limited by their small sizes, poor design, and retrospective nature. Favorable therapeutic benefit of cytoreductive surgery was limited largely to case reports until recently.[52,53] In recent years, the role of cytoreductive surgery for PCNSL has been reintroduced. ▶ Table 26.6 presents a summary of the literature review.

Table 26.6 Summary of literature of surgical treatment outcomes, ordered by level of evidence and reverse chronological date of publication

Study	Design	Primary outcomes	Interpretation	Overall
Level IIb evidence				
Weller et al[54]	IIb: secondary analysis of prospective randomized control trial (2000–2009), n = 516	PFS (mo); median OS (mo) Biopsy: 6; 18 Resection: 11; 32: • Subtotal 15; 31 • Gross total 11; 32	Statistically significant between biopsy and resection PFS (p = 0.005) and OS (p = 0.024). Statistically significant between subtotal and total PFS (p = 0.023) but not OS (p = 0.218)	Favorable
DeAngelis et al[55]	IIb: retrospective analysis of prospective cohort (1985–1988), n = 26	Morbidity Resection: 40% Biopsy: 0%	Suggests high complication rates when attempting resection	Unfavorable
Level IIIb evidence				
Rae et al[56]	IIIb: retrospective pooled cohort (NCDB: 2004–2013; SEER: 1995–2013; MSKCC: 2000–2017), n = 13,488	Median OS (mo) NCDB; MSKCC single center • Biopsy: 11.0; 24.7 • Resection: 19.5; 46.0 SEER database • Biopsy: 10.0 • Resection: ○ Subtotal: 24.0 • Grand total: 29.0	Improved survival with craniotomy resection by 8.5 mo (p <0.001, NCDB) No statistically significant survival benefit seen between groups in MSKCC single-institute analysis (n = 132) SEER database demonstrated statistically significant difference in OS with both subtotal and grand total resections, with a trend toward increasing survival benefit with extent of resection	Favorable
Yun et al[57]	IIIb: retrospective pooled cohort (1998–2013), n = 95	Morbidity Biopsy: 23.16% Resection: 20.59%	No statistical difference in operative complications between biopsy and resection groups (p = 0.458)	Favorable
Level IVb evidence				
Jahr et al[58]	IVb: retrospective single center cohort (2003–2014), n = 27	PFS (mo); median OS (mo) Biopsy: 7.7; 11.7 Resection: 12.6; 28.6	Not statistically significant difference in PFS or OS, between groups, extent of resection also not found to be significant	Unfavorable
Villalonga et al[59]	IVb: retrospective single center cohort (1994–2015), n = 50	Median OS (mo) Biopsy: 14.5 Resection: 31	Significant difference (p = 0.016) between groups, lost when factoring immune status (p = 0.07)	Favorable
Cloney et al[60]	IVb: retrospective single center cohort (2000–2015), n = 129)	Morbidity Resection: 17.2% Biopsy: 28.2%	Equivalent to GBM cohort, in overall, regional and neurological complication rates. Higher systemic complication rate in PCNSL cohort	Favorable
Jelicic et al[61]	IVb: retrospective single center cohort (2002–2013), n = 27	Median OS (mo) Partial tumor reduction/biopsy: 23 Total tumor reduction; not reached	Statistically significant difference in OS (p = 0.014)	Favorable
Kellogg et al[62]	IVb: retrospective single center cohort (2005–2012), n = 51	Morbidity Biopsy: 8.1% Resection: 16.7%	Significant morbidity associated with resection; study limited by sole surgical intent of palliative debulking mass effect	Unfavorable
Shibamoto et al[63]	IVb: retrospective pooled cohort (1995–2004), n = 207	1995–1999 median OS (mo) Biopsy/subtotal resection: 29 Total resection: 26 2000–2004 median OS (mo) Biopsy/subtotal resection: 24 Gross total resection: 23	No statistically significant difference in median OS found in either group (p = 0.99 and 0.45).	Unfavorable
Bataille et al[64]	IVb: retrospective multi-center cohort (1980–1995), n = 248	1-year OS (%) Resection: Complete: 56.6% Partial: 48.6% Biopsy: 48.6%	Cox multivariate analysis suggests partial resection to have an unfavorable impact on survival (p = 0.040)	Unfavorable
Hayakawa et al[65]	IVb: retrospective multi-institution cohort (1970–1989), n = 102	Morbidity Biopsy: 6.0%, Resection: 0%	Postbiopsy intratumoral hemorrhage with resultant 3 deaths were reported, which comprised the only complications recorded throughout	Favorable

(Continued)

Table 26.6 (*Continued*) Summary of literature of surgical treatment outcomes, ordered by level of evidence and reverse chronological date of publication

Study	Design	Primary outcomes	Interpretation	Overall
Pollack et al[66]	IVb: retrospective single-center cohort (1976–1986), n = 27	*Morbidity* Biopsy: 8.3% Resection: 0%	1 postbiopsy severe intratumoral hemorrhage was reported, which comprised the only complication recorded throughout	Favorable
Henry et al[67]	IVb: retrospective single center cohort (prior to 1974), n = 43	*Median OS (mo)* "Supportive care alone": 3.3 "Surgical intervention": 4.6	Unclear what constitutes surgical intervention. No statistical analysis provided	Unfavorable

Abbreviations: GBM, glioblastoma; MSKCC, Memorial Sloan Kettering Cancer Center; NCDB, National Cancer Database; OS, overall survival; PCNSL, primary central nervous system lymphoma; PFS, progression-free survival, SEER, Surveillance, Epidemiology, and End Results.

Note: Exclusion criteria: studies with n < 25 or nonextractable data or data irrelevant to OS, PFS, and morbidity. Levels of evidence were defined according to the 2011 Oxford Centre for Evidence-Based Medicine guidelines.

The first study to definitively challenge the traditional view that surgical intervention should be limited to debulking was a prospectively collected, retrospectively analyzed, German phase III randomized controlled trial done in 2012.[54] When controlled for both age and KPS, the study demonstrated improved PFS and OS in patients who underwent subtotal resection or gross total resection, compared to the biopsy-only cohort.[54] All patients received recommended adjuvant therapy. The hazard ratio of biopsy compared to surgical resection was unchanged for PFS, but was slightly worse for OS.[54] Although the study accounted for a number of lesions as a confounding factor, it did not specify or account for depth of lesion(s). Of note, there was no difference between rates of PFS between subtotal and grand total resection groups. The extent of resection has further been postulated to have some survival benefit by Rae et al as well, but these results showed a trend only without statistical significance.[56] In a large retrospective cohort study using two large national databases, Rae et a demonstrated improved median OS with resection when compared to biopsy alone.[56]

In the absence of prospective randomized data evaluating the role of surgery for PCNSL, critical examination of the available literature is crucial. Available data are biased toward single-center studies, retrospective design, and cytoreductive operative strategies for candidates who were younger, in better overall health, with superficial target lesions, and with fewer comorbidities.[54,56] Notwithstanding these limitations, recent literature suggests there could be survival benefit derived from careful selection of operative candidates with a low burden of superficial disease and planned adjuvant therapy. Further research is required to direct surgical intervention definitively.

26.8 Authors' Recommendations

- All patients with a suspected diagnosis of PCNSL require systemic investigation for non-Hodgkin's lymphoma with secondary CNS lymphoma. This also includes investigation for immunodeficiency including HIV serology.
- Given stereotactic brain biopsy is relatively safe and the diagnostic yield of lumbar puncture is low, *early* stereotactic brain biopsy remains the gold standard in diagnosis and can avert detrimental diagnostic delay.
- Where clinically possible, steroids should be avoided prior to tissue diagnosis in order to minimize risk of nondiagnostic yield. However, in a neurologically deteriorating patient in whom corticosteroids cannot be avoided, emerging literature still suggests a high yield from subsequent tissue diagnosis, so biopsy should not be delayed.
- Formal histopathology is required as intraoperative rapid frozen section can distort the cells and lead to misdiagnosis of glioma.
- Early referral to medical oncology is strongly advised as the mainstay of treatment is HD-MTX induction therapy and consolidative chemotherapy with either WBRT or autologous stem cell transplant.
- The deep brain location in many PCNSLs results in greater morbidity with attempted resection. For these complex tumors, diagnostic stereotactic brain biopsy should be the mainstay of neurosurgical management. However, if tumor location allows for safe surgical resection, this should be performed in line with increasing evidence of survival benefit of cytoreductive surgery in PCNSLs.

References

[1] Louis DN, Ohgaki H, Wiestler OD, Cavenee WK, World Health Organization, International Agency for Research on Cancer. WHO classification of tumours of the central nervous system. Revised 4th ed. Lyon: International Agency for Research on Cancer; 2016:408

[2] Greenberg MS. 2016

[3] Scott BJ, Douglas VC, Tihan T, Rubenstein JL, Josephson SA. A systematic approach to the diagnosis of suspected central nervous system lymphoma. JAMA Neurol. 2013; 70(3):311–319

[4] Coté TR, Manns A, Hardy CR, Yellin FJ, Hartge P, AIDS/Cancer Study Group. Epidemiology of brain lymphoma among people with or without acquired immunodeficiency syndrome. J Natl Cancer Inst. 1996; 88(10):675–679

[5] Shiels MS, Pfeiffer RM, Besson C, et al. Trends in primary central nervous system lymphoma incidence and survival in the U.S. Br J Haematol. 2016; 174(3):417–424

[6] Mendez JS, Grommes C. Treatment of primary central nervous system lymphoma: from chemotherapy to small molecules. Am Soc Clin Oncol Educ Book. 2018; 38:604–615

[7] Mendez JS, Ostrom QT, Gittleman H, et al. The elderly left behind-changes in survival trends of primary central nervous system lymphoma over the past 4 decades. Neuro-oncol. 2018; 20(5):687–694

[8] Kaye AH. Essential Neurosurgery. 3rd ed. Malden, MA: Blackwell; 2005

[9] Han CH, Batchelor TT. Diagnosis and management of primary central nervous system lymphoma. Cancer. 2017; 123(22):4314–4324

[10] Abrey LE, Batchelor TT, Ferreri AJ, et al. International Primary CNS Lymphoma Collaborative Group. Report of an international workshop to standardize baseline evaluation and response criteria for primary CNS lymphoma. J Clin Oncol. 2005; 23(22):5034–5043

[11] Morell AA, Shah AH, Cavallo C, et al. Diagnosis of primary central nervous system lymphoma: a systematic review of the utility of CSF screening and the role of early brain biopsy. Neurooncol Pract. 2019; 6(6):415–423

[12] Haldorsen IS, Espeland A, Larsson EM. Central nervous system lymphoma: characteristic findings on traditional and advanced imaging. AJNR Am J Neuroradiol. 2011; 32(6):984–992

[13] Hegde U, Filie A, Little RF, et al. High incidence of occult leptomeningeal disease detected by flow cytometry in newly diagnosed aggressive B-cell lymphomas at risk for central nervous system involvement: the role of flow cytometry versus cytology. Blood. 2005; 105(2):496–502

[14] Baraniskin A, Schroers R. Modern cerebrospinal fluid analyses for the diagnosis of diffuse large B-cell lymphoma of the CNS. CNS Oncol. 2014; 3(1):77–85

[15] Hoang-Xuan K, Bessell E, Bromberg J, et al. European Association for Neuro-Oncology Task Force on Primary CNS Lymphoma. Diagnosis and treatment of primary CNS lymphoma in immunocompetent patients: guidelines from the European Association for Neuro-Oncology. Lancet Oncol. 2015; 16(7):e322–e332

[16] Choi JY, Kafkala C, Foster CS. Primary intraocular lymphoma: a review. Semin Ophthalmol. 2006; 21(3):125–133

[17] Cerqua R, Balestrini S, Perozzi C, et al. Diagnostic delay and prognosis in primary central nervous system lymphoma compared with glioblastoma multiforme. Neurol Sci. 2016; 37(1):23–29

[18] Mathew BS, Carson KA, Grossman SA. Initial response to glucocorticoids. Cancer. 2006; 106(2):383–387

[19] Pirotte B, Levivier M, Goldman S, Brucher JM, Brotchi J, Hildebrand J. Glucocorticoid-induced long-term remission in primary cerebral lymphoma: case report and review of the literature. J Neurooncol. 1997; 32(1):63–69

[20] Bakshi R. Neuroimaging of HIV and AIDS related illnesses: a review. Front Biosci. 2004; 9:632–646

[21] Toh CH, Castillo M, Wong AM, et al. Primary cerebral lymphoma and glioblastoma multiforme: differences in diffusion characteristics evaluated with diffusion tensor imaging. AJNR Am J Neuroradiol. 2008; 29(3):471–475

[22] Ogawa T, Kanno I, Hatazawa J, et al. Methionine PET for follow-up of radiation therapy of primary lymphoma of the brain. Radiographics. 1994; 14(1):101–110

[23] Palmedo H, Urbach H, Bender H, et al. FDG-PET in immunocompetent patients with primary central nervous system lymphoma: correlation with MRI and clinical follow-up. Eur J Nucl Med Mol Imaging. 2006; 33(2):164–168

[24] Ambady P, Fu R, Netto JP, et al. Patterns of relapse in primary central nervous system lymphoma: inferences regarding the role of the neuro-vascular unit and monoclonal antibodies in treating occult CNS disease. Fluids Barriers CNS. 2017; 14(1):16

[25] Ferreri AJ, Blay JY, Reni M, et al. Prognostic scoring system for primary CNS lymphomas: the International Extranodal Lymphoma Study Group experience. J Clin Oncol. 2003; 21(2):266–272

[26] Abrey LE, Ben-Porat L, Panageas KS, et al. Primary central nervous system lymphoma: the Memorial Sloan-Kettering Cancer Center prognostic model. J Clin Oncol. 2006; 24(36):5711–5715

[27] Ferreri AJ, Batchelor T, Zucca E, Cavalli F, Armitage J. International Collaborative Group against Primary CNS Lymphomas. J Clin Oncol. 2003; 21(8):1649–1650

[28] Levine AM, Sullivan-Halley J, Pike MC, et al. Human immunodeficiency virus-related lymphoma. Prognostic factors predictive of survival. Cancer. 1991; 68(11):2466–2472

[29] Baumgartner JE, Rachlin JR, Beckstead JH, et al. Primary central nervous system lymphomas: natural history and response to radiation therapy in 55 patients with acquired immunodeficiency syndrome. J Neurosurg. 1990; 73(2):206–211

[30] Janavs JL, Aminoff MJ. Dystonia and chorea in acquired systemic disorders. J Neurol Neurosurg Psychiatry. 1998; 65(4):436–445

[31] Bayraktar S, Bayraktar UD, Ramos JC, Stefanovic A, Lossos IS. Primary CNS lymphoma in HIV positive and negative patients: comparison of clinical characteristics, outcome and prognostic factors. J Neurooncol. 2011; 101(2):257–265

[32] Norden AD, Drappatz J, Wen PY, Claus EB. Survival among patients with primary central nervous system lymphoma, 1973–2004. J Neurooncol. 2011; 101(3):487–493

[33] Bullis CL, Maldonado-Perez A, Bowden SG, et al. Diagnostic impact of preoperative corticosteroids in primary central nervous system lymphoma. J Clin Neurosci. 2020; 72:287–291

[34] Porter AB, Giannini C, Kaufmann T, et al. Primary central nervous system lymphoma can be histologically diagnosed after previous corticosteroid use: a pilot study to determine whether corticosteroids prevent the diagnosis of primary central nervous system lymphoma. Ann Neurol. 2008; 63(5):662–667

[35] Binnahil M, Au K, Lu J-Q, Wheatley BM, Sankar T. The influence of corticosteroids on diagnostic accuracy of biopsy for primary central nervous system lymphoma. Can J Neurol Sci/Journal Canadien des Sciences Neurologiques. 2016; 43(5):721–725

[36] O'Neill BP, O'Fallon JR, Earle JD, Colgan JP, Brown LD, Krigel RL. Primary central nervous system non-Hodgkin's lymphoma: survival advantages with combined initial therapy? Int J Radiat Oncol Biol Phys. 1995; 33(3):663–673

[37] von Baumgarten L, Illerhaus G, Korfel A, Schlegel U, Deckert M, Dreyling M. The diagnosis and treatment of primary CNS lymphoma. Dtsch Arztebl Int. 2018; 115(25):419–426

[38] Herrlinger U, Küker W, Uhl M, et al. Neuro-Oncology Working Group of the German Society. NOA-03 trial of high-dose methotrexate in primary central nervous system lymphoma: final report. Ann Neurol. 2005; 57(6):843–847

[39] Pels H, Schmidt-Wolf IG, Glasmacher A, et al. Primary central nervous system lymphoma: results of a pilot and phase II study of systemic and intraventricular chemotherapy with deferred radiotherapy. J Clin Oncol. 2003; 21(24):4489–4495

[40] Juergens A, Pels H, Rogowski S, et al. Long-term survival with favorable cognitive outcome after chemotherapy in primary central nervous system lymphoma. Ann Neurol. 2010; 67(2):182–189

[41] Gavrilovic IT, Hormigo A, Yahalom J, DeAngelis LM, Abrey LE. Long-term follow-up of high-dose methotrexate-based therapy with and without whole brain irradiation for newly diagnosed primary CNS lymphoma. J Clin Oncol. 2006; 24(28):4570–4574

[42] Omuro AM, Ben-Porat LS, Panageas KS, et al. Delayed neurotoxicity in primary central nervous system lymphoma. Arch Neurol. 2005; 62(10):1595–1600

[43] Omuro AMP, DeAngelis LM, Karrison T, et al. Randomized phase II study of rituximab, methotrexate (MTX), procarbazine, vincristine, and cytarabine (R-MPV-A) with and without low-dose whole-brain radiotherapy (LD-WBRT) for newly diagnosed primary CNS lymphoma (PCNSL). J Clin Oncol. 2020; 38(15):2501

[44] Kumar R, Laack N, Pollock BE, Link M, O'Neill BP, Parney IF. Stereotactic radiosurgery in the treatment of recurrent CNS lymphoma. World Neurosurg. 2015; 84(2):390–397

[45] Ferreri AJM, Illerhaus G. The role of autologous stem cell transplantation in primary central nervous system lymphoma. Blood. 2016; 127(13):1642–1649

[46] Ferreri AJM, Cwynarski K, Pulczynski E, et al. International Extranodal Lymphoma Study Group (IELSG). Whole-brain radiotherapy or autologous stem-cell transplantation as consolidation strategies after high-dose methotrexate-based chemoimmunotherapy in patients with primary CNS lymphoma: results of the second randomisation of the International Extranodal Lymphoma Study Group-32 phase 2 trial. Lancet Haematol. 2017; 4(11):e510–e523

[47] Alnahhas I, Jawish M, Alsawas M, et al. Autologous stem-cell transplantation for primary central nervous system lymphoma: systematic review and meta-analysis. Clin Lymphoma Myeloma Leuk. 2019; 19(3):e129–e141

[48] Labak CM, Holdhoff M, Bettegowda C, et al. Surgical resection for primary central nervous system lymphoma: a systematic review. World Neurosurg. 2019; 126:e1436–e1448

[49] Skolasky RL, Dal Pan GJ, Olivi A, Lenz FA, Abrams RA, McArthur JC. HIV-associated primary CNS lymorbidity and utility of brain biopsy. J Neurol Sci. 1999; 163(1):32–38

[50] Sugita Y, Terasaki M, Nakashima S, Ohshima K, Morioka M, Abe H. Intraoperative rapid diagnosis of primary central nervous system lymphomas: advantages and pitfalls. Neuropathology. 2014; 34(5):438–445

[51] Koriyama S, Nitta M, Shioyama T, et al. Intraoperative flow cytometry enables the differentiation of primary central nervous system lymphoma from glioblastoma. World Neurosurg. 2018; 112:e261–e268

[52] Davies KG, Cole GC, Weeks RD. Twenty-year survival following excision of primary CNS lymphoma without radiation therapy: case report. Br J Neurosurg. 1994; 8(4):487–491

[53] Sonstein W, Tabaddor K, Llena JF. Solitary primary CNS lymphoma: long term survival following total resection. Med Oncol. 1998; 15(1):61–65

[54] Weller M, Martus P, Roth P, Thiel E, Korfel A, German PCNSL Study Group. Surgery for primary CNS lymphoma? Challenging a paradigm. Neuro-oncol. 2012; 14(12):1481–1484

[55] DeAngelis LM, Yahalom J, Heinemann MH, Cirrincione C, Thaler HT, Krol G. Primary CNS lymphoma: combined treatment with chemotherapy and radiotherapy. Neurology. 1990; 40(1):80–86

[56] Rae AI, Mehta A, Cloney M, et al. Craniotomy and survival for primary central nervous system lymphoma. Neurosurgery. 2019; 84(4):935–944

[57] Yun J, Yang J, Cloney M, et al. Assessing the safety of craniotomy for resection of primary central nervous system lymphoma: a nationwide inpatient sample analysis. Front Neurol. 2017; 8:478

[58] Jahr G, Da Broi M, Holte H, Jr, Beiske K, Meling TR. The role of surgery in intracranial PCNSL. Neurosurg Rev. 2018; 41(4):1037–1044

[59] Villalonga JF, Alessandro L, Farez MF, et al. The role of surgery in primary central nervous system lymphomas. Arq Neuropsiquiatr. 2018; 76(3):139–144

[60] Cloney MB, Sonabend AM, Yun J, et al. The safety of resection for primary central nervous system lymphoma: a single institution retrospective analysis. J Neurooncol. 2017; 132(1):189–197

[61] Jelicic J, Todorovic Balint M, Raicevic S, et al. The possible benefit from total tumour resection in primary diffuse large B-cell lymphoma of central nervous system: a one-decade single-centre experience. Br J Neurosurg. 2016; 30(1):80–85

[62] Kellogg RG, Straus DC, Karmali R, Munoz LF, Byrne RW. Impact of therapeutic regimen and clinical presentation on overall survival in CNS lymphoma. Acta Neurochir (Wien). 2014; 156(2):355–365

[63] Shibamoto Y, Tsuchida E, Seki K, et al. Primary central nervous system lymphoma in Japan 1995–1999: changes from the preceding 10 years. J Cancer Res Clin Oncol. 2004; 130(6):351–356

[64] Bataille B, Delwail V, Menet E, et al. Primary intracerebral malignant lymphoma: report of 248 cases. J Neurosurg. 2000; 92(2):261–266

[65] Hayakawa T, Takakura K, Abe H, et al. Primary central nervous system lymphoma in Japan: a retrospective, co-operative study by CNS-Lymphoma Study Group in Japan. J Neurooncol. 1994; 19(3):197–215

[66] Pollack IF, Lunsford LD, Flickinger JC, Dameshek HL. Prognostic factors in the diagnosis and treatment of primary central nervous system lymphoma. Cancer. 1989; 63(5):939–947

[67] Henry JM, Heffner RR, Jr, Dillard SH, Earle KM, Davis RL. Primary malignant lymphomas of the central nervous system. Cancer. 1974; 34(4):1293–1302

27 Natural History and Management Options of Normal-Pressure Hydrocephalus

Bob Homapour and Chris Xenos

Abstract

Normal pressure hydrocephalus is a form of communicating hydrocephalus that generally affects the elderly population. Clinically, it is characterized by the triad of gait apraxia/ataxia, urinary incontinence, and dementia. The natural history is not clear, although limited available data have suggested a progressive clinical decline over time. The results of ventriculoperitoneal shunt placement typically depend on the strength of the clinical evaluation, appropriate work-up, and treatment indication.

Keywords: hydrocephalus, communicating hydrocephalus, ventriculoperitoneal shunt, dementia

27.1 Introduction

Several population-based studies have attempted to determine the prevalence of idiopathic normal-pressure hydrocephalus (iNPH). The most accurate estimate will most likely be represented by surveys carried out on selected patients based on both clinical examination and radiographic assessment.[1,2] Generally, the prevalence is accepted at a range of 0.5 to 1.5% of the population over the age of 60 years. This figure may be rising for several reasons such as improved diagnostic modalities, disease awareness, and changes in the age distribution pyramid. The incidence increases with age; however, patients between the ages of 70 and 79 years should receive the most attention. They have a higher incidence than those in their 60 s and also have a better risk-to-benefit ratio for surgical measures related to the diagnosis.[3]

The proposed theory regarding the pathophysiology of iNPH is based on Greitz's description of the hydrodynamic theory after the appreciation of the Windkessel effect, that is, the elastic reservoir of blood vessels. In the elderly population, especially in the presence of arteriolosclerosis, the Windkessel effect may not occur as the vessel elastin fragments diminish. As the wall of the basilar arteries become more rigid, the systolic pulse waveform is not absorbed by the elasticity of the vessels and is transmitted unimpeded into the capillary bed of the parenchyma. The arterial pulse wave flows unimpeded through the entire parenchyma. This leads to a short-lived increase in parenchymal volume during systole. In the subarachnoid space, this can be compensated for by discharging cerebrospinal fluid (CSF) through the foramen magnum. This does not happen for the parenchyma adjacent to the ventricles and an increased counter pressure occurs. A gradual degeneration of the parenchyma surrounding the ventricle occurs resulting in a passive widening of the caliber of the ventricle without the need for an increase in ventricular pressure.[4]

The cardinal symptoms of the disease include gait disturbance, dementia, and incontinence. This is often referred to as Hakim's triad. The components may be present concurrently or at different times. Most symptoms, if present, will progress with time. This progression can show variability in its time course. Typically, the condition occurs in patients older than 60 years. All three symptoms will present simultaneously in about one-half of the patients.[3] Gait disturbance is almost always present, whereas incontinence or dementia alone caused by iNPH is extremely rare. The gait disturbance is often the first feature noted and is described as a gait apraxia. There is decreased velocity with shorter and more variable strides. Step height is reduced and the dorsiflexion of the foot is insufficient (magnetic gait). The arm swing is preserved distinguishing it from Parkinson's disease.[5] Urinary dysfunction starts as frequency and urgency and may progress to incontinence in advanced stages. Fecal incontinence is also a late feature. Due to the age of this cohort, 90% have other significant comorbidities. Except for evidence of gait, balance, and cognitive dysfunction, the neurological examination in iNPH patients is often normal and any lateralizing sign should raise suspicion of an alternative secondary diagnosis.[6]

Magnetic resonance imaging (MRI) is the preferred modality to confirm the absence of a secondary cause and the presence of CSF pathway communication. The Evans ratio is often found to be greater than 0.3. Characteristic morphological features on MRI include frontal and parietal narrowing of the subarachnoid space, upward bowing of the corpus callosum, and marked dilatation of the Sylvian fissure[3] (▶ Fig. 27.1). The mismatch between the narrowing of the subarachnoid space at the high convexity with the widening of the Sylvian fissure on fluid-attenuated inversion recovery (FLAIR) sequences seems to have a strong positive predictive value (PPV).[7] In Japanese papers, this is described as Disproportionately enlarged subarachnoid space hydrocephalus (DESH). DESH may have a high predictive value in demonstrating shunt responsiveness, but its negative predictive value was not found to be as useful in excluding patients from surgery.[8] Periventricular white mater lesions on FLAIR are common, but if positioned more peripherally, may represent chronic ischemic changes.[9]

Gait disturbances react most extensively to treatment; therefore, gait tests are of high clinical significance. Some symptoms are subtle and subjective, so it is important to consider patient and relative reports regarding everyday life.[10] Gait speed is generally assessed by the time taken to cover a 10-m distance. In addition, a 3-m timed up and go (TUG) test is performed. The TUG test has been shown to be a reliable quantitative test for predicting improvements in gait in patients 12 months after surgery.[11] This assessment also includes recording step length and the quality of the gait.

After the initial recording of the gait parameters, the test is repeated the same day after a tap test. The lumbar puncture is performed with an 18- to 20-gauge spinal needle. CSF is taken for analysis and the opening pressure is measured. The average opening pressures in NPH studies range from 8.8 ± 1.3 to 14.62 ± 1.5 mm Hg. In the cases where the opening pressure is greater than 18 mm Hg, further investigations are needed to exclude

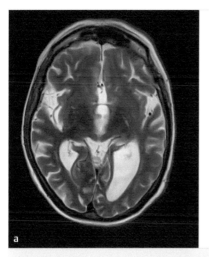 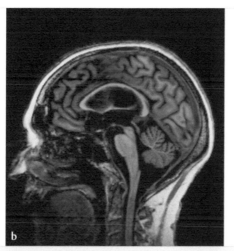 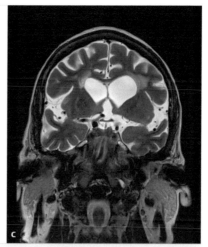

Fig. 27.1 Magnetic resonance imaging (MRI) of a 77-year-old lady with classical symptoms of iNPH. **(a)** T2 axial image demonstrating enlarged Sylvian fissures contrasted with the narrow interhemispheric cerebrospinal fluid (CSF) space in the coronal T2 image in **(c)**. **(b)** The upward bowing of the corpus callosum is evident. This image also shows a patent aqueduct of Sylvius.

secondary causes.[12] Approximately 30 to 50 mL of CSF is allowed to drain off and after a brief period of rest on the short stay ward, the gait assessment is repeated by the same assessor. If the tap test is negative, the patient is given the option of repeating the gait test or insertion of a lumbar drain for 48 to 72 hours. The drainage system is monitored to produce an effusion rate of CSF of about 5 to 10 mL per hour and ideally a total drainage of greater than 300 mL.[13] The gait tests are recorded before, during, and after the drainage period.

Other invasive diagnostic modalities include intracranial pressure (ICP) monitoring and lumbar infusion test. During ICP monitoring, the presence of B waves has been noted to be associated with NPH due to presumed lower compliance. This involves ICP oscillations with a frequency of 0.3 to 3 per minute and amplitudes of up to 50 mm Hg. False positives are relatively common. Increased pulse pressure amplitude during sleep has a much stronger correlation with NPH. This correlation with shunt responsiveness varies from 50 to 90%. Unfortunately, these studies are limited by a paucity of aged-matched control data.[14] This phenomenon has also been demonstrated in lumbar infusion tests. As iNPH is communicating, the ICP monitoring can be done through a lumbar drain, needle, or intracranial device.[15] In the infusion test, the ICP is measured during an infusion of artificial CSF at a constant rate between 0.76 and 2 mL/min.[16] This typically involves infusion through one spinal needle and pressure measurement through a second needle. The increased CSF pressure generated by the infusion is registered and once a new steady state for pressure is achieved, the infusion is discontinued. At the point when the newly set plateau is achieved, it is assumed that the reabsorption rate is equal to the infusion rate. The infusion usually takes about 40 to 60 minutes to achieve the plateau in pressure. Outflow resistance R_{out} (Torr/mL/min) is a measure of the pressure increase following a bolus injection. By calculating outflow resistance, the quantitative extent of a disruption of reabsorption or disruption of passage of CSF can be determined. ICP increases with increasing

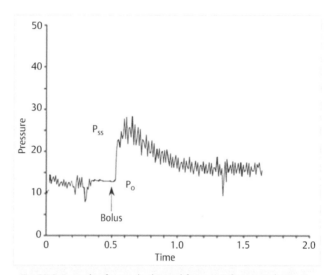

Fig. 27.2 Example of a graph obtained from an infusion study. P_{SS} is the steady state pressure, P_0 is the opening pressure, and I_{INF} is the infusion rate of the bolus set by the clinician.

outflow resistance in a nonlinear fashion.[17] Outflow resistance is calculated with the following formula and considered abnormal above a value of 13 (▶ Fig. 27.2):

$$R_{out} = P_{SS} - P_0/I_{INF}.$$

The PPV of the tap test is reported to be between 73 and 100%, with sensitivity at 26 to 62% and specificity of 33 to 100%. The PPV of external lumbar drainage is reported as 80 to 100%, with sensitivity of 50 to 100% and specificity of 60 to 100%. The infusion test has a higher sensitivity than the tap test (57–100%), but a similar predictive value of 75 to 92%. Some authors advocate combining the tap test with other modalities such as those mentioned earlier to increase the PPV.[18,19] Trial of lumbar drainage for a number of days has the highest negative predictive value and PPV.[12]

27.2 Selected Papers on the Natural History of Idiopathic Normal Pressure Hydrocephalus

- Scollato A, Tenenbaum R, Bahl G, Celerini M, Salani B, Di Lorenzo N. Changes in aqueductal CSF stroke volume and progression of symptoms in patients with unshunted idiopathic normal pressure hydrocephalus. AJNR Am J Neuroradiol 2008;29(1):192–197
- Razay G, Vreugdenhil A, Liddell J. A prospective study of ventriculo-peritoneal shunting for idiopathic normal pressure hydrocephalus. J Clin Neurosci 2009;16(9):1180–1183
- Savolainen S, Hurskainen H, Paljärvi L, Alafuzoff I, Vapalahti M. Five-year outcome of normal pressure hydrocephalus with or without a shunt: predictive value of the clinical signs, neuropsychological evaluation and infusion test. Acta Neurochir (Wien) 2002;144(6):515–523, discussion 523
- Pfisterer WK, Aboul-Enein F, Gebhart E, Graf M, Aichholzer M, Mühlbauer M. Continuous intraventricular pressure monitoring for diagnosis of normal-pressure hydrocephalus. Acta Neurochir (Wien) 2007;149(10):983–990, discussion 990

27.3 Natural History

The natural history of iNPH is not clear and the evidence to support the treatment is not of high quality. There is no gold standard test for diagnosis. If shunt placement were offered solely on the basis of history, examination, and presence of ventriculomegaly on imaging, only 46 to 61% of patients would benefit from surgery. Only very few studies include iNPH patients who did not undergo shunting and include the criteria of diagnosis and an objective method of outcome assessment.[20] Six studies are listed in ▶ Table 27.1, which include the inclusion criteria and outcome of 102 patients who were diagnosed iNPH and did not undergo shunt insertion surgery. The follow-up period ranges from 3 months to 7.2 years.[18,21,22,23,24,25] ▶ Table 27.2[21,22]

shows two studies that looked into the outcome of unshunted probable iNPH patients with no added confounding factor. Both show that unshunted patients progressively worsen over time. ▶ Table 27.3[24,25] shows the results of patients thought to benefit from shunting based on selection with a prognostic test. Since none of these tests are 100% specific or sensitive, the unshunted group might include some true iNPH patients. The rest might represent patients with other diagnoses or advanced iNPH. The natural history of patients thought to be unlikely to benefit from shunt surgery is unknown. Some patients did improve, demonstrating iNPH is not a universally progressive condition. However, the contribution of improvement from the temporary lumbar drainage of CSF is not clear. A significant number of patients showed evidence of clinical stabilization of one or more components of the triad. All studies demonstrate an improvement in either clinical assessment or outcomes score in the shunted patients. The patients who did not undergo shunting were excluded because either they did not meet the criteria set by the authors or the patients refused surgery. Each study has a different diagnostic assessment and inclusion criteria for shunting. Follow-up periods vary and each study presents outcome data in a different way. The percentage of patients who either do not change, or worsened clinically, is significantly higher in the unshunted group. No trial has yet compared the placement of a shunt versus conservative management in a randomized controlled manner. Although the level of evidence for these studies is classed at 4, collectively it is possible to draw reasonable conclusions. The majority of unshunted patients deteriorate without surgery and shunt insertion does improve outcome. The deterioration in the iNPH can occur as early as 3 months after initial assessment. In a study in which shunting was delayed due to hospital-related administrative issues, the magnitude of improvement after surgery was not affected by the length of preoperative delay, which shows reversibility even when treated late. The final outcome of surgery is often linked to the severity of preoperative symptoms. However, the delay in treatment resulted in progression of comorbidities, and the proportion of patients able to

Table 27.1 Summary of studies looking at outcomes of shunted versus unshunted patients

Study	Year	Number	Follow-up	Diagnostic criteria	Outcome assessment	Comparison to shunt
Savolainen et al[24]	2002	26	12 mo	ICP monitoring	Clinical review of symptoms	Shunted patients performed better in all components of triad
Eide and Brean[23]	2006	15	12 mo	Ventriculomegaly, symptoms of triad, ICP monitoring	Stein–Langfitt scale	Shunted patients had significantly improved scores
Pfisterer et al[25]	2007	26	7.2 y	ICP monitoring and infusion study	Dutch Classification	Shunted patients performed better in all components of triad
Scollato et al[21]	2008	9	20 mo	Ventriculomegaly, symptoms of triad	MMSE, incontinence scale, gait scale	None
Brean and Eide	2008	12	12 mo	Symptoms of triad, infusion study, and measurement of Rout	NPH grading scale	Unshunted patients remained the same or worsened
Razay et al[22]	2009	14	4 mo	Ventriculomegaly, symptoms of triad, cisternography, and CSF flow stasis	CIBIC-plus rating Scale, MMSE, timed up and go, 10-m walk test	Shunted patients performed better in all components of triad

Abbreviations: CIBIC-plus, clinician interview-based impression of change, plus caregiver interview; CSF, cerebrospinal fluid; ICP, intracranial pressure; MMSE, Mini-Mental State Examination; NPH, normal-pressure hydrocephalus.

Table 27.2 Studies that looked at outcome of unshunted patients who were diagnosed based on radiology and clinical findings

Study	Follow-up	Gait	Cognition	Urinary symptoms
Scollato et al[21]	24 mo	Worsened 89%	Worsened 100%	Worsened 100%
Razay et al[22]	4 mo	Worsened 64%	Worsened 57%	–

Table 27.3 Studies that looked at outcomes in unshunted patients where the diagnosis was based on a prognostic test

Study	Follow-up	Gait	Cognition	Urinary symptoms
Savolainen et al[24]	5 y 9 patients died	Worsened 65% Unchanged 35% Improved none	Worsened 77% Unchanged 18% Improved none	Worsened 59% Unchanged 35% Improved none
Pfisterer et al[25]	7.2 y 5 patients died	Worsened 25% Unchanged 60% Improved 15%	Worsened 55% Unchanged 36% Improved 9%	Worsened 36% Unchanged 45% Improved 18%

live independently was significantly lower in the delayed group.[26] From a health economic perspective, shunt surgery is cost-effective and reduces caregiver burden.[27]

27.4 Selected Papers on the Treatment Options of Idiopathic Normal Pressure Hydrocephalus

- Malm J, Kristensen B, Stegmayr B, Fagerlund M, Koskinen LO. Three-year survival and functional outcome of patients with idiopathic adult hydrocephalus syndrome. Neurology 2000;55(4):576–578
- Black PM. Idiopathic normal-pressure hydrocephalus. Results of shunting in 62 patients. J Neurosurg 1980;52(3):371–377
- Tisell M, Hellström P, Ahl-Börjesson G, et al. Long-term outcome in 109 adult patients operated on for hydrocephalus. Br J Neurosurg 2006;20(4):214–221

27.5 Treatment Options

Although there have been studies to suggest lumboperitoneal shunting is a safe and beneficial option, because of their higher failure rates, the ventriculoperitoneal (VP) shunt is usually considered the treatment of choice.[28,29] There is some evidence to suggest that clinical improvement is significantly better with a low opening pressure of the shunt. However, this has to be balanced with the increased risk of overdrainage. Therefore, the addition of an antisiphon device is usually recommended. The condition of patients typically deteriorates even with a patent shunt; therefore, adjustability of the opening pressure of the shunt may offer some advantage at this stage. Initial valve

adjustments are not necessary for at least 6 weeks to 3 months after the placement of a shunt. This is because of the chronic nature of the disease and the slow pace at which clinical symptoms can vary.[30] Although there are no specific data showing the superiority of one valve over another in this condition, our surgeons use almost exclusively the Miethke ProGav 2.0 programmable shunt with reservoir and a patient appropriate shunt-assistant antisiphon unit. The other commonly used system is the Codman Hakim programmable valve with Siphonguard as the antisiphon device. To select the valve opening pressure, the following equation can be used to achieve normal ICPs:

$$ICP = GD - HPD + VOP + IAP,$$

where HPD is the hydrostatic pressure difference between the abdomen and the head, VOP is the valve opening pressure, IAP is the intra-abdominal pressure, and GD is the setting for the gravitational unit. The average ICP in the lying position has been found to be approximately 13 cm H_2O and the average IAP is between 7 and 10 cm H_2O. HPD is generally taken to be zero in these calculations. Variations can exist when patients tend toward obesity or extremes of height. As mentioned earlier, it is advantageous to be able to adjust VOP to match deterioration in symptoms with time or changes in body habitus resulting in changes in IAP.[31]

However, downregulating the pressure improves drainage in the horizontal position but increases risks associated with overdraining. In this situation, adjustability of the gravitational device may be more advantageous. All shunt configurations used for NPH in our unit contain an adjustable valve, an antisiphon device either integrated in the valve or as an in line add-on gravitational valve, a reservoir, and antibiotic impregnated catheters (▶ Fig. 27.3). Adjustable gravitational units (ProSA, Aesculap) are used only in special circumstances or following complications. The Dutch Normal-Pressure Hydrocephalus study in 1999 demonstrated better outcomes in the course of the disease with lower set differential pressure valves. Unfortunately, the lower valve settings had a 73% overdrainage rates compared to 34% for the intermediate-pressure range.[32]

Endoscopic third ventriculostomy (ETV) has been used for iNPH, but the results are inferior to the results of ETV in obstructive hydrocephalus. There is at least one randomized control trial comparing ETV versus VP shunt. This was stopped early due to the poor results of the ETV.[33]

For the follow-up period after surgery, all of our patients receive an X-ray shunt series as a baseline image. There is also a computed tomography (CT) of the head to demonstrate baseline conditions immediately after surgery for the position of the ventricular catheter, ventricular gauge, and the absence of space-occupying subdural collections or intraventricular hemorrhage. Patients can then be reviewed in the outpatient department at 1, 3, and 6 months after surgery. The first visit is to assess for wound problems, shunt failure, or symptoms of overdrainage. At later reviews, the effect of the shunt can be determined. After 6 weeks to 3 months, enough time has elapsed to say that any effect in the patient is from the shunt function rather than the CSF drained during surgery. At 6 months, a CT would be useful in ensuring there is no overdrainage problem and the ventricles can be remeasured to gauge whether there is adequate drainage. Adjustments can be made in the valve settings to improve the patient's symptoms if

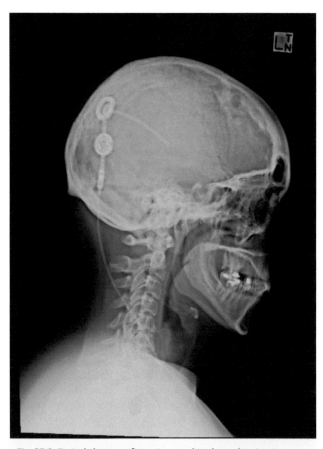

Fig. 27.3 Typical shunt configuration used in the authors' unit demonstrating a unitized reservoir, adjustable valve, and an antisiphon device.

necessary.[34] The setting at the time of insertion for the Miethke ProGav 2.0 valve is usually set at 10.0. This is then gradually reduced over a period of time titrated against symptom response in the patient. If at any point the patients show a negative response, one can investigate with a scan to ensure there is no overdrainage or shunt failure. Shunt failure (including infection) is investigated and treated as per any hydrocephalus case. Failure of the shunt usually presents as the sudden or gradual return of original symptoms and is rarely an emergency. Once revised, most patients continue with their original clinical progress. However, worsening symptoms may also represent worsening of the pathology itself or coexistent comorbidities. As the valve setting is lowered, there is a gradual increase in potential risk of overdrainage. This can manifest clinically as orthostatic headaches, imbalance, and development of subdural hygromas and even hematomas. The evidence for the presence of overdrainage comes from the Dutch Normal-Pressure Hydrocephalus study. Clinical improvement was found in 74% of patients with a low-pressure valve and 53% with a medium- to high-pressure valve. The results were not statistically significant. Subdural effusions occurred in 71% of the low-pressure group and in 34% in the medium- to high-pressure group.[32] These results were reproduced in another study by Meier.[35] For this reason, in the authors' unit, a programmable valve is used with an antisiphon component and the pressures are reduced gradually with concurrent scans to reduce the rate of hygromas

and overdrainage symptoms. The main aim is to achieve clinical improvement and not a reduction in ventricular size, which can remain large even in the setting of a well-functioning shunt. Ventricles that remain large are not an indication to lower the opening pressure of the valve. In the event of overdrainage symptoms or a significant hygroma (> 5 mm on scan), the opening pressure setting of the valve can be increased or the antisiphon device can be replaced to be more flow limiting. This can be fixed or programmable (e.g., Miethke ProSa).[36]

27.6 Treatment Outcomes

An assessment of the individual symptoms is needed to determine not only the diagnosis but also the likely chance of improvement after surgery. The Black grading scale is well suited for iNPH and is an evaluation of the effects of shunting. This scale is, however, limited by the lack of subcategorization of each symptom in the Hakim triad.[30] The Kiefer grading takes into account the severity of the individual symptoms including headaches and dizziness.[37] The scale ranges from 0 to 25 (maximum severity of disease). The Kiefer score can then be used to calculate the NPH recovery rate:

NPH recovery rate = NPH grade post-op – NPH grade pre-op/NPH grade post-op.

The NPH recovery rate shows good correlation with the Black grading scale for shunt assessment.[38] This condition is often diagnosed in elderly patients who have a significant chance of comorbidity. There is also a significant coexistence of other dementing conditions. It is important to recognize certain patients have such severe coexisting conditions that the operation carries a low likelihood of altering the quality of life for the individual. Kiefer and Unterberg[39] therefore created a comorbidity index (CMI) for quantification of this additional risk. The CMI ranges from 0 to 23 points. The reported incidence of comorbidities in NPH can be as high as 43%. Vascular encephalopathy is a very common concurrent pathology. This same study group described an indirect correlation between CMI and potential for recovery and overall outcome. A CMI of 3 has been determined to be the threshold for a favorable outcome. Above this value, patients show a significant decline in percentage demonstrating good recovery. In patients with a CMI of ≥ 6, the prognosis after shunting is particularly poor.[40]

The results of surgery, as per any condition, depend on the strength of the indications for treatment and the quality of the evaluation. There have been studies to find predictors of response. The presence of dementia, particularly for longer than a year, is considered by some researchers as a negative predictor. Advanced age, male gender, and comorbidities also constitute negative predictors.[41] Ataxia, however, particularly upon improvement after a tap test, has a much better predictive value. As mentioned earlier, lumbar drainage of CSF for more than 48 hours may increase the predictive value of this phenomenon. Others have used the drainage resistance (R_{out}) in the intrathecal infusion test as a predictive tool. Patients with early-stage disease (no brain atrophy) and a R_{out} values of 15 Torr/mL/min, or patients with late-stage disease (with brain atrophy) and R_{out} values of more than 20 Torr/mL/min may have a positive prognosis.[42] ICP monitoring in contrast has not been found to be a useful predictor. Response to shunting can vary a great deal depending on the study and can range from 40 to 90% improvement. Each individual symptom of the triad may show differences in degrees of improvement in the same patient. Long-term studies of over 5 years do show a marked reduction in improvement after shunting with time, but gains can still be as high as 60%.[40] Recurrence and deterioration after initial improvement of symptoms have been reported in up to 40% in some studies. The short-term improvement was severely attenuated after 1 year. The reason for this may be shunt dysfunction, progression of disease, or comorbidities. Secondary deterioration attributable to shunt failure requiring revision has been shown to be as high as 20%. There has also been a difference noted with regard to age. There seems to be a clear difference in long-term improvements in patients under the age of 75 years (64%) compared with those older than 75 years (11%).[43] The long-term follow-up studies after shunting in iNPH, with at least 3 years of follow-up, are shown in ▶ Table 27.4.[29,44,45,46,47,48,49,50,51,52,53] These studies show an overall improvement of 43 to 91%, with one study showing 40% were unchanged and 13% worsened after 3 years. With the use of programmable shunts, once shunt failure has been ruled out, the opening pressure can be lowered as the patient's disease progresses with time. In our practice, we have seen a modest benefit in gradually lowering the shunt setting over a several year period.

The European iNPH multicentre study aimed to determine the sensitivity, specificity, PPV and negative predictive value of the tap tests, and R_{out}, for the outcome of shunting. All 115 patients had a programmable shunt and 12 months follow-up with the modified Rankin Scale (MRS) and a newly modified iNPH scale. There was no correlation of the two tests with outcome measured with either domain. Only an increase in the gait task after tap test correlated significantly with improvement of scores. The PPV of both tests was greater than 90% and the negative predictive value was less than 20%. R_{out} of greater than 12 had an overall accuracy of 65% and the CSF tap test 53%; combining the two tests did not improve their predictive power. No correlation was found between R_{out} and the results of the tap test. The authors conclude that the tap test and R_{out} can be used to select patients for shunt surgery but were not of value for excluding patients from treatment. Improvement rate after surgery in patients diagnosed without the use of supplementary tests is generally considered to be 50%, whereas studies that apply various supplementary tests and in particular CSF pulse amplitudes have reported improvements rates of up to 90%. One-third of patients had shunt adjustments because of over- or underdrainage. There was a dramatic reduction of patients not able to live independently from 47% before surgery to 18% afterward.[13,54] Comorbidity, disability, and frailty are recognized as independent markers of surgical risk in the elderly. There is a lack of evidence to support a surgical selection process based on preoperative comorbidities. D'Antona et al[55] conducted a study to look at preoperative risk factors and early postoperative morbidity of patients with NPH using the standardized postoperative morbidity survey (POMS). Cardiac comorbidities were most frequent, affecting 57% of the patients. The most common postoperative morbidity after shunt insertion was found to be nausea and a decline in mobility. There was no correlation between preoperative morbidity, early postoperative outcomes, and postoperative length of stay. There was, however, a correlation between the length of stay and the mobility scores of the patient. The POMS data were more sensitive than traditional outcome measures in detecting postoperative morbidity (28 vs. 7%).[55]

The main cause of death in most studies relating to iNPH is cardiovascular or cerebrovascular ischemia. It is doubtful that shunt responders gain a normal annual mortality rate. The overall risk of death in a patient with iNPH seems to be 3.3 times higher than that in the healthy age-matched population. The survival plot for patients with their first-ever stroke is almost identical to the survival curve corresponding to the shunted patient with iNPH. Survival in the untreated iNPH patient is substantially reduced, with a hazard ratio for death of 3.8 compared to the general population. In treated patients, a relative risk for death of 3.3 and a standardized mortality of 2.5 have been calculated in single-center studies. Risk factors for cerebrovascular disease are common, but it is unknown to what

Table 27.4 Long-term follow-up studies after shunting in iNPH, with at least 3 years of follow-up

Study	Year	Number	Follow-up (y)	Results and general comments	Deaths
Greenberg et al[46]	1977	28	3	43% improvement	4
Black[47]	1980	62	3	47% improvement, 40% unchanged, and remainder worsened	5
Malm et al[45]	2000	42	3	26% improved gait and 28% improved cognition	12
Savolainen et al[24]	2002	25	5	47% improved gait, 38% improved cognition, and 29% improved urinary function	8
Aygok et al[48]	2005	50	3	75% improved gait, 80% improved cognition, and 80% improved urinary function	4
Raftopoulos et al[49]	2006	23	5	91% improved	12
Spagnoli et al[50]	2006	66	4.3	60% improved	16
Tisell et al[51]	2006	109	4.2	55% improved	29
Kahlon et al[52]	2007	23	5	40% improved gait	28
Pujari et al[53]	2008	55	2.5	83% improved gait, 84% improved cognition, and 77% improved urinary function	–
Andren et al[44]	2020	979	5.9	Study of survival of shunted patients vs. controls	362

Abbreviation: iNPH, idiopathic normal pressure hydrocephalus.

extent they influence survival.[44] The association between severity of symptoms and survival has not been extensively studied and whether the degree of improvement post shunting influences survival is largely unknown. A large study of 979 shunted patients showed a 1.8 times increased (hazard ratio) risk of death for iNPH compared to 4,890 controls. The follow-up period was 5.9 years. More pronounced symptomology before shunt surgery was associated with a higher mortality. This applied to all tested domains, with gait and cognition being the most important domains. The patients who improved in their gait and postoperative MRS survived longer. Only heart disease as a comorbidity was found to be associated with survival. Unresponsive patients had a substantially higher mortality than patients with improved scores. Deaths related to shunt surgery itself was rare with a 0.5% 30-day postoperative mortality. There were no sex or age differences. In iNPH, the prevalence of risk factors for cerebrovascular disease is higher than in controls.[44,45]

The future of treating this condition should be directed at early diagnosis when ataxia is the only symptom and the younger age and lower rates of comorbidities will result in improved outcome. Education of medical personnel and the public can be a key point in improving overall care in these patients as there may be a significant rate of underdiagnosis. Potentially as high as 80% of the cases of NPH may go unrecognized.[56] The involvement of a physician or neurologist early in the process is also desirable. This is not only to assess the extent of coexistence of dementing conditions but also to take over care, usually within 3 to 5 years, when the effects of shunting have worn off and the chronic nature of the disease prevails.[39]

27.7 Authors' Recommendations

- Patients suspected for iNPH should be screened clinically for Hakim's triad.
- If any of the symptoms of the triad are present, then an MRI should be arranged.
- Patients should be reviewed by a neurologist to rule out other conditions that may mimic iNPH.
- Any features of secondary hydrocephalus should be ruled out.
- Patients with positive symptoms and MRI features should be offered a tap test.
- Patients should have gait assessment by an independent clinician before and after CSF drainage.
- If the tap test is positive, then the option of shunting can be discussed. If the tap test is negative, then CSF drainage by lumbar drain can be considered.
- Calculate the CMI for each patient prior to discussing surgery with the family.
- A programmable VP shunt with antisiphon device is the preferred surgical option.
- Reassess the patient at intervals following surgery and make adjustments to the opening pressure of valve while titrating to clinical response.
- Opening pressure should be set at a high or moderately high level prior to reduction over time.
- Any return of symptoms should be investigated as shunt failure or overdrainage before diagnosing progression of disease.

- As the shunt setting is lowered, a CT scan should be considered to rule out complications of overdrainage.

References

[1] Iseki C, Kawanami T, Nagasawa H, et al. Asymptomatic ventriculomegaly with features of idiopathic normal pressure hydrocephalus on MRI (AVIM) in the elderly: a prospective study in a Japanese population. J Neurol Sci. 2009; 277 (1–2):54–57

[2] Tanaka N, Yamaguchi S, Ishikawa H, Ishii H, Meguro K. Prevalence of possible idiopathic normal-pressure hydrocephalus in Japan: the Osaki-Tajiri project. Neuroepidemiology. 2009; 32(3):171–175

[3] Relkin N, Marmarou A, Klinge P, Bergsneider M, Black PM. Diagnosing idiopathic normal-pressure hydrocephalus. Neurosurgery. 2005; 57(3) Suppl: S4–S16, discussion ii–v

[4] Greitz D. The hydrodynamic hypothesis versus the bulk flow hypothesis. Neurosurg Rev. 2004; 27(4):299–300

[5] Stolze H, Kuhtz-Buschbeck JP, Drücke H, et al. Gait analysis in idiopathic normal pressure hydrocephalus: which parameters respond to the CSF tap test? Clin Neurophysiol. 2000; 111(9):1678–1686

[6] Nutt JG, Marsden CD, Thompson PD. Human walking and higher-level gait disorders, particularly in the elderly. Neurology. 1993; 43(2):268–279

[7] Williams MA, Relkin NR. Diagnosis and management of idiopathic normal-pressure hydrocephalus. Neurol Clin Pract. 2013; 3(5):375–385

[8] Craven CL, Toma AK, Mostafa T, Patel N, Watkins LD. The predictive value of DESH for shunt responsiveness in idiopathic normal pressure hydrocephalus. J Clin Neurosci. 2016; 34:294–298

[9] Hashimoto M, Ishikawa M, Mori E, Kuwana N, Study of INPH on neurological improvement (SINPHONI). Diagnosis of idiopathic normal pressure hydrocephalus is supported by MRI-based scheme: a prospective cohort study. Cerebrospinal Fluid Res. 2010; 7:18

[10] Podsiadlo D, Richardson S. The timed "Up & Go": a test of basic functional mobility for frail elderly persons. J Am Geriatr Soc. 1991; 39(2):142–148

[11] Yamada S, Ishikawa M, Miyajima M, et al. Timed up and go test at tap test and shunt surgery in idiopathic normal pressure hydrocephalus. Neurol Clin Pract. 2017; 7(2):98–108

[12] Wikkelsø C, Hellström P, Klinge PM, Tans JT, European iNPH Multicentre Study Group. The European iNPH Multicentre Study on the predictive values of resistance to CSF outflow and the CSF Tap Test in patients with idiopathic normal pressure hydrocephalus. J Neurol Neurosurg Psychiatry. 2013; 84(5): 562–568

[13] Kosteljanetz M. Intracranial pressure: cerebrospinal fluid dynamics and pressure-volume relations. Acta Neurol Scand Suppl. 1987; 111:1–23

[14] Nornes H, Rootwelt K, Sjaastad O. Normal pressure hydrocephalus. Long-term intracranial pressure recording. Eur Neurol. 1973; 9(5):261–274

[15] Marmarou A, Shulman K, LaMorgese J. Compartmental analysis of compliance and outflow resistance of the cerebrospinal fluid system. J Neurosurg. 1975; 43(5):523–534

[16] Eklund A, Smielewski P, Chambers I, et al. Assessment of cerebrospinal fluid outflow resistance. Med Biol Eng Comput. 2007; 45(8):719–735

[17] Brean A, Eide PK. Assessment of idiopathic normal pressure patients in neurological practice: the role of lumbar infusion testing for referral of patients to neurosurgery. Eur J Neurol. 2008; 15(6):605–612

[18] Kahlon B, Sundbärg G, Rehncrona S. Comparison between the lumbar infusion and CSF tap tests to predict outcome after shunt surgery in suspected normal pressure hydrocephalus. J Neurol Neurosurg Psychiatry. 2002; 73(6):721–726

[19] Marmarou A, Black P, Bergsneider M, Klinge P, Relkin N, International NPH Consultant Group. Guidelines for management of idiopathic normal pressure hydrocephalus: progress to date. Acta Neurochir Suppl (Wien). 2005; 95: 237–240

[20] Toma AK, Stapleton S, Papadopoulos MC, Kitchen ND, Watkins LD. Natural history of idiopathic normal-pressure hydrocephalus. Neurosurg Rev. 2011; 34(4):433–439

[21] Scollato A, Tenenbaum R, Bahl G, Celerini M, Salani B, Di Lorenzo N. Changes in aqueductal CSF stroke volume and progression of symptoms in patients with unshunted idiopathic normal pressure hydrocephalus. AJNR Am J Neuroradiol. 2008; 29(1):192–197

[22] Razay G, Vreugdenhil A, Liddell J. A prospective study of ventriculo-peritoneal shunting for idiopathic normal pressure hydrocephalus. J Clin Neurosci. 2009; 16(9):1180–1183

[23] Eide PK, Brean A. Intracranial pulse pressure amplitude levels determined during preoperative assessment of subjects with possible idiopathic normal pressure hydrocephalus. Acta Neurochir (Wien). 2006; 148(11):1151–1156, discussion 1156

[24] Savolainen S, Hurskainen H, Paljärvi L, Alafuzoff I, Vapalahti M. Five-year outcome of normal pressure hydrocephalus with or without a shunt: predictive value of the clinical signs, neuropsychological evaluation and infusion test. Acta Neurochir (Wien). 2002; 144(6):515–523, discussion 523

[25] Pfisterer WK, Aboul-Enein F, Gebhart E, Graf M, Aichholzer M, Mühlbauer M. Continuous intraventricular pressure monitoring for diagnosis of normal-pressure hydrocephalus. Acta Neurochir (Wien). 2007; 149(10):983–990, discussion 990

[26] Andrén K, Wikkelsø C, Tisell M, Hellström P. Natural course of idiopathic normal pressure hydrocephalus. J Neurol Neurosurg Psychiatry. 2014; 85(7):806–810

[27] Kameda M, Yamada S, Atsuchi M, et al. SINPHONI and SINPHONI-2 Investigators. Cost-effectiveness analysis of shunt surgery for idiopathic normal pressure hydrocephalus based on the SINPHONI and SINPHONI-2 trials. Acta Neurochir (Wien). 2017; 159(6):995–1003

[28] Kazui H, Miyajima M, Mori E, Ishikawa M, SINPHONI-2 Investigators. Lumboperitoneal shunt surgery for idiopathic normal pressure hydrocephalus (SINPHONI-2): an open-label randomised trial. Lancet Neurol. 2015; 14(6):585–594

[29] Miyajima M, Kazui H, Mori E, Ishikawa M, on behalf of the SINPHONI-2 Investigators. One-year outcome in patients with idiopathic normal-pressure hydrocephalus: comparison of lumboperitoneal shunt to ventriculoperitoneal shunt. J Neurosurg. 2016; 125(6):1483–1492

[30] Meier U, Kiefer M, Neumann U, Lemcke J. On the optimal opening pressure of hydrostatic valves in cases of idiopathic normal-pressure hydrocephalus: a prospective randomized study with 123 patients. Acta Neurochir Suppl (Wien). 2006; 96:358–363

[31] Lemcke J, Meier U, Müller C, et al. Safety and efficacy of gravitational shunt valves in patients with idiopathic normal pressure hydrocephalus: a pragmatic, randomised, open label, multicentre trial (SVASONA). J Neurol Neurosurg Psychiatry. 2013; 84(8):850–857

[32] Boon AJ, Tans JT, Delwel EJ, et al. Dutch Normal-Pressure Hydrocephalus Study: the role of cerebrovascular disease. J Neurosurg. 1999; 90(2):221–226

[33] Pinto FC, Saad F, Oliveira MF, et al. Role of endoscopic third ventriculostomy and ventriculoperitoneal shunt in idiopathic normal pressure hydrocephalus: preliminary results of a randomized clinical trial. Neurosurgery. 2013; 72(5):845–853, discussion 853–854

[34] Kiefer M, Eymann R, Steudel WI. Outcome predictors for normal-pressure hydrocephalus. Acta Neurochir Suppl (Wien). 2006; 96:364–367

[35] Meier U. The grading of normal pressure hydrocephalus. Biomed Tech (Berl). 2002; 47(3):54–58

[36] Meier U, Lemcke J. The influence of co-morbidity on the postoperative outcomes of patients with idiopathic normal pressure hydrocephalus (iNPH). Acta Neurochir Suppl (Wien). 2008; 102:141–144

[37] Meier U, Stengel D, Müller C, et al. Predictors of subsequent overdrainage and clinical outcomes after ventriculoperitoneal shunting for idiopathic normal pressure hydrocephalus. Neurosurgery. 2013; 73(6):1054–1060

[38] Sprung C, Schlosser HG, Lemcke J, et al. The adjustable proGAV shunt: a prospective safety and reliability multicenter study. Neurosurgery. 2010; 66(3):465–474

[39] Kiefer M, Unterberg A. The differential diagnosis and treatment of normal-pressure hydrocephalus. Dtsch Arztebl Int. 2012; 109(1–2):15–25, quiz 26

[40] Black PM, Ojemann RG, Tzouras A. CSF shunts for dementia, incontinence, and gait disturbance. Clin Neurosurg. 1985; 32:632–651

[41] Chang S, Agarwal S, Williams MA, Rigamonti D, Hillis AE. Demographic factors influence cognitive recovery after shunt for normal-pressure hydrocephalus. Neurologist. 2006; 12(1):39–42

[42] Meier U, König A, Miethke C. Predictors of outcome in patients with normal-pressure hydrocephalus. Eur Neurol. 2004; 51(2):59–67

[43] Mirzayan MJ, Luetjens G, Borremans JJ, Regel JP, Krauss JK. Extended long-term (> 5 years) outcome of cerebrospinal fluid shunting in idiopathic normal pressure hydrocephalus. Neurosurgery. 2010; 67(2):295–301

[44] Andrén K, Wikkelsø C, Sundström N, et al. Survival in treated idiopathic normal pressure hydrocephalus. J Neurol. 2020; 267(3):640–648

[45] Malm J, Kristensen B, Stegmayr B, Fagerlund M, Koskinen LO. Three-year survival and functional outcome of patients with idiopathic adult hydrocephalus syndrome. Neurology. 2000; 55(4):576–578

[46] Greenberg JO, Shenkin HA, Adam R. Idiopathic normal pressure hydrocephalus– a report of 73 patients. J Neurol Neurosurg Psychiatry. 1977; 40(4):336–341

[47] Black PM. Idiopathic normal-pressure hydrocephalus. Results of shunting in 62 patients. J Neurosurg. 1980; 52(3):371–377

[48] Aygok G, Marmarou A, Young HF. Three-year outcome of shunted idiopathic NPH patients. Acta Neurochir Suppl (Wien). 2005; 95:241–245

[49] Raftopoulos C, Massager N, Balériaux D, Deleval J, Clarysse S, Brotchi J. Prospective analysis by computed tomography and long-term outcome of 23 adult patients with chronic idiopathic hydrocephalus. Neurosurgery. 1996; 38(1):51–59

[50] Spagnoli D, Innocenti L, Bello L, et al. Impact of cerebrovascular disease on the surgical treatment of idiopathic normal pressure hydrocephalus. Neurosurgery. 2006; 59(3):545–552, discussion 545–552

[51] Tisell M, Hellström P, Ahl-Börjesson G, et al. Long-term outcome in 109 adult patients operated on for hydrocephalus. Br J Neurosurg. 2006; 20(4):214–221

[52] Kahlon B, Sjunnesson J, Rehncrona S. Long-term outcome in patients with suspected normal pressure hydrocephalus. Neurosurgery. 2007; 60(2):327–332, discussion 332

[53] Pujari S, Kharkar S, Metellus P, Shuck J, Williams MA, Rigamonti D. Normal pressure hydrocephalus: long-term outcome after shunt surgery. J Neurol Neurosurg Psychiatry. 2008; 79(11):1282–1286

[54] Klinge P, Hellström P, Tans J, Wikkelsø C, European iNPH Multicentre Study Group. One-year outcome in the European multicentre study on iNPH. Acta Neurol Scand. 2012; 126(3):145–153

[55] D'Antona L, Blamey SC, Craven CL, et al. Early postoperative outcomes of normal pressure hydrocephalus: results of a service evaluation. J Neurosurg Anesthesiol. 2019

[56] Conn HO. Normal pressure hydrocephalus: a case report by a physician who is the patient. Clin Med (Lond). 2007; 7(3):296–299

227

Index

Note: Page numbers set **bold** or *italic* indicate headings or figures, respectively.